ASX 4922

1

MAGNETIC RESONANCE IMAGING
OF THE CENTRAL NERVOUS SYSTEM

Magnetic Resonance Imaging of the Central Nervous System

Editors

Michael Brant-Zawadzki

David Norman

Department of Radiology
University of California, San Francisco
San Francisco, California

Raven Press ❧ **New York**

Raven Press, 1185 Avenue of the Americas, New York, New York 10036

Made in the United States of America

Library of Congress Cataloging-in-Publication Data

Magnetic resonance imaging of the central nervous
   system.

   Includes bibliographies and index.
    1. Central nervous system—Diseases—Diagnosis.
2. Magnetic resonance imaging. I. Brant-Zawadzki,
Michael. II. Norman, David.
RC361.5.M34 1986   616.8'04757   86-15476
ISBN 0-88167-240-8

9 8 7 6 5 4 3 2 1

To Hans Newton
for his inspiration, guidance, and friendship

PREFACE

This introductory text on magnetic resonance imaging (MRI) of the central nervous system, spine, nasopharynx, and neck is intended for the individual for whom the clinical applications of MRI are fairly new.

Because the development of magnetic resonance is ongoing, the material herein represents a necessarily transient state in that evolution. Nevertheless, because the majority of the clinical indications for magnetic resonance studies have involved the regions covered, a great deal of experience has already been garnered by the authors in this setting. The manner in which the basic principles are explained, and the applications of those principles to image interpretation, have been tested in the tutorial setting. Given the diversity of journal literature on MRI, the befuddled practitioner understandably often requests a distillation in one reference volume of the major practical points of interest; this book is a response to that request.

The contributors to this volume are all highly experienced, frequent practicing users of MRI with documented ability to transmit knowledge to their colleagues in a simple and organized fashion. Magnetic Resonance Imaging of the Central Nervous System presents a pragmatic approach to the use of MRI in the clinical settings of neurology, neurosurgery, otolaryngology, and orthopedics.

Other, more thorough reference texts will become available as MRI matures. Nevertheless, the clinical use of this technique is growing rapidly, and this volume is intended to fill the existing needs of residents and practicing radiologists, as well as interested clinicians, in understanding the basic concepts and major clinical applications of magnetic resonance imaging.

ACKNOWLEDGMENTS

Many people contributed to the effort that this volume represents. The excellent fellows in the Neuroradiology department at University of California, San Francisco, who helped monitor the patient studies illustrated herein include Gordon Sze, Keith McMurdo, William Keyes, Patricia Rhyner, Wallace Peck, and Walter Olsen. Our appreciation of their help in this endeavor and in our daily workload during the production of this book cannot be overstated. Our administrative assistants, especially Yolanda Eldred, deserve our sincere gratitude for the word processing work that was involved. The help of our publisher, in the personna of Mary Rogers, is not to be underestimated. As the editors, we would also like to acknowledge a great debt to the fine authors whom we were lucky enough to cajole into this task. And, needless to say, we appreciate the support of our families whose time with us was sacrificed for the sake of this volume. Finally, the foresight of our chairman Alexander R. Margulis, in projecting those fuzzy magnetic resonance images of rats in the 1970s to their eventual clinical potential of the 1980s, must be acknowledged. Without his vision and faith in his faculty, this book would not have been possible.

CONTENTS

CONTRIBUTORS

Robert A. Bell, Ph.D.   *Consultant, Science Applications International Corporation, 1257 Tasman Drive, Sunnyvale, California 94089*

Isabelle Berry, M.D.   *Department of Radiology, University of California School of Medicine, Los Angeles, California 90024*

Larissa T. Bilaniuk   *Department of Radiology, Hospital of the University of Pennsylvania, Philadelphia, Pennsylvania 19104*

William G. Bradley, Jr., M.D.   *Magnetic Resonance Imaging Laboratory, Huntington Medical Research Institutes; and Department of Radiology, Huntington Memorial Hospital, Pasadena, California 91105*

Michael Brant-Zawadzki, M.D.   *Department of Radiology, University of California, San Francisco, California 94143; Current address: Department of Radiology, Newport Harbor Radiology—Hoag Memorial Hospital, Newport Beach, California 92660*

Wil M. Chew, B.S.   *School of Pharmacy, Department of Pharmaceutical Chemistry, University of California, San Francisco, California 94143*

Jack DeGroot, M.D., Ph.D.   *Department of Anatomy, S1334, University of California, San Francisco, California 94143*

William P. Dillon, M.D.   *Department of Radiology, Veterans Administration Medical Center, 4150 Clement Street, San Francisco, California 94121*

Burton P. Drayer, M.D.   *Division of Neuroradiology, Barrow Neurological Institute, Phoenix, Arizona 85013*

William N. Hanafee, M.D.   *Department of Radiology, University of California School of Medicine, Los Angeles, California 90024*

Betsy Holland, M.D.   *Department of Radiology, University of California School of Medicine, 513 Parnassus Avenue, San Francisco, California 94143*

Thomas L. James, Ph.D.   *School of Pharmacy, Department of Pharmaceutical Chemistry, University of California, San Francisco, California 94143*

William M. Kelly, M.D.   *David Grant Medical Center, Radiology Department, Travis Air Force Base, [city], California 94535*

Bent O. Kjos, M.D.   *Department of Radiology, Alta Bates Hospital, Berkeley, California 94705*

Walter Kucharczyk, M.D.   *Department of Radiology, Toronto General Hospital, Toronto, Ontario MSG 1L7 Canada*

Robert B. Lufkin, M.D. *Department of Radiology, University of California School of Medicine, Los Angeles, California 90024*

Michael T. McNamara, M.D. *Service of Magnetic Resonance Imaging, Centre Hospitalier Princesse Grace, Principaute de Monaco*

Michael E. Moseley, Ph.D. *Department of Radiology, University of California School of Medicine, 513 Parnassus Avenue, San Francisco, California 94143*

Thomas P. Naidich, M.D. *Department of Radiology, Children's Memorial Hospital, 2300 Children's Plaza, Chicago, Illinois 60614*

David Norman, M.D. *Department of Radiology, University of California School of Medicine, 513 Parnassus Avenue, San Francisco, California 94143*

David D. Stark, M.D. *Department of Radiology, Massachusetts General Hospital; and Harvard Medical School, Boston, Massachusetts 02115*

Gordon Sze, M.D. *Department of Radiology, Memorial Sloan-Kettering Cancer Center, 1275 York Avenue, New York, New York 10021*

Robert A. Zimmerman, M.D. *Department of Radiology, Hospital of the University of Pennsylvania, Philadelphia, Pennsylvania 19104*

CHAPTER 1

Magnetic Resonance Imaging Principles: The Bare Necessities

Michael Brant-Zawadzki

The intent of this chapter is to provide the practicing radiologist with a conceptual basis for the underlying principles of magnetic resonance imaging (MRI). The complexity of this new procedure induces anxiety even in those with an above average background in physics and mathematics. However, just as one need not understand thoroughly the physics of the xenon detector or the advanced mathematics of reconstruction algorithms to properly utilize computed tomography (CT) in the daily practice of radiology, so too can one learn to perform and interpret MRI studies with confidence in everyday practice, provided a conceptual framework of certain crucial fundamentals is learned. The goal of what follows is to provide the reader with this conceptual framework in a relatively facile manner. By design, some repetition and certain oversimplifications will be used, and the experts might argue that accuracy is stretched by this approach. Needless to say, the interested and more advanced reader should refer to the more complete treatises on MRI principles referenced subsequently. It should be pointed out, however, that even the experts still debate some of the most fundamental aspects of MRI, and that the rapid evolution of knowledge regarding MRI principles, instrumentation, and imaging techniques makes even their most ambitious treatment obsolete by the time it is printed. Nevertheless, the rapid dissemination of this technology in the clinical arena necessitates that most radiologists, at this point in time, need at least a conceptual model of the fundamentals with which to approach MRI, and need eventually to enrich their understanding through hands-on experience and further study. Providing a working conceptual model is the limited goal of this chapter.

MRI AND CT: SIMILARITIES AND DIFFERENCES

Both MRI and CT provide cross-sectional, *digital* images of the body. The phrase "digital image" implies that the visible depiction of the anatomy is based on a numerical, computerized representation of certain physical properties of the tissue. In X-ray CT, the cross section of anatomy is initially represented by an array or grid of numbers in computer memory. Each of those numbers represents the X-ray attenuation of a finite volume of tissue in the plane through which the X-ray beam has passed. The array of numbers is called a matrix; the finite volume of tissue represented by each number is the voxel. Spatial resolution depends on slice thickness, the cross-sectional area ("field of view") covered by the matrix, and the dimensions of each voxel. The more voxels per given area—i.e., the bigger the matrix—the smaller the dimension of each voxel and the better the spatial resolution.

In CT, the numerical value of each voxel correlates directly with the X-ray attenuation (a physical property) of the tissue that the voxel represents. By assigning a shade of gray to the voxels, the greater the numerical value the brighter the shade of gray assigned, the image processor of the CT scanner reproduces the matrix of voxels in the section scanned as a pictorial representation of that section in "black and white." Visual contrast between different regions is seen as differences in the shades of gray, and directly reflects the differences in X-ray attenuation of disparate tissue voxels in the section studied. Of note in CT is the fact that contrast on the resulting images is absolute in the sense that those tissues with relatively great X-ray attenuation properties will always be represented by relatively higher numbers (and brighter shades of gray) than tissues with relatively low X-ray attenuation properties.

MRI shares most of these basic aspects of CT in that it, too, provides a cross-sectional image based on a matrix of numbers each assigned a shade of gray, and each representing a physical property of the tissue voxel it subtends. The major difference, of course, is that the physical property represented by the digital values in the magnetic resonance (MR) images is entirely different to that sampled by X-ray attenuation, and is obtained by a completely different set of interactions between energy and matter. The ultimate numerical value assigned to each voxel (and subsequently assigned a shade in the gray scale) represents the *intensity* of a radiowave signal emanating from the tissue in which hydrogen nuclei have been perturbed by a characteristic radiofrequency (RF) pulse. Contrast on the MR image, therefore, depends on differences in signal intensity from disparate tissues, differences represented by shades of gray on the image. Of major importance are two further inherent divergences from CT imaging. The first is that this intensity of signal recorded from any given tissue will have a characteristic decay envelope; that is, the intensity of the signal diminishes from its initial level over time. The second is that both this initial level of intensity and its rate of decay each depend on somewhat different and unique physical properties of tissues (in contrast to CT, where X-ray attenuation depends primarily on the *single* physical property of tissue electron density).

These two conceptual breaks from CT imaging have major implications. Appropriate use of the MR instrument provides the ability to emphasize or highlight in the observed signal intensity the contribution of each of the several physical properties of the tissues being imaged. By varying the time between excitations the operator can choose to maximize or minimize the differences in the initial signal intensity from distinct tissue types. By sampling not only the initial value of the signal intensity, but also its value at several points along its decay envelope, the operator can observe further differences in the diverse tissues being excited in the MRI sequence. Again, such differences of signal intensity at any single sampling of the entire section are expressed in terms of the shades of gray on the ensuing image of that section. Therefore, contrast in any acquired MR image is a consequence of difference in signal intensity emanating from disparate tissues. Because one tissue type may start with a very strong signal (on account of certain properties) but that signal decays very rapidly (because of other properties), such tissue may be seen as a very bright region compared to neighboring tissue with less initial signal on an early sampling of the signal. However, a later sampling will show this initially intense but

rapidly decaying tissue as dark compared to its neighbor, whose lower initial signal may decay very slowly as a result of characteristic physical properties. This reversal of intensity relationships or contrast between two tissues—based simply on choice of instrument parameters (in this case, sampling interval) by the operator—is unlike anything in X-ray CT work, where contrast between tissue types is stable and depends on absolute differences in the single physical property of X-ray attenuation ("bright" tissues attenuate X-rays more than "dark" tissues). At first such variability of contrast in MRI is befuddling. But it is this very feature of MRI that allows much greater sensitivity to differences in tissue composition, and hence gives this procedure its superior diagnostic capability.

To more fully appreciate how the signal is produced with MRI and how the multifactorial tissue properties influence its intensity over time necessitates at least an intuitive appreciation of the basics of MRI principles. Such an appreciation will help the neophyte to change the appropriate instrument parameters for a particular study, and to interpret the resulting images.

BASIC PRINCIPLES OF PROTON MRI: AN OVERVIEW

Two major theories can be used to explain the physics of MRI (1–5). Just as the physics of light can be explained either by the waveform or by the particulate theory, the principles of MRI can be elucidated either by

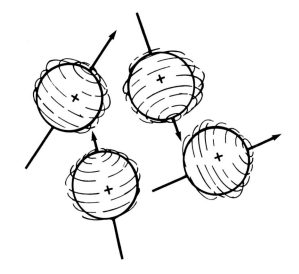

FIG. 1. The spinning hydrogen nuclei are essentially positively charged protons. The magnetic vector they generate is directed through the center of their spin, and randomly oriented before placement in a magnetic field.

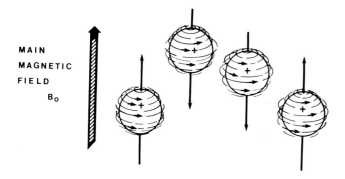

FIG. 2. Two possible states of alignment for the spinning protons exist when placed in a powerful magnetic field, B_0. The alignment with the direction of B_0 confers a lower energy state.

classical (Newtonian) or by quantum mechanical tenets. Because each theory explains certain aspects best, both will be drawn upon in this simplified overview.

Charged particles which move through space generate a magnetic field. The most common example of this is the electron moving through a length of wire, the basis of electromagnetism. A hydrogen nucleus is composed of a single proton; thus it has a positive charge. This nucleus (henceforth also called a proton) spins on its axis; therefore, as a charged particle moving in space, it generates a magnetic field. In the case of the spinning proton, the magnetic field can be described as a vector (i.e., a quantity with magnitude *and* direction) through the center of the spin. This vector or moment is randomly directed under normal circumstances (Fig. 1). But when such spinning protons find themselves in a powerful magnetic field, their magnetic moments tend to align in that superimposed, external magnetic field.

The theory of quantum mechanics dictates only two possible states of alignment for the protons' magnetic moments. They can align either with (parallel to) or directly against (antiparallel to) the direction of the external magnetic field. Alignment with the magnetic field confers a lower energy state on those protons so aligned when compared to those aligned in the opposite direction (Fig. 2). This difference in energy between the two states of alignment is the crux of MRI.

As is common to most phenomena in nature, the lower energy state is preferred. Therefore, given a large group of protons placed in a powerful magnetic field, after a certain period of time a slightly greater number of protons have their magnetic moments aligned parallel to the magnetic field than the number of protons with moments aligned antiparallel (Fig. 3). This alignment for each proton is not static, of course. Any source of energy in the system can raise a proton's state from the lower (parallel) to the higher one (antiparallel to the magnetic field). For instance, a random thermal interaction of the low energy proton with a nearby molecule may allow an infusion of energy to the proton, thus raising its state, or vice versa. In any case, when one has a sample in the powerful magnetic field and observes the group of protons in their environment or "lattice," one can see that each individual proton fluctuates between the high energy and the low energy states over time. However, because the lower energy state is preferred, there is a tendency for more and more protons to exist in the lower energy state at any instant in time following the placement of the sample in the magnetic field (Fig. 3).

This tendency is not linear. If one were to sum all the individual protons' magnetic vectors together, the high energy (antiparallel) subtracted from the low energy (parallel with the field) sum would yield a net vector or

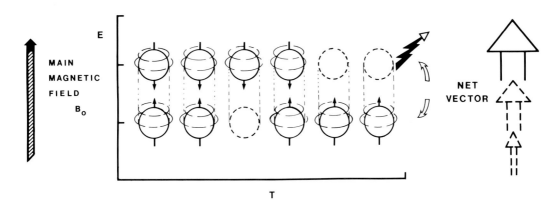

FIG. 3. Alignment of protons in a magnetic field over time. Random thermal energy interactions allow flipping of individual protons from one energy state to the other. Because the lower energy state is preferred, more and more protons tend to exist in that state given some time in the magnet. Therefore, a net magnetization vector (sum vector of the individual proton vectors) grows with time, in the direction of the magnetic field (see text). E, energy; T, time.

moment, the magnitude of which would represent the balance of protons pointing with and against the field. Given the preference for the lower energy state, that sum vector would have the same direction as the magnetic field (parallel), and its magnitude would grow with time as more and more protons would tend to be present in the lower energy state. This growth of the net vector represents what is called the magnetization of the proton sample. However, as mentioned above, the growth of this vector is not linear, but exponential. Initially, the rate of its growth is fast, but, with time, this rate of magnetization slows and flattens out (Fig. 4). An analogy can be drawn to loading charge in a capacitor. At first packing charge (in the form of electrons) into one plate of the capacitor is easy; but as the charge builds, the process gets more and more difficult.

As one might intuitively gather, this rate of growth of the sum vector, i.e., the ability of the hydrogen nuclei (protons) to align with the external field of magnetization, is different for different tissue types. Because the process depends on the ability of the protons to exchange energy with their environment (or lattice), that environment is a strong determinant of the rate of magnetization (also called spin–lattice relaxation). Some tissues allow their protons to exchange thermal energy quickly; in others the rate of this energy exchange, which determines the rate of magnetization, is slower. This process, which is represented by the time constant T1, is therefore tissue specific. One T1 period is that amount of time by which 63% of the total magnetization (i.e.,

63% of the growth of the sum vector) for a particular sample has been achieved, and thus three T1 periods allow almost complete magnetization (95%) (Fig. 4). Liquids, especially pure water, will have a long T1. One can conceptualize this by thinking of the relatively widely dispersed H_2O molecules in pure water, a homogeneous substance, and the relatively small chance those hydrogen nuclei have to exchange energy with other molecules in their environment—hence the relatively long time (T1) for their magnetization. Other tissues with more compact and complex environments allow more readily the exchange of energy between protons and their lattice, thus faster magnetization (i.e., shorter T1 relaxation). It should be pointed out that other factors influence the ability of protons to undergo spin–lattice relaxation, and not only proximity of other molecules or particles in the environment. For example, a major factor is the motion or tumbling rate—a property of all molecules. Thus temperature and even the field strength of the magnet, both of which may influence the molecular motion of a given substance, will affect the energy exchange capability of protons (T1 relaxation) within their molecular environment (6,7). The tissue-specific rate of magnetization (T1 relaxation) can be easily used to differentiate between disparate tissues on the MR image because of the crucial concept that *the initial signal intensity observed from a sample following an RF excitation is directly related to the degree of magnetization* (i.e., the magnitude of the net vector) *achieved.* Thus, an MR image based on an immediate

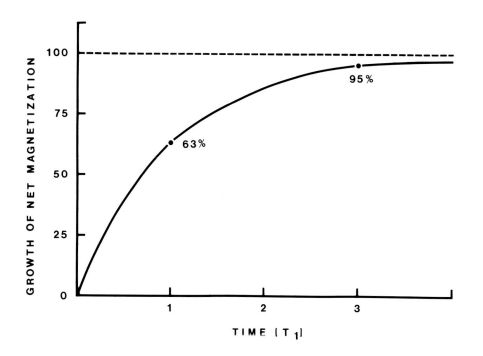

FIG. 4. Rate of growth of the sum vector (see Fig. 3) with time. Note that the experimental nature of the curve is described by the T1 relaxation time. One T1 is that amount of time needed to achieve 63% of the vector's ultimate growth. That amount of time is a characteristic property of the protons' tissue environment (i.e., their ability to exchange thermal energy therein).

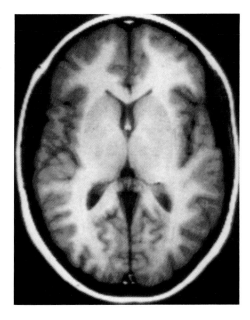

FIG. 5. Normal brain, T1-weighted (TR 600 msec, TE 24 msec) image. Signal intensity reflects degree of alignment (magnetization) achieved by disparate tissues in the 600 msec interval. Note slow alignment (long T1) in the CSF compared to gray matter, with faster alignment (shorter T1) in the white matter and subcutaneous fat. Signal intensity in this image reflects the T1 properties of the tissue (see Fig. 6).

sampling of intensity shows those tissues with rapid rates of magnetization (short T1 values) as having high intensity (i.e., bright pixel regions), whereas those tissues with slow rates (long T1) appear as low intensity or dark regions (Figs. 5 and 6). Therefore, contrast between such disparate regions is perceived in terms of, and in this example is based on, T1 influence on signal intensity ("T1-weighted" contrast). Returning to the example of water, which we noted had a long T1 (its protons not being efficient in exchanging energy with the environment), it would be seen as dark (little intensity) compared to more solid tissue which "magetized" faster and yields greater intensity of signal with the same excitation. Indeed, because water is such a ubiquitous source of hydrogen nuclei (protons) in biologic tissue (the body being approximately 75% water), the content of water in different tissues very strongly influences their T1 relaxation values, and hence contrast on "T1-weighted" images. Having briefly considered one of the major influences on signal intensity, let us next turn to how the signal itself is generated from the proton sample, and combine what we now know regarding its initial intensity with those properties of tissue which influence the signal decay. Let us return to our protons fluctuating randomly between two possible energy states within the magnetic field, with a tendency for more to be present in the lower energy state, given some time in that field through the T1 relaxation mechanisms described above. We can generate a signal of electromagnetic radiation in the RF range from the protons as follows. By adding energy to the sample via RF irradiation which precisely matches the energy difference between the two states of alignment, all the protons are raised to the higher energy state and drop back down between the bursts of energy delivery, and are made to fluctuate between the two

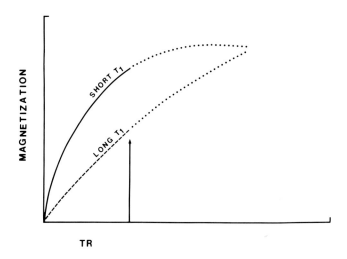

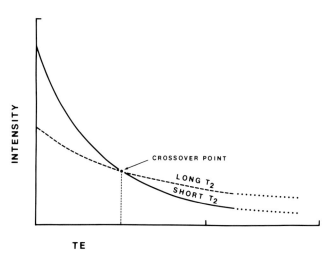

FIG. 6. Signal intensity observed, as a function of magnetization rate and sampling time, in a T1-weighted image (e.g., Fig. 5). Given the short time between excitations, TR, the tissue with short T1 yields greater signal intensity (brighter pixels), especially if sampled early (TE) in the decay period (e.g., white matter versus gray, or edematous versus normal).

energy states ("flip") *in unison.* This phenomenon is called coherent resonance. It is this unified drop of all the protons from the high energy state to the lower one which releases energy strong enough to be detected. Prior to the RF irradiation, when individual protons would give up energy and drop to the lower energy state (Fig. 3) that energy was likely to be taken up by the molecular lattice (and perhaps infused into another proton, raising it to a higher energy state). However, when *all* the protons in a sample drop to a lower state and give up energy *in unison,* a sufficiently strong packet of energy is released out of the lattice that it can be detected (Fig. 7). Because the energy so released precisely matches that difference in the two energy levels for the protons dictated by the magnetic field strength, it is of the same RF as the excitation pulse and can be detected with an RF antenna placed around the region of interest.

To reiterate the earlier discussion, the actual intensity of the energy so generated from the resonating protons depends not only on their number, but also on how much magnetization (T1 relaxation) was achieved prior to the sample's excitation. Indeed, the RF excitation, which itself generates the signal, abolishes the magnetization as no differential energy states exist during the excitatory RF pulse. Therefore, the initial intensity of the energy observed from the excited sample depends on how much alignment has occurred since the previous excitatory pulse was turned off. Again, those tissues which allow ready exchange of energy between their protons and lattice will give off relatively greater signal intensity with each periodic RF excitation than tissues with less optimal capacity for energy exchange. The two can therefore be differentiated on the basis of the *initial* signal intensity—high intensity tissue represented by assigned pixels with bright shades of gray.

A somewhat different physical effect operates in tissues to cause the generated RF signal to decay and die out over time. This other aspect or property of tissues can also be used to differentiate distinct tissue subtypes, and enhances the ability of MRI to provide contrast discrimination between disparate tissues. Consider again the protons immediately at the point when the RF excitation ceases. Giving off maximum signal by flipping back and forth in unison, they immediately begin to experience subtle inhomogeneities in their micro-magnetic environment which disrupt their abilities to keep up with their colleagues. As other charged nuclear or molecular species "tug" on a particular proton or repel it differentially from its colleagues, it no longer keeps pace with them. In this manner, the unison or coherence of the resonating proton sample begins to dissipate. As it was this coherence which allowed the emission of a sufficient signal intensity, so the rate of loss of coherence dictates the rate of signal loss. Obviously, the more inhomogeneous (in terms of magnetic moment interactions) a tissue environment that the proton sample experiences, the faster will be the loss of flip unison or coherent resonance for that sample, and the faster will the signal decay. Not surprisingly, different tissues have different degrees of magnetic homogeneity in their microenvironments. Even assuming equal numbers of protons and equal rates of thermal energy exchange (T1 relaxation or "magnetization") for two distinct tissues which would yield equal signal intensity at time $t = 0$ from both tissues, the signal would decay at different rates for the two populations of protons if their microenvironment's magnetic homogeneities were distinct. Thus, an image based on sampling the signal at some time point after $t = 0$ would distinguish that tissue with a relatively homogeneous microenvironment, as the signal intensity decay would be slow (and therefore

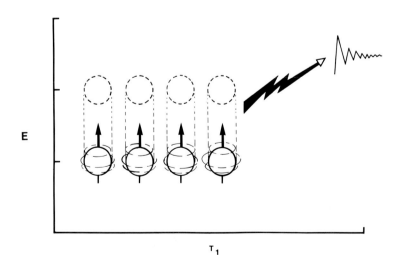

FIG. 7. Unified drop of proton ensemble from the higher to the lower energy state induced by an RF excitation pulse (see text) releases observable energy producing an RF signal. A random fluctuation of a single proton to the lower state would not produce a sufficient signal (see Fig. 3).

the signal still relatively high) when compared to the more inhomogeneous tissue in which the more rapid signal intensity loss would be seen as low intensity pixel values (depicted visually as darker shades of gray).

Returning to the earlier example, water, one would predict the relatively slow decay of signal from such a homogeneous structure where the relatively sparse molecular density allows little chance for dissipation of coherent resonance. Thus, although relatively little *initial* signal may be generated by successive RF excitations of water because of its protons' relative difficulty in exchanging thermal energy within the lattice (i.e., long T1 relaxation), that signal which will be produced persists over a long period. Hence, if one samples the signal from heterogeneous biological tissue relatively late after excitation, the watery regions will show the greatest level of signal. The solid, inhomogeneous regions, having lost coherent resonance (i.e., signal intensity) much more quickly, will appear dark despite their much brighter appearance than water on images obtained soon after excitation. It should be mentioned that the magnets of MR instruments provide some inherent inhomogeneity of the magnetic field in the tissues being sampled. This inhomogeneity induces an instrument-related T2 decay (T2*) over and above that caused by the inherent tissue inhomogeneity. The instrument-induced decay can be canceled out by using refocusing pulses which give an "echo" of the signal, the intensity of which more accurately reflects only the tissue's contribution to the decay of coherent resonance. The interval of time between the original excitatory RF pulse and the detection of this echo is called TE. Multiple refocusing pulses can be applied after each excitation to generate multiple samplings of signal intensity (echoes) after each excitation. The first such sampling generally shows the intensity as most influenced by proton density and T1 effects. The subsequent ones detail the decay of signal intensity. Of course, some decay (T2 relaxation) influences even the first echo sampling, as the refocusing pulse takes a few milliseconds to generate, and the effects of tissue inhomogeneity have that amount of time to cause some loss of coherence.

It should be more clear now, given the above, that in MRI the gray scale image contrast between disparate tissues is relative: on a given set of samplings following an RF excitation a tissue may go from being brighter than its neighbors (based on high initial intensity due to rapid T1 relaxation) to being darker because of rapid signal decay (T2 relaxation). In fact, disparate tissues may show identical signal intensity at the crossover time point, which, if sampled, will not allow their distinction (Fig. 6). Therefore judicious use of excitation intervals (TR) and intervals between excitation and sampling is necessary to optimize contrast between one normal tis-

sue and another, or between normal and pathologic tissues. This requires an understanding of the compositions of normal and pathologic tissues, and the values of T1 and T2 relaxation at the field strength of the instrument used.

For instance, if one is faced with separating two tissues, one with relatively long T1 and T2 values compared to the other, one can overcome the danger of sampling at the crossover point by allowing sufficient time between excitations (TR) for both to "magnetize" fully. Because the T1 process is exponential, a tissue with long T1 relaxation will "catch up" to the degree of magnetization achieved by one which had fully relaxed earlier. Provided the RF excitation interval chosen is sufficiently long to allow this, the signals obtained from both will be maximized, and only the decay differences will be operative in providing intensity differences between the two. The image contrast in such an instance can be said to be "T2-weighted," as the T1 influences have been minimized by the long TR—the intensity profile being all beyond the crossover point (Fig. 8).

Obviously, some *a priori* knowledge of how long it takes biological tissues to relax dictates the choice of TR and T1. It turns out that in the brain and spinal cord tissue (but not the cerebrospinal fluid), one T1 (63% "magnetization" of the sample) takes approximately 400 to 900 msec, depending on the field strength—the higher fields having the longest values because of their effects on the differential between the protons' resonant frequency and the molecular tumbling rates (8). Therefore, an interval of 1,500 to 2,700 msec between excitations would be necessary to allow at least three T1 periods (i.e., 95% "magnetization"). This choice of TR will generally minimize the degree of T1 relaxation differences between tissues of the CNS. On the other hand, signal decay is much faster, and in general most signal from tissue is lost within 100 msec after excitation, with the exception of signals from pure liquids. (This effect is essentially independent of field strength.) Therefore, the differentiation of T2 relaxation values from disparate tissues requires rapid intervals between excitation and sampling.

Of course, subtle differences in the constitutions of tissues will affect the relaxation values, thus understanding of tissue structure and make-up is crucial. The choice of water in earlier examples was premeditated, and based on the fact that this substance is the richest source of protons in the tissues of the CNS, making up 82% of the gray matter and 70% of the white matter. Also, most disease processes that affect the brain will increase the water content of the affected tissue. In fact, most if not all of the contrast in the CNS is based on differences in bulk water content between distinct tissue types. As mentioned above, free water, called "bulk"

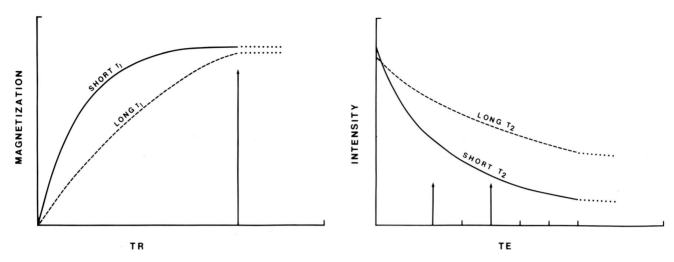

FIG. 8. Signal intensity observed over time in a T2-weighted image. Given a sufficiently long interval between excitations (TR), the total magnetization of a tissue with long T1 "catches up" to that of the tissue with short T1 (*left*). The resulting signal intensity following an RF excitation is equal initially from the two different tissue types. Their intensity distinction (contrast) at sample intervals (TE) is based on decay (T2 relaxation) differential (*right*). Effectively, the approach cancels out their T1 differences (compared with Fig. 6).

water by many, will have very long T1 and T2 relaxation values. However, as proteins or other complex molecular species are added to a water sample, some of the water molecules adhere to the added structure, and exchange of energy between the protons and their environment occurs more easily. Therefore, T1 relaxation is faster for the more complex sample, representing an averaged T1 of the still free "bulk" water molecules and the relatively "bound" water molecules (9). Also, the added inhomogeneity induces faster loss of coherent resonance (i.e., T2 relaxation), leading to more rapid signal decay. When looking at the biochemical differences between the gray and the white matter, it is the difference in bulk water content and resultant T1/T2 characteristics that provide the different signal intensities (contrast) on MR images. Optimizing that contrast is dependent on appropriate choice of instrument parameters. The T1 relaxation times of gray and white matter are approximately 550 and 450 msec, respectively, at 0.35 tesla (T) (with an approximate 40–50% increase at 1.5 T). Therefore, use of a TR interval of the order of 500 msec will allow a clear distinction of the two tissues, the white matter being well over 63% magnetized, and the gray at least 50 msec below that percentage (Figs. 5 and 6). Both tissues are still in the early, steep portion of the magnetization curve, making their distinction easier. Note that at higher field strengths the steepness of the initial portion of the T1 curve is not as great, resulting in lengthening of T1 for both tissues; therefore the TR may be longer and still provide good T1 differentiation. As it takes 800 to 900 msec to get to 63% magnetization at

high field strength, a 1,000 msec TR may be used and will still provide T1 differentiation.

Conversely, if one wants to negate the influence of T1 relaxation, a TR long enough to provide at least three T1 periods for the gray matter is needed, e.g., 2,000 msec. This permits over 95% magnetization in gray matter, and allows it essentially to catch up to that achieved by the white matter, both now together on the distal flat end of the T1 curve. Again, a longer TR may be necessary for this result at the higher field strength (2,500–3,000 msec). The signal generated with use of such long TRs would be equal for both tissues were it not for the proton density and T2 characteristics. Having more free water, the gray matter has more protons resonating, thus a stronger signal will be seen. Also, the slower decay of signal will add to the greater relative intensity of the gray matter compared to the white, even on the first echo which provides a small amount of T2 decay (Figs. 8 and 9). As later echoes are obtained, the slower decay of the signal from the gray matter will further accentuate its relatively greater signal compared to white matter (though in absolute terms the signal from both is decaying).

It is important to reiterate that even the long TR (2,000–3,000 msec) used to allow almost complete magnetization of the brain's various soft tissues is not sufficient to allow cerebrospinal fluid (CSF) even one T1 (63% magnetization). Therefore this relatively pure liquid will have relatively little signal intensity on the early sampling (echo) compared to the rest of the brain. As later and later echoes are obtained, the very slow

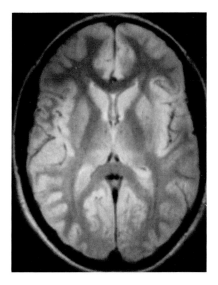 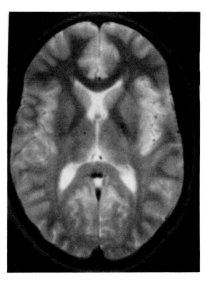

FIG. 9. Same axial section as shown in Fig. 5, but obtained with T2-weighted sequences (TR 2,000 msec, TE 40, 80 msec). The two images are samples of signal intensity at 40 msec (*left*) and again at 80 msec (*right*) after an RF excitation delivered every 2 sec. Note that gray–white matter contrast has reversed compared to Fig. 5. The gray matter is brighter because it is losing signal more slowly (longer T2 relaxation), having more water. Note that "pure water," CSF, is initially of lower intensity, then gains relative to brain on the 80 msec image (see Fig. 10).

decay of the CSF signal will become evident as relatively more signal will be seen from it when compared to the more rapidly decaying soft tissues (Figs. 9 and 10). As one adds large amounts of protein to CSF, e.g., infected or malignant fluid, the T1 and T2 relaxation values shorten, and the signal changes begin to approach those of very hydrated solid tissues.

Returning to more solid brain tissue, any insult of that tissue which induces an increase in water content will produce the types of prolongation of T1 and T2 relax-

ation that are evident when comparing the gray to the white matter. Clearly, a set of TR and TE parameters can be unfortunately chosen which can allow both T1 and T2 effects to influence signal intensity in such a way that, at the time sampled, the intensities from two different tissues, one "wetter" than the other, will be the same. For example, an infarct may produce a slight increase in water content sufficient to lengthen T1 relaxation slightly. If a short TR is used to study the lesion, it would show a lower intensity in the infarct, but because

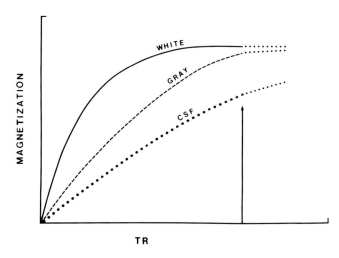 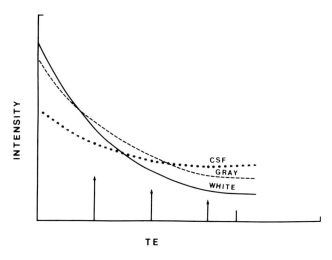

FIG. 10. Signal intensity differences between brain and CSF on T2-weighted (e.g., TR 2,000 msec) image. The very long T1 relaxation of pure water does not allow its magnetization to "catch up" to that of gray or white matter despite the relatively long TR used. Therefore, the initial signal intensity after the RF excitation of CSF is low, but its very slow decay eventually produces greater signal compared to the more rapidly decaying brain tissues (see Fig. 0).

the T2 relaxation is also longer, the slow decay of signal from the infarct compared to the more rapid decay from normal surroundings over the time it takes to do the sampling may counteract the long T1 effect at the sampling point and produce an isointense signal for both—i.e., no contrast (Fig. 11). This opposite effect of T1 and T2 prolongations on intensity in any tissue which has elevated water content can be overcome in one of two ways. Use of delayed sampling (long TE) times will allow the domination of signal intensity by T2 factors, but at the price of overall lower signal to noise.

Alternatively, use of long TR settings to optimize magnetization (and signal) in all tissues minimizes T1 differences seen early in the T1 curves for disparate tissues, and allows the T2 prolongation and increased proton density of "wet" tissues to dominate the signal intensity. An associated advantage of the long TR sequences is the ability to image more slices. Given the 2,000 msec interval between successive excitations at each slice location, and the signal sampling time of only 100 msec or so, 1,900 msec of "dead time" occurs at each slice. The instrument can perform the excitation and sampling procedure at several successive levels during that 1,900 msec before returning to the original slice 2,000 msec after the first excitation occurred there for the next excitation. Approximately 20 consecutive slices can be obtained with TRs of 2,000 msec, whereas shorter TRs provide less time for exciting and sampling successive slices.

To this point the fundamental concepts of MRI in the CNS have been illustrated by stressing the signal characteristics of water and its admixture with solid tissue.

Obviously, other tissue constituents contain hydrogen, and the reader may be perplexed by the treatment to this point. The hydrogen nuclei of fat can resonate and produce signal, as seen in extraneural tissue, including the orbital fat, that in the scalp's subcutaneous tissue, and that in the bone marrow of the cranium. Indeed, strong signal is seen from these tissues because of rapid magnetization (easy thermal energy exchange, short T1) of protons in these lipids, especially on T1-weighted sequences. In fact, 16% of the white matter and 6% of the gray is composed of lipid. Why then, do we not see that component of the signal from the CNS parenchyma? The major reason is the category of fat with which we are dealing. One-half of the white matter's dry weight is represented by myelin, which contains almost all of its fat. Myelin is a complex, structural lipoprotein which binds its hydrogen nuclei within such a heterogeneous environment that resonance decays very quickly and little signal is seen from this component, leaving the water nuclei to dominate the signal profile (given the 70% water content of white matter) in the manner described previously (10). It is interesting to speculate that with demyelination some of the lipid byproducts would be detectable, but the loss of myelin allows a significant increase in the water content which overpowers any small signal which might have appeared from residual myelin breakdown products. One can observe lipid constituents in the gray and white matter with spectroscopic methods which include various water suppression techniques, methods which will offer important breakthroughs in understanding brain metabolism—as discussed elsewhere in this volume.

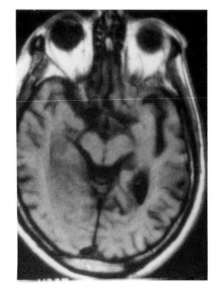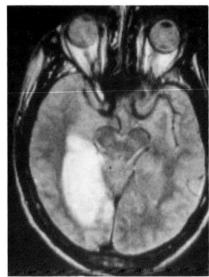

FIG. 11. Acute (8-hr-old) infarct. CT shows subtle changes in the distribution of the right posterior cerebral artery in this patient with acute left homonymous hemanopsia. A T1-weighted MR image (TR 500 msec, TE 30 msec) indicates minimal decrease in signal intensity in the abnormal region because of prolongation of T1 and T2 relaxation values (i.e., intensity sampled at the crossover point—see Fig. 6). Obviously higher intensity as a consequence edema in the infarcted region is seen on the T2-weighted image (TR 2,000 msec, TE 60 msec). The differential T1 relaxation effects were canceled by use of the long TR (see Fig. 8).

An additional point is raised by this inability of routine MRI to detect signal from the protons of brain lipids. The quantification of proton density by MRI instruments, as reported in the literature, suffers from this lack of brain lipid signal detection. When basic biochemical methods are used to determine the concentration of hydrogen, the gray and the white matter are bound to contain essentially equal amounts of this atom (11). However, MRI studies mention a 15 to 20% greater protein density in the gray matter than in the white matter (12). This discrepancy is explained by MRI's inability to "count" the protons in myelin. These points explain the obvious correlation between MRI's quantification of proton density differences and the known water concentration differences between gray and white matter; that is, only the water protons are accounted for in the MRI signal.

Having come this far, a rather simple distillate remains for us. Most conditions which affect the brain will result in edema, i.e., a raised water content. The slow magnetization of the water protons leads to *lower* signal on T1-weighted sequences compared to dry tissue if the sample point is sufficiently early to avoid the crossover point discussed earlier. On the other hand, the increase in free water means more protons to resonate and give signal and slow signal decay, the two phenomena combining to produce *high* signal on T2-weighted images. The sensitivity of MRI to even small increases in water content is great. However, this sensitivity has a price. Because most damage to brain tissue either is a consequence of an elevated water content or results in a raised water content in the affected tissue compared to normal, the signal characteristics of many diverse brains may be similar.

As is the case for CT, the ability to differentiate between various insults which produce edema in the brain relies heavily on the morphologic appearance of the lesion, its location, and our knowledge of disease presentation and pathophysiology in the CNS. It must be remembered at this point that other distinct biochemical alterations besides simple changes in tissue water content are operative in MRI, and their understanding improves one's ability to interpret MRI studies. Perhaps the other most important pathologic factor in the depiction of CNS disease on MRI is hemorrhage.

Some of the iron-containing molecules like hemoglobin, methemoglobin, hemosiderin, and ferritin may dramatically shorten the T1 and/or T2 relaxation values of nearby hydrogen nuclei. The amount of associated free water produced with hemorrhage, the type and perhaps configuration of the iron-containing molecule, its distribution (intra- versus extracellular; homogenous versus irregular), and the field strength of the MR images all strongly influence the degree of relaxation effect that

may be seen. These effects are discussed in depth elsewhere in this volume. To briefly introduce this topic, it suffices to say that certain molecules intrinsic to biological tissues (and ones which can be introduced intentionally) significantly shorten the ability of hydrogen nuclei to exchange energy with their lattice, and alter the magnetic homogeneity of the environment. T1 and T2 relaxation values may both be shortened by these substances. For example, when red cells lyse after a hemorrhage, and their hemoglobin is altered into methemoglobin, the T1 relaxation of nearby protons is drastically shortened; that is, they magnetize much more quickly, leading to a much stronger signal from affected tissues on T1-weighted images. Another example is that of hemosiderin, found in phagocytic cells in sites of previous hemorrhage. This compound disrupts local magnetic homogeneity, causing some loss of coherent resonance and signal intensity from nearby protons. The effect is more evident at higher magnetic fields and leads to signal void (dark pixels) (13). This preferential T2 shortening may also be seen in acute hemorrhage in which deoxyhemoglobin within red cells is the responsible substance.

The former effect (T1 shortening produced by certain paramagnetic substances like methemoglobin) has been exploited in the production of contrast-enhancing moieties to be injected when identification of otherwise isointense tissues is needed. Accumulation of the contrast agent in one of the two tissues (presumably the abnormal one) would shorten that tissue's T1 relaxation time, leading to a higher signal being seen. As discussed in the chapter on contrast agents, the concentration of these substances is critical. Too high a concentration can produce unwanted T2 relaxation shortening, akin to that observed in sites of hemosiderin accumulation, and signal will be lost.

Calcium deposits, be they dystrophic or metastatic, are alterations seen in the tissues of the CNS which affect MRI signal intensity. The more calcium in a region of interest, the less hydrogen, and, by extension, the less signal elicited. CT is very sensitive to the presence of calcium in tissues; MRI is not. When focal signal void is evident, calcium deposition can be inferred, but partial volume effects make detection of calcium difficult. On the other hand, if the tissue harboring the calcium is abnormal, its hydrogen nuclei still behave in the pathologic patterns described above. Therefore, calcified tumors, such as astrocytomas, are more easily separated from benign calcification with MRI than with CT, where the neoplastic component may appear isodense, with only the calcification being seen.

Finally, flow strongly influences the appearance of certain structures as shown by MRI. The complexity of flow phenomena necessitate a separate treatment of this topic elsewhere in this volume. Both blood and CSF motions can provide important data on MRI.

REFERENCES

1. Bradley W, Newton T, Crooks LE. Physical properties of NMR. In: Newton TH, Potts DG, eds. *Modern Neuroradiology,* Vol. 2, *Advanced imaging techniques.* San Francisco: Clavadel Press, 1983:15–61.
2. Young IR, Burl M, Clarke G, et al. Magnetic resonance properties of hydrogen: imaging the posterior fossa. *AJR* 1981;137:895–901.
3. Gore JC, Emergy EW, Orr JS, et al. Medical nuclear magnetic resonance imaging—I. Physical principles. *Invest Radiol* 1981;16:269–74.
4. Pykett IL. NMR imaging in medicine. *Sci Am* 1982;246(5):78–88.
5. Crooks LE, Mills CM, Davis PL, et al. Visualization of cerebral and vascular abnormalities by NMR imaging—the effects of imaging parameters on contrast. *Radiology* 1982;144:843–52.
6. Crooks LE, Arakawa M, Hoenninger J, et al. Magnetic resonance imaging: effects of magnetic field strength. *Radiology* 1984;151:127–33.
7. Koenig SH, Brown RD, Adams D. Magnetic field dependence of 1/T1 of protons in tissue. *Radiology* 1984;19:76–81.
8. Johnson G, Herfkens R, Brown M. Tissue relaxation time: *in vivo* field dependence. *Radiology* 1985;156:805–10.
9. Fullerton G, Cameron I, Ord V. Frequency dependence of magnetic resonance spin–lattice relaxation of protons in biological materials. *Radiology* 1984;151:135–8.
10. Kjos B, Ehman R, Brant-Zawadzki M, et al. Reproducibility of relaxation times and spine density calculated from routine MR imaging sequences: clinical study of the CNS. *AJNR* 1985;6:271–6.
11. Brooks R, Di Chiro G, Keller M. Explanation of cerebral white-gray contrast in computed tomography. *J Comput Assist Tomogr* 1980;4:489–91.
12. Wherli F, Breger R, MacFall J, et al. Quantification of contrast in clinical MR brain imaging at high magnetic field. *Invest Radiol* 1985;20:360–9.
13. Gomori J, Grossman R, Goldberg H, et al. Intracranial hematomas: imaging by high field MR. *Radiology* 1985;157:87–94.

CHAPTER 2

Magnetic Resonance Instrumentation

Robert A. Bell

Magnetic resonance (MR), while opening new vistas to diagnostic medicine, utilizes equipment that is unfamiliar to most clinicians. Beyond learning to cope with new terms, such as *spin–echo, T1, T2,* and *spin density,* health care professionals are faced with the inclusion of magnetic and radiofrequency effects in their facilities produced by a complex array of devices. It is the purpose of this chapter to outline the components of an MR imaging system, to discuss their functions, and to note the variations in equipment commercially available.

Although basic MR physics is discussed thoroughly in another chapter, a review of fundamental concepts may aid our understanding of these devices.

1. A magnetic field is necessary to establish the two "spin" energy states available to hydrogen nuclei (parallel to the external magnetic field and antiparallel; up and down).

2. Radiofrequencies (RF) are used to "excite" the nuclei. Some absorb this energy and flip to the higher energy state, yielding a distribution of spins different from normal conditions (equilibrium).

3. Once the RF pulse ceases, the spins begin to flip back to the lower energy state (relax) to reattain their normal equilibrium distribution. To do so, they give up the energy they have taken on by emitting an RF signal. These signals are detected and processed into images or spectra.

4. The frequencies (W_0) at which nuclei may absorb or reemit energy, the process known as *resonance,* are strictly specified by the type of constituents within the nucleus (gyromagnetic ratio) and the magnetic field (B_0) they experience ($W_0 = \gamma B_0$). Only those nuclei that fulfill certain conditions may receive or give RF signals.

A block diagram of generic components found in a modern MR system is shown in Fig. 1. The dominant feature is the magnet, which generates the main external or "static" magnetic field. Within its bore are located the shim, gradient, and RF coils. Shim coils correct small irregularities in the static field. Gradient coils are necessary to spatially encode the image information. Radiofrequency coils are the antennae used in the transmission of RF pulses and in the reception of weak signals

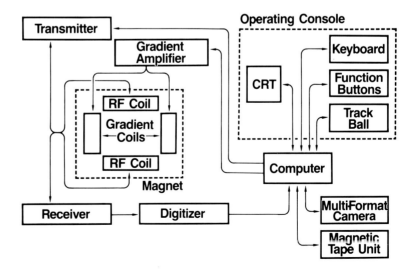

FIG. 1. Block diagram for generic MR system.

produced by the tissue. A computer controls the RF transmitter and gradient power supplies to generate proper pulse sequences. It also enables the receiver to listen at the appropriate time for RF signals, which are then processed into digitized images. The image data are displayed on the operator's console from which it may be filmed or stored on magnetic disks or tape.

An MR system may be divided into five main areas: (a) magnet, (b) gradient system, (c) RF system, (d) computer, and (e) ancillary devices. Each shall be examined in detail. (See refs. 1 and 2 for further reading.)

MAGNETS

The magnet provides the main field (B_0) for orienting the nuclei. As the magnetic field is increased, the energy separation between the two energy states in which the nuclei are aligned (Zeeman splitting) is increased. This results in greater population differences between these states, which gives rise to more signal. There are, however, varying sources of noise in each system, so optimal field strength remains controversial.

The four major types of magnets are permanent, resistive, hybrid, and superconducting. Wide variations in cost, construction, and technical specifications produce no clear choice for all imaging applications. Each is discussed with regard to advantages and shortcomings.

Permanent Magnet

This is the well-known bar, horseshoe, or refrigerator magnet. An iron core can retain a permanent magnetic field through ferromagnetic alignment of iron nuclei. Because the iron itself provides a return pathway for magnetic flux, there is at most a negligible external magnetic field. Thus, some siting problems may be reduced (magnetic interactions with equipment or intrusions into public areas). Permanent magnets do not require electric power to produce their magnetic fields nor do they need cryogens (liquified gases) or large volumes of cooling water. The orientation of the field, transverse to the bore, allows the use of solenoidal RF coils, which may offer some advantages in signal-to-noise (S/N) considerations (3).

Present designs are, however, not without disadvantages. Currently, permanent systems are limited to a field strength of approximately 0.3 tesla (T) [3,000 gauss (G)] for full-bore instruments. These magnets weigh approximately 100 tons (200,000 lbs), thereby posing some unique siting demands. Field homogeneity is critically dependent on design and to a lesser degree on the temperature stability of the room. Should inexpensive higher field materials become available (e.g., rare earth ceramics), permanent systems may be more attractive.

Resistive Magnet

Electric current flowing through a wire produces a magnetic field that circulates about the wire. Wrapping wire into coils and stacking them as shown in Fig. 2 produces a magnetic field down the bore (common centers). Such air-core toroidal resistive magnets employ well-known technology and inexpensive materials and allow assembly on site. They require no cryogens, are relatively light weight (~5 tons) and can be shut down when not in use. However, since the copper windings present some resistance to the passage of electric current (hence the name), significant amounts of electricity are continuously needed to produce the field. In this process, heat is produced that must be removed by relatively large volumes of cooling water. Practical limitations on power consumption and cooling water have yielded maximum magnetic fields of approximately 0.2 T (2,000 G). These systems also exhibit the sensitivity of their field homogeneity to fluctuations of temperature seen with permanent magnets.

Hybrid Magnet

An attempt to combine the positive features of permanent and resistive magnets has resulted in various hybrid designs. Most incorporate an iron core, with resistive electromagnets augmenting the field. Thus, higher magnetic fields may be attained with lower power, cooling, or weight requirements than those of standard permanent or resistive systems. At present, two such systems are commercially available. One is designed for mobile operation, has a field strength of 0.3 T (3,000 G) and weighs approximately 35 tons (70,000 lbs). The other weighs approximately 15 tons and operates at 0.4 T (4,000 G).

Although the iron core is not sufficient to absorb fully the total external magnetic flux, the external field is still smaller than an equivalent resistive or superconducting

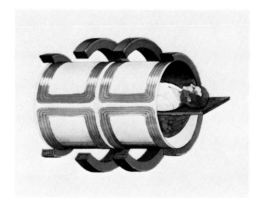

FIG. 2. Air-core toroidal magnet.

design. Electricity and cooling water are necessary to operate the magnet. Again, sensitivity of field homogeneity to variations in ambient temperature may be of concern.

Superconducting Magnet

Certain alloys and other materials lose all resistance to the passage of electric current when they are chilled below a critical temperature (4,5). Magnet coils made of niobium/titanium wire, one such alloy, and cooled with liquid helium (4.2°K) may be energized much as a battery is charged. Electric current, necessary to produce the designed magnetic field, is circulated through these coils. The power supply is then disconnected via a superconducting switch, and the trapped electricity produces a constant field without additional energy.

Superconducting whole-body systems have generated the strongest fields yet obtained, up to 2 T (20,000 G). They have a high degree of homogeneity and stability and low-temperature sensitivity. Although the magnet does not require additional electricity, cryogens (liquified gases) are needed to keep the coils below their critical temperature. With larger magnetic fields comes the possibility of increased siting concerns. The superconducting wire and the dewars (vacuum-enclosed bottles that hold the coils and cryogens) increase the cost of manufacture, service, and installation. Although the field is almost always kept on, shut-down, if needed, may involve substantial cryogen consumption.

Shim Coils

As yet, no magnet produces a sufficiently homogeneous field by itself to be used for MR imaging or spectroscopy (Table 1). A set of coils called shims are used to adjust portions of the static field by adding or subtracting small bits of magnetism where appropriate. These are placed directly inside the bore of the magnet. When the magnet is installed, the field is measured, and the

TABLE 1. *The four major types of magnets*

Magnet		Characteristic
Permanent	Positive	Reduced external magnetic fields
		No cryogen or electric power needed
		Low-cost materials
		Transverse field allows solenoidal coils
	Negative	Field strength limited to 0.3 T
		Heavy (~100 tons); may require structural reinforcing
		Temperature sensitive
		Field homogeneity highly dependent on pole design
Resistive	Positive	Well-known technology (manufacture, service, installation)
		No cryogens needed
		Relatively lightweight (~5 tons)
		Easy to shut down field
	Negative	Large amounts of electricity needed
		Heat produced must be removed with cooling water
		Limited to 0.2 T at present
		Temperature sensitive
Hybrid	Positive	Lower weight than permanent (~35 tons)
		No cryogens needed
		Small fringe field
		Transverse design allows solenoidal coils
	Negative	Electricity and cooling water required
		Low field at present (0.3 T)
		Temperature sensitive
		Heavier than resistive or superconducting
Superconducting	Positive	Higher fields attainable (up to 2.0 T)
		Field more homogeneous
		Field less temperature sensitive
		No electricity needed after energizing
	Negative	More expensive
		Stronger fields may require magnetic shielding
		Cryogens are necessary
		Shut-down, if needed, may involve substantial cryogen loss

shims are set. Once set they need not be altered unless the magnet is moved or unless there are substantial changes in the magnet location or the amount of iron around the magnet. This procedure, known as active shimming, is of critical importance to establish the homogeneity characteristics of the system on which imaging depends.

Minor field adjustments may also be accomplished through the careful placement of small pieces of iron on the magnet. This technique, known as passive shimming, may be used in conjunction with active shimming to remove the effects of large metal objects (e.g., structural steel) close to the magnet.

GRADIENT SYSTEM

The Larmor equation, $W_0 = \gamma B_0$, states that the resonant frequency (W_0) equals the product of the gyromagnetic ratio (where γ is a constant specific for each nucleus; e.g., ^1H, ^{31}P) and the external magnetic field (B_0). Small changes in the magnetic field that the particular nucleus in the tissue experiences will result in small but observable changes in the frequency at which its RF absorption or emission will occur. We can exploit this property by adding a weak changing (gradient) magnetic field to the static field. The previously mentioned shim coils are used to add or subtract small bits of magnetism from the main field to produce greater homogeneity. In like fashion, gradient coils, which lie inside the shim coils, can add and subtract magnetism to give an evenly increasing magnetic field as a function of distance.

Consider a coil, wound as shown in Fig. 3, which yields +25 G at one end tapering to zero field at the center and dropping smoothly to −25 G at the other end. When operated in the bore of a 15,000-G superconducting magnet, the total field would be 15,025 G at one end, 15,000 G in the center, and 14,975 G at the far end. Protons at 15,000 G normally resonate (give or receive RF) at approximately 63.9 megahertz (MHz). In this field gradient, however, only those in the middle of the magnet will resonate at this frequency; those at the higher field end will respond to slightly higher frequency (64.0 MHz) and those at the lower field end to lower frequency (63.8 MHz). Therefore by choosing the appropriate frequency, we can selectively excite a particular slice of tissue. Slice thickness is specified by a combination of gradient strength and transmitter frequency bandwidth (amount of variation about the transmitted frequency).

Field gradients may also be established down the remaining directions (vertical and horizontal). These are used while the signal from the tissue is being received. Just as the transmission gradient down the longitudinal direction was used to select the slice, these field gradients provided X, Y coordinates for the pixels in the image.

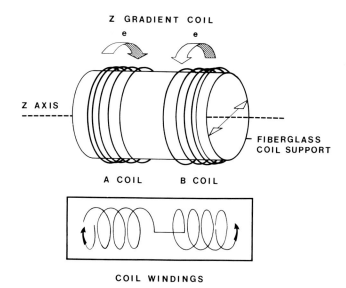

FIG. 3. Gradient coil design.

Individual volume elements of tissue (voxels) are thereby related to picture elements (pixels) on the image. One direction is frequency encoded; the magnetic variation induced by the field gradient over the tissue slice is matched with a group frequency. Each voxel gives a different frequency signal so it can be correlated with the location of a pixel in an image. The strength of this signal becomes a measure of the brightness of that pixel.

Since two different frequencies cannot be received simultaneously from the same voxel of tissue, the second image direction is phase encoded. If two spins are precessing together at the same frequency, they are said to be "in phase," as shown in Fig. 4. If the magnetic field gradient is turned on, the spin in the higher field will precess faster and get ahead of the other spin, generating a "phase difference," which can be detected. Since phase is the product of frequency times the length of time the gradient is on (or the magnitude of the gradient), we can calculate the frequency once the phase is determined. Therefore, using X and Y gradients alternately, we can encode both image directions, one with frequency and the other with phase.

Gradient coil design is a critical feature of an MR system. Various parameters have a strong impact on image quality and system flexibility:

1. *Homogeneous volume.* Standard "Golay" coils (saddle type) produce sufficient homogeneity for imaging over only approximately 60% of coil volume. Because space is very limited within the magnet bore, the smaller the homogeneous volume the greater the constraint on imaging volume.

2. *Linearity.* A lack of precision in the gradients will produce dark areas around the edge of images or distor-

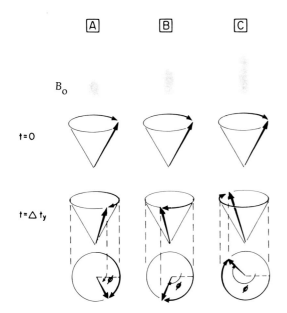

FIG. 4. Principle of phase encoding. At the beginning of the phase-encoding period ($t = 0$), all nuclear magnetic moments have the same relative phase. Since the field increases from left to right (y gradient), the nucleus in voxel C precesses faster than the nucleus in voxel A. At the end of the phase-encoding period, the nucleus in voxel C, therefore, has built up a phase angle that is larger than that for a nucleus in voxel A. It is evident that the phase angle in this case is uniquely related to the position of the nucleus along the y axis.

tions of anatomical features. Linearity is a measure of evenness.

3. *Gradient magnitude and flexibility.* The strength (magnitude) of the gradient field impacts slice thickness and field of view (FOV). If variable, different FOVs are available and offer the operator selectable levels of spatial resolution (FOV divided by matrix equals spatial resolution). Since the matrix is one determinant of acquisition time, such variation can result in substantial time savings. Magnitude and flexibility are characteristics of the gradient power amplifier.

4. *Gradient risetime.* The speed with which gradients attain their operational values determines in large part how fast echoes may be obtained. This impacts the system's future applications using short echo-delay times (sodium imaging, cartilage, and fibrous tissue, etc.).

Gradient coils are typically wound as a single assembly that contains coils for all three directions ($X, Y,$ and Z axes) and fits in the magnet bore inside of the shim coils. They are energized individually over a short time interval (a few milliseconds) to create additional magnetic fields within the static field. Because magnets attract or repel each other, the coil attempts to move in the static field, thus generating the "knocking" noise common to MR images. Sound-insulating materials and

modifications of gradient pulse shape can be used to reduce this noise.

Summary

The gradient system may be used in conjunction with choice of frequency and bandwidth; the transmission gradient establishes slice location and thickness. During signal collection, the remaining two gradients give X, Y coordinates to image pixels. Critical design features include (a) homogeneous volume, which impacts on volume available for imaging and should be at least 90%; and (b) linearity, which measures "evenness" of gradient; deviations should not exceed 2%. In magnitude and variability, it impacts slice thickness and FOV view, and should be variable from 0.3 G/cm to at least 1.0 Gauss/cm (3–10 mT/m). The risetime impacts the speed at which echoes may be sampled; this should be approximately 1 msec.

RADIOFREQUENCY SYSTEM

Radiofrequencies are necessary to promote spins from the lower energy state (parallel) to the higher (antiparallel). The RF subsection of an MR system is comprised of a transmitter, power amplifier, antenna coils, receiver, and low-noise signal amplifiers used in the receiver circuit. As shown in the block diagram of Fig. 1, the antenna coils are located within the magnet bore. Various parameters are now discussed.

1. *Frequency response.* Magnetic resonance active elements differ in their gyromagnetic ratios. Hence, they resonate at different frequencies in the same magnetic field. Table 2 lists some representative nuclei at 1.5 T (15,000 G). Multinuclear capability requires both a transmitter and a receiver that operate over a wide range of frequencies. Fixed-frequency systems can only observe a single element and only at the designated magnetic field (e.g., 21 MHz selects hydrogen at 0.5 T).

2. *Noise.* S/N ratios are of critical importance in MR; this technique is starved for signal. Therefore, all possible efforts must be taken to maximize signal and mini-

TABLE 2. *NMR data for nuclei of biological interest*

Nucleus	Spin	Abundance (%)	At 1.5 T (MHz)
^{1}H	1/2	99.99	63.85
^{13}C	1/2	1.11	16.05
^{19}F	1/2	100.00	60.06
^{23}Na	3/2	100.00	16.89
^{31}P	1/2	100.00	25.84

mize noise. Electronic noise from amplifier stages is one source. RF coil design also has an impact by improving signal. Whereas the largest noise source at field strength of 0.3 T and above is the patient within the instrument, noise contributions from amplifiers and RF coils must be controlled (6).

3. *Linearity and stability.* Because slice location and thickness are determined by RF frequency and bandwidth, the constancy of RF transmitter response over the frequency range is important. The receiver circuitry must also properly amplify appropriate signals over the same range to assure that pixel intensities properly represent differing tissues.

4. *Power.* Optimal signal requires full excitation of the selected tissue slice by transmitted RF. Because humans vary in shape, weight, and tissue ratios, the absorption of transmitted RFs will also vary. Heavier patients require more RF power than thinner patients.

5. *RF coil design.* Perhaps no aspect of MR will undergo as many changes in the next few years as the coils used to transmit and receive the radio signals. Already there are saddle coils, solenoidal coils, slotted resonators, surface coils, and a variety of other types. The highly competitive and proprietary nature of this area makes it a priority for manufacturers and research institutions. One measure of coil performance, Q (quality factor), is often quoted for comparison. Such figures may, however, be assessed with the coil unloaded (empty) or loaded (with patient in place). Clearly, the loaded Q is more relevant to clinical use.

6. *Quadrature detection and/or excitation.* The MR signal returning from the patient has two components: so-called absorption and dispersion modes (real and imaginary parts). Modern systems utilize quadrature detection to collect both modes, which provides S/N enhancement of $\sqrt{2}$ over single-component detection (7).

Transmission of RF energy into the patient can be accomplished in one of two ways. Linear excitation uses linearly oscillating (polarized) magnetic and electric fields. This means that these fields rise and fall within single planes that are oriented 90° to one another. The linear behavior of the magnetic field can be pictured mathematically through two vectors rotating like clock hands in opposite directions. When these are aligned, the magnetic field is at a maximum; when they are opposed, the field drops to zero. This is shown in Fig. 5. The hydrogen nuclei precess in only one direction. Therefore, under linear excitation the MR technique makes use of only one of these two vectors; half of the RF power is wasted. Quadrature excitation places the entire RF energy into a single rotating magnetic field vector (circular polarization). No power is wasted. Two major advantages over linear excitation are (a) the production of a much more evenly rotating magnetic field

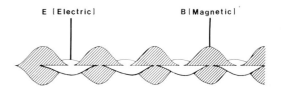

RADIOFREQUENCY PROPAGATION

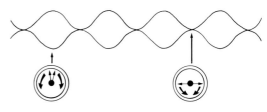

LINEARLY POLARIZED
B-VECTOR

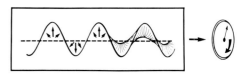

CIRCULARLY POLARIZED
[QUADRATURE]
B-VECTOR

FIG. 5. Linear and quadrature excitation.

(better RF homogeneity and improved images), and (b) a reduction in power deposition by a factor of 2. The latter is especially useful in multislice, multiecho body imaging of very heavy patients at high field (8).

COMPUTER

The computing system is usually the second most expensive component in an MR system. As a technique heavily dependent on numerical methods, MR requires powerful and versatile computers. Poor design in this section can produce major operational difficulties or expensive delays if new processors are needed. Architecture, hardware/software, and storage capabilities should be considered with regard to utility, flexibility, and upgrade potential.

Architecture

The various approaches to MR data processing offer a spectrum of advantages and drawbacks. Some manufacturers prefer interlinked processors for system functions (data collection, system coordination, image processing, etc.); others prefer a large control unit that shares time among the functions. Whatever the design, there are important questions.

1. Is the system capable of processing the large amount of data inherent in MR in an efficient manner? This can be evaluated by noting the reconstruction time of a multislice, multiecho acquisition. A modern MR system should process $(256)^2$ images in less than 10 sec per image, and times of less than 5 sec are achievable.

2. Does operation of one part of the system exclude operation of other parts? If image reconstruction or tape archiving precludes data collection, substantial time may be lost in operation.

3. Is the pulse programmer (subsystem responsible for coordinating the RF pulses and gradient fields) flexible enough to accommodate new pulse sequences that surely will appear? System flexibility can be measured to a large degree by the range of scan protocols it encompasses. Different choices of echo delay time (TE) and pulse repetition time (TR) produce various ratios of T1, T2 and hydrogen density and therefore different images. Limited spans for TE and TR result in limited access to information that is important to diagnosis. What ranges are available? When will increased ranges appear? What guarantees are manufacturers willing to give? All good questions.

Hardware/Software

The evaluation of the computing portion of an MR system should be based on a number of factors. Processing speed in certainly important, but we must also consider the expertise of the manufacturer, the opportunity for upgrades, the flexibility and acceptance of the languages available, and the ability to network various instruments. Even service policies should be examined, because the purchaser could be trapped in a squabble between the medical equipment manufacturer and his computer supplier (who may hold the responsibility for computer repair). Many hours have been lost in finger-pointing.

Upgradeability is of special importance and merits individual comment. Without question, new pulsing sequences and computational algorithms will appear. Can the system adjust to those changes without major component changes or inordinate downtime? To what degree can the user program critical operational parameters? Does the manufacturer provide a schedule for promised software upgrades? Are guarantees explicit? Is the manufacturer sensitive to users' suggestions for system improvement?

Storage Capability

Magnetic resonance is more information intensive than other techniques such as computed tomography (CT). In large part this is due to the increased number of images created. Consider a typical case: a 20-slice, two-echo acquisition taken in two different planes (e.g., axial and sagittal) yields 80 images. If utilizing a 256×256 matrix, this represents a minimum of 10 megabytes of image information, excluding patient data or raw acquisition data. If 12 to 20 patients are scanned each day, the accumulated data would rapidly approach 200 megabytes of required storage. Archiving more than once a day can require inordinate technologist time and have a negative effect on system economics by decreasing efficiency. In future, raw data storage may also be important for advanced techniques, such as spectroscopy and restrospective image synthesis, further straining marginal storage capability. Consider system storage capability carefully.

ANCILLARY CONCERNS

Console

The design of the operator's console contributes to MR efficiency. The speed with which scan setups are completed, images processed and photographed, and the degree of confidence technologists feel with an instrument can have a marked impact on the number and quality of examinations. These are worth consideration:

Display. Larger displays offer advantages for diagnosing from the console. Higher resolution monitors yield better images.

Upgrade policy. MR, as a technique in transition, will experience many changes in the next 10 years. What provisions have been made for such changes?

Versatility. Are some system functions locked out when others are in use?

Special features. Multi-image display; operator instructions available in display; automatic prescan procedures; intercom to patient; graphic prescription relating subsequent images to a localizer; cine-mode, etc.

Radiofrequency Shielding

All efforts must be made to protect the weak signal originating in the patient from interfering RF sources in the environment. MR imaging is an S/N-starved technique; other signals, such as television and radio transmissions, computer noises, pager transmitters, can seriously degrade images. Some form of RF shielding is required.

Radiofrequency shielding works by "grounding" electrical signals coming from the outside. External or "room" shielding consists of copper or specially treated aluminum sheets on all walls, floor, and ceiling and a special door to seal against leakage. Internal or "wave-guide" shielding is usually a conductive tube that is pulled out from the bore of the magnet to elongate the patient tube. Radio signals that enter the ends are grounded as they bounce down the tube.

Shield effectiveness is rated in decibels (dB). Every 10 dB is a *factor* of 10 in the attenuation or reduction of RF noise. The difference in attenuation between 60 and 100 dB is 10,000, not 40. Ratings should be at or above the expected operating frequency; 60 dB at 20 MHz is approximately 55 dB at 60 MHz. Most MRI manufacturers recommend room shielding as insurance against future RF noise sources and to reduce patients' feelings of claustrophobia.

Magnetic Shielding

Magnetic resonance imaging has brought strong magnetic fields into the hospital. Other instruments, particularly those that use electron beams (CT, X-ray, image intensifiers, TV monitors, etc.), as well as people with cardio- or neurostimulating devices may be affected if placed too close to the field. Conversely, large metal objects, such as automobiles, girders, plates, or trash carts, may perturb the homogeneity of the field and degrade imaging. For these reasons, magnetic shielding has been developed.

Iron absorbs magnetism much as a sponge absorbs water. Hence, magnetic shielding entails placing sufficient amounts of iron around a magnet to pull in the field to match site requirements. At the same time, the shield should by no means restrict the imaging or spectroscopic capabilities of the system. Customers who require magnetic shields are well advised to obtain strong operational guarantees from the designers. Shields are moderately expensive; mistakes in design can result in far more expensive delays.

Shields are usually custom designed and built, owing to the unique characteristics of individual sites. Many sites with room to spare require no magnetic shielding at all. Certainly this is preferable from an instrumental viewpoint but with the realities of real estate costs, proximity within the hospital, and other site issues, it can be comforting to know solutions are available.

Patient Comfort and Safety

One of the characteristics of MR is its noninvasive nature. Patients are comforted by the absence of needles, contrast agents, and radioisotopes. However, since patients must be placed into the magnet to be imaged, some experience a degree of claustrophobia. This can be minimized through instrument design: widening the bore of the system, opening the head coil so that patients can see out, lighting the magnet bore, and providing ventilation have all been used. One should take the time to experience all systems under consideration from the patient's vantage.

Patient safety must also be considered. Imagine the case of a patient who has a heart attack while undergoing an MR scan. The crash team may have difficulty operating resuscitation equipment near the bore of the magnet, so most manufacturers have made provision for removing the patient to a "crash area" of low magnetic field. Some employ a removable table; others have a pallet on which the patient is carried. Discuss these features carefully to prepare for any untoward events.

Service Consideration

Never has there been so complicated a device in hospitals as the MR scanner. It not only incorporates the complexity of modern computer equipment (disk and tape drives, array processors, etc.) but also powerful yet precise RF transmitters, receivers, power supplies, and gradient systems. These require specially trained and equipped service personnel. There are also instrument features that can augment their effectiveness.

1. *Quality assurance procedures.* Daily checks of critical performance parameters such as S/N, linearity, field uniformity, slice thickness, contrast ratios, and resolution.
2. *Service diagnostic software incorporated into the operating system.* The computer can be used to monitor system performance.
3. *Component access.* Design of cabinets, consoles, etc., to allow rapid service.
4. *Autotuning.* Automatic control of frequency tuning, pulse angle, precision shimming, and other critical adjustments.

Extended Features

A wide variety of special features are available that can add to data analysis and broaden the patient base. We may wish to consider some of the following:

1. *Cardiac gating.* Data acquisition is linked to cardiac phase, allowing images of various points in the heart cycle (9).
2. *Respiratory motion compensation.* MR imaging acquisitions take minutes in general and as such are subject to image degradation from motion. Various techniques are offered to correct for these (10).
3. *Flow imaging.* MR imaging has great potential for some aspects of vascular imaging, offering not only visualization but also direction and magnitude (11,12).
4. *T1/T2 measurement.* Tissue characterization may become increasingly important for specificity and contrast optimization (13).
5. *Synthetic imaging.* If accurate T1, T2, and spin density values can be extracted for a slice of tissue, any image protocol may be computer synthesized. This gives

promise to the development of a standard protocol for patient exam in which the choices are slice location, thickness, number, and matrix. Later, the radiologist may synthesize the appropriate images by his selection of TR and TE (or TR/T1 for inversion recovery) (14).

6. *Chemical shift imaging.* Allows imaging of selected chemical species (e.g., fat images or water images); also can be used to remove chemical shift artifacts (15,16).

7. *Surface coils.* Specialized RF coils designed to maximize S/N in various anatomical regions (orbit, knee, breast, etc.) (17).

8. *Spectroscopy.* MR is capable of yielding chemical information as well as images. These chemical data may, in future, be used to diagnose disease or discriminate between degrees of malignancy in tumors (18,19).

Mobile Operation

Magnetic resonance imaging units have been placed in vans to service larger areas. New technical challenges have been met, but we should consider possible trade-offs.

1. As in fixed systems, the most important aspect of mobile MR is the magnet. Superconducting systems require special internal reinforcing against road vibration. Permanent systems at this time appear to be too heavy for mobile operation, but hybrid designs will accommodate federal highway weight limits.

2. Vibration strengthening in superconducting magnets entails greater heat leakage into the dewars. Thus, cryogen consumption is substantially greater than in fixed systems. Additional cryogen is lost in ramping procedures (the magnet must be deenergized before and reenergized after each move). Most superconducting mobile MR systems employ on-board refrigeration to minimize these losses, but we may still expect greater cryogen use than in fixed systems.

3. RF shielding is built directly into the body of the van.

4. Magnetic shielding, if necessary, is available in the form of iron "garages" into which the van can be parked.

5. Carefully evaluate any compromises imposed upon an MR system by mobile configuration. Question manufacturers in detail and request performance specifications.

REFERENCES

1. Bradley WG, Newton TH, Crooks LE. In: Newton TH, Potts DG, eds. *Modern radiology, Vol. 2.* San Anselmo, California: Clavadel Press, 1983:15–61.
2. Mansfield P, Morris PG. *NMR imaging in biomedicine.* New York: Academic Press, 1982.
3. Arakawa M, Crooks LE, McCarten B, Hoenninger JC, Kaufman L. Abstracts of the Society of Magnetic Resonance in Medicine meeting, Aug 13–17, New York, 1984:10.
4. Geballe TH, Hulm, JK. *Sci Am* 1980;243:138.
5. Geballe TH, Hulm JK, Matthias BT. *Science* 1980;208:881–7.
6. Hoult DI, Lauterbur PC. *J Mag Res* 1979;34:425.
7. Mansfield P, Morris PG. *J Mag Res* 1979;34:28.
8. Glover GH, Hayes CE, Pelc NJ. *J Mag Res* 1985;64:255–70.
9. Higgins CB, et al. *Radiology* 1985; 155:671–9.
10. Bailes DR, et al. *JCAT* 1985;9:835–8.
11. O'Donnell M. *Med Phys* 1985;12:59–64.
12. Wehrli FW, MacFall JR, Axel L, et al. *Non-Invasive Med Imag* 1984;1:127–136.
13. Bottomley PA, Foster TH, Argersinger RE, Pfeifer LM. *Med Phys* 1984;11:425–48.
14. Bobman SA, Riederer SJ, Lee JN, et al. *Am J Neuroradiol* 1985;6:265–9.
15. Dixon NT. *Radiology* 1984;153:189.
16. Bottomley PA, et al. *Proc Natl Acad Sci USA* 1984;81:6856–60.
17. Edelstein WA, et al. *JAMA* 1985;253:828.
18. Bottomley PA, et al. *Proc Natl Acad Sci USA* 1985;82:2148–52.
19. Bottomley PA, et al. *J Mag Res* 1984;59:338–42.

CHAPTER 3

Pathophysiologic Correlates of Signal Alterations

William G. Bradley, Jr.

Magnetic resonance (MR) is a nonionizing imaging technique capable of producing cross-sectional images, as does its predecessor, X-ray computed tomography (CT). Unlike CT, however, MR can provide images directly in the transverse axial, coronal, and sagittal planes, as well as in various oblique orientations. Like CT, MR provides computer-generated images comprised of pixels of a specific intensity. The pixel intensity in CT is based on the X-ray attenuation coefficient, which in turn depends on the electron density, whereas the pixel intensity in MR is a complex function of proton density, T1 and T2 relaxation times, and flow which can be approximated (1) as follows:

$$I = N(H)f(v)e^{-TE/T2}(1 - e^{-TR/T1})$$

where I is the intensity of the pixel, $N(H)$ is the proton density, $f(v)$ is a function of flow, "e" is the base of the natural logarithm (approximately 2.7), and TE and TR are the programmable sequence parameters, the echo delay time and the repetition time, respectively. Thus although the intensity of a pixel on a CT image is a monotonic function of electron density, the intensity of the pixel in an MR image is a variable function of four independent parameters. Notice also that the intensity depends on the programmable sequence parameters TR and TE. Thus the intensity of a given pixel in an MR image is partially determined by the proton density, T1, T2, and flow characteristics of the substance, and is partially determined by sequence parameters chosen for the particular acquisition (2). By proper selection of these imaging parameters, contrast between suspected pathology and background can be enhanced.

Certain combinations of TR and TE on spin echo images are useful in distinguishing between different normal tissues and in maximizing contrast between certain lesions and the normal background (3). Images acquired with short TR and TE times enhance the differences in the T1 relaxation times of different substances.

These are referred to as T1-weighted images (Fig. 1). Images with long repetition times (TR) allow essentially total T1 recovery between repetitions. In such cases, there is little T1 influence on the image. If the echo delay time TE is kept short, the image reflects differences in proton density. As the echo delay time TE is prolonged, differences in the tissue T2 relaxation times are brought out. Images of the brain or spinal cord where the CSF is more intense than neural tissue are referred to as "heavily T2-weighted" images (Fig. 2). Images acquired in which the CSF and brain or spinal cord are isointense

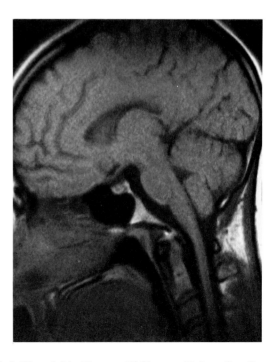

FIG. 1. T1-weighted image. Midline sagittal section through the brain with short TR/short TE technique produces good contrast between brain and CSF (TR = 0.5 sec, TE = 28 msec).

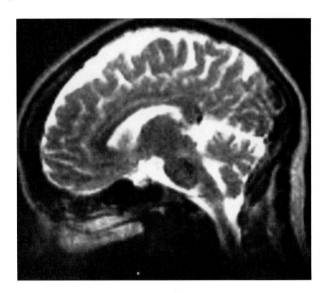

FIG. 2. Heavily T2-weighted image. Midline sagittal section through the brain with long TR/long TE technique produces images with CSF brighter than brain (TR = 3.0 sec, TE = 150 msec).

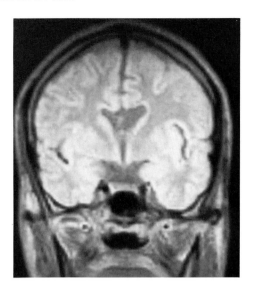

FIG. 4. Mildly T2-weighted image in patient following corpus callosum sectioning. The relatively long TR provides gray–white differentiation on the basis of differences in proton density. A relatively short TE keeps the long-T2 CSF relatively less intense than brain. (*Note:* A proton density-weighted image would have a similar appearance; however, most scanners commercially available today are unable to provide echo delay times short enough to provide a true proton density weighted image). (TR = 2.0 sec, TE = 28 msec.)

are referred to as "moderately T2-weighted" images (Fig. 3). Images in which there is gray–white differentiation (based on differences in proton density) and where CSF is less intense than brain (Fig. 4) are variously referred to as "proton density-weighted" images or "mildly T2-weighted" images (2).

Tissue characterization in MR images is based on differences in T1 and T2 relaxation times and, to a lesser extent, on differences in mobile proton density. The

"mobile" modifier in this case refers to the fact that there is no MR-visible lipid within the normal brain. Although lipid is obviously present in myelin, it is tightly membrane-bound and essentially in the solid

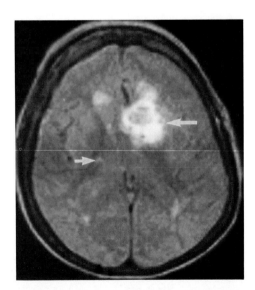

FIG. 3. Moderately T2-weighted image. At intermediate values of TR and TE, brain and CSF become isointense, facilitating visualization of periventricular lacunar infarcts (arrowhead). Note also hypertensive bleed (arrow) (TR = 2.0 sec, TE = 56 msec).

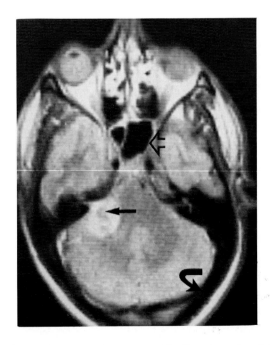

FIG. 5. Low intensity tissues on MR. Note low signal from cortical bone (curved arrow), calcification in acoustic neuroma (arrow), and air in sinuses (open arrow).

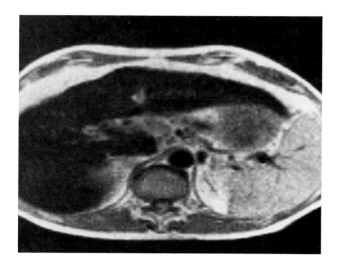

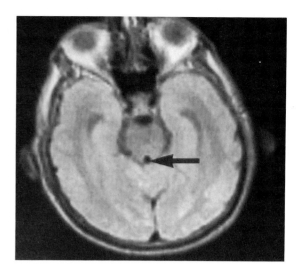

FIG. 6. Hemochromatosis. Magnetically susceptible hemosiderin produces region of locally intense magnetic field. Subsequent dephasing of locally diffusing protons results in T2 shortening (TR = 1.0 sec, TE = 28 msec).

FIG. 8. Aqueductal flow void sign. Pulsatile motion of CSF through the aqueduct produces dephasing and signal loss (arrow). Signal loss may be correlated with ventricular compliance (TR = 2.0 sec, TE = 28 msec).

phase. Thus, it has a very short T2 relaxation time, which prevents it from being visualized on MR images, even those acquired with the shortest echo delay times in the 20 msec range. This lack of visibility of lipid has been demonstrated by proton spectroscopy as well (4).

Tissues that appear dark on MR images generally have little hydrogen, a long T1, and a short T2, or they are in motion during signal acquisition. Examples of low intensity because of low hydrogen density include calcification, cortical bone, and air (Fig. 5). Skeletal muscle has a long T1 and a short T2 relaxation time and thus appears relatively dark on MR images. As discussed below, both solid and magnetically susceptible substances such as tissue iron (Fig. 6) cause extreme T2

shortening with subsequent loss of signal. This can be observed in acute hematomas (5) and in regions where hemosiderin is deposited in the normal or degenerated brain. Such magnetic susceptibility effects are particularly noticeable on high field images. Low signal as a consequence of motion is observed in rapid, turbulent blood flow through arteries (6,7) and in arteriovenous malformations (AVMs) (Fig. 7), as well as in pulsatile flow of CSF (8) through the cerebral aqueduct (Fig. 8).

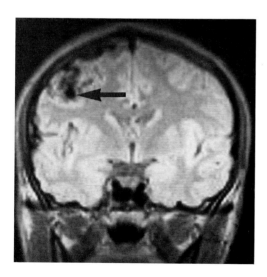

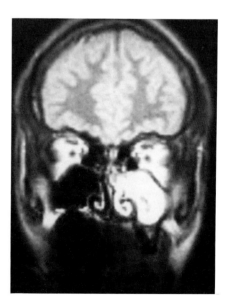

FIG. 7. Arteriovenous malformation. Signal loss is produced by high velocity, turbulent, "disturbed" flow through AVM (arrow).

FIG. 9. High intensity tissues on MR. Mucus in the maxillary sinus appears bright, as does the fat in the orbit, marrow, and subcutaneous soft tissues (TR = 2.0 sec, TE = 56 msec).

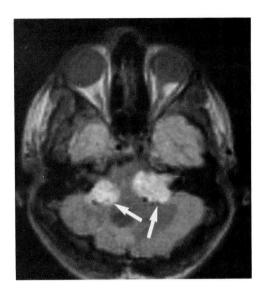

FIG. 10. Paramagnetic contrast-enhanced MR image. High signal intensity is noted following administration of Gd-DTPA in neurofibromotosis patient with bilateral acoustic neuromas (arrows). The short TR/short TE, T1-weighted pulsing sequence brings out the T1 shortening produced by the paramagnetic agent (TR = 0.5 sec, TE = 28 msec).

High signal intensity is found in hydrogen-containing, stationary substances with short T1 and long T2 relaxation times (Fig. 9). These include paramagnetic substances in aqueous solution such as the methemoglobin

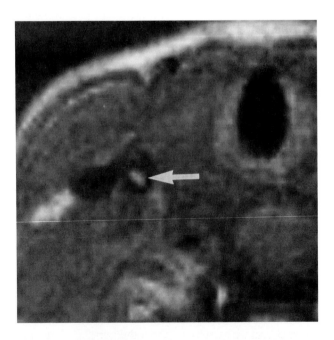

FIG. 11. Flow-related enhancement. High signal intensity is demonstrated in first slice of multislice imaging volume as inflowing, fully magnetized, unsaturated protons yield high signal intensity relative to partially saturated stationary protons in adjacent tissues. Thus, high signal intensity in common carotid artery (arrow) is normal flow phenomenon rather than thrombus (TR = 1.5 sec, TE = 28 msec).

in subacute hemorrhage (9) and gadolinium-DTPA (Gd-DTPA) (10,11), the intravenous MR contrast agent (Fig. 10). Fat has relatively short T1 and long T2 relaxation times and generally appears bright. Slow venous flow can produce high signal. "Flow-related enhancement" (7) occurs when slowly flowing blood enters the first slice of a multislice imaging volume (Fig. 11). "Even echo rephasing" (12) is also seen in slow flow on even echo images (Fig. 12).

When the fundamentals of MR contrast are understood and the sequence parameters properly applied, tissues can often be better characterized by MR than by CT, allowing a more specific diagnosis to be made. In some cases, CT and MR are complementary and both may be required to provide the best noninvasive diagnosis (13).

WATER

While it is strictly true that all mobile protons are capable of contributing to the MR signal detected from a voxel of tissue, water is by far the greatest contributor. In normal tissues, 80% of the signal originates in the cytosol and 20% originates from the extracellular space (14). When the concentration of water is increased locally, e.g., because of brain edema, the magnetic relaxation times are altered in a predictable manner. Specifically, the T1 and T2 relaxation times become prolonged as the water content increases (15). Thus on T1-weighted images an edematous lesion will appear less intense than brain, whereas on T2-weighted images an edematous lesion will appear more intense than brain.

The molecular environment of water has a significant influence on its magnetic relaxation characteristics. "Pure" water (sometimes referred to as "bulk phase" water) like CSF has very long T1 and T2 relaxation times (16). T1 relaxation is most efficient when the natural motional frequencies of the molecule are similar to the operating (Larmor) frequency of the MR imager (17). Water, being a very small molecule, translates, vibrates, and rotates at much higher frequencies than the Larmor frequencies routinely used for MR imaging, i.e., 6 to 65 MHz. Thus bulk phase water is inefficient at T1 relaxation and thus has a long T1 relaxation time. Similarly, protons attached to slowly tumbling macromolecules have natural frequencies much lower than the Larmor frequency and are equally inefficient at T1 relaxation. These molecules also have long T1 relaxation times. When protein is added to pure water, some of the water molecules are attracted to the charged, or polar, hydrophilic side groups of the protein (Fig. 13). These water molecules are arranged in hydration layers around the slowly tumbling protein and their natural motion is between the high frequencies of bulk phase water and the very low motional frequencies of the protein itself.

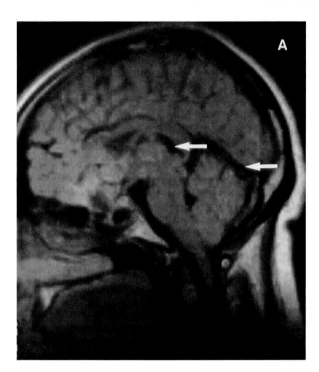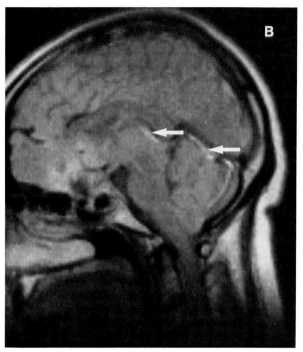

FIG. 12. Even echo rephasing. **A:** First echo image demonstrates dephasing and low signal intensity (arrows) in internal cerebral vein and straight sinus (TR = 1.0 sec, TE = 28 msec). **B:** Even echo rephasing with resultant increased signal intensity (arrows) is noted in internal cerebral vein and straight sinus (TR = 2.0 sec, TE = 56 msec).

As the protein concentration of an aqueous solution increases, an increasing percentage of the water molecules moves at or near the Larmor frequency; the water molecules thus become very efficient at T1 relaxation (16). The T1 relaxation time of proteinaceous solutions is thus much shorter than the T1 of pure water. In fact, the relaxation *rate* (1/T1) can be shown to

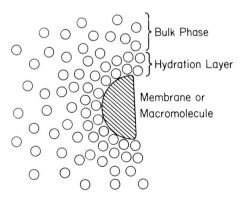

FIG. 13. Molecular environment of water. Water protons in the bulk phase have natural motional frequencies much higher than the Larmor frequency and thus have a long T1 relaxation time. When attracted to hydrophilic side groups of large macromolecules like proteins, the natural motional frequencies are slowed, approaching the Larmor frequency. More efficient T1 relaxation decreases the T1 relaxation time.

increase in direct proportion to the protein concentration (16).

The concepts of "hydration layer" and "bulk phase" water are useful in the clinical context (18). Although cystic astrocytomas may not have densities significantly different from CSF on CT, the T1 relaxation time of the proteinaceous cyst fluid is always shorter than that of CSF on MR. Thus, when a lesion appears to be entirely cystic on CT, MR is sensitive in the distinction of lesions containing only CSF (e.g., arachnoid cysts) from those with higher protein content (Fig. 14) (e.g., cystic astrocytomas or arachnoid cysts which have been complicated by hemorrhage or infection). Similarly, hydromyelia, i.e., CSF in the central canal of the spinal cord, can be distinguished from cord cavitation associated with a tumor on the basis of differences in protein content. The tumor cyst has greater protein content, more hydration layer water, and therefore greater intensity than simple hydromyelia (Fig. 15).

Figure 16 demonstrates encephalomalacia resulting from an old infarct. On a moderately T2-weighted image, there is abnormal high intensity separating the normal brain parenchyma from the peripheral atrophic region with CSF intensity. Both abnormal areas are considered to be "encephalomalacia" on CT. The high intensity portion bordering the normal parenchyma appears as multiple small cysts when viewed microscopically (19). This is known pathologically as "microcystic encephalomalacia." In this abnormal region of the

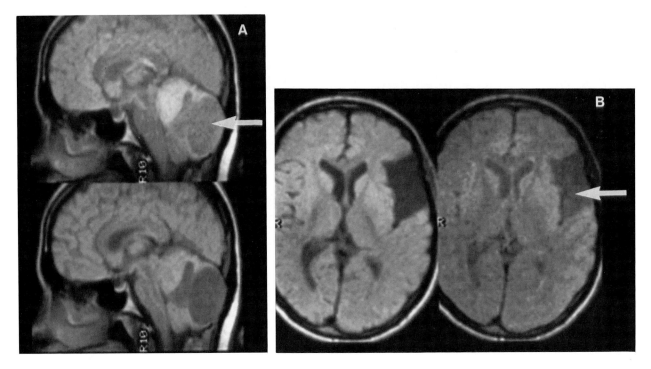

FIG. 14. Differentiation of cystic cerebral masses. **A:** Cystic astrocytoma. Cyst fluid has higher intensity than CSF, indicating higher protein content (TR = 1.0 sec, TE = 28 and 56 msec). **B:** Arachnoid cyst. Intensity of cyst is identical to that of CSF (TR = 1.0 sec, TE = 28 and 56 msec).

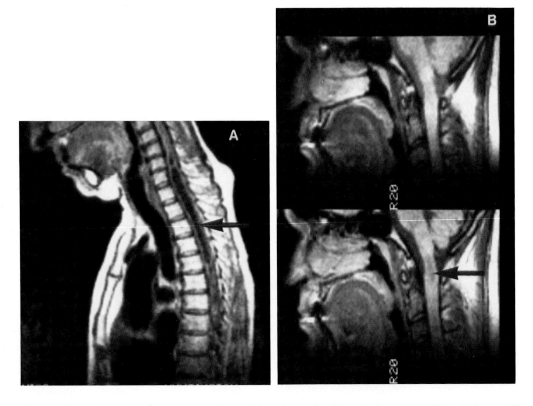

FIG. 15. A: Hydromyelia. Central cystic structure (arrow) has intensity identical to CSF (TR = 0.5 sec, TE = 28 msec). **B:** Syringomyelia associated with tumor. Higher intensity (arrow) is noted within a cystic lesion, indicating higher protein content which is associated with neoplasia (TR = 1.0 sec, TE = 28 and 56 msec).

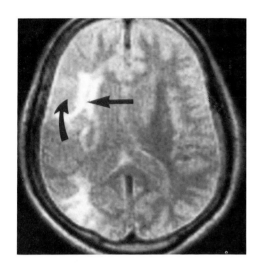

FIG. 16. Encephalomalacia following chronic infarct. Central high intensity (straight arrow) region ("microcystic encephalomalacia") has higher percentage of hydration layer water (with shorter T1) than peripheral zone of "macrocystic encephalomalacia" (curved arrow) where bulk phase water predominates.

brain, the water is found in multiple small cysts interspersed within the brain parenchyma. Because the water in such cysts is always close to a membrane or protein surface, the majority of it is in hydration layers. Such water is expected to have a relatively short T1 relaxation time, yet the T2 relaxation time remains relatively long. Thus there is increased intensity on the moderately T2-weighted image. Peripherally the water is found in larger cystic spaces (which are difficult to distinguish from the enlarged adjacent sulci in the subarachnoid space). This region is known as "macrocystic encephalomalacia" and there is a larger percentage of water in the bulk phase, which thus appears more like CSF (19). Consequently, the abnormal region of brain which we refer to

only as "encephalomalacia" on CT can be divided into two regions ("microcystic" and "macrocystic" encephalomalacia) on MR. It has been speculated that the amount of microcystic encephalomalacia in an infarct reflects the degree of mass effect which was present during the period of acute infarction (19). Such high intensity is also noted in association with gliosis (which itself is fibrotic and therefore has low MR intensity) as a result of previous trauma, surgery, inflammation, hemorrhage, or demyelination (Fig. 17).

BRAIN EDEMA

Brain edema can be classified under three headings: vasogenic, cytotoxic, and interstitial (18,20). Vasogenic edema is the most common form of edema and is produced by blood-brain barrier breakdown. Cytotoxic edema is a result of ischemia and is found in association with acute infarcts. Interstitial edema is found in the periventricular region as a result of transependymal spread of CSF in obstructive hydrocephalus.

Vasogenic edema is found in association with primary and metastatic tumors, hemorrhage, infarction, inflammation, and trauma. When the tight junctions of the blood-brain barrier are disrupted, a protein-rich filtrate of plasma enters the extracellular space of the brain. Vasogenic edema tends to spread along white matter tracts as "finger-like" projections from the inciting lesion, generally sparing the gray matter which is more tightly integrated (Fig. 18).

Because there is increased water content, the T2 relaxation time is increased, thus, vasogenic edema is best appreciated on T2-weighted images (Fig. 18). Using such techniques, MR is more sensitive in the detection of vasogenic edema than CT. This is particularly true at

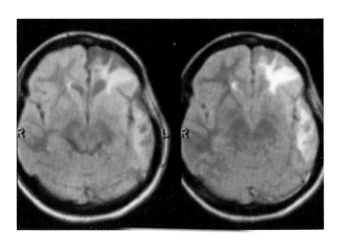

FIG. 17. Postoperative gliotic encephalomalacia following trauma (TR = 2.0 sec, TE = 28 and 56 msec).

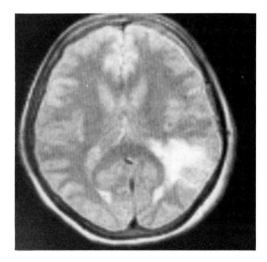

FIG. 18. Vasogenic edema. High intensity edema spreads along white matter tracts in finger-like projections from inciting lesion (in this case, a meningioma).

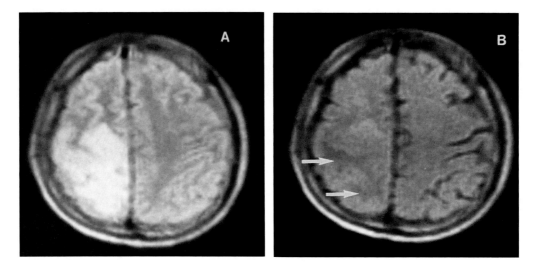

FIG. 19. Relative advantages of T1- and T2-weighted images. **A:** T2-weighted image is *sensitive* to the presence of vasogenic edema but may *mask* underlying lesion. Single edematous lesions seen on T2-weighted image, thus favored diagnosis is glioma. **B:** T1-weighted image indicates two lesions, changing the favored diagnosis to probable metastatic disease.

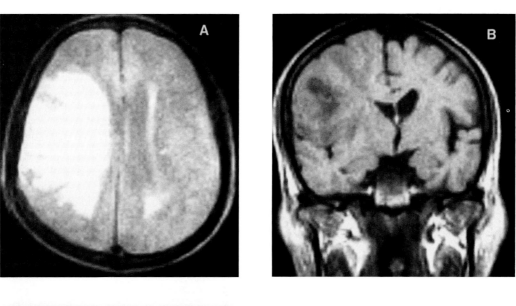

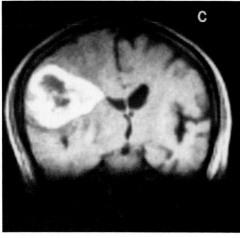

FIG. 20. Gadolinium-enhanced glioblastoma multiforme. **A:** T2-weighted image shows edema but masks underlying tumor margins (TR = 2.0 sec, TE = 56 msec). **B:** T1-weighted precontrast image demonstrates mass effect; lower intensity regions represent tumor and necrosis. **C:** Following administration of Gd-DTPA, viable portions of the tumor are enhanced. Gd-DTPA may be useful for stereotactic biopsy and to follow tumor size through chemotherapy and radiation therapy.

the vertex and in the middle and posterior cranial fossae, where CT is relatively degraded by beam hardening bone artifact. Although MR is generally considered more *sensitive* in the detection of vasogenic edema than CT, it may not be possible to make a *specific* diagnosis (21). Without the benefit of the clinical history, it may be very difficult to distinguish between vasogenic edema associated with tumors, abscesses, or even large demyelinated plaques. When lesions are small and have no discernable mass effect, it may be very difficult to distinguish periventricular MS plaques from deep white matter infarcts or, in the brainstem, MS plaques from vertebrobasilar infarcts or small tumors (13).

Although the presence of vasogenic edema certainly increases the sensitivity of MR in the detection of many disease processes, the high intensity from the edema may mask an underlying lesion. In Fig. 19, a T2-weighted image demonstrates a single parenchymal lesion whereas the T1-weighted image (which mutes the vasogenic edema) demonstrates two separate lesions (3). On the T2-weighted image, the diagnosis of primary brain tumor was favored while the T1-weighted image suggested multiple lesions and therefore metastases.

Vasogenic edema may also obscure the exact location of an underlying tumor, knowledge of which may be required prior to stereotactic biopsy. Although heavily T1- and T2-weighted images may occasionally distinguish the tumor from surrounding edema, areas of necrosis and cyst formation may also be mistaken for tumor; thus, intravenous contrast may be required. Although it is likely that the portion of a tumor which is enhanced by iodinated contrast is smaller than the actual lesion (22), the enhanced portion still provides a target for biopsy and is useful to follow through radiation and chemotherapy. The most promising MR contrast agent, Gd-DTPA dimeglumine, behaves like an iodinated contrast agent (e.g., meglumine diatrizoate) in CT (10). Gd-DTPA demonstrates blood-brain barrier

breakdown, probably with greater sensitivity than contrast-enhanced CT. In a recent collaborative study (23), MR with gadolinium was found to be capable of detecting 15% more metastases than unenhanced MR. (By comparison, unenhanced MR had been shown previously (21) to detect 30% more lesions than enhanced CT.) However, although gadolinium has been shown to be useful in distinguishing between tumor and edema (Fig. 20), it is not generally available at this time; therefore contrast-enhanced CT is still required in this clinical setting. By 1987, it is expected that Gd-DTPA will be generally available and, at that time, gadolinium-enhanced MR should be more sensitive and more specific for this application than CT. Early indications are that gadolinium is also safer than iodinated contrast (23).

Although it may be useful to separate the enhanced portion of the tumor from surrounding vasogenic edema, a more clinically appropriate separation would be viable tumor from surrounding edema. There have been some interesting, albeit preliminary, results using ^{23}Na MR to distinguish between tumor and surrounding vasogenic edema. Using a very short spin echo technique (e.g., 0.6 msec TE), Hilal et al. claim to be able to separate intracellular and extracellular Na in animals and humans (24). Although as yet unproven, their reasonable contention is that the intracellular Na signal corresponds to the viable tumor, whereas the large, extracellular Na signal corresponds to the surrounding vasogenic edema (24). Should this be verified with subsequent histologic correlation, Na MR imaging may well become the only noninvasive technique capable of distinguishing between tumor and edema.

Cytotoxic edema increases the intracellular water content, producing cellular swelling in response to ischemia. As the oxygen supply to a cell is decreased, the ATP level falls, the Na–K pump fails, and Na and water enter the cell, resulting in cellular swelling (18). Simultaneously, the extracellular space is decreased. Cytotoxic

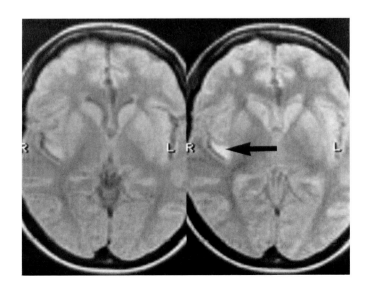

FIG. 21. Acute infarct. Twenty-four hours following onset of symptoms, CT is normal and well marginated, high intensity (arrow) is noted in the right insula secondary to acute infarct. The high intensity represents a combination of vasogenic and cytotoxic edema. The sharp margination is caused by cytotoxic, swollen cells at the periphery of the infarct which tend to confine the vasogenic edema produced centrally.

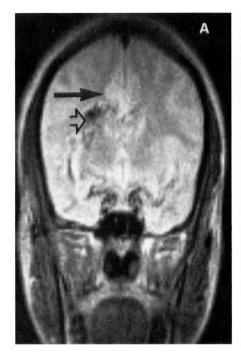
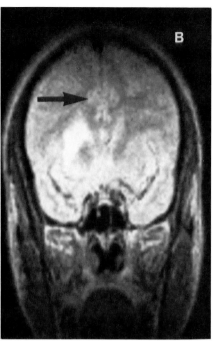

FIG. 22. Cytotoxic edema associated with arteriovenous malformation. A: High intensity (arrow) is noted in the adjacent cingulate cortex because of presumed vascular steal phenomenon from high flow AVM (open arrow). B: Following immobilization of AVM, intensity of the cingulate cortex has returned to normal, coinciding with return to normal function. The involvement of gray matter and subsequent return to normal intensity and function are evidence for reversible cytotoxic rather than vasogenic edema. Note complicating infarction in the basal ganglia following embolization.

edema is the earliest manifestation of ischemia and, therefore, an impending infarct. As the ischemia–infarction progresses, cytotoxic edema is found at the border between normal brain and the more damaged tissue centrally. The vasogenic edema produced centrally is therefore dammed up by the cytotoxic swollen cells at the periphery, resulting in the sharp margins of an acute infarct (Fig. 21). Unlike vasogenic edema, cytotoxic edema involves gray matter and white matter; they are both potentially reversible. Thus if the oxygen supply to an ischemic region is reestablished, cytotoxic cells can presumably recover both structure and function. This has been observed in a patient with ischemic deficits secondary to vascular steal phenomena from a high flow AVM. Prior to embolization, cytotoxic edema, i.e., high intensity and mass effect, was noted in cortical gray matter adjacent to a large AVM. Following embolization, the ischemic deficits referable to this area (and the high intensity and mass effect) resolved (Fig. 22).

Interstitial edema results from transependymal spread of CSF when the intraventricular pressure is elevated (18). The result is a smooth, high intensity border around the lateral, and occasionally third, ventricles. The high intensity border is always seen on T2-weighted images in acute cases of obstructive or communicating hydrocephalus (Fig. 23). As compensation occurs, the intraventricular pressure decreases and the interstitial edema is resorbed. Thus with total compensation there is no evidence of interstitial edema (Fig. 24). This finding can be of some clinical utility in determining which patients should be shunted for elevated CSF pressure.

Although interstitial edema is actually CSF in the interstitial space of the periventricular tissues, the molecu-

lar environment of the CSF water has changed significantly, resulting in an altered appearance. CSF within the ventricle is in the bulk phase, with the usual long T1 relaxation time of pure water. When CSF is in the interstitial periventricular space, much of the water is in hy-

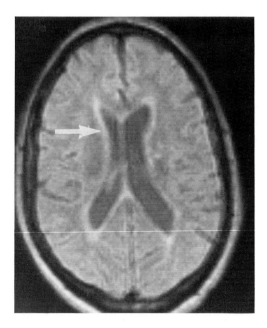

FIG. 23. Interstitial edema. Smooth, high intensity border is noted surrounding dilated lateral ventricles in patient with acute obstructive hydrocephalus. The high intensity border represents transependymal spread of CSF out of the ventricles under a pressure gradient. In the new environment, the CSF becomes interstitial edema and has a shorter T1 relaxation time (while maintaining a long T2 relaxation time) because of the greater amount of hydration layer water (TR = 2.0 sec, TE = 28 msec).

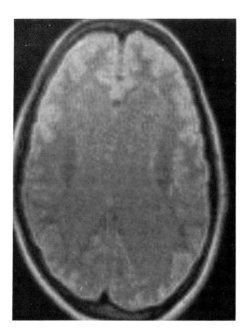

FIG. 24. Twenty-four-year-old patient with hydrocephalus without interstitial edema (compensated congenital aqueductal stenosis). Although the ventricles are dilated, there is no evidence of interstitial edema, nor was there clinical evidence of elevated CSF pressure (TR = 2.0 sec, TE = 56 msec).

dration layers around the proteins in the myelin, which results in T1 shortening and, therefore, increased MR intensity.

Although the smooth border of high intensity is always seen in cases of acutely elevated intraventricular pressure, the converse is not true, i.e., the smooth border may not disappear following shunting. After interstitial edema has been present for a period of several weeks, the myelin lipids are leached out, resulting in increased water content of these tissues (20). Until remyelination can occur, increased intensity may remain around the lateral ventricles for an indefinite period of time.

HEMORRHAGE

The earliest reports of intracranial hemorrhage (25,26) suggested a relatively intense MR appearance of the hemorrhage relative to surrounding brain. This was attributed to the short T1 of presumably paramagnetic, iron-containing hemoglobin. Figure 25 illustrates this appearance in a patient imaged 1 week after rupture of an anterior communicating artery aneurysm with resultant intraparenchymal hematoma and subarachnoid hemorrhage. The short T1 character of the lesion is enhanced relative to surrounding brain on a T1-weighted spin echo image.

As experience was gained, subsequent reports (27,28) indicated that acute intracranial hemorrhage could be much more difficult to detect on MR images. This was attributed by Sipponen et al. to a lack of T1 shortening

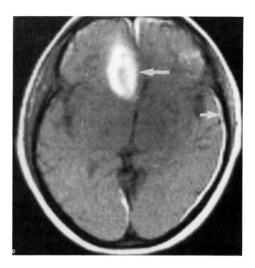

FIG. 25. Subacute subarachnoid hemorrhage. Intraparenchymal hematoma (arrow) and subarachnoid hemorrhage (arrowhead) noted 1 week following rupture of anterior communicating artery aneurysm. The contrast between the lesions and the surrounding brain is enhanced on this T1-weighted spin echo image (TR = 0.5 sec, TE = 28 msec).

during the acute phase; however, no explanation of this phenomenon was attempted (27). Acute subarachnoid hemorrhage in particular was said to be difficult to detect, especially by comparison with CT (28). Although DeLaPaz et al. (28) agree with Sipponen et al. (27) that acute intracranial hemorrhage is difficult to detect on MR images, they disagree as to the mechanism of the later MR-intense appearance. The data of Sipponen et al. (27), Bailes et al. (25), Bydder et al. (26), and Bradley et al. (9) suggest a T1-shortening process, whereas the data of DeLaPaz et al. (28) suggest no change in T1 but rather a prolongation of T2, both of which would increase the intensity on spin echo images. Recently Gomori et al. have described the short T2 appearance of an acute intracranial hematoma at 1.5 tesla (T) (5). They note that the subsequent intensity increase in the hematoma reflects a shortening of T1 *and* a prolongation of T2.

It now seems that there is agreement on the *appearance* of intracranial hemorrhage; however, the biochemical mechanisms for this appearance continue to be a matter of some debate. Not only does the MR appearance of intracranial hemorrhage change over time, but it depends on the field strength of the particular MR imaging system being used. A working understanding of this complex topic requires a basic knowledge of MR relaxation mechanisms.

MECHANISMS OF PROTON RELAXATION ENHANCEMENT

The mechanisms of proton relaxation enhancement (PRE) have been described in detail previously (29,30).

In biological substances, the dipole–dipole interaction between nuclear magnetic moments is the principal mechanism for T1 and T2 relaxations. The magnitude of these nuclear magnetic moments is small and requires an odd number of neutrons or protons (or both) in the nucleus (1). This is referred to as "nuclear paramagnetism." The hydrogen nucleus has a magnetic moment because it consists of a single, unpaired proton. This property is the basis of all clinical proton MR imaging. The dipole–dipole interaction between hydrogen nuclei is dependent upon their proximity and falls off as the sixth power of the distance between them. The electron has a magnetic moment which is 700 times greater than that of the proton, primarily as a consequence of its smaller size. Only the unpaired electrons contribute to the magnetic moment of a given atom. This is called "electronic paramagnetism," although the modifier "electronic" is usually dropped in MR imaging literature. The greater the number of unpaired electrons, the greater the magnetic moment of the particular atom. Unpaired electrons in the outer shell of an atom are constantly flipping "up" and "down" (in a quantum mechanical sense) relative to the main magnetic field. This results in temporal change in the electronic magnetic moment which is called the "electron spin relaxation time." How rapidly the unpaired electrons flip back and forth is a major determinant of the magnetic influence of the paramagnetic substance on the water protons in the environment (9). Since the interaction between the dipole of the electron and that of a local hydrogen nucleus falls off as the sixth power of the distance between them, hydrogen nuclei must be able to approach to within a few angstroms of the paramagnetic center (5) or there will be no enhancement of proton relaxation. The paramagnetic center produces local magnetic "turbulence," enhancing the return to equilibrium magnetization (i.e., shortening the T1 and T2 values) of all accessible water protons.

When discussing the properties of paramagnetic substances, it is useful to consider the reciprocals of the T1 or T2 relaxation times, called the R_1 and R_2 *relaxation rates,* respectively (31). Adding a paramagnetic substance to an aqueous solution affects the R_1 and R_2 relaxation *rates* to the same degree, i.e.,

$$R_{net} = R_{substance} + R_{paramagnetic\ agent}$$

where $R = R_1$ or R_2. The effect on the T1 or T2 relaxation *times,* however, differs markedly. For example, if a substance has a T1 of 600 msec and a T2 of 50 msec, then, $R_1 = 1/T1 = 1.66\ sec^{-1}$ and $R_2 = 1/T2 = 20\ sec^{-1}$. If the paramagnetic agent increases both relaxation rates by 1 sec^{-1}, then $R_{1net} = 2.66\ sec^{-1}$ and $R_{2net} = 21\ sec^{-1}$. The resultant T1 = 1/2.66 = 376 msec, and the resultant T2 = 1/21 = 48 msec. Thus T1 has decreased by 37.4% while T2 has decreased by only 4%, despite the "equal" effect on the *relaxation rates.*

This relation applies to proton–electron dipole–dipole interactions when the water protons in an aqueous solution have access to the paramagnetic center. Since the T1 of most biologic tissues is significantly longer than the T2, the effect of adding a paramagnetic agent is initially one of T1 shortening and, as the concentration increases, T2 shortening (2). The effect of T1 shortening, of course, is to increase the intensity, particularly on T1-weighted spin echo images. At higher concentrations, however, the effect of T2 shortening is to decrease the intensity because of increased dephasing and loss of coherence (2).

When considering paramagnetic substances in aqueous solutions, T1 shortening always occurs to a greater degree and at lower concentration than T2 shortening. There are other mechanisms of relaxation, however, by which T2 can be selectively shortened without affecting T1 (5). The T2 relaxation time of a substance reflects the randomly fluctuating internal magnetic fields which lead to irreversible loss of phase coherence (1). The fixed nonuniformities in the main (static) magnetic field cause even greater loss of coherence in the free induction decay (FID) at a rate T2* (1). The loss of coherence because of these fixed nonuniformities, however, can be reconstituted by the 180° radiofrequency pulse of a spin echo sequence. Several additional examples of dephasing (and subsequent spin echo signal loss) have appeared in the MR imaging literature. Autodiffusion through a magnetic field gradient causes dephasing, decreasing the intensity of the spin echo (32). Thus T2 values of fluids (with high autodiffusion coefficients) calculated from MR images (obtained with slice-selecting, phase-encoding, and read-out gradients) will be lower than T2 values calculated from spectrometers which do not use gradients (32). When blood in a vessel flows slowly through a gradient, signal is lost because of dephasing (12). If flow through the gradient continues slowly (i.e., is laminar) for a multiecho sequence, then the even echoes will demonstrate rephasing, and thus increased intensity (12). The dephasing in these cases has been shown to be proportional to the square of the local magnetic field gradient (33).

Recently an additional cause of dephasing has been described in tissues with high magnetic susceptibility (5). Iron-containing, paramagnetic substances such as hemosiderin become strongly magnetized when placed in a magnetic field, i.e., they have a high magnetic susceptibility. (The magnetic susceptibility is the ratio of the *induced* to the *applied* magnetic fields.) Paramagnetic substances will cause both T1 and T2 shortening, but only if there is free access of water protons to the paramagnetic center. If water protons are unable to approach to within several angstroms of the paramagnetic center, however, there will be no enhanced proton relaxation. When paramagnetic deoxyhemoglobin is free in solution, for example, it does not enhance proton relaxation, i.e., there is neither T1 nor T2 shortening (34). When deoxyhemoglobin is contained within an intact red blood cell, however, the strong induced magnetic field changes direction quite slowly, creating regions of locally increased magnetic field (5). Diffusion of water molecules through these regions causes dephasing which is proportional to the square of the local magnetic field gradient (33). It should be emphasized that this is not the magnetic gradient used to provide spatial information but rather that caused by local magnetic nonuniformity, induced in the magnetically susceptible substance by the main magnetic field. Thus, the dephasing which results increases with the square of the applied static magnetic field. The dephasing, of course, only results in T2 shortening, T1 remaining unchanged. This T2 shortening effect is more noticeable at higher field strengths (e.g., 1.5 T), although it has been noted at intermediate field strengths as well (31). T2 shortening has also been reported for paramagnetic hemosiderin in macrophages (5) and for ferritin, which is deposited in various structures in the brain, namely, the globus pallidus, the red nucleus, the reticular portion of the substantia nigra, the putamen, and the dentate nucleus of the cerebellum (35). The effect has also been noted in the liver in patients with hemochromatosis (Fig. 6).

OXIDATION OF HEMOGLOBIN

In order to understand the variable MR appearance of intracranial hemorrhage, the structure of hemoglobin and its various breakdown products must be considered in some detail. In its circulating form, hemoglobin alternates between the oxy and deoxy forms as oxygen is exchanged during transit through the high oxygen environment of the lungs and low oxygen environment of the capillary circulation. In order to bind oxygen reversibly, the iron in the hemoglobin (the "heme iron") must be maintained in the reduced ferrous (Fe^{2+}) state (36). To do this, the red cell maintains several metabolic pathways to prevent various oxidizing agents from converting its heme iron to the nonfunctional ferric (Fe^{3+}) state. When removed from the circulation, these metabolic pathways fail and the hemoglobin begins to undergo oxidative denaturation.

The heme iron is normally suspended in a nonpolar crevice in the center of the hemoglobin molecule. It is held in this position by a covalent bond with a histidine at the so-called F8 position of the globin chain and by four planar hydrophobic van der Waals' bonds with various nonpolar groups on the globin molecule. The sixth coordination site of the heme iron is occupied by molecular oxygen in the oxyhemoglobin and is vacant in deoxyhemoglobin (Fig. 26). As oxidative denaturation of hemoglobin proceeds, the ferrous heme iron is oxidized to the ferric state and paramagnetic methemoglobin is formed (9). Although the five bonds to the

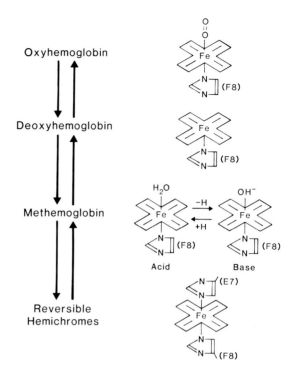

FIG. 26. Oxidative denaturation of hemoglobin. In the circulating oxy- and deoxyhemoglobin forms, the heme iron is in the reduced, ferrous state which can reversibly bind molecular oxygen. Following oxidation to the paramagnetic, ferric form as methemoglobin, the heme iron can no longer bind oxygen and is thus nonfunctional. Continued oxidative denaturation produces hemichromes which are ferric compounds with the sixth coordination site occupied by a ligand from the now denatured globin chain.

globin molecule are unchanged, the sixth coordination site is now occupied by a water molecule at physiologic pH. With continued oxidative denaturation, methemoglobin is converted to derivatives known as hemichromes (36). Although the iron in these compounds remains in the ferric state, alteration of the tertiary structure of the globin molecule occurs such that the sixth coordination site of the heme iron is occupied by a ligand from within the now-denatured globin molecule (most likely the distal histidine at E7).

The magnetic properties of blood were first evaluated by Faraday 140 years ago (37). However, he only considered blood in the dried, solid state; it was not until 90 years later that Pauling and Coryell (38) considered the magnetic properties of blood in the fluid state. By using a capillary tube filled with either oxy- or deoxyhemoglobin suspended between the poles of an electromagnet, they were able to determine that deoxyhemoglobin was paramagnetic, i.e., attracted to the stronger part of the magnetic field, whereas oxyhemoglobin was diamagnetic, i.e., repelled from the stronger part of the magnetic field. Stated differently, deoxyhemoglobin has a high magnetic susceptibility, i.e., a stronger local magnetic field is induced in deoxyhemoglobin than in (low magnetic susceptibility) oxyhemoglobin when an external magnetic field is applied. These observations led them to describe the various electron spin states of oxy- and deoxyhemoglobin. In deoxyhemoglobin, the heme iron is in the "high spin" ferrous state, characterized by six electrons in the outer *d* shell, four of which are unpaired. When oxygen is added, one of the electrons is partially transferred to the oxygen molecule, resulting in a low spin form with a single, unpaired electron in the outer shell (36).

Although the static susceptibility test performed by Pauling and Coryell demonstrates that deoxyhemoglobin is paramagnetic, this does not ensure a proton paramagnetic enhancement effect in aqueous solution. Such an effect was originally described by Bloembergen et al. (29) and requires not only that a paramagnetic center be present, but also that it is accessible to surrounding water protons. As noted above, the quantitation of this effect requires consideration of the magnitude of the magnetic moment of the paramagnetic dipole (i.e., the number of unpaired electrons), the electron spin relaxation rate, the concentration of paramagnetic dipoles, the average distance from surrounding water protons, and the relative motion of the proton and paramagnetic centers (9,29,30). Such theories of proton relaxation by paramagnetic solute ions are based on translational diffusion and the distance of closest approach of the proton and paramagnetic ions which determines an "outer sphere" of influence (39). It has also been shown that there can be a contribution to the relaxation from exchange between solvent and water ligands in the first coordination sphere of the paramagnetic ion, i.e., "inner sphere effects" (39). Thus deoxyhemoglobin is considered "paramagnetic" from static susceptibility experiments (38), but the T1 relaxation times of aqueous solutions of oxy- and deoxyhemoglobin do not demonstrate a difference in the proton paramagnetic relaxation effects (34). Methemoglobin, on the other hand, causes significant T1 shortening in aqueous solution because of a combination of "inner sphere" and "outer sphere" effects (39). Thus T1 relaxation by methemoglobin is caused by a combination of ligand exchange effects (from the water molecule at the sixth coordination site) and outer sphere diffusional effects, perhaps by virtue of increased access of solvent protons to the heme iron through the nonpolar crevice (39).

SUBARACHNOID HEMORRHAGE

Figure 27A illustrates the rather subtle increased intensity present in acute subarachnoid hemorrhage 17 hr post ictus. One week following the acute bleed, the intensity is significantly greater (Fig. 27B). Possible causes for this temporal change in the MR intensity of subarachnoid hemorrhage are now discussed.

To begin, one must evaluate the possible interactions between water protons in the CSF and the iron-containing hemoglobin within the red cell. A trivial explanation for the observed T1 shortening which occurs over a matter of days following subarachnoid hemorrhage might be red cell lysis, which can certainly occur as a result of exposure to phospholipases in the CSF. Obviously water molecules are already allowed access to the hemoglobin by virtue of rapid transit across the red cell membrane (29,40). Bradley and Schmidt (9) mod-

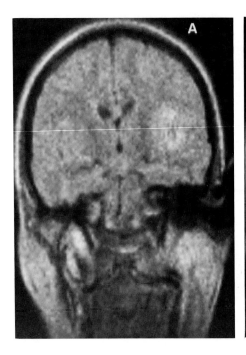
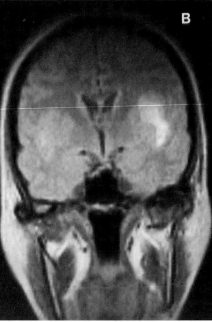

FIG. 27. Subarachnoid hemorrhage. **A:** Seventeen hours post ictus. Coronal section demonstrates minimally increased intensity in the left sylvian cistern on this TR = 1.5 sec, TE = 28 msec. **B:** One week post ictus. Intensity of the CSF in the left sylvian cistern has increased significantly.

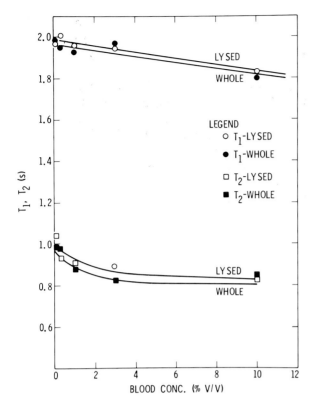

FIG. 28. Change in magnetic relaxation times (20 MHz) as a function of red cell concentration in CSF and red cell lysis. A 10% decrease in the T1 (**above**) and T2 (**below**) times is noted as a function of increasing concentration of red cells in the CSF from concentration of pure CSF to 10% (by volume) red cells in CSF. There is no significant effect of red cell lysis on T1 or T2.

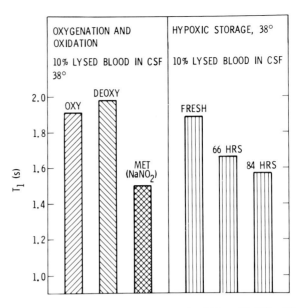

FIG. 29. Relaxation times for blood in CSF at 10 MHz. The T1 times for oxy- and deoxyhemoglobin are similar. The T1 time for methemoglobin (produced by treatment with $NaNO_2$) is significantly less than that of oxy- and deoxyhemoglobin. The T1 time of the 10% solution of lysed blood and CSF is followed over a period of 84 hr during hypoxic storage and is seen to decrease.

eled subarachnoid hemorrhage *in vitro* by the addition of fresh venous human blood to artificial CSF and mixing. The effects of red cell concentration and of lysis on T1 and T2 were evaluated using a spectrometer operat-

ing at 20 MHz. These effects were found to be small or negligible (Fig. 28). Thus, such a mechanism for enhanced proton relaxation can be excluded.

One might then consider changes which occur during the course of oxidative denaturation of hemoglobin as an explanation for the changing MR appearance of subarachnoid hemorrhage. Oxy- and deoxyhemoglobin were produced *in vitro* by bubbling oxygen or nitrogen, respectively, through fresh solutions of bloody CSF.

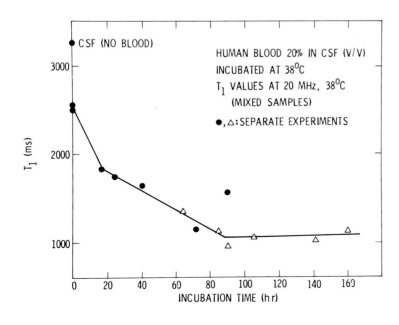

FIG. 30. Change in T1 relaxation time during subarachnoid hemorrhage. Changing T1 relaxation time for solution of 20% whole blood in CSF is followed for 160 hr and is seen to decrease to a plateau value at approximately 90 hr.

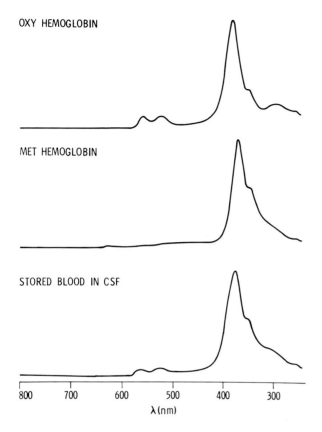

OXY HEMOGLOBIN

MET HEMOGLOBIN

STORED BLOOD IN CSF

800   700   600   500   400   300

λ(nm)

FIG. 31. Spectrophotometry of oxy- and methemoglobin and hypoxically stored blood in CSF. Strong absorption is noted near 400 nm (Soret band) which is nonspecific. The specific absorption for methemoglobin is perceptible at 630 nm in both the methemoglobin and the unknown bloody CSF solution.

Methemoglobin was produced by treatment with $NaNO_2$. Figure 29 demonstrates that the T1 measurements of oxy- and deoxyhemoglobin are quite similar, confirming what has been reported previously (34). Methemoglobin, however, is seen to have a significantly

shorter T1 value than oxy- or deoxyhemoglobin. No significant T2 difference was found among oxy-, deoxy-, and methemoglobin at 20 MHz (0.47 T). Figure 29 also shows temporal decrease in T1 for a 10% "unknown" solution of lysed red cells in CSF stored hypoxically over 84 hr of measurement. Figure 30 demonstrates T1 shortening of a 20% solution of whole red cells in CSF stored hypoxically for 160 hr. The T1 value continues to shorten for 90 hr and then plateaus.

UV–visible spectrophotometry of the known solutions of oxy-, deoxy-, and methemoglobin and of the two unknown solutions of bloody CSF demonstrate absorption at 360 nm (the "Soret band") (Fig. 31). Strong absorption is present for all forms of hemoglobin in this region; thus it is not specific. The portion of the spectrum which is most specific for methemoglobin is the 630 nm region; this is illustrated in Fig. 32. Here temporal increase in a broad peak is observed in the unknown solutions; this increase corresponds to increasing methemoglobin concentration. (Although there is a significant difference in the heights of the 630 nm and 360 nm peaks, this reflects differences in the extinction coefficients rather than differences in concentration. Thus, by comparison to known standards, the peak observed at 92 hr at 631 nm corresponds to 90% methemoglobin.) This experiment thus demonstrated that methemoglobin could be a cause of progressive T1 shortening *in vitro* over several days. *In vivo* methemoglobin has now been demonstrated spectroscopically in a subacute subdural hematoma in this laboratory. Thus methemoglobin formation is now felt to be the principal determinant of T1 shortening during evolving subarachnoid hemorrhage.

INTRAPARENCHYMAL HEMATOMA

The MR appearances of intraparenchymal hematomas (IPHs) have been described by several authors

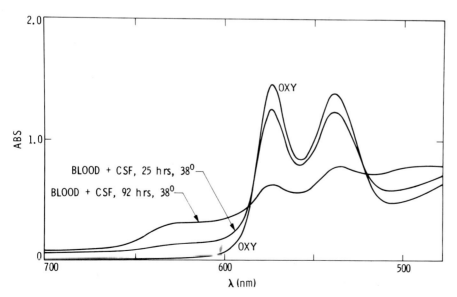

2.0

ABS   1.0

OXY

BLOOD + CSF, 25 hrs, 38°

BLOOD + CSF, 92 hrs, 38°

OXY

0

700   600   500

λ (nm)

FIG. 32. Spectrophotometry at 630 nm. Oxyhemoglobin is seen to have no absorption at 630 nm. During hypoxic storage of a solution of blood and CSF, a broad-based peak develops at 630 nm. By comparison with known standards, the peak at 92 hr was shown to correspond to 90% methemoglobin. (Differences in peak heights reflect differences in extinction coefficients.)

TABLE 1. *MR appearance of intraparenchymal hematomas*

	Acute	Subacute	Chronic
T1-weighted images			
Inner core	0	0	+
Outer core	0	++	++
Rim	NP	NP	NP
Reactive brain	−	−	0
T2-weighted images (0.35 T/1.5 T)			
Inner core	−/−−	−/−−	+/+
Outer core	−/−−	++/++	++/++
Rim	NP/NP	NP/−	−/−−
Reactive brain	++/++	++/++	0/0

Scale: ++, much more intense than brain; +, more intense than brain; 0, isointense with brain; −, less intense than brain; −−, much less intense than brain; NP, not present.

(25–28) and more recently by Gomori et al. (5). When describing an IPH, it is useful to consider four separate factors (31): the age of the hematoma, separate zones within and surrounding the hematoma, the MR technique (i.e., T1 or T2 weighted), and the strength of the imaging field (Table 1). Three stages in the evolution of a hematoma can be described: acute (0–2 days), subacute (2–14 days), and chronic (more than 2 weeks). Four zones can be detected: inner core, outer core, rim, and reactive brain. Acutely (0–2 days) the hematoma consists of deoxyhemoglobin within intact red cells (Fig.

33). This has been demonstrated by Gomori et al. (5) in material aspirated from an acute IPH. Over the subacute period from 2 to 14 days, the deoxyhemoglobin undergoes oxidative denaturation, forming methemoglobin, first at the periphery (outer core) and then in the center (inner core) (5). During this phase, red cell lysis occurs as well (Fig. 34). At the end of the first 2 weeks, modified macrophages have begun to remove the iron from the hemoglobin within the hematoma (41). This marks the beginning of the "chronic" phase. The heme iron is deposited at the periphery as a rim of hemosiderin within (Fig. 35) the macrophages surrounding the hematoma (5,41). The center of the hematoma (41) is left with a noniron-containing, nonparamagnetic heme pigment called "hematoidin." During the acute phase, the hematoma is surrounded by vasogenic edema; this edema is gradually resorbed during the subacute phase and is essentially absent during the chronic phase.

On T1-weighted images, the hematoma is acutely isointense with brain whereas the reactive vasogenic edema is somewhat less intense than brain because of its longer T1 value. In the subacute phase, as the deoxyhemoglobin is initially oxidized to methemoglobin in the outer core, T1 is markedly shortened, resulting in increased intensity on T1-weighted images (Fig. 25) (9). During the chronic stage, the deoxyhemoglobin in the inner core is also oxidized to methemoglobin and the vasogenic edema is resorbed (5).

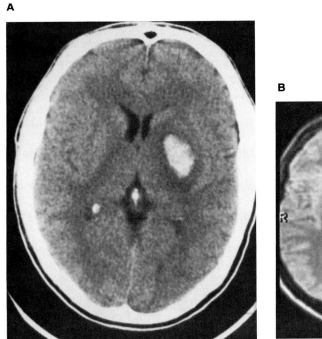

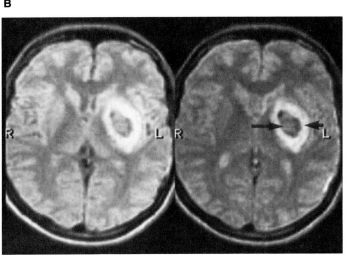

FIG. 33. Acute parenchymal hematoma. **A:** Unenhanced CT scan demonstrates high density in left basal ganglia with surrounding low density due to vasogenic edema. **B:** T2-weighted MR study demonstrates decreasing intensity within hematoma (*arrow*) as TE is prolonged, indicating T2 shortening. (*Left:* TR − 2.0, TE − 28. *Right:* TR = 2.0, TE = 56.) This reflects presence of paramagnetic deoxyhemoglobin within intact red cells. Surrounding rim of vasogenic edema has high intensity (*arrowhead*).

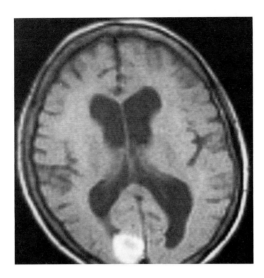

FIG. 34. Subacute hemorrhage. Focal right occipital hematoma noted one week following bleed. High intensity reflects T1 shortening due to presence of paramagnetic methemoglobin. (TR = 1.0, TE = 28.)

On T2-weighted images, the appearance of an evolving hematoma depends to a greater extent on the field strength of the MR imaging system (5,31). Acutely, there is decreased intensity centrally, particularly at higher fields (5) (Figs. 9–11). This reflects T2 shortening as a consequence of the presence of the highly magnetically susceptible deoxyhemoglobin within intact red cells (5). The dephasing (T2 decay) which occurs as a result of the local magnetic nonuniformities increases as the square of the local field gradients. Since the induced magnetic field in magnetically susceptible, paramagnetic substances depends on the strength of the applied magnetic field, T2 shortening also increases as the

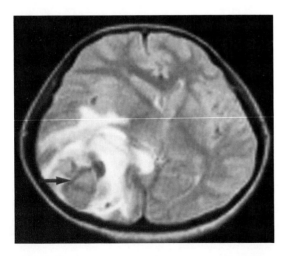

FIG. 35. Chronic hemorrhage. Rim of low intensity noted surrounding chronic hematoma (*arrow*) due to presence of magnetically susceptible hemosiderin within macrophages. (TR = 2.0, TE = 56.)

square of the applied (static) magnetic field. Thus the low intensity appearance in the center of an acute hematoma is more obvious at 1.5 T than at 0.35 T (5). Vasogenic edema surrounding the hematoma in the acute and subacute stages results in a high intensity appearance on T2-weighted images (Figs. 9–11).

In the subacute stage, the red cells in the outer core have lysed and methemoglobin has formed. This results in shortening of T1 and lengthening of T2, both of which will increase the intensity of the hematoma on T2-weighted images (Fig. 10). As long as deoxyhemoglobin is still present within intact red cells in the inner core, the central low intensity persists.

In the chronic stage, hemosiderin is found within macrophages in the rim surrounding a hematoma (41). Like deoxyhemoglobin, the intracellular, magnetically susceptible, paramagnetic hemosiderin causes preferential T2 shortening (5) (Fig. 10). Since this is also a magnetic susceptibility effect, the low intensity rim is much more noticeable at higher fields. The persistent low intensity center in chronic hemorrhage may reflect the removal of paramagnetic iron by the macrophages, leaving hematoidin centrally (41).

SUBDURAL AND EPIDURAL HEMATOMAS

Subdural hematomas (SDHs) have three distinct stages of evolution and three distinct appearances on MR. Acute subdurals contain deoxyhemoglobin within intact red cells. As noted above, this results in T2 shortening. Thus acute SDHs will have low intensity on T2-weighted images, particularly at higher fields (5). They will be isointense with brain on T1-weighted images.

During the subacute stage (CT isointense), the red cells lyse and deoxyhemoglobin becomes oxidized to methemoglobin. These changes tend to shorten the T1 and lengthen the T2, which will increase the intensity on either T1- or T2-weighted images (Fig. 36).

Chronic SDHs (i.e., at least 3 weeks old) have decreased MR intensity. Continued oxidative denaturation of methemoglobin forms hemichromes, which are low spin, nonparamagnetic, ferric compounds (36). The T1 values of such compounds are decreased relative to that of paramagnetic methemoglobin; thus the intensity of chronic SDHs (Fig. 12) is decreased relative to that of subacute SDHs, particularly on T1-weighted images (18). As the chronic SDH continues to age over many years, the protein content of the fluid decreases, approaching that of CSF.

Epidural hematomas age in a manner similar to SDHs. They are distinguished from SDHs by the low intensity appearance of the fibrous dura between the hematoma and the brain (Fig. 37). Like an acute SDH, an acute epidural hematoma will have deoxyhemoglo-

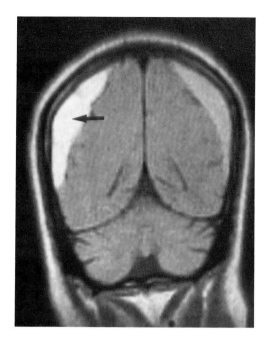

FIG. 36. Bilateral subdural hematomas. CT demonstrated isodense subacute subdural hematoma on the right side and chronic subdural hematoma on the left side. The intensity of the subacute subdural hematoma (*arrow*) is greater than that of the chronic subdural due to presence of methemoglobin on the right side. (TR = 1.0, TE = 28.)

bin within intact red blood cells resulting in T2 shortening and low intensity on T2-weighted images, particularly at high fields. At higher fields in fact, it may be difficult to separate the low intensity dura from the low

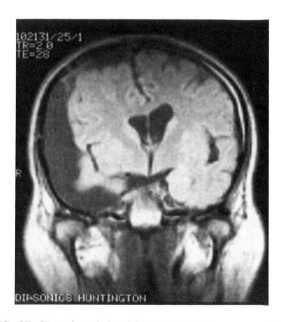

FIG. 37. Chronic subdural hematoma. Many years following trauma, large extraaxial fluid collection is noted with CSF intensity, presumed secondary to chronic subdural hematoma. A subdural hygroma and arachnoid cyst would have a similar appearance. (TR = 2.0, TE = 28.)

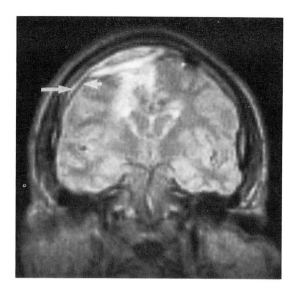

FIG. 38. Epidural hematoma. Following surgery, there is a high intensity (*arrow*) epidural fluid collection which is distinguished from subdural collection by low intensity dura (*arrowhead*). (TR = 2.0, TE = 56.)

intensity hematoma acutely and accurately to distinguish a subdural from an epidural collection (Fig. 38). In the subacute phase of an epidural hematoma, methemoglobin is formed and the diagnosis is obvious on both T1- and T2-weighted sequences, regardless of field strength.

ACKNOWLEDGMENTS

I thank Jay Mericle, Terry Andrews, and Leslee Watson for technical assistance, and Kaye Finley for manuscript preparation.

REFERENCES

1. Bradley WG, Crooks LE, Newton TH. Physical principles of NMR. In: Newton TH, Potts DG, eds. *Modern neuroradiology,* Vol. 2, *Advanced imaging techniques.* San Francisco: Clavadel Press, 1983;15–61.
2. Bradley WG. Fundamentals of MR image interpretation. In: Bradley WG, Adey WR, Hasso AN, eds. *Magnetic resonance imaging of the brain, head and neck: a text atlas.* Rockville, Md: Aspen, 1985.
3. Bradley WG. Effect of magnetic relaxation times on magnetic resonance image interpretation. *Noninvasive Med Imaging* 1984;1:193–204.
4. Rosen BR, Pykett IL, Brady TJ. NMR chemical shift imaging. In: James TL, Margulis AR, eds. *Biomedical magnetic resonance.* San Francisco: Radiology Research and Education Foundation, 1984.
5. Gomori JM, Grossman RI, Goldberg HI, et al. Intracranial hematomas: imaging by high field MR. *Radiology* 1985;156:99–103.
6. Bradley WG, Waluch V, Lai K, et al. The appearance of rapidly flowing blood on magnetic resonance images. *AJR* 1984; 143:1167–74.
7. Bradley WG, Waluch V. Blood flow: magnetic resonance imaging. *Radiology* 1985;154:443–50.
8. Bergstran G, Berstrom M, Nordell B, et al. Cardiac gated MR imaging of CSF flow. *J Comput Assist Tomogr* 1985;9:1003–6.

9. Bradley WG, Schmidt PC. Effect of methemoglobin formation on the MR appearance of subarachnoid hemorrhage. *Radiology* 1985;156:99–103.

10. Graif M, Bydder GM, Steiner RE, et al. Contrast-enhanced MR imaging of malignant brain tumors. *AJNR* 1985;(6):855–62.

11. Claussen C, Laniado M, Schorner W, et al. Gadolinium-DTPA in MR imaging of glioblastomas and intracranial metastases. *AJNR* 1985;(5):669–74.

12. Waluch V, Bradley WG. NMR even echo rephasing in slow laminar flow. *J Comput Assist Tomogr* 1984;8:594–8.

13. Bradley WG. MRI of the posterior fossa and brainstem. *Semin Neurol,* In press.

14. Hazelwood CF. A view of the significance and understanding of the physical properties of cell-associated water. In: Drost-Hansen W, Clegg J, eds. *Cell associated water.* New York: Academic Press, 1979;165–259.

15. Brant-Zawadzki M. NMR imaging: the abnormal brain and spinal cord. In: Newton TH, Potts DG, eds. *Modern neuroradiology,* Vol. 2, *Advanced imaging techniques.* San Francisco: Clavadel Press, 1983;159–86.

16. Fullerton GD, Cameron IL, Ord VA. Frequency dependence of magnetic resonance spin–lattice relaxation of protons in biological materials. *Radiology* 1984;151:135–8.

17. Farrar TC, Becker ED. *Pulse and Fourier transform NMR: introduction to theory and methods.* New York: Academic Press, 1971.

18. Bradley WG. Magnetic resonance imaging of the central nervous system. *Neurol Res* 1984;6:91–106.

19. Flannigan BD, Bradley WG, Kortman KE, et al. MRI of cerebral infarction. *Semin Neurol,* In press.

20. Fishman RA. Brain edema. *NEJM* 1975;293:706.

21. Bradley WG, Waluch V, Yadley RA, et al. Comparison of CT and MR in 400 patients with suspected disease of the brain and cervical spinal cord. *Radiology* 1984;152:695–702.

22. Daumas-Duport C, Meder JF, Monsaingeon V, Missir O, Aubin ML, Szikla G, *J Neuroradiol* 1983;10:51–80.

23. Bradley WG, Brant-Zawadzki M, Brasch RC, et al. Initial clinical experience with Gd-DTPA in North America: MR contrast enhancement of brain tumors. *Radiology* 1985;157(P):125.

24. Hilal SK, Ra JB, Silver AJ, et al. *In vivo* sodium imaging using a very short echo time: potential for selective imaging in intracellular sodium and extracellular space. *Radiology* 1985;157(P):188.

25. Bailes DR, Young IR, Thomas DJ, et al. NMR imaging of the brain using spin-echo sequences. *Clin Radiol* 1982;33:395–414.

26. Bydder GM, Steiner RE, Young IR, et al. Clinical NMR imaging of the brain: 140 cases. *AJR* 1982;139:215–36.

27. Sipponen JT, Sepponen RE, Sivula A. Nuclear magnetic resonance (NMR) imaging of intracerebral hemorrhage in the acute and resolving phases. *J Comput Assist Tomogr* 1983;7:954–9.

28. DeLaPaz RL, New PFJ, Buonanno FS, et al. NMR imaging of intracranial hemorrhage. *J Comput Assist Tomogr* 1984;8:599–607.

29. Bloembergen N, Purcell E, Pound E. Relaxation effects in nuclear magnetic resonance absorption. *Phys Rev* 1948;73:679–712.

30. Wolf GL, Burnett KR, Goldstein EJ, et al. Contrast agents for magnetic resonance imaging. In: Kressel HY, ed. *Magnetic resonance annual 1985.* New York: Raven Press, 1985;231–66.

31. Bradley WG. MRI of intracranial hemorrhage. In: Partain CL, Price RR, Patton JA, et al., eds. *Magnetic resonance imaging,* 2nd ed. Philadelphia: WB Saunders, in press.

32. Wesbey GE, Moseley ME, Ehman RL. Translational molecular self-diffusion in magnetic resonance imaging: effects and applications. In: James TL, Margulis AR, eds. *Biomedical magnetic resonance.* San Francisco: Radiology Research and Education Foundation, 1984;63–78.

33. Packer KJ. The effects of diffusion through locally inhomogeneous magnetic fields on transverse nuclear spin relaxation in heterogeneous systems: proton transverse relaxation in striated muscle tissue. *J Magn Reson* 1973;9:438–43.

34. Singer JR, Crooks LE. Some magnetic studies of normal and leukemic blood. *J Clin Engng* 1978;(3):237–43.

35. Drayer BP, Burger P, Payne C, et al. MR mapping of brain iron. II. Basal ganglia disorders. *Radiology* 1985;157(P):290.

36. Wintrobe MM, Lee GR, Boggs DR, et al. *Clinical hematology.* Philadelphia: Lea & Febiger, 1981;88–102.

37. Pauling L, Coryell C. The magnetic properties and structure of hemoglobin, oxyhemoglobin and carbonmonoxyhemoglobin. *Proc Natl Acad Sci USA* 1936;22:210–16.

38. Pauling L, Coryell C. The magnetic properties and structure of the hemochromogens and related substances. *Proc Natl Acad Sci USA* 1936;22:159–63.

39. Koenig SH, Brown RD, Lindstrom TR. Interactions of solvent with heme region of methemoglobin and fluoro-methemoglobin. *Biophys J* 1981;(34):397–408.

40. Brooks RA, Battocletti JH, Sances A, et al. "Nuclear magnetic relaxation in blood: *IEEE Trans Biomed Engng* 1975;1:12–18.

41. Whisnant JP, Sayer GP, Milikan CH. Experimental intracerebral hematoma. *Arch Neurol* 1963;9:586–92.

CHAPTER 4

Image Artifacts and Technical Limitations

William M. Kelly

The swift temporal progression of magnetic resonance imaging (MRI) from experimental prototype design to sophisticated instrument production can be sharply contrasted to the more protracted time course that characterized the development of X-ray computed tomography (CT). Most notably, the current generation of CT scanners represents the product of more than a decade of design innovation and technologic improvement, punctuated by the introduction of a whole new "generation" of CT scanners at periodic intervals.

The more rapid evolutionary changes unique to MRI have been permitted by the greater abundance of sophisticated technologic expertise and necessitated by economic considerations, especially the desire to avoid premature obsolescence. Quite clearly, "state-of-the-art" MRI units available today are intended to remain state of the art for many years into the future.

In clinical trials, MRI has proved particularly efficacious for evaluation of suspected neurologic disease, prompting neuroradiologists to welcome this new non-invasive diagnostic tool with unprecedented enthusiasm. In early reports, the lack of ionizing radiation, apparent absence of significant biological hazards, and "elimination" of artifacts were all acclaimed as major technical advantages (1–4). Now, as this diagnostic modality is undergoing widespread dissemination and a large body of clinical experience begins to accumulate, increasing attention is being focused on the limitations of MRI.

The pace of scientific developments has often outstripped the ability of the radiologist to absorb and comprehend fully both technical and clinical aspects of MRI, an especially challenging task for those with a limited background in physics. For instance, when confronted with a magnetic resonance (MR) image of the head, few radiologists would have difficulty identifying a major zone of signal abnormality. Frequently, the presence of a lesion is patently obvious, and an appropriately ordered differential diagnosis can often be

generated merely on the basis of lesion topography and morphology, integrated with clinical factors. However, in order to realize more fully and consistently the true diagnostic potential of MRI, while mitigating potential for diagnostic errors, a much greater scope of understanding and depth of involvement is required.

The participation of the radiologist begins at the point of patient selection wherein familiarity with the proven clinical utility of various diagnostic applications is desirable, and awareness of certain absolute and relative contraindications to MRI is mandatory. Next, a specific pulse sequence or series of pulse sequences must be designed, often tailored for a particular anatomic region and sometimes modified during the course of an examination. This process involves considerably more than the mere selection of repetition time (TR) and echo time (TE) values. The rather extensive list of operator-selected instrument parameters presented in Table 1 must be programmed for each pulse sequence performed. Many of these factors are interrelated, and their individual as well as combined effects on image quality [signal-to-noise ratio (SNR), contrast resolution, spatial resolution, and artifact production] and acquisition time must be understood if MRI is to be used in a clinically efficacious and cost-effective manner.

A proficient level of diagnostic expertise in the interpretation of MR images requires, at its foundation, familiarity with the physical principles of MRI. This essential fund of knowledge should include a basic understanding of MR pulse-sequencing techniques, the multiparametric determinants of MR signal intensity represented by tissue variables (T1, T2, resonant proton density, flow factors) as well as MR signal acquisition and reconstruction methods. Armed with this framework of technical knowledge, the radiologist is better equipped to proceed intelligently with pulse sequence selection in a manner most likely to optimize image quality, suppress artifacts, and maximize the conspicuity of abnormalities. A technically informed radiolo-

TABLE 1. *MR imaging parameters: Relative effects of operator-dependent choices*

Parameter	Option	Advantage	Disadvantage
TR	Increase	Increased magnetization (potential signal amplitude) exponentially related to T1 Increased number of multislice images feasible	Increased acquisition time Decreased T1 contrast Decreased time-of-flight effect (flow-related enhancement)
	Decrease	Decreased acquisition time Increased T1 contrast Increased time-of-flight effect (flow-related enhancement)	Decreased magnetization (potential signal amplitude) exponentially related to T1 Decreased number of slice locations available
TE	Increase	Increased T2 contrast Increased time-of-flight effect (high-velocity signal loss)	Decreased SNR
	Decrease	Reduced signal decay exponentially related to T2	Decreased T2 contrast Decreased time-of-flight effect (high-velocity signal loss)
No. of averages (data sets)	Increase	Increased SNR by square-root factor Potentially reduced motion artifact (image-averaging effect)	Increased acquisition time
	Decrease	Decreased acquisition time	Decreased SNR by square-root factor Propensity for increased visibility of image harmonics (motion artifact)
Matrix size	Increase	Increased spatial resolution	Decreased SNR Increased acquisition time
	Decrease	Increased SNR Decreased acquisition time	Decreased spatial resolution
Slice thickness	Increase	Increased SNR Increased volume of tissue imaged	Increased partial volume averaging Decreased time-of-flight effects
	Decrease	Decreased partial volume averaging Increased time-of-flight effects	Decreased SNR Decreased volume of tissue imaged
Interslice gap	Increase	Decreased cross-excitation artifact Increased coverage of anatomic region orthogonal to image plane	Increased chance of "missing" pathology situated within interslice gap
	Decrease	Decreased chance of "missing" pathology situated within interslice gap	Increased cross-excitation artifact Decreased coverage of anatomic region orthogonal to image plane
FOV	Increase	Increased SNR Decreased aliasing artifact Increased coverage of anatomic region parallel to image plane	Decreased spatial resolution
	Decrease	Increased spatial resolution	Decreased SNR Increased aliasing artifact Decreased coverage of anatomic region parallel to image plane
Receiver coil	Surface	Increased SNR within sensitive volume Decreased motion artifact from distant sources (vessels) Decreased aliasing artifact potential	Inhomogeneous sensitivity profile Decreased FOV range
	Volume	Homogeneous sensitivity Increased FOV range Increased SNR for deeply situated anatomy	Decreased SNR for superficial anatomy Increased motion artifact from vessels within excited volume Increased aliasing artifact potential

gist is also more likely to identify accurately a variety of persistent artifacts or signal aberrations unique to MRI that can either obscure anatomy or simulate pathology.

MOTION-RELATED SIGNAL ALTERATIONS

The effects of various types of gross anatomic and physiologic motion on MR signal acquisition are numerous, exceedingly complex, and difficult to comprehend fully. Yet the ability to recognize motion-induced signal alterations and confidently separate such artifacts from pathology is an essential skill required for accurate interpretation of MR images.

Most radiologists adept with the pattern-recognition method of CT scan interpretation are able to identify quickly both increased edge blurring and streak artifacts as the major detrimental effects of motion on CT scans. Unfortunately, the impact of motion on MR images is fundamentally different and substantially more complicated than with CT.

In order to deal effectively with the diagnostic challenges posed by the effects of motion on MR images, the radiologist must first become familiar with a variety of technical issues. Only then can we proceed to prescribe imaging protocols and select pulse sequence parameters judiciously from a confusing assortment of procedural options. These efforts are aimed in part at (a) reducing or eliminating controllable sources of skeletal motion and suppressing the adverse effects of physiologic motion; (b) minimizing the potential for diagnostic errors due to misinterpretation of motion artifact as pathology; and (c) gaining insight into the potential diagnostic utility of certain signal alterations modulated by physiologic motion (specifically vascular and CSF flow phenomena) that can be elicited or modified by operator-controlled instrument variables.

Technical Considerations

Macroscopic motion of an imaged volume or component substructure during an MR pulse sequence results in MR signal alterations that can be considered in terms of flow phenomena and true motion artifacts. In the context of neuroimaging, flow phenomena are applicable to both the vascular system as well as the CSF circuit and can be categorized as either "time-of-flight" effects or "spin-phase" changes.

Time-of-flight effects are operative whenever the fluid channel is oriented perpendicular to the plane of sectioning and include the competing effects of flow-related enhancement (FRE) and high-velocity signal loss (HVSL) (5). At flow rates exceeding approximately 10 cm/sec, HVSL is the dominant mechanism. At slower flow rates, FRE may account for paradoxically increased signal, depending on a variety of factors, includ-

TABLE 2. *Instrument and physiologic variables governing intraluminal signal intensity of blood vessels on routine spin-echo images*

Instrument parameter	Physiologic factors
TR value	Vessel orientation
TE value	Direction of blood flow
Echo number (odd vs. even)	Velocity
Echo type (symmetric/ asymmetric)	Velocity profile
Single slice vs. multislice acquisition	Acceleration
Multislice section position	Acceleration profile
Multislice excitation order	Laminar vs. turbulent flow
Section thickness	Pseudogating/cardiac phase
Interslice gap thickness	
ECG gating/cardiac phase	

ing the direction of flow and the order of a slice within a multislice volume.

Spin-phase changes occur whenever fluid motion traverses gradient fields such that individual protons, moving at differential velocities or acceleration rates, experience slightly different magnetic field strengths (6). As a result, an ensemble of mobile protons acquires a distribution of phase angles that are not completely refocused following a 180° detection phase. [An exception occurs in the case of laminar fluid motion, wherein coherence is reestablished following each complete 360° rotation, assuming the use of symmetrical echo pulses. Hence, the term even-echo rephasing (7).] Because gradient fields are on at one time or another in all three coordinate dimensions during an MR pulse, dephasing occurs with respect to both perpendicular flow and in-plane flow. Signal loss due to spin-phase changes is particularly pronounced on images wherein fluid motion is parallel to and confined to the plane of the MR section such that time-of-flight effects do not occur. This is especially true for rapid or pulsatile flow characterized by marked spatial and temporal changes in velocity.

Although blood and CSF have markedly different T1 and T2 magnetic relaxation times (relatively short and long, respectively), their MR signal intensities in the dynamic state within the cerebral vasculature and CSF pathways are modified focally in similar fashions by the composite effects of the three flow phenomena described above. The interaction of these mechanisms is decidedly complex, and the relative contribution of each is dependent on the partial list of instrument and physiologic variables presented in Table 2.

Most routine MR images display both normal arteries and veins as areas of signal void, owing to the dominant effects of HVSL and spin-phase changes. Conspicuous exceptions occur secondary to FRE, even-echo rephasing, and diastolic pseudogating. The occasional presence of increased intraluminal signal, as a result of these flow phenomena, can be regarded as a potential pitfall, nuisance artifact, or potentially valuable physiologic information, depending on the experience of the observer.

Among these signal-augmenting flow effects, FRE is most frequently observed, generally on short-TR images and within the first few sections encountered by slowly flowing blood (5). The underlying mechanism of FRE can be explained as follows: During each TR interval, fully magnetized flowing protons from outside the excited volume enter a slice. These protons, having achieved equilibrium remagnetization, emit paradoxically bright signal, especially when compared to surrounding stationary and partially saturated tissue that has experienced a prior history of slice-selective excitation pulses. This effect is most pronounced at the minimum velocity that permits complete replacement of an intravascular channel with inflowing protons during each TR interval. Two governing parameters under direct operator control include Δz, the section thickness, and the TR interval. These factors are related by the equation, $v = \Delta z/TR$. The interdependence of these factors as determinants of FRE is shown in Table 3.

As the flow velocity begins to exceed $\Delta z/TR$, HVSL becomes the dominant time-of-flight effect. Signal loss caused by HVSL is also related to the slice-selective nature of 90° excitation and 180° refocusing pulses. At the downstream edge of a voxel that incorporates an arterial lumen, protons respond to a 90° excitation pulse and acquire transverse magnetization; but because these protons exit the section before the slice selective 180° pulse ($\frac{1}{2}$ TE later), refocusing does not occur, and these protons fail to contribute signal. On the upstream side of the voxel, flowing protons that entered the section in the time interval between the slice-selective 90° and 180° pulses (again, $\frac{1}{2}$ TE) do not acquire transverse magnetization and hence do not emit signal, even though they respond to the 180° pulse. The net effect of these signal-losing mechanisms is total signal void achieved at velocity $v = \Delta z/\frac{1}{2}$TE. The interdependence of these factors as determinants of HVSL is shown in Table 4.

Besides flow phenomena considered in the preceding discussion and developed in more detail in another chapter, we must contend with inherent motion artifacts present to some extent in virtually all MR images. This statement is at variance with assertions made in the early MR literature that discounted the issue of motion artifacts or even erroneously claimed that MR produces no motion artifact (3,4). There are two manifestations of motion artifact in MRI: (a) image blurring (indistinctness of native anatomic interfaces); and (b) the occurrence of image harmonics (in the phase-encoded direction), resulting in the production of ghost artifacts.

Although the overall study time of a typical MR examination is comparable to an equivalent CT study, it must be emphasized that using currently employed multislice techniques, signal data at each individual slice location are generated and collected throughout an entire pulse sequence. In other words, individual MR images are acquired in the time frame of minutes (typically 3–20 min), whereas individual CT slices are obtained in several seconds (typically 2–4 sec using fourth-generation CT scanners). As a result, MR is vulnerable to image degradation from various types of patient motion that occur during the relatively protracted acquisition time of the pulse sequence. Physiologic motion, especially that related to cardiac activity, respiration, and peristalsis of the alimentary tract, represents a frustrating impediment to high-quality body MR. Consequently, equipment vendors have targeted considerable scientific resources toward developing satisfactory solutions to the artifacts engendered by physiologic motion. Several clever techniques have already been applied with mixed results (8,9).

For instance, simple respiratory gating enables "acquisition registration" of thoracoabdominal anatomy, but only if the patient's respiratory pattern varies mini-

TABLE 3. *Interdependent relationship of flow-related enhancement on velocity, TR, and section thickness*[a]

TR (sec)	Maximal FRE velocities (cm/sec) at varying section thicknesses (cm)		
	0.3	0.5	1.0
0.150	2.00	3.33	6.67
0.200	1.50	2.50	5.00
0.300	1.00	1.67	3.33
0.400	0.75	1.25	2.50
0.500	0.60	1.00	2.00
0.600	0.50	0.83	1.67
0.800	0.38	0.63	1.25
1.000	0.33	0.50	1.00

[a] The velocity at which flow-related enhancement achieves its maximal effect depends on the TR and section thickness. Different velocities are shown for multiple combinations of TR and section thickness.

TABLE 4. *Interdependent relationship of high-velocity signal loss on velocity,*[a] *interpulse value ($\frac{1}{2}$TE), and section thickness*

Interpulse value $\frac{1}{2}$TE (msec)	Maximal HVSL velocities (cm/sec) at varying section thicknesses (cm)		
	0.3	0.5	1.00
10.0	30.0	50.0	100.0
12.5	24.0	40.0	80.0
15.0	20.0	33.3	66.7
20.0	15.0	25.0	50.0
30.0	10.0	16.7	33.3
45.0	6.7	11.1	22.2
60.0	5.0	8.3	16.7

[a] The velocity at which high-velocity signal loss achieves its maximal effect depends on the interpulse value of the echo sample ($\frac{1}{2}$TE) and the section thickness. Different velocities are shown for multiple combinations of $\frac{1}{2}$TE and section thickness.

mally throughout the pulse sequence. Even relaxed patients seldom maintain uniform and reproducible excursion of the diaphragm with each respiratory cycle (10). More important, the variable success of respiratory gating is gained only at the expense of decreased patient throughput. The time penalty of respiratory gating can amount to an approximate doubling of imaging time (11,12).

Echo planar imaging involving the use of low flip angles and gradient recalled echo samples enable very rapid multislice data acquisition that can be completed in a single breathhold. Although this strategy is appealing from the standpoint of artifact reduction, the technique suffers from reduced SNR and produces proton density-weighted images that to date have unproved utility in screening applications, at least for cerebral MRI.

Pharmacologic aids have been advocated both for sedation and analgesia. Such measures are indicated for the pediatric age group, claustrophobic individuals, and patients who may develop postural discomfort during the course of an MR examination. The use of glucagon may also be of value in suppressing bowel motion artifact (13,14). These techniques may successfully reduce or eliminate artifact originating from skeletal motion or peristalsis, but when used independently, they fail to address other sources of motion.

Still other motion compensation schemes involve real time or postprocessing computer techniques ranging from relatively simple operations, such as image averaging, to sophisticated methods of signal filtration.

Gross Head/Spine Motion

Ghost images constitute the most obvious artifact resulting from gross modulus motion of the head or spine, especially if the motion is repetitive and periodic. These artifacts usually appear as curvilinear crescents of signal and represent partial copies of native anatomic interfaces that are reproduced at periodic intervals along the phase-encoded direction (Fig. 1). This type of artifact is unique to the two-dimensional Fourier transform method of data acquisition/reconstruction wherein spatial data are phase encoded along one coordinate dimension of the image plane (horizontal or vertical axis) and frequency encoded along the opposite direction. Phase encoding is accomplished by switching on a variable amplitude/duration gradient shortly after the 90° excitation pulse of each pulse cycle. Frequency encoding is achieved by the brief application of a fixed gradient in the opposite coordinate direction later in the pulse cycle, encompassing the moment of echo sampling when signal is emitted due to reestablished coherent precession.

The two-dimensional Fourier transform method of image reconstruction used in MRI is a departure from the back-projection technique utilized in CT scanning.

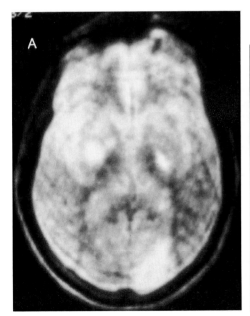 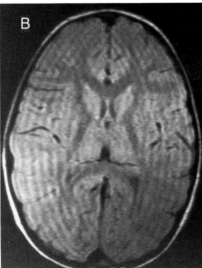

FIG. 1. Phase-encoded artifact from gross head motion. **A:** Acquired immunodeficiency syndrome (AIDS) patient with CNS toxoplasmosis and intractable hiccoughs. Periodic motion of the head causes parallel curvilinear ghost artifacts distributed along the vertical axis of the displayed image. The alignment of these ghost images corresponds to the phase-encoded axis of the two-dimensional Fourier transform image (TR = 2,000 msec, TE = 56 msec). **B:** Excessive head motion resulting from inadequate sedation of uncooperative child. This examination was performed on a different imager than the study shown in **A.** Note the distribution of alternating hypo- and hyperintense curvilinear ghosts (corresponding to reinforcement and cancellation phenomena) are distributed along the horizontal axis of this displayed image, again, corresponding to the phase-encoded axis (TR = 2,000 msec, TE = 35 msec). Repetitive, and especially periodic, motion often results in image harmonics or ghost artifacts as the dominant adverse effect of motion.

This difference accounts in part for the significantly altered appearance of motion artifact on MR images when compared to CT. If in fact, multiple phase-encoded angle views were acquired for back-projection reconstruction of MR images, the effect of motion might more closely resemble the streak or starburst patterns common to CT.

Intermittent motion occurring during an MR pulse sequence gives rise to image harmonics or ghosts, which appear only in the phase-encoded direction regardless of the direction of motion. The latter observation is readily apparent on routine clinical images, that exhibit motion artifact. For instance, rotatory motion, such as rapid eye movement, produces ghosts only across the phase-encoded direction. Because the orientation of phase versus frequency encoding is arbitrary and without an industry-wide convention, the directional projection of ghosts may be rotated 90° when comparing results obtained from one commercial unit to the results of a competing manufacturer (Fig. 1). Also, equipment manufacturers usually provide a means of switching gradient orientations either directly by computer command or indirectly by intentionally indicating an incorrect patient anatomical position to the computer; for instance, indicating a decubitus position when in fact the patient is supine (Fig. 2).

The crescents of phantom signal distributed along the phase-encoded direction of a MR image are incomplete copies of native anatomy because of reinforcement and cancellation phenomena. It has been demonstrated experimentally that the spacing between a high-contrast interface and its derivative ghosts is a function of the TR interval and the rate of reciprocal motion (15). An increase in either the TR value or the frequency of motion increases the spacing between parent signal and daughter ghosts. An increase in the amplitude of motion increases edge blurring (of both native anatomy and ghosts) but does not otherwise alter the appearance of image harmonics.

Efforts to eliminate ghost artifacts are appropriately directed toward ensuring that the patient remains stationary during data acquisition. In adults, claustrophobic reactions commonly lend to motion artifact but can usually be avoided by careful patient preparation and counselling. Occasionally, psychotropic drugs may be needed in order to enable an adequate level of patient cooperation. Certain patients may have difficulty maintaining a stationary supine position because of muscle spasms or radicular pain (as may occur from discogenic disease or other forms of spinal axis pathology), necessitating analgesic medication. Routine sedation is appropriate for infants and younger children up to ages 6 to 8 years, depending on their level of cooperation. The use of orally administered chloral hydrate (50–75 mg/kg, up to 1,000 mg, given 10–15 min prior to examination) is safe and convenient for this purpose, especially in an outpatient environment. Alternatively, intramuscular medication, such as pentobarbital (5–6 mg/kg, i.m.), may be utilized.

Intravascular Flow Effects

VASCULAR GHOSTS

Image harmonics originating from laminar flow within venous structures are usually identified easily as such, especially if the parent vessel is aligned parallel to

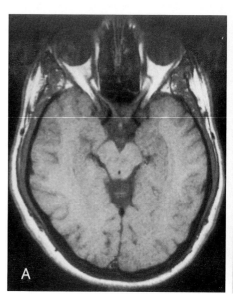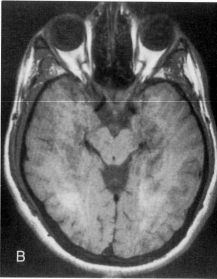

FIG. 2. Ghost artifact from rapid eye movement. The effect of switching the phase- and frequency-encoded axes is demonstrated. A: "Routine" image with phase-encoded direction along the x axis. Rotatory motion of the globes leads to the production of ghost artifacts that are particularly obvious lateral to either globe (TR = 600 msec, TE = 25 msec). B: This image was obtained in a fashion similar to A, except that the patient's anatomic reference was entered falsely intentionally as decubitus while maintaining the patient supine. As a result, the phase-encoded direction now corresponds to the vertical axis of the displayed image. Note the appearance of "noise" distributed along the vertical projection of either globe. This represents phase-encoded artifact not present at the same location in A (TR = 600 msec, TE = 25 msec).

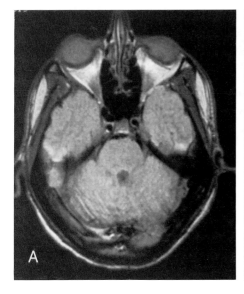
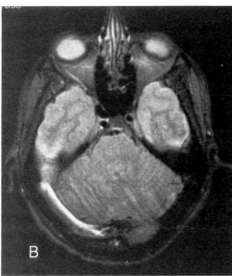

FIG. 3. Ghost artifact from physiologic motion of blood flow in transverse sinus. **A:** A first echo image shows faint alternating crescents of hypo- or hyperintensity distributed across the posterior aspect of the posterior fossa (TR = 2,000 msec, TE = 35 msec). **B:** The second echo image highlights the right transverse sinus due to even-echo rephasing and clearly identifies this vascular channel as the source of the ghost images. These crescents of signal aberration conform in contour to, and represent partial copies of, the transverse sinus (TR = 2,000 msec, TE = 70 msec).

the plane of sectioning. These curvilinear artifacts conform to the morphologic contour of the static vessel and are distributed at periodic intervals along the phase-encoded direction (Fig. 3). Adjustment of window/level settings at the monitor will confirm that the ghost images are replicated across the entire display matrix, extending peripheral to the scalp surface. On even-echo images, the originating venous structure is often highlighted due to the phenomenon of even-echo rephasing (Fig. 3).

Recognition of ghosts originating from pulsatile arterial flow can be more difficult. Predictably, these artifacts are more commonplace on images that incorporate the basal cisterns and circle of Willis (Fig. 4). The basilar artery and parasellar carotid arteries (in addition to surrounding mobile CSF) in particular frequently produce ghosts that are usually projected through either temporal lobe on axial images. Reinforcement and cancellation phenomena may result in the appearance of a single, or at least a dominant, hyperintense ghost that

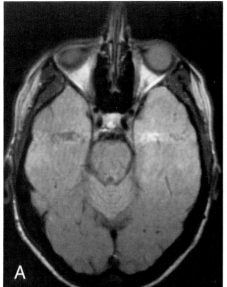
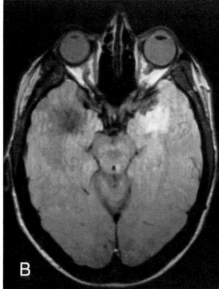
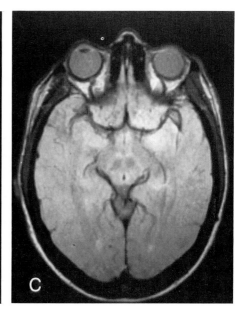

FIG. 4. Ghost artifacts from physiologic motion of blood flow (and surrounding CSF) in basilar and suprasellar cisterns. **A:** A hypointense "cancellation" ghost is projected horizontally through the right temporal lobe while a mirror image "reinforcement" ghost is projected through the opposite temporal lobe. These are due to physiologic motion within the basilar cistern. The focal hyperintensity in the midline at the posterior aspect of the sella represents fat-like signal normally seen in the posterior pituitary gland (TR = 2,000 msec, TE = 35 msec). **B:** On this image, at a slightly higher level, broader zones of reinforcement and cancellation ghost artifact are due to inclusion of a broader area of flow-containing structures in the suprasellar cistern (TR = 2,000 msec, TE = 35 msec). **C:** At the level of the optic chiasm, the dominant reinforcement artifact overlying the uncus of the left hippocampal gyrus simulates a true signal abnormality (TR = 2,000 msec, TE = 35 msec).

can closely simulate parenchymal brain pathology. In such cases, several procedural options may help avoid diagnostic errors. A supplemental pulse sequence obtained using a different TR value will change the character and distribution of the ghosts, enabling differentiation of image harmonics from true pathology. The supplemental pulse sequence may also be obtained by using a different slice orientation (e.g., sagittal versus axial versus coronal) in order to distribute the suspected ghost artifact through a different anatomic region (Fig. 5). Finally, the directions of phase versus frequency encoding may be rotated 90° in order to achieve a similar result (Fig. 2).

The brainstem is perhaps the most frequent site of vascular ghosts that mimic pathology. We have encountered focal signal artifact originating from the petrous carotid artery, jugular bulb, sigmoid sinus, and vertebral basilar system (and/or surrounding CSF) that, to an unwary observer, can closely simulate CSF spread of tumor, intrinsic brainstem neoplasia, demyelinating disease, or even subacute hemorrhage. Clues to the artifactual nature of such signal aberrations include:

1. hyperintensity on a first echo image that either does not change appreciably or shows unlikely, inexplicable change on a subsequent echo (Fig. 6);

2. focal hyperintensity at a location that fails to show any discernible abnormality on an image obtained with a different TR value or slice orientation (Fig. 7);

3. a multiplicity of ghosts, especially a combination of cancellation and reinforcement artifacts, causing alternating hypo- and hyperintensity, resulting in a linear alignment of ghosts across the phase-encoded axis;

4. spurious signal "abnormality" that extends across unlikely anatomic boundaries or tissue compartments (Fig. 8); and

5. the uniform and conspicuous absence of either mass effect or focal atrophy in relation to suspected phase-encoded artifacts.

FLOW-RELATED ENHANCEMENT

On routine MR pulse sequences, most vascular channels, especially arterial structures, are displayed with intraluminal flow void, owing to the dominant effects of

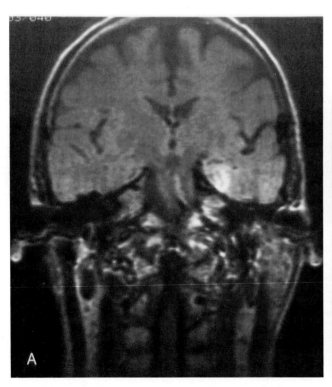
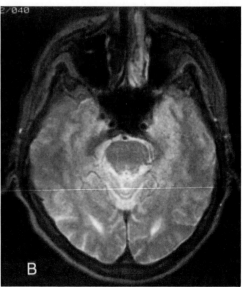

FIG. 5. Vascular ghost artifact: diagnostic value of supplemental pulse sequence obtained using a different slice orientation and TR value. **A:** Direct coronal image shows a focal hyperintensity in the medial aspect of the left temporal lobe unassociated with mass effect. This signal aberration represents ghost artifact distributed at this site from physiologic motion in and about the pontine cistern on this image obtained with a horizontal phase-encoded axis (TR = 2,000 msec, TE = 35 msec). **B:** Supplemental transaxial image obtained through the temporal lobes. There is clearly no evidence of either true signal abnormality or ghost artifact within the left temporal lobe. The ghost artifact was successfully eliminated by a combination of a change in slice orientation (intended to exclude the presumed source of motion artifact from the anatomic section) and lengthening of the TR value (TR = 2,000 msec, TE = 70 msec).

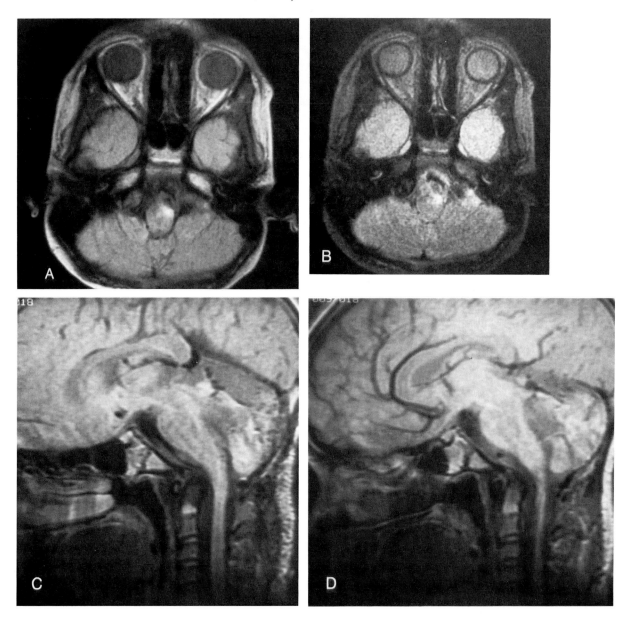

FIG. 6. Confusing flow-related ghost artifact at surface of medulla in child with known cerebellar astrocytoma. **A:** On this image alone, the focal hyperintensity at the anterior surface of the medulla on the left could be confused with CSF spread of tumor (TR = 2,000 msec, TE = 35 msec). **B:** The second echo image fails to show relative hyperintensity (as would characteristically be expected from T2 prolongation), thus discounting the possibility that this finding represents CSF tumor spread and favoring flow-induced ghost artifact originating from vicinity of the vertebral arteries (TR = 2,000 msec, TE = 70 msec). **C, D:** Adjacent T2-weighted images obtained sagittally near the midline show the partially resected tumor near the superior vermis but no evidence of signal abnormality at the level of the medulla, confirming the artifactual nature of the signal aberration shown on the axial views (TR = 2,000 msec, TE = 80 msec).

HVSL and turbulent dephasing; however, paradoxically increased signal due to FRE may occur, especially on short-TR images. This phenomenon is most commonly seen on sections near the edge of a selectively excited volume that receives inflowing (fully magnetized) venous blood. The signal produced may be overlooked, misinterpreted as a pathologic finding, or correctly identified as a potentially important physiologic parameter of blood flow that can aid in the overall assessment

of structural lesions and contribute meaningfully toward an accurate vascular diagnosis (Fig. 9).

At slice locations situated more deeply within a multislice volume, FRE is less commonly encountered, in keeping with the governing physical principles reviewed earlier; however, an exception to this general rule seems to occur when a multislice pulse sequence is prescribed with a wide interslice gap (approximately 50% or more of the section thickness) or an interleaved technique is

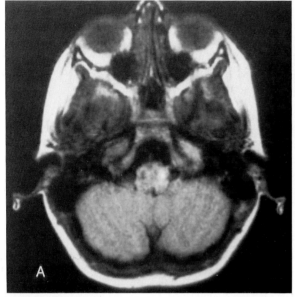
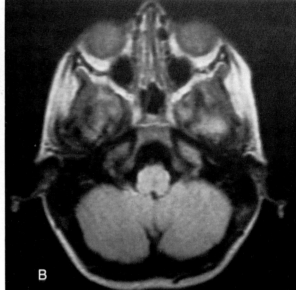
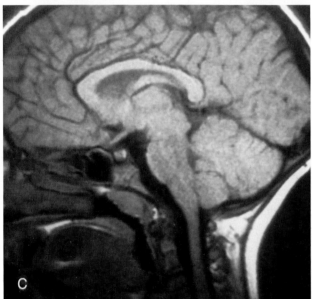

FIG. 7. Ghost artifact from flow identified by using pulse sequence with different TR value. **A:** Routine T1-weighted image through the level of the lower brainstem shows focal hyperintensity at the left medulla. Note mirror-image hypointensity in the right medulla. This pattern suggests ghost artifact from physiologic motion of flow (TR = 600 msec, TE = 25 msec). **B:** A T2-weighted pulse sequence at the time same slice location shows no evidence of signal abnormality within or about the medulla, discounting the likelihood of a true signal abnormality (TR = 2,000 msec, TE = 35 msec). **C:** Direct sagittal image through the brainstem confirms the absence of signal abnormality using pulse sequence parameters identical to those in image **A** (TR = 600 msec, TE = 25 msec).

utilized. In either case, the gap of unperturbed tissue between intervening sections presumably serves as a sanctuary zone that effectively prolongs the time available for remagnetization of flowing protons that traverse the gap. As a result, depending on the specific dynamics of flow, we may observe a confusing augmentation of FRE deep within an excited volume, even on the center slice. For instance, using a multislice partial saturation pulse sequence, the unexpected presence of increased signal within a midline structure, such as the straight sinus, could be misconstrued as evidence of sinus thrombosis (Fig. 10).

Diastolic Pseudogating

Chance synchronization of a radiofrequency (RF) pulse cycle with the patient's cardiac cycle may result in paradoxically increased signal within an arterial lumen. This phenomenon occurs when (a) the TR value is equal to, or an integer multiple of, the R–R interval; and (b) the MR signal (echo) is sampled in late diastole, corresponding to the period of reduced flow. Under such conditions, virtually motionless intra-arterial blood is "captured" and depicted as bright signal (on short TR images) due to the relatively short T1 of blood (Fig. 11). The magnitude of this effect is less pronounced with respect to intracranial arteries because of the reduced pulse pressure within the cerebral arteries, resulting in nearly constant antegrade flow.

CSF Motion Effects

Motional characteristics and flow patterns present at various locations along the CSF circuit are dependent

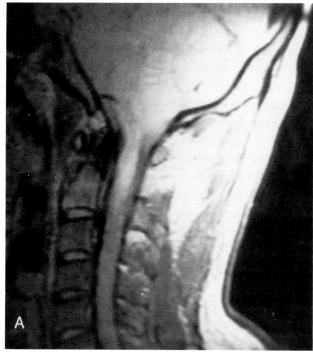

FIG. 8. Cervical cord lesion in young adult with upper motor neuron disease. **A:** A T2-weighted sagittal image through the upper cervical cord shows a nonspecific elliptical zone of signal abnormality that could represent a primary tumor or demyelinating disease. A multiplicity of lesions is mimicked by confusing flow artifacts in and about the fourth ventricle (TR = 2,500 msec, TE = 40 msec). **B:** At the level of the fourth ventricle, a first echo transaxial image suggests an abnormal hyperintense focus subependymally at the left side of the fourth ventricle. Note also subtle low signal intensity adjacent to the subependymal aspect of the fourth ventricle on the right, as well as a linear alignment of multiple crescentric flow artifacts projected across the plane of the sigmoid sinuses (TR = 2,000 msec, TE = 35 msec). **C:** The second echo image better demonstrates the margins of the fourth ventricle (due to increased relative hyperintensity of CSF). The mirror-image hyper- and hypointense ghost artifacts from flow clearly bridge an unlikely anatomic barrier (the ependymal surface of the fourth ventricle), thus confirming the artifactual nature of this finding (TR = 2,000 msec, TE = 70 msec).

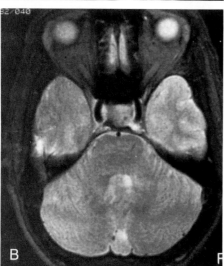

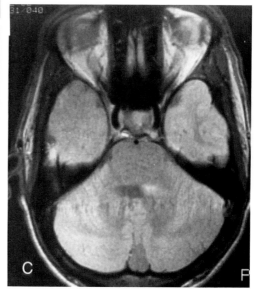

on complex physioanatomic relationships. Especially important for MRI are the effects of transmitted cardiovascular pulsations on CSF dynamics.

Spatially dependent MR signal differences can be observed routinely along the ventricular pathway as well as within the extraventricular CSF compartments (16). Initial speculation as to the cause of the signal differences has focused on the known slight gradient increase in protein concentration when comparing intraventricular CSF (0–10 mg/dl protein concentration) to extraventricular CSF (15–25 mg/dl protein concentration) (17); however, subsequent *in vitro* experiments have suggested that more substantial concentrations of protein are required in order to significantly reduce the T1 relaxation time of static fluid collections such that visible signal differences will occur (18).

Rather than being related to any modest differences in protein concentration, focal CSF signal alterations are modulated by pulsatile and vibratory forces initiated with each systolic impulse. The resulting signal changes are analogous to the intravascular flow phenomena described previously.

HIGH-VELOCITY SIGNAL LOSS

CSF achieves relatively high linear flow rates only within the aqueduct of Sylvius, where the caliber of the ventricular pathway is markedly narrowed. The reduced cross-sectional diameter of the aqueduct is accompanied by an acceleration of CSF flow that is periodically augmented by each cardiosynchronous pulsation of the

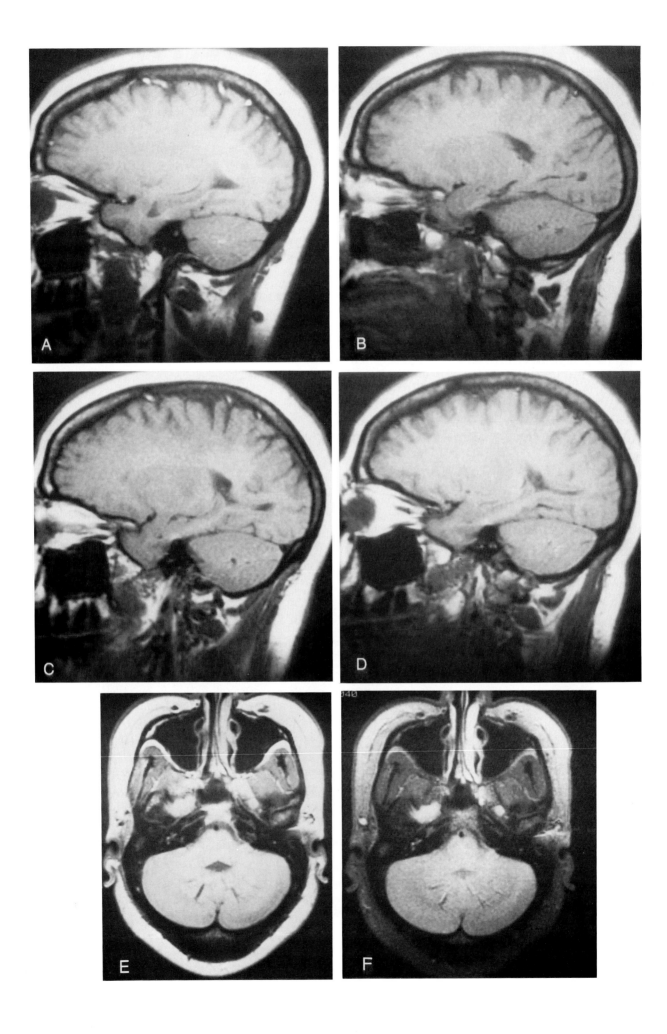

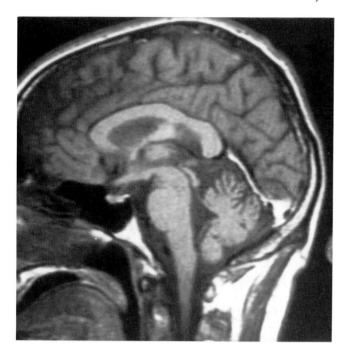

FIG. 10. Center slice flow-related enhancement within straight sinus-simulating sinus thrombosis. Linear hyperintensity is present throughout the straight sinus extending from the posterior aspect of the splenium of the corpus callosum into the torcula. Usually, an end-slice phenomenon, flow-related enhancement was present on this center slice due to the "sanctuary effect" of a wide interslice gap, allowing increased time for remagnetization of flowing protons dependent on the orientation of central draining veins and flow dynamics (TR = 600 msec, TE = 25 msec, six-slice acquisition). A transaxial spin-echo pulse sequence documented normal flow void within the straight sinus.

ventricular system. On transaxial head images, the phenomenon of HVSL may contribute to the depiction of the aqueduct as a focus of signal void, especially if pseudosystolic gating occurs (Fig. 12). This phenomenon is also contributed to by dephasing effects resulting from the random motion of CSF protons. Bradley et al. (19) have described an increased frequency of aqueductal HVSL in patients with normal pressure hydrocephalus, a finding attributed to reduced compliance (and hence increased CSF flow) of the expanded ventricular system.

In patients with a pattern of ventriculomegaly suggestive of aqueductal stenosis (large third and lateral ventricles; small or normal size fourth ventricle), conspicuous absence of HVSL within the aqueduct may provide an important physiologic cycle that complements the structural findings encountered in this disorder (Fig. 13).

FLOW-RELATED ENHANCEMENT

Flow-related enhancement of CSF is often visible on the most cephalic transaxial image of a multislice cervi-cal or thoracic spine study (Fig. 14). The underlying mechanism is related to the bulk caudal flow of CSF that occurs with each systolic impulse. The fluid dynamics responsible for this effect can be appreciated fluoroscopically during the performance of a C1–C2 puncture cervical myelogram wherein injected iodinated contrast material can be observed to stream caudally within the subarachnoid space. During the MR pulse sequence, in the time interval between slice-selective 90° excitation pulses, fully magnetized CSF protons are propelled into the most cephalic slice location. More caudal sections contain CSF that has experienced the prior history of 90° excitation pulses, resulting in partially saturated protons that emit comparatively less signal. At the lumbar level, the absence of a significant component of bulk CSF flow precludes a similar phenomenon.

Rarely, FRE of CSF may be observed on the most caudal transaxial slice of a multisection volume, usually at the level of the fourth ventricle (Fig. 15). This phenomenon is probably due to diastolic pseudogating and retrograde flow or to refluxing eddy currents of fully magnetized CSF that enter the most caudal slice location during each TR interval.

FIG. 9. Subtle artifact-like flow-related enhancement of venous angioma; a finding of diagnostic value. Images **A** and **D** represent end-slice images from the left and right sides of a nine-slice-location sagittal pulse sequence (TR = 600 msec, TE = 25 msec). Images **B** and **C** were obtained contiguous to **A** and **D**, respectively. **A:** Subtle punctate foci of increased signal are seen in the mid-left cerebellum. **B:** Several foci of discrete hypointensity (flow void) are seen at similar locations on the adjacent slice. **C:** Near the right side of the excited volume, punctate areas of flow void are also seen within the right cerebellum. **D:** The most rightward image shows several punctate foci of increased signal similar to those demonstrated in the left cerebellum. The appearance of FRE on either "end slice" of the excited volume and flow void on the immediately contiguous slice suggests a bilateral vascular lesion with venous flow rates and central drainage. **E, F:** First (**E**) and second (**F**) echo images from a transaxial pulse sequence confirms the presence of a symmetrical "caput medusae" venous angioma with tributary veins in either cerebellar hemisphere showing even-echo rephasing phenomenon on the second echo image (TR = 2,000 msec, TE = 25/50 msec).

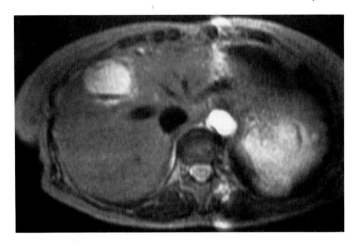

FIG. 11. Diastolic pseudogating of abdominal aorta. Flow void normally expected within the midabdominal aorta is replaced with homogeneous hyperintensity. This phenomenon is due to diastolic pseudogating such that the TR interval was an integral multiple of the patient's R-R interval, and selective excitation of this slice coincided with the diastolic phase of the patient's cardiac cycle. Center slice positioning of this section (a ten-location multislice pulse sequence) excludes flow-related enhancement, and the conspicuous presence of ghost images projected vertically (along the phase-encoded axis) confirms patency of the abdominal aorta (TR = 800 msec, TE = 50 msec).

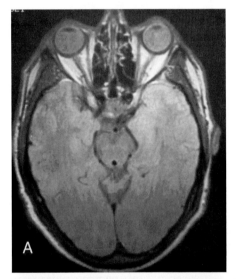

FIG. 12. Normal time-of-flight effects within patent aqueduct of Sylvius. **A, B:** On first (**A**) and second (**B**) echo transaxial images, high-velocity signal loss within the aqueduct of Sylvius produces signal void similar in appearance to the basilar artery anteriorly. In this plane, the flow void is produced both by the section transition effects of rapidly flowing CSF protons entering and exiting the slice during the interpulse interval, as well as the dephasing effects of turbulent CSF flow perpendicular to the plane of sectioning (TR = 2,000 msec, TE = 35/70 msec). **C:** A midline sagittal image shows relative flow void within the aqueduct blending proximally with the mid-third ventricle and caudally with the upper fourth ventricle. Because CSF flow is now parallel to and contained within the plane of sectioning, time-of-flight effects are eliminated, and the aqueductal flow void is accounted for solely by turbulent dephasing (random differential flow of individual CSF protons through gradient fields) (TR = 600 msec, TE = 25 msec).

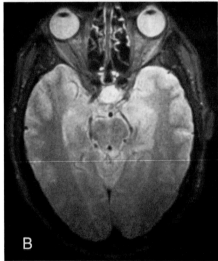

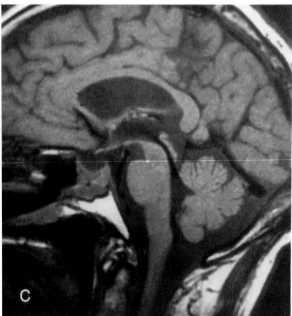

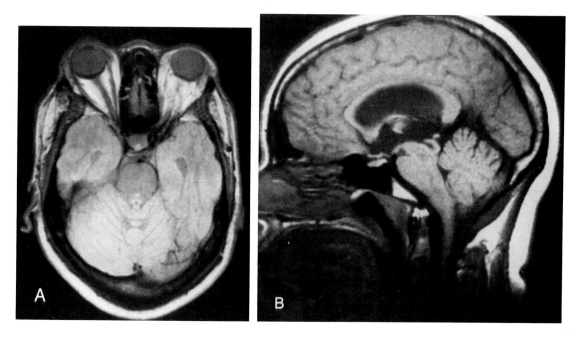

FIG. 13. Absence of aqueductal high velocity signal loss and dephasing in aqueductal stenosis. **A:** Transaxial image through the midbrain shows aqueductal signal equivalent to static CSF in other locations (temporal horns, pontine cistern). Note the similarity between the aqueduct posteriorly and the basilar artery anteriorly (TR = 2,000 msec, TE = 35 msec). **B:** Midline sagittal view shows an absence of dephasing effects within the aqueduct. The absence of time-of-flight effects and dephasing in conjunction with the typical pattern of ventricular dilatation helps secure the diagnosis of benign aqueductal stenosis in this patient (TR = 600 msec, TE = 25 msec).

TURBULENT DEPHASING

Time-of-flight effects (HVSL and FRE) are not applicable when fluid motion is parallel to and confined within the plane of sectioning. Under these circumstances, the effects of flow-induced spin-phase changes are isolated. Focal CSF signal loss from dephasing is most pronounced at sites of rapid or pulsatile flow characterized by marked spatial and temporal changes in velocity (6). A typical example is a sagittal image of the aqueduct of Sylvius, where focal signal loss results from the pulsatile and turbulent flow of CSF contained within the section (Fig. 12). As they approach the aqueduct, CSF protons are accelerated at varying rates. The differential movement of these individual spins through the gradient fields creates a time-varying distribution of phase angles within each pixel. With respect to in-plane flow, it is this process that nullifies the refocusing effects of a 180° pulse and causes focally diminished signal.

Signal loss from spin-phase changes may also be observed on transaxial images of the head. Enlarged ventricles often exhibit concentric rings of decreased signal, especially in the vicinity of the trigones, a finding attributable to cardiosynchronous vibratory forces transmitted by choroidal pulsations. In a somewhat similar fashion, a dilated inferiorly expanded third ventricle may exhibit decreased signal (due to spin-phase changes) from turbulent to-and-fro motion caused by pulsations

transmitted from either the circle of Willis or propulsive CSF flow (Fig. 16).

Within the pontine cistern, a peribasilar ring of decreased CSF signal may simulate a fusiform aneurysm (Fig. 17). This deceptive appearance of CSF surrounding the basilar artery is most commonly seen in children and young adults with nonatherosclerotic vessels. Again, the mechanism is turbulent in-plane motion of CSF and spin-phase changes caused by gross movement of the basilar artery with each systolic impulse.

Although flow through the aqueduct produces the most striking example of signal loss from turbulent dephasing, spin-phase changes significantly reduce the signal of subarachnoid CSF on sagittal images of the cervical or thoracic spine. This effect is present routinely in normal patients and may be difficult to appreciate except at the thoracolumbar junction, where a gradient of increased signal from CSF in the lumbar cistern can be seen (Fig. 18). The increased signal yielded from the more caudal CSF is attributable to a relative lack of significant motion effects and hence elimination of spin-phase changes.

The motion-dependent dephasing of CSF normally present in the cervical or thoracic region can be demonstrated with clarity when the subarachnoid space is bordered by a static, sequestered collection of CSF, such as within a pseudomeningocele (Fig. 19). In such cases, relative hyperintensity of the immobile fluid collection

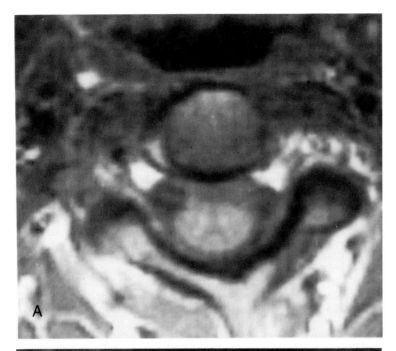

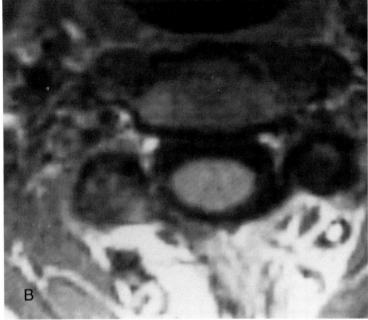

FIG. 14. Flow-related enhancement of CSF in cervical subarachnoid space (entry-slice phenomenon). **A:** End-slice image shows relative hyperintensity of the subarachnoid space compared to subadjacent levels. This phenomenon is attributable to propulsive caudal flow of fully magnetized CSF between successive slice selective excitations at this section location level. This effect could potentially mimic discogenic disease or other forms of pathology (TR = 1,000 msec, TE = 25 msec). **B:** A subjacent transaxial image displays CSF with relatively less signal due to the absence of flow-related enhancement. CSF contained within this section, as well as more caudal slices, contains protons that have experienced a prior history of excitation pulses, thus reducing potential for flow-related enhancement (TR = 1,000 msec, TE = 25 msec).

might initially suggest an elevated protein concentration; however, our experience to date includes three examples of hyperintense cysts (compared to adjacent subarachnoid space CSF) wherein fluid aspirates revealed protein concentrations less than 25 mg/dl (CSF normal range, 0–25 mg/dl). These laboratory data support the view that sagittal images routinely depict normal subarachnoid CSF with substantially reduced signal due to spin-phase changes. This conclusion is further supported by the observation that ECG-synchronized images have shown an augmentation of signal from cervical CSF on relatively short TR images when data col-

lection is triggered for late diastole, thereby capturing CSF in an immobile state.

The presence of an epidural lesion, causing a subarachnoid block, may also result in augmentation of CSF signal below the level of obstruction (Fig. 20). Because CSF pulsations can no longer be transmitted directly to CSF below the block, dephasing related to flow is virtually eliminated. This physiologic effect, when recognized, can lend diagnostically important information to the assessment of epidural lesions, possibly obviating the need for myelographic evaluation.

Finally, specialized pulse sequences can aid in the dif-

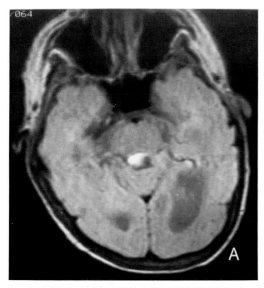

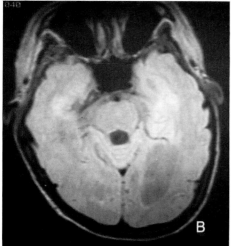

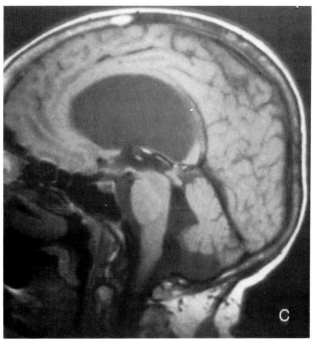

FIG. 15. Flow-related enhancement of CSF within the fourth ventricle due to diastolic pseudogating and retrograde pulsatile CSF flow. **A:** The most caudal image of a multislice pulse sequence shows discrete hyperintensity of CSF within the fourth ventricle caused by flow-related enhancement. This effect is due to cardiosynchronous excitation of this slice in diastole, resulting in the "capture" of fully magnetized retrograde currents of CSF moving cephalad during diastole (TR = 2,000 msec, TE = 35 msec). **B:** A repeat pulse sequence was performed using similar instrument parameters, except that the level of the fourth ventricle is now situated centrally within the excited volume. Note the absence of flow-related enhancement within the fourth ventricle, which is now depicted as homogeneously low signal intensity, slightly less than occipital horn CSF due to dephasing effects (TR = 2,000 msec, TE = 35 msec). **C:** T1-weighted midsagittal image shows diffuse ventriculomegaly and confirms the absence of signal abnormality or tissue within the expanded fourth ventricle in this patient with communicating hydrocephalus (TR = 600 msec, TE = 25 msec).

ferentiation of static CSF containing lesions from more actively flowing CSF compartments. Specifically, we have utilized a short-TR spin-echo pulse sequence (TR = 150 msec, TE = 20 msec), with a nonselective 180° pulse, in order to map the distribution of static CSF, either within or surrounding suspected cysts (Fig. 21). Using such a pulse sequence, normal CSF, which has a T2 time constant in the range of 150 msec [at 1.5 tesla (T)], will maintain measurable transverse magnetization between successive pulse cycles, provided that no significant turbulent dephasing occurs from motion. Mobile CSF, though, is displayed with low signal, due to the combined effects of dephasing and its relatively long T1 relaxation time.

CSF GHOSTS

Given that CSF signal loss from motion-induced spin-phase changes is common at numerous sites along the CSF circuit, it follows that phase-encoded motion artifacts are common as well. The physical explanation for these artifacts is identical to the image harmonics phenomena that account for the presence of vascular ghosts. In either case, the underlying mechanism is cardiosynchronous motion and its unique effect on the two-dimensional Fourier transform image acquisition/reconstruction technique commonly employed in MRI. The ghost images that are distributed across the phase-encoded image axis can usually be identified as partial

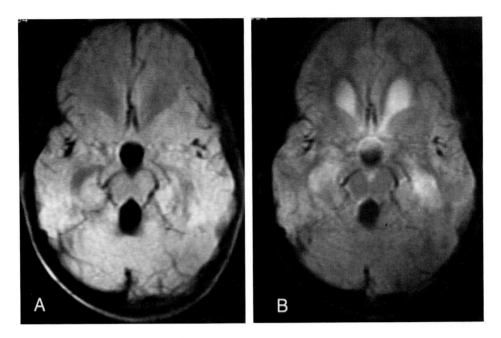

FIG. 16. Turbulent dephasing of third and fourth ventricular CSF in patient with communicating hydrocephalus. **A:** First echo image through the base of the brain shows homogeneous low signal intensity of third and fourth ventricular CSF compared to CSF contained within the temporal or frontal horns. This effect is due to turbulent propulsive flow of CSF related either to circulatory dynamics of CSF or arterial pulsations transmitted by vessels near the circle of Willis (TR = 2,000 msec, TE = 40 msec). **B:** The second echo image of the same pulse sequence shows persistence of dephasing effects within both the expanded third and fourth ventricle. Note relative augmented signal intensity of less mobile CSF within the temporal and frontal horns (TR = 2,000 msec, TE = 80 msec).

copies of a CSF compartment, thus confirming the artifactual nature of the signal pattern produced, as well as its originating source (Fig. 22).

In many instances, though, especially in the posterior fossa, consistent and accurate recognition of CSF flow artifacts is a challenging task. At the level of the fourth ventricle, or perimedullary cistern, phase-encoded flow artifacts often masquerade as pathologic findings (Figs. 6 and 7). Also, it is often not entirely clear whether flowing vascular spaces, mobile CSF, or both types of motion account jointly for certain artifacts near the foramen magnum due to the juxtaposition of neurovascular anatomy amid variable CSF currents.

Varying with the direction of phase-encoding, sagittal images of the craniocervical junction region may show peculiar, yet somewhat distinctive, patterns of motion artifact. Using an anteroposterior (AP) dimension phase gradient, the brainstem will often appear to be "noisy" due to the projection of basilar artery as well as peribasilar CSF ghosts through the pons and medulla. Some-

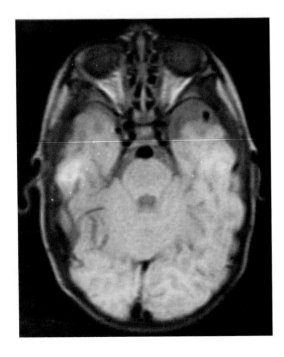

FIG. 17. Turbulent dephasing of peribasilar CSF simulating fusiform aneurysm. Transaxial image through the pons shows a large ovoid area of hypointensity corresponding to the expected location of the basilar artery within the pontine cistern. This appearance may suggest a fusiform aneurysm of the basilar artery; however, the basilar artery is seen as a subtle focus of intermediate signal centrally. This effect is most commonly observed in younger patients and is due to gross movement of the basilar artery with each systolic impulse. Peribasilar CSF undergoes turbulent motion resulting in dephasing and focally diminished signal (TR = 2,000 msec, TE = 35 msec).

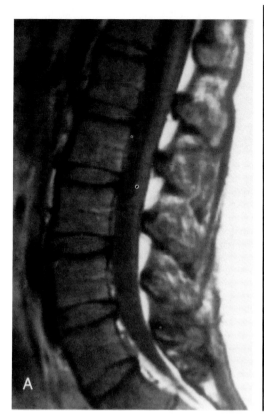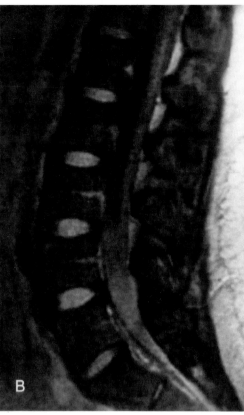

FIG. 18. Differential dephasing of thoracolumbar CSF. **A:** T1-weighted sagittal image (first echo) of the lumbar spine shows slight difference in signal between CSF at the thoracolumbar junction compared to relatively hyperintense CSF in the caudal lumbar cistern (TR = 1,000 msec, TE = 20 msec). **B:** T2-weighted sagittal image (second echo) at the same location further accentuates the differential dephasing of thoracolumbar CSF. The increased mobility (cardiosynchronous to-and-fro motion) of CSF contained in the thoracic subarachnoid space compared to relatively stagnant CSF situated in the caudal thecal sac causes differential dephasing resulting in the signal changes shown. Predictably, this phenomenon is most pronounced on images that exhibit the effects of pseudosystolic gating (TR = 1,000 msec, TE = 70 msec).

what low in the cervical region, less rapid and predominantly longitudinal motion of subarachnoid CSF may cause replication of a linear ghost within the cord that closely resembles the appearance of a syrinx cavity (Fig. 23). Anticipation of these problems, familiarity with the underlying technical principles, and skillful interactive pulse-sequence prescription help ensure optimal image quality while reducing the potential for diagnostic errors.

SYSTOLIC PSEUDOGATING

CSF attains maximal linear velocity shortly after transmission of the systolic impulse to the ventricular, cisternal, and subarachnoid compartments. The fluid dynamics of CSF also vary considerably at different locations along the CSF circuit depending on anatomic factors as well as individual patient physiology and homeostatic mechanisms. Nevertheless, it appears reasonable to assume that in general, bulk flow, as well as turbulent motion of CSF, peaks or at least demonstrates a plateau coincident with each systolic impulse, proba-

bly persisting into the midportion of the cardiac cycle. This periodic pulsatile motion is followed by diastolic slowing, stagnation, and perhaps a component of retrograde flow (depending on the level being considered) immediately prior to the subsequent cardiac contraction.

Although peak systolic flow rates at the aqueduct of Sylvius might result in decreased signal due to HVSL (on axial images), the dominant signal-loss effect of CSF motion is accounted for by turbulent dephasing. Based on the foregoing discussion, it follows that the qualitative effect of turbulent dephasing is also a cardiosynchronous event, exerting its maximal signal-loss effect during the systolic portion of the cardiac cycle. This cyclic nature of turbulent dephasing, combined with the effects of pseudogating, can produce a confusing alternation of CSF signal intensity on anatomically ordered sections acquired using a nonsequential selective excitation scheme. This complicated phenomenon is demonstrated in Fig. 24 and is best explained and understood in the context of an axial sequence of the spine. Recall

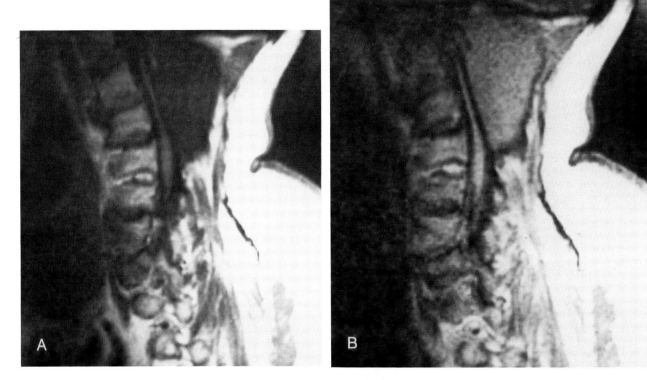

FIG. 19. Normal CSF within cervical pseudomeningocele contrasted by dephased hypointensity of subarachnoid CSF. **A:** T1-weighted parasagittal view shows a triangular configuration postoperative pseudomeningocele posterior to an atrophic cervical spinal cord surrounded by subarachnoid CSF. Note slight differential signal intensity between relatively hyperintense pseudomeningocele fluid and subarachnoid CSF (TR = 600 msec, TE = 25 msec). **B:** A more heavily T2-weighted image further exaggerates signal differences between the pseudomeningocele and subarachnoid CSF. Relative hyperintensity of the pseudomeningocele is not due to protein elevation. The pseudomeningocele fluid was percutaneously aspirated, and chemistries revealed protein concentration of 22 mg/dl, less than subarachnoid CSF. Sequestration of CSF within the pseudomeningocele and isolation from the CSF circuit eliminate the dephasing effects that account for comparatively less signal emitted from the normal subarachnoid CSF (TR = 2,000 msec, TE = 40 msec).

first that multislice imaging entails selective excitation and signal recording of individual slices. The "cycle time" required for each slice selective "train" consisting of a 90° excitation pulse and one or more 180° refocusing pulses (each followed by an echo sample) is on the order of 50 to 100 msec. The remainder of the TR interval is "dead time" for any particular slice; time needed for recovery of longitudinal magnetization prior to the next of 128 or 256 total slice-selective "pulse trains," each distinguished only by a slightly different phase-encoding gradient settings. During this dead time, other sections of the multislice volume can be excited, thus realizing the temporal efficiency of multislice imaging.

It might initially appear logical to sequentially excite slices (administer pulse trains) in anatomic order, that is, section 1, followed by section 2, followed by section 3, etc.; however, an important technical advantage, reduction of cross-excitation artifact (see below), can be gained by utilizing a nonsequential selective excitation order (20). For instance, the 15-section pulse sequence, partially illustrated in Fig. 23, was completed by first exciting the odd-numbered slice locations (1, 3, 5, . . . ,

15), followed by the even-numbered slice locations (2, 4, 6, . . . , 14). Using this nonsequential excitation method, the undesired impact of cross-excitation (partial excitation of tissue in adjacent sections due to an inherently imperfect slice profile) is reduced by effectively prolonging the time available for recovery of tissue in the next slice (compared to a sequential excitation order). However, if pseudogating occurs (TR interval equal to an integral multiple of the R-R interval), several consecutive odd-numbered sections might temporally coincide with systole and demonstrate turbulent dephasing of CSF, resulting in diminished signal. Intervening even-numbered sections would have been obtained $\frac{1}{2}$TR later in the cardiac cycle, corresponding to diastole and resulting in stagnant CSF showing comparatively greater signal. Both of these alternating effects are shown in Fig. 24.

CHEMICAL SHIFT ARTIFACT

A very slight but significant difference in resonant frequency exists when comparing hydrogen nuclei

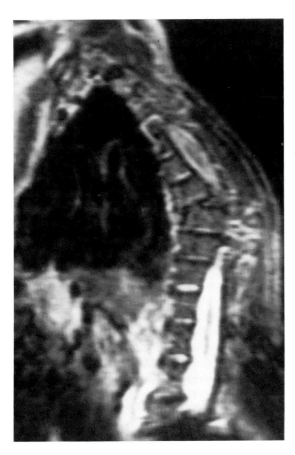

FIG. 20. Augmentation of CSF signal inferior to spinal epidural block (elimination of dephasing effects). This patient has metastatic disease with vertebral body destruction and subluxation in the midthoracic level, resulting in an epidural mass and thecal sac compression. Note the markedly increased signal emitted from the more caudal CSF contained within the subarachnoid space inferior to the block compared to CSF contained within the subarachnoid space above the block (TR = 2,000 msec, TE = 70 msec).

bound in water molecules to those bound in lipid molecules. The degree of resonant proton frequency shift attributable to the two chemical and unique micromagnetic environments (water versus fat) is approximately 3.25 parts per million (ppm). Because this effect is proportional to the operating strength of the main magnetic field, the exact magnitude of the frequency shift is significantly greater at 1.5 T (63.8 MHz Larmor frequency × 3.25 ppm = 208 Hz) than at 0.35 T (15 MHz Larmor frequency × 3.25 ppm = 48 Hz). It also follows that unless corrective measures are taken, the degree of chemical shift misregistration artifact visible on images produced using high-strength systems will be more pronounced than at lower operating field strengths (21). What is the effect of this chemical shift phenomenon and how is the resulting artifact manifest on images?

Most MR systems currently utilize a two-dimensional Fourier transform acquisition/reconstruction technique wherein the spatial data of each slice is phase encoded along one coordinate dimension and frequency encoded along the opposite orthogonal dimension (horizontal and vertical axes of the displayed image). Frequency encoding is achieved by the application of a linear magnetic gradient, referred to as the readout gradient, during acquisition of the signal generated by a spin-echo. Precise linear modification of the main magnetic field along the direction of the readout gradient is intended to produce a predictable linear incrementation in resonant (Larmor) frequencies, which in turn enables accurate spatial localization of detected signal along the same dimension. The linear spectrum of proton resonant frequencies then is a direct function of the strength of the frequency-encoding gradient. For instance, many instruments use gradient fields in the range of 1 G/cm or 1.0 mT/m. Assuming in-plane pixel dimensions of 1 mm × 1 mm [as would be achieved using a 256 × 256 image matrix and 25 cm × 25 cm field of view (FOV)], such a gradient field produces an increment in resonant proton frequency of 42.58 Hz/pixel at B_0 = 1.5 T. At this same field strength of 1.5 T, the chemical shift of 208-Hz resonant frequency between water- and fat-bound protons results in a spatial misregistration of several pixel widths.

The computer records a spectrum of frequencies generated at the moment of spin-echo signal sampling. The Fourier transform reconstruction algorithm is not able to distinguish a frequency shift produced by chemical factors from the distribution of frequencies produced by the readout gradient. As a result, the chemical, tissue-based frequency shift is misinterpreted by the computer algorithm as a difference in spatial location along the instrument-based frequency-encoded dimension. Displacement of fat-generated signal creates an artifactual gap of signal void at one edge of a tissue interface and an artifactual overlap of augmented signal on the opposite edge (Fig. 25).

It must be understood that the coordinate directions (x or y) selected for phase versus frequency encoding are arbitrary and usually programmed in software provided by the equipment vendor. Thus, depending on the manufacturer, chemical shift may appear either across the horizontal or vertical axes of a displayed image, varying with the direction of the frequency gradient. Also, using the same instrument, the direction of the frequency-encoding gradient (and chemical shift artifacts) can be rotated 90° or reversed 180° either by operator selection or by placing the patient in a decubitus or feet-first position (compared to head and feet first, respectively) within the magnet gantry.

Chemical shift misregistration artifact is readily visible at the interfaces between well-hydrated structures and fat, especially on high field strength images. The juxtaposition of these two tissue compartments is more

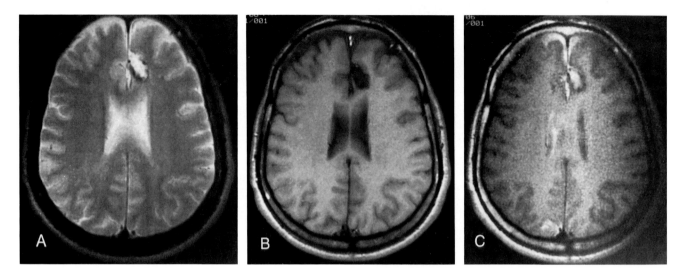

FIG. 21. Absence of dephasing effects in CSF containing left frontal lobe cyst demonstrated by using specialized pulse sequence. **A:** Routine T2-weighted transaxial image shows an ovoid zone of hyperintensity in the medial left frontal lobe bordered by a circumscribed perimeter of relative hypointensity. **B:** Routine T1-weighted axial image obtained by using selective 90° and selective 180° RF pulses shows hypointensity of the cyst contents similar in appearance to the lateral ventricles and subarachnoid space. (TR = 600 msec, TE = 25 msec). **C:** Specialized single slice-location pulse sequence obtained by using extremely short-TR value (150 msec) with selective 90° and nonselective 180° RF pulses displays static CSF collections with relative hyperintensity due to persistence of transverse magnetization between successive excitations and reduction of dephasing effects (TR = 150 msec, TE = 25 msec).

commonplace in the body (kidney/perirenal fat, liver/omentum) than in the central nervous system; however, chemical shift misregistration artifact is normally and routinely seen in the orbit or spine, where fat normally borders soft tissue structures. Also, certain lipomatous lesions, including congenital tumors such as lipomas and dermoids, may demonstrate confusing patterns of chemical misregistration artifact. Specifically, the artifactual gap of signal void at one edge of a fat deposit could be misinterpreted as a punctate or crescentic focus of calcium, whereas the opposite edge might simulate the appearance of edematous or even neoplastic tissue (Fig. 26).

It is technically feasible to eliminate chemical shift artifact entirely by utilizing any of a variety of compensation methods that isolate either the water or fat image or reregister the two, creating an artifact-free composite image (22–24).

FERROMAGNETIC HAZARDS AND ARTIFACTS

Biomedical Concerns

The absence of ionizing radiation is a widely acclaimed advantage of MRI, an advantage that is obviously not shared by alternative X-ray-based imaging methods, such as CT or angiography. The elimination of the known carcinogenic risk associated with the use of X-rays has evoked an enthusiastic response from the medical community; however, even among otherwise zealous proponents of MRI, the prevailing opinion with regard to health risks appropriately falls short of complacency. Potentially adverse biomedical effects of MRI are known to exist and have prompted the Food and Drug Administration to issue guidelines pertaining to the use of MR equipment. Legitimate concern has also been expressed about the possibility of yet undetermined deleterious biomedical effects of the electromagnetic fields used in MRI.

For these reasons, regulatory efforts address specifically each of the three electromagnetic fields required to facilitate proton alignment, localization, and excitation. The FDA has mandated that the main magnetic field (B_0), used for proton alignment, shall not exceed 2.0 T. This threshold level is considered empirically safe because no reproducible adverse biologic effects have been observed in systems operating below this level.

Changing magnetic fields of lesser magnitude are used to enable accurate spatial localization of the MR signal. The FDA has indicated that these gradient fields should not exceed 3 T/sec in order to avoid safely impairment of either myocardial or peripheral nerve conduction. Time-varying magnetic fields may also cause malfunction of cardiac pacemakers. Consequently, all such patients should be carefully screened and excluded from the magnet area. Of somewhat less concern, magnetic

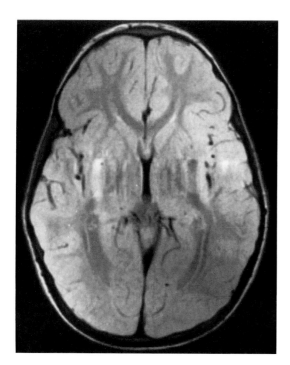

FIG. 22. Third ventricular ghosts. Transaxial image through the level of the thalamus shows hypointensity within the third ventricle due to dephasing effects indicative of CSF motion. Concomitantly, phase-encoded artifacts consisting of alternating bands of hypo- and hyperintensity (corresponding to cancellation and reinforcement image harmonics artifacts, respectively) are distributed across the horizontal (phase-encoded) direction. Note that these artifacts, attributable to physiologic motion of CSF, are confined to the band-like zone of tissue demarcated by the horizontal projection of the third ventricle (TR = 2,000 msec, TE = 35 msec).

phosphenes can be produced (resulting in visual scotomata), and normal bone healing processes may be disturbed at levels above 3 T/sec.

Current FDA guidelines stipulate that RF power deposition (specific power absorption), resulting from electromagnetic pulses used for proton excitation, shall not exceed 0.4 W/kg. This threshold level is intended to limit heating effects to the physiologic range maintained by normal metabolic processes. Experimental evidence suggests that more stringent guidelines may be appropriate for certain clinical situations. For instance, laboratory studies have demonstrated significant local temperature elevations generated by conducting pathways between two hip prostheses immersed in a conducting solution and exposed to RF fields similar to those used under clinical conditions (25).

Ferromagnetic Hazards

The presence of metal objects about and especially within the patient is a separate issue of major concern,

both from the standpoint of patient safety as well as artifact production. As a general safety precaution, the entire magnet area should be designed, equipped, decorated, and maintained with attention given to the imperative exclusion of ferromagnetic articles from the imaging room. This rule applies especially to such items as writing instruments, clip boards, needles, and hand tools, which may be carried inadvertently into the room by patients, technologists, physicians, or service personnel. These articles have been known to leave the grasp of the individual carrying them. Rapid acceleration of these objects toward the magnet portal obviously jeopardizes the safety of anyone in their path. Similar restrictions apply to resuscitation equipment maintained usually in an area adjacent to the magnet room. Wheelchairs, guerneys, intravenous stands, oxygen cylinders, ECG monitors, defibrillators, and other support devices, if not constructed of aluminum or nonferrous metal alloys, should be kept away from the magnet. Several vendors have responded to these constraints by developing mobile patient tables that can dock or separate from the magnet housing quickly. Thus, if necessary, a patient can be transferred rapidly to an adjacent room designated for emergency treatment and equipped with standard resuscitation devices.

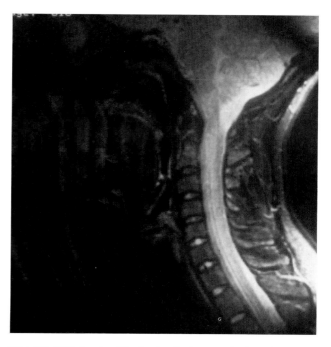

FIG. 23. CSF ghost artifacts simulating cervical cord syrinx. Sagittal T2-weighted image of cervical spine in normal patient shows multiple curvilinear foci of bright signal. This artifact is replicated across the phase-encoded (horizontal) axis of the displayed image and is attributable to pulsatile cardiosynchronous motion of CSF in the subarachnoid space. Superimposition of this artifact over the spinal cord can simulate a syrinx cavity (TR = 2,000 msec, TE = 70 msec).

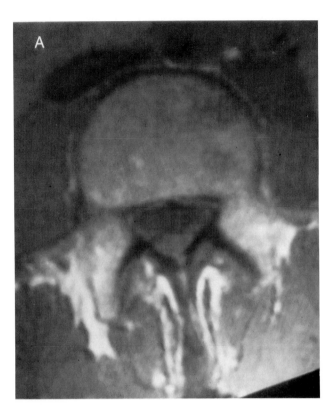 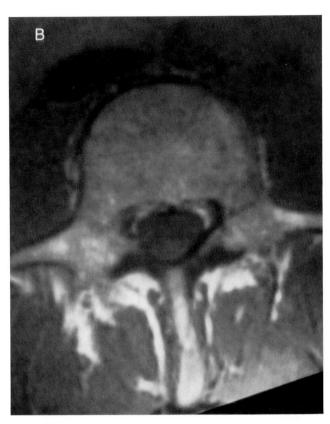

FIG. 24. Alternating hypointensity of subarachnoid CSF due to dephasing effects of systolic pseudogating and the use of a nonsequential excitation order. **A–E:** The first five (most superior) transaxial images of the lumbar spine show relative hypointensity of supernatant CSF compared to dependent nerve roots on images **A, C,** and **E,** corresponding to the first, third, and fifth images. The data for these images were acquired during systole (systolic pseudogating), resulting in dephasing effects and diminished signal of CSF. The intervening slices (**B, D**) were acquired in diastole, wherein the absence of CSF motion results in comparatively increased CSF signal. This phenomenon is due to a nonsequential excitation order (implemented to reduce cross-excitation artifact) such that odd-number images are excited first (1, 3, 5, . . .), followed by even number sections (2, 4, 6, . . .) (TR = 1,000 msec, TE = 20 msec, 15-slice location multislice pulse sequence). **F:** A midsagittal T1-weighted image of the lumbar spine shows uniform signal intensity of subarachnoid CSF in the lumbar region (TR = 1,000 msec, TE = 20 msec).

Individual patients must also be carefully screened for the presence of metal within their bodies. Patients harboring metallic objects internally may be at risk for local heating effects, malfunction of electromechanical devices (such as cardiac pacemakers), or potentially harmful motion of the object itself. Ferromagnetic implants or foreign bodies can respond to longitudinal and torque forces produced by the gradient and static fields. Quite clearly, the presence of a ferromagnetic cerebral aneurysm clip represents a contraindiction for MRI because of the potential for clip dislodgement, with resulting subarachnoid hemorrhage. The multitude of cerebral aneurysm clips in current or past usage tends to reduce one's confidence level in determining that any particular implanted clip is not ferromagnetic. Hence, at most centers, liability concerns dictate the prudent policy that patients with a history of cerebral aneurysm surgery be categorically excluded from consideration for MRI. Fur-

ther impetus for a conservative approach on this matter derives from the observation that certain metal alloys acquire ferromagnetic properties only after tooling or deformation effected by surgical placement, thus discounting the reliability of ferromagnetic determinations based on experimental data. It is interesting that a great many patients with known ferromagnetic "hemostatic" clips (various types of stainless steel alloy clips commonly used in chest, abdomen, and vascular surgery) have undergone MRI with no untoward effects reported to date. Presumably, such clips are fastened securely and tethered indirectly to rigid anatomy such that any magnetic forces experienced are inconsequential clinically.

At least one instance of a hemorrhagic complication resulting from ferromagnetically induced motion of an internally situated foreign body has been documented (26). In that reported case, unilateral blindness from a vitreous hemorrhage occurred secondary to magnetic

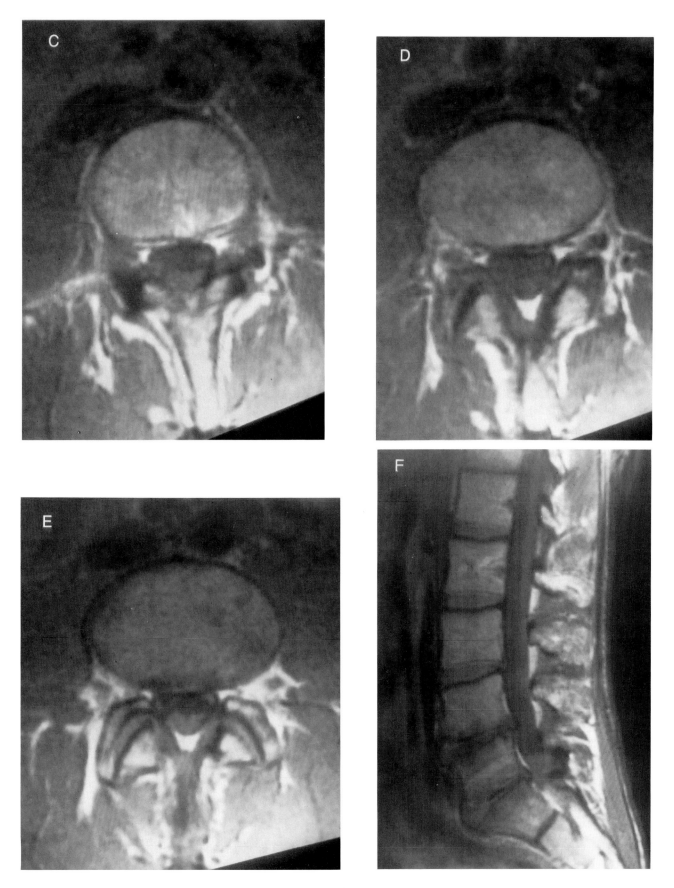

FIG. 24. *(Continued)*

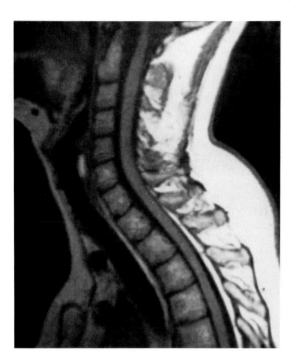

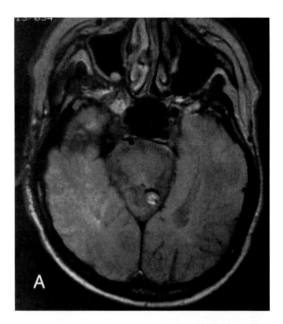

FIG. 25. Chemical shift artifact on normal cervical spine image at high field strength (1.5 T). Midsagittal T1-weighted image of the cervical spine. Note the asymmetric appearance of superior and inferior end plates at each vertebral level. This is caused by a 2–3-pixel inferior shift of the "fat" image (relative to the "water" image) in the direction of negative polarity of the frequency-encoding gradient. As a result, there is "chemical" misregistration of the composite image, a finding that is readily visible at fat/water interfaces. The exaggerated thickness of the superior end plate is due to the additive effect of artifactual signal void while overlap of fat-containing marrow at the inferior margin of each vertebral body causes obscuration of the inferior end plates. This effect is field-strength dependent and can produce clinically undesired and diagnostically confusing depiction of anatomic or pathologic structures unless compensatory maneuvers are employed (TR = 600 msec, TE = 25 msec).

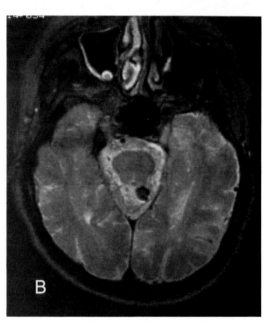

torquing or deflection of an iron filing (foreign body) situated in the posterior globe (Fig. 27). This incident occurred despite vigorous screening procedures, underscoring the need to consider clinically and historically occult metal deposits when scheduling patients. As an initial procedure, each candidate for MRI should be questioned for the presence of various metal implants and prostheses listed in Table 5. The potential significance of any prior surgical history or traumatic injury should be evaluated and pertinent occupational histories as well as military service records elicited. Persistence in these areas might help to identify the possibility of a significant metallic foreign body from a variety of surgical, work-related (welding, tool and dye work, lathe operation), recreational, or even wartime injuries.

If sufficient uncertainty exists about the presence of metal, and no prior X-ray studies are available, plain

FIG. 26. Chemical misregistration artifact of lipoma simulating nonhomogeneous signal intensity. **A:** The first echo image of a T2-weighted pulse sequence shows focal hyperintensity in the left quadrigeminal plate cistern corresponding in location to a lipoma visible at this site on CT scan. Note the crescent of hypointensity at the anterior aspect of the lesion as well as the crescent of hyperintensity at the opposite (posterior) aspect of the lesion. These chemical shift artifacts (always seen in the frequency-encoded direction) could be misconstrued as either calcification or edematous tissue (TR = 2,000 msec, TE = 35 msec). **B:** The second echo image shows signal changes centrally within the lesion equivalent to the diminished signal intensity of subcutaneous fat, corroborating the impression of lipoma. Note that the opposing crescents of signal gap and signal overlap artifact (due to chemical shift) persist (TR = 2,000 msec, TE = 70 msec).

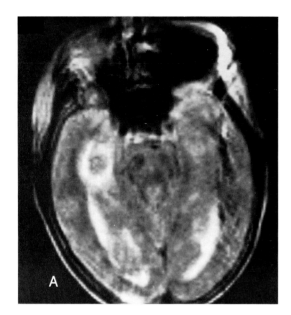

FIG. 27. Ferromagnetic artifact obliterating left globe in patient who was unilaterally blinded by vitreous hemorrhage from ferromagnetically induced motion of a metallic foreign body near the left disc margin. **A:** T2-weighted transaxial image shows signal void obliterating much of the left orbit demarcated by a rim of hyperintensity that fades peripherally. This pattern is highly suggestive of ferromagnetic artifact. A lesion is incidentally noted in the right temporal horn, as well as interstitial edema surrounding the ependymal surface of the occipital horns. This patient experienced sudden-onset left-sided blindness as the patient cradle was withdrawn from the magnet gantry. Incidentally, note aliasing artifact near occiput on right due to "wraparound" of anterior facial anatomy (nose) onto the opposite edge of the displayed image. This artifact may occur whenever patient anatomy extends peripheral to the FOV (TR = 2,000 msec, TE = 56 msec). **B:** Contrast-enhanced CT scan shows a hyperdensity at the posterior aspect of the left globe. Repeat thin-section CT displayed at bone windows confirmed metal, accounting for this density. Intracranially, well-circumscribed hyperdense lesions are visible in the right temporal horn as well as the periaqueductal brainstem. **C:** The patient died 1 month later from sepsis related to metastatic disease. Gross cross section of the enucleated left globe shows a hemosiderin-stained scar near the left disc margin from which a 2 × 4 mm rusted iron filing was extracted (see *inset*). Although the patient had had a methyl methacrylate lens implant 2 years previously, the metal filing presumably originated from the patient's occupation as a lathe operator/sheet-metal worker. (From ref. 26.)

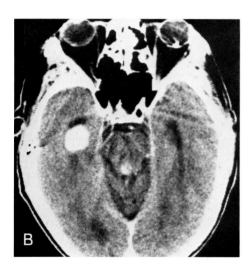

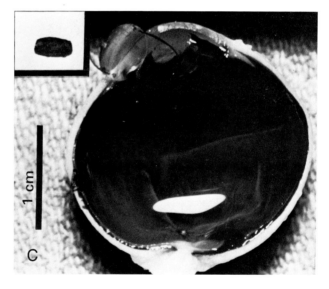

film radiography of the skull, orbits, or spine may occasionally be of value for screening purposes.

It is interesting that the presence of even large zones of ferromagnetic artifact on clinical images does not reliably predict the presence of radiographically visible metal at the corresponding location on either plain film or CT scan. We have observed this phenomenon in several different settings, including ferromagnetic metallic pigment contained in cosmetic preparations (such as cobalt-based eyeliner) (Fig. 28) and minute, radiographically invisible steel particles retained in calvarial burr holes (Fig. 29). The latter artifact is probably caused by microscopic metal shavings from either the high-speed

drill bit or metal sucker used for burr-hole placement. Either of these instruments will demonstrate scored surfaces at their tips following multiple usages. If plain films or comparison CT studies are not available, the rather extensive artifact sometimes seen in relation to burr holes (or even osteotomies at other skeletal sites) is often incorrectly assumed to represent artifact from a hemostatic clip that is not in fact present.

The use of magnetometers or metal detectors has been suggested as a sensitive method of detecting metal objects or implants imbedded within patients (27). Although these devices are expensive (thousands of dollars), the need to screen MRI candidates safely and

TABLE 5. *Potentially significant metal implants and metallic artifact sources*

Cardiac pacemaker
Neural stimulator (Tens unit)
Hearing aids
Cerebral aneurysm clips
Hemostatic clips
Prosthetic heart valves
Insulin pump
Electrodes
Intrauterine device
CSF shunts (spinal or ventricular)
Joint prosthesis
Extremity prosthesis
Orthopedic plates, pins, screws, or wires
Harrington rods
Wire mesh implants
Wire sutures
Braces
Dentures
Schrapnel
Imbedded metal fragments

accurately for metal implants is of paramount importance both ethically and from a medicolegal perspective.

Ferromagnetic and Nonferromagnetic Conductor Artifacts

Ferromagnetic implants produce artifact proportional to the degree of ferromagnetism and the mass of the object (28). On two-dimensional Fourier transform images, which incorporate the implant, this type of artifact is usually evident as a round zone of signal void bordered by a circumscribed halo of hyperintensity that fades peripherally (Fig. 27). Common sources include stainless steel dental hardware (braces, permanent bridges, root canal pins), shunt-tube hardware (valves, connectors, and shunt tips), wire mesh, wire sutures, hemostatic clips (usually stainless steel), and metallic foreign bodies. Recognition of the resulting signal aberration as ferromagnetic artifact is usually straightforward when viewing a set of multislice images; however, if the metal substance is not incorporated into a section, the image distortion produced may be less distinctive and may perhaps simulate a tissue abnormality. Similarly, if the ferromagnetic implant is in an unusual or unexpected location, resulting signal changes could mimic, and be misinterpreted as, various types of pathology, including calcification and hemorrhagic residua (Fig. 30). Obviously, knowledge of the presence of a metal implant and familiarity with the expected patterns of ferromagnetic artifact help reduce the likelihood of a diagnostic error.

Although most manufacturers no longer utilize backprojection image-reconstruction algorithms on MRI,

the appearance of ferromagnetic artifact is different and considerably more extensive on such images (28).

Metal implants that fail to demonstrate measurable ferromagnetic properties can produce image artifact very similar to, although less extensive than, ferromagnetic material of comparable mass. This phenomenon occurs because nonferromagnetic conductors induce local eddy currents in response to changing magnetic fields (gradients). These small currents in turn produce their own electromagnetic fields that sufficiently distort the main magnetic field to degrade image quality focally.

MISCELLANEOUS TECHNICAL ARTIFACTS

Inhomogeneous RF Signal Reception

Radiofrequency antennae used for routine head or body imaging are generally cylindrical in shape due to the saddlelike configuration of the coil elements. Be design, this type of coil achieves uniform signal collection throughout its sensitive volume; however, significant artifactual inhomogeneities in the levels of detected signal can result from a variety of sources. Especially detrimental are the nonuniform flip angles (often in excess of

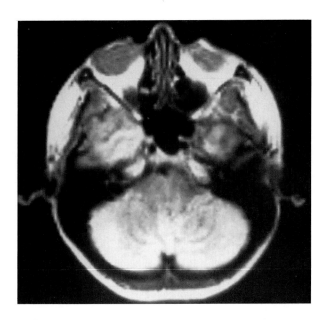

FIG. 28. Ferromagnetic artifact from metal-containing cosmetic preparation. Transaxial MR image through the orbits shows a nonspherical configuration of either globe due to ferromagnetic artifact anteriorly, in this case due to ferromagnetic cobalt pigment contained within eyeliner. The artifact is more obvious on the left, where signal void (due to distortion of the local magnetic field) obliterates the anterolateral globe. A characteristic transition of hyperintensity is seen medially. This pattern can also be produced by various other cosmetic preparations containing "metal-flake" compounds (TR = 2,000 msec, TE = 28 msec).

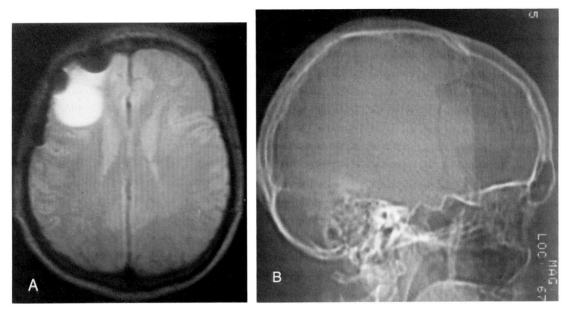

FIG. 29. Ferromagnetic artifact from radiographically occult microscopic metal filings deposited in burr-hole tracts. **A:** T2-weighted postoperative MRI shows characteristic crescents of ferromagnetic artifact in relation to calvarial burr holes overlying and partially obscuring a hyperintense right frontal lobe cyst. This type of artifact is often presumed to be secondary to hemostatic stainless steel clips (TR = 2,000 msec, TE = 40 msec). **B:** Lateral scout view digital radiograph of same patient shows frontal craniotomy site without any radiographically detectable evidence of metal in vicinity of burr holes; however, small microscopic deposits may be left along the burr-hole tracts due to scoring and separation of metal from the high-speed drill bit or the metallic tip of the suction device.

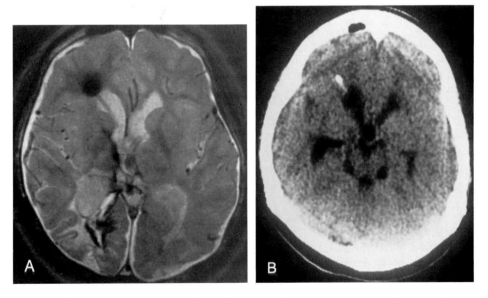

FIG. 30. Ferromagnetic artifact from ventricular shunt tip simulating hemorrhagic residua. **A:** A transaxial high-field-strength T2-weighted image shows hyperintensity in the peripheral subarachnoid space due to subacute subarachnoid hemorrhage. A thrombosed/hemorrhagic arteriovenous malformation is seen in the right occipital lobe with characteristic central hyperintensity (methemoglobin effect) and peripheral hypointensity due to a preferential T2 proton relaxation enhancement effect of hemosiderin. A somewhat similar hypointensity in the right frontal lobe could potentially be misinterpreted as hemosiderin effect; however, partial visualization of a shunt tube coursing through the right frontal horn (diminished signal of CSF within the shunt tube compared to ventricular CSF confirms patency and active function of the shunt device) suggests the possibility of ferromagnetic artifact (TR = 2,000 msec, TE = 70 msec). **B:** Noncontrast CT scan confirms the presence of a metal tip shunt device embedded within the right frontal lobe, confirming a ferromagnetic artifact accounting for the signal aberration seen at this location on MRI.

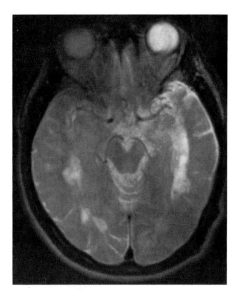

FIG. 31. Inhomogeneous signal reception using cylindrical head coil. Transaxial T2-weighted image through the level of the midorbit in a known multiple sclerosis patient shows multiple white-matter plaques intracranially. Marked hypointensity of the right vitreous compared to the left globe is not pathologic and is accompanied by diminished signal intensity from the surrounding periorbital anatomy on the right. This artifact is known as "shading" and is commonly seen with linear drive excitation schemes wherein nonuniform flip angles (often in excess of 90°) may result in diminished signal from various portions of the image. This problem can be further aggravated by coil malfunction and insufficiently precise tuning of the shim coils (TR = 2,000 msec, TE = 70 msec).

90°) achieved by using a linear drive RF excitation method (Fig. 31). This artifact can be further accentuated by a lack of precise tuning of the shim coils used to compensate for inhomogeneities in the main magnetic field. The equipment manufacturers have addressed this problem with several approaches, including the use of quadrature coils and techniques aimed at stabilizing the B_0 field.

The use of surface coils has gained widespread acceptance as a method of augmenting SNRs of MR images. The basic strategy is to place a specially shaped, usually flat antenna in close proximity to the source of signal emission. Such coils enable high-resolution thin-section images using relatively short acquisition times. These advantages help explain the extensive use of surface coil imaging for specialized study of superficial anatomic regions, such as the spine and orbit. However, unlike volume coils, surface coils are characteristically inhomogeneous signal receivers. The variation in intensity of a particular coil depends on several factors including size and shape of the coil, the location of the image plane relative to the coil surface, and the orientation of the image plane both to the surface coil and the main mag-

netic field. Generally, the sensitivity profile of a surface coil varies in relation to the depth of tissue from the coil surface. Besides the inherent but predictable inhomogeneous sensitivity profile orthogonal to the plane of the surface coil, focally diminished signal may result from the metallic components of the coil itself (29). These areas of signal void or lines of null sensitivity are seen when the field of view (FOV) exceeds the coil dimensions and can potentially simulate pathology (Fig. 32).

Gibbs Phenomena (Edge Effect)

The profile of signal strength across certain high-contrast interfaces is predictably defined by abrupt transitions in signal magnitude; however, the Fourier trans-

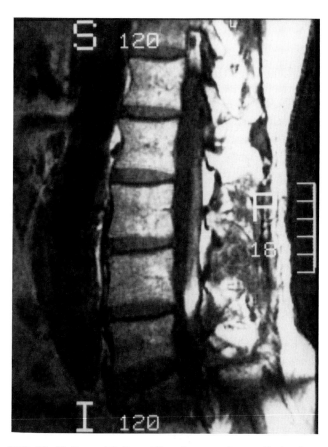

FIG. 32. Null sensitivity artifact from surface coil simulating fibrous tract in patient with tethered-cord syndrome. T1-weighted sagittal image of lumbar spine in patient with bowel and bladder dysfunction shows caudal extension of the spinal cord to the L4 level where a lipoma tethers the neural placode to a dysraphic defect dorsally. The ill-defined low-signal-intensity band extending from the caudal thecal sac to the skin surface represents a null-sensitivity artifact, not a fibrous tract. This artifact is caused by the metallic conductor within the wire loop of the receiver and is produced circumferentially about the receiver coil (the superior artifact is not contained within this FOV) (TR = 600 msec, TE = 25 msec).

formation, which reconstructs image data across such high-contrast anatomic boundaries, reproduces object contrast with only limited precision. Rather than faithful duplication of a sharp interface, a variable oscillation in signal intensity occurs (30). This artifact can be considered as an alternating overshoot/undershoot approximation of true signal and tends to blur and accentuate high-contrast interfaces (Fig. 33). The conspicuity of this artifact fades rapidly in a direction perpendicular to the high-contrast boundary. It can be differentiated from motion artifact by the absence of associated ghost images. Both the wavelength and amplitude of the oscillations that produce Gibbs artifact can be reduced by decreasing the pixel size (expanding the matrix while maintaining FOV constant); however, this strategy is effective only to a certain degree in that approximately 10% contrast overshoot will persist regardless of pixel dimensions (29).

The presence of Gibbs artifact can be anticipated in most anatomic areas, given the somewhat predictable differential intensities of bordering structures contained within a particular section; however, in conditions of pathologic alteration or in regions of unfamiliar anatomy, the juxtaposition of high-contrast tissues of uncertain composition can be associated with Gibbs artifact, which could be misconstrued as a component of true signal abnormality, chemical shift, or even nonspecific flow phenomenon (Fig. 34).

Crosstalk (Cross-Excitation)

The major determinants of MR signal intensity can be considered in terms of intrinsic tissue variables (T1, T2, proton density, flow effects) and operator-controlled instrument variables. In the latter category, alterations in the TR or TE settings produce a dominant effect on the depiction of biologic tissue. Still other less familiar technical choices can influence dramatically the appearance of an MR image: for instance, when using a multislice-selective excitation technique, the interdependent relationships among interslice gap, slice profile, and cross-excitation is an important concept that warrants careful consideration when designing an MR pulse sequence.

Ideally, selective 90° and 180° RF pulses should excite uniformly a section or block of tissue defined by a given thickness (Δz). The slice thickness is determined by the frequency bandwidth (BW) of the excitation pulse and the strength of the slice-defining gradient (G_z). The location of a slice relative to the remainder of an excited volume is determined by the center frequency of the excitation pulse. The section thickness may be reduced by either narrowing the BW or increasing G_z. Both maneuvers are limited by design constraints and technical tradeoffs. More important (with respect to the

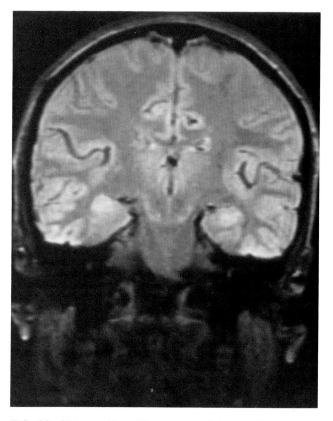

FIG. 33. Gibbs artifact. Direct coronal image through the temporal lobe shows margins of artifactually increased signal near either temporal lobe surface inferiorly (*arrows*). This artifact is intrinsic to the two-dimensional Fourier transform reconstruction method wherein depiction of high-contrast interfaces is inherently inaccurate. The representation of bordering compartments with markedly different signal intensities is only approximated and accompanied by overshoot/undershoot artifact at their junction. The severity of this artifact varies in proportion to pixel dimensions (TR = 2,000 msec, TE = 35 msec, acquisition matrix = 128 × 128).

phenomenon of crosstalk), in order to excite uniformly a block of tissue with discrete margins, an RF pulse must approximate a rectangular shape when described in the frequency domain. Such a pulse would be represented by a (sin z)/z or sinc function in the time domain characterized by a dominant sinusoidal component at isocenter and multiple 0 crossings of lesser amplitude that extend out infinitely to either side. Although the shape of the central component determines section thickness in a gross fashion, an increased number of 0 crossings adds sharpness to the definition of slice thickness, thereby producing a more sharply defined slice profile. Unfortunately, the need to confine the duration of an RF pulse to 10 msec or less necessitates truncation of the time domain 0 crossings to about 8 to 16. As a result, the ideal "square" excitation is only approximated and compromised by a frequency domain that shows ta-

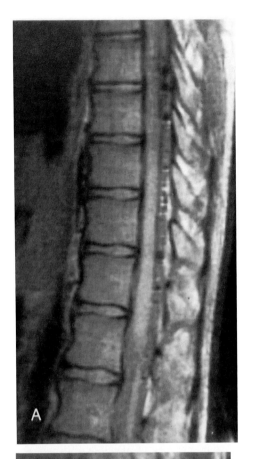

FIG. 34. Gibbs artifact in thoracic epidural space simulating vascular malformation in patient with myelopathic symptoms following epidural anesthesia. **A:** First echo sagittal image of the thoracic spine shows bead-like foci of low signal in the posterior epidural space circumscribed by rings of increased signal (TR = 2,000 msec, TE = 35 msec). **B:** The second echo image at the same slice location serves to accentuate the curvilinear hyperintensity bordering the small rounded foci of signal void within the fluid-filled posterior epidural space (TR = 2,000 msec, TE = 70 msec). **C:** Transaxial CT scan confirms the presence of air iatrogenically introduced within the epidural space from a preceding epidural anesthesia procedure. Specialized flow sequences failed to reveal any evidence of a vascular lesion or fat-containing signal (as might be suggested by images **A** and **B**) simulated by the high-contrast juxtaposition of air and fluid.

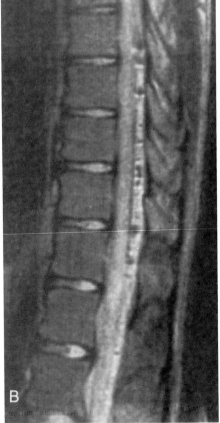

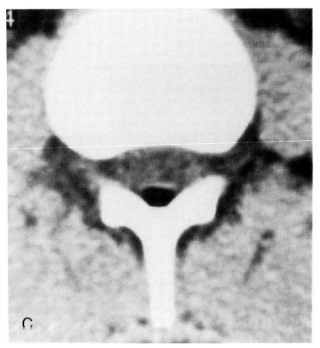

pered side lobes of frequency components (Fig. 35). These stray frequency components produce the undesired effect of partially exciting tissue peripheral to the intended slice margins. Depending on the width of the interslice gap, a significant volume of tissue in the adjacent slices (on either side) may respond to the "slice-selective" excitation to a degree proportional to the satisfaction of resonant conditions. Cross-excitation effectively reduces the time available for recovery (longitudinal remagnetization) and introduces T1 contrast. This effect is especially pronounced on long-TR, long-TE images obtained contiguously or with a relatively narrow interslice gap, wherein significant loss of signal and diminished T2 contrast may be observed (Fig. 35).

The problem of cross-excitation can be alleviated partially or wholly by using one or more of several approaches. An interleaved technique essentially eliminates cross-excitation but requires the completion of two separate pulse sequences offset by one section thickness in the slice-defining dimension. The penalty incurred consists of a doubling in the imaging time. Although the total number of sections that may be acquired is doubled, this advantage yields little practical benefit compared to a single long-TR pulse sequence that can accommodate up to 20 or more slice locations depending on the specific TR value. Alternatively, the use of an interslice gap of approximately 40% to 50% section thickness effectively eliminates most cross-excitation effects (Fig. 36). In clinical applications wherein high-quality T2-weighted images 5 mm in thickness are a priority concern (such as parenchymal brain imaging), a 2 to 2.5-mm interslice gap is acceptable in that the improvement in image quality probably outweighs the risk of "missing" a small focal lesion (un-

associated with regional mass effect or perifocal edema) wholly contained in an interslice gap. Such a pulse sequence has less utility, however, as a primary screening technique for detection of small extra-axial lesions. In the sella region for instance, high-resolution, thin, contiguous T1-weighted images (less affected by cross-excitation) have gained favor over T2-weighted imaging for screening purposes.

Yet another adjunctive procedure that helps reduce the adverse effect of cross-excitation on T2-weighted images entails nonsequential slice excitation (20). This method works by timing the excitation of a particular slice to coincide with the mid-pulse-cycle ($\frac{1}{2}$TR later) of its neighbors. Thus, the recovery time available for partially excited tissue in adjacent slices is prolonged compared to sequential excitation of slices at 100-msec intervals or less. Such a scheme can be implemented in combination with an interslice gap and might typically involve excitation of odd-number slice locations, followed by the intervening even-number slice locations.

Partial Volume Averaging

The MR image, in its final displayed form, is a two-dimensional representation of a three-dimensional section of tissue. Each picture element, or pixel, of the analog image can be defined by its linear dimensions along the x and y coordinates within the image plane. The precise volume of tissue represented by each pixel is delimited by an additional third dimension, the slice thickness. Altogether, these three measurements describe a volume element, or voxel, of tissue. The actual gray-scale level of any individual pixel is determined by

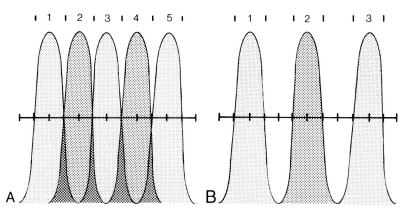

FIG. 35. Dependency of cross-excitation (cross-talk) on slice profile and interslice gap. **A:** Design constraints and technical limitations preclude an ideal "square" slice profile. As a result, each slice-selective excitation pulse contains side lobes of frequency components that serve to excite and partially saturate tissue in the adjacent slices, shown as overlapping *shaded areas* below full-width half-maximum (FWHM). Cross-excitation reduces the time available for remagnetization of tissue in the adjacent slice locations, resulting in decreased SNRs and the introduction of undesired T1 contrast on T2-weighted images. This effect is especially pronounced on contiguous images obtained without an interslice gap. **B:** Cross-excitation effects can be eliminated by using a wide interslice gap such as the 100% section thickness gap shown here. If desired, the intervening gaps can be imaged by using an interleaved technique although a time penalty would be incurred.

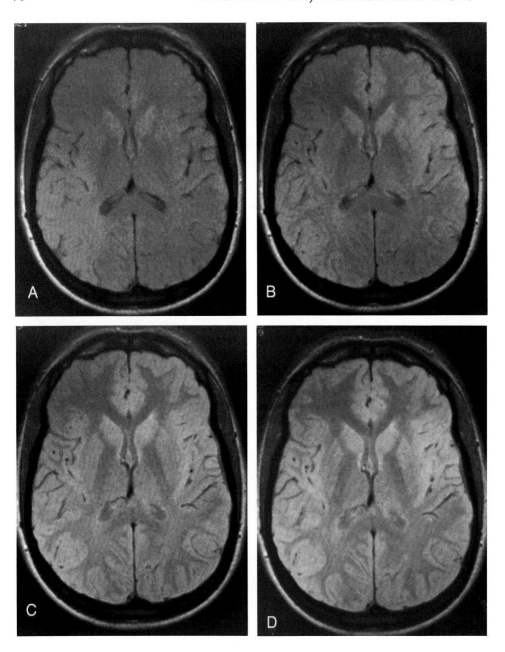

FIG. 36. Dependency of cross-excitation on interslice gap: effects on clinical images. **A–D:** These images were obtained at the same transaxial slice location by using four separate multislice pulse sequences; each pulse sequence was performed using identical instrument parameters except for the use of four different interslice gaps: (**A**) 0% interslice gap; (**B**) 20% interslice gap; (**C**) 50% interslice gap; (**D**) 100% interslice gap. Note the improved SNR and T2 contrast obtained by using an increasingly thick interslice gap (maximal at 100% section thickness; all images obtained using TR = 2,000 msec, TE = 35 msec).

the average signal intensity of the various tissue constituents or anatomic compartments contained within the corresponding voxel. Therefore, voxels containing predominantly one type of tissue (such as gray matter, white matter, or CSF) are accurately depicted as pixels that faithfully record the signal levels returned from the relatively homogeneous voxel constituents. However, when objects or tissues with widely disparate MR properties are incorporated within a voxel, the signal intensity of the pixel represents their average and is not necessarily characteristic of any particular component. This phenomenon is referred to as partial volume averaging (PVA) and is common to other cross-sectional imaging modalities such as ultrasound and CT (31).

The extended contrast range of MRI as well as the unique and variable gray-scale differentiation of bordering tissues (vascular structures vs CSF or neural tissue) engender potentially misleading PVA effects. For these reasons, the possibility of PVA must be taken into account routinely when interpreting MR images. For instance, PVA of a vascular channel can create an especially confusing pattern on MRI owing to the intraluminal signal void of most vascular structures (Fig. 37).

Normal asymmetry of the structural architecture of the brain or an equivalent effect due to tilting of the patient's anatomy may also contribute toward PVA, which can simulate the appearance of a lesion (Fig. 38). In such cases, careful evaluation of adjacent slices may

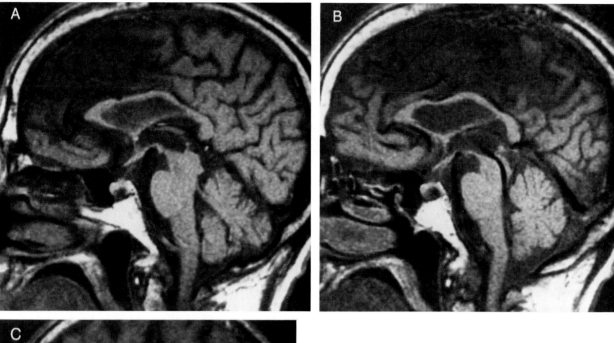

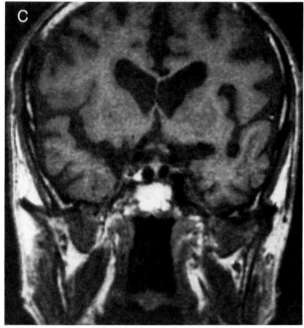

FIG. 37. Partial volume averaging of cavernous carotid arteries simulating pituitary adenoma. **A, B:** Contiguous thin-section parasagittal T1-weighted images of the head suggest the presence of a hypointense lesion at the inferior aspect of the pituitary gland (TR = 600 msec, TE = 25 msec). **C:** A coronal plane image shows an elevated and effaced pituitary gland due to medial bowing of the dolichoectatic cavernous carotid arteries. Parital volume averaging of pituitary tissue above and carotid artery below simulated the appearance of a microadenoma, even near the midline on parasagittal images. The appearance of partial volume averaging effects may vary considerably on MR compared to CT due to new and unique contrast differences of bordering tissues and anatomic compartments (TR = 600 msec, TE = 25 msec).

help identify the spurious artifactual nature of such "suspected" lesions. If doubt remains, a supplemental pulse sequence can be obtained with the image plane oriented perpendicular to the anatomic boundary suspected of causing PVA.

Aspect Ratio Distortion

The Fourier transformation reconstructs image data that are phase encoded in one coordinate dimension and frequency encoded in the opposite dimension. The spatial encoding process is facilitated by the application of time-varying magnetic field gradients oriented along the coordinate dimensions. The aspect ratio (height and width) of the reconstructed image is influenced heavily by the relationship between the phase- and frequency-encoding gradients. In order to ensure that anatomic proportions are maintained, the gradient parameters (amplitude and duration) in the phase and frequency directions must be adjusted together. Otherwise, if the phase and frequency gradients are not properly matched, the aspect ratio of the reconstructed image will be affected adversely, and the image will no longer convey 1:1 anatomic proportions. Such an image appears to

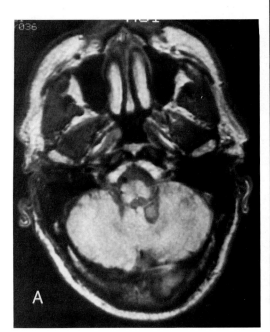 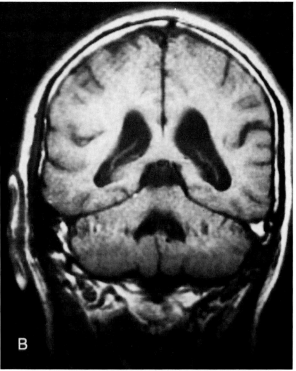

FIG. 38. Partial volume averaging of normal variant asymmetric tonsils simulating left cerebellar lesion. **A:** Transaxial image obtained low through the posterior fossa shows asymmetric signal intensity when comparing structures on either side of the inferior vermis. The appearance of a medial left cerebellar lesion is suggested by a 1-cm zone of intermediate signal intensity bordered by a circumscribed ring of less intense signal. The possibility of a vascular lesion or calcified mass cannot be excluded on this image alone (TR = 2,000 msec, TE = 35 msec). **B:** Direct coronal image shows asymmetry in the height of the right and left cerebellar tonsils forming the floor of the fourth ventricle. A transaxial image obtained near the floor of the fourth ventricle would thus include predominantly tonsillar tissue to the right of midline and only partial volume average the superior tip of the left cerebellar tonsil circumscribed by a "moat" of low-intensity CSF on this T1-weighted image (TR = 600 msec, TE = 25 msec).

be distorted due to relative "stretching" or "compression" of spatial characteristics along one coordinate dimension (Figs. 39 and 40).

Aliasing (Wraparound)

Patient anatomy that extends peripherally to the FOV may be redisplayed or "wrapped around" onto the opposite edge of a cross-sectional image (Fig. 27). This effect is technically referred to as aliasing, a phenomenon that can occur in either the phase- or frequency-encoded directions whenever the MR signal is sampled (N is the number of pixels) at less than the optimal Nyquist rate, which for frequency encoding is determined by the product of bandwidth and sampling time (T_s) (29). The value of T_s is constrained to about 10 msec

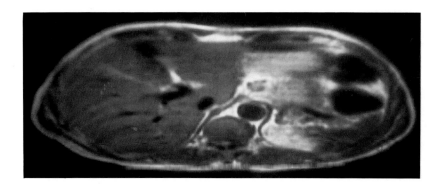

FIG. 39. Gross aspect ratio distortion. Transaxial image of the abdomen shows marked "compression" of anatomical features in the AP dimension. This is due to unbalanced power of the phase- and frequency-encoding gradients (TR = 1,500 msec, TE = 35 msec).

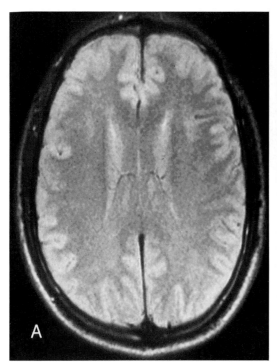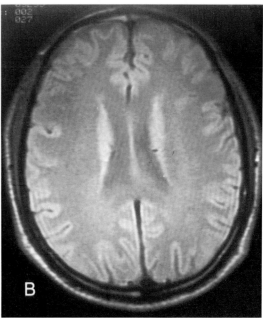

FIG. 40. Subtle aspect ratio distortion visible on results obtained using two different imaging systems (same patient). **A:** An intermediate field strength transaxial image through the roof of the lateral ventricles distorts the anatomic features and simulates a slight dolichocephalic appearance of the head due to relative "stretching" of anatomy in the AP direction (TR = 2,250 msec, TE = 52 msec). **B:** A transaxial high-field-strength image obtained at the same level more accurately portrays true anatomic proportions. Subtle degrees of aspect ratio distortion may become apparent when comparing results obtained from one manufacturer's unit to another. These can generally be avoided by performing routine phantom studies (most often daily), which would reveal the need for technical adjustments in gradient settings (TR = 2,000 msec, TE = 25 msec).

or less due to the sharp temporal peak of the spin-echo and the effect of differential T2 decay. The FOV can be made larger (and the image "unwrapped") in this direction by increasing the bandwidth or decreasing the frequency gradient strength. In the phase-encoded direction, a similar effect is achieved by increasing the number of pixels while maintaining pixel dimensions constant.

When using a cylindrical coil for head or body imaging, a FOV that accommodates the entire cross-sectional circumference must be selected if aliasing is to be avoided. For this reason, most routine axial images of the head or spine are performed using FOVs in the range of 20 to 24 cm and 32 to 40 cm, respectively. However, for certain specialized applications, such as pituitary imaging, a smaller FOV may be desired in order to improve spatial resolution (reduce pixel dimensions while maintaining matrix size constant) or reduce acquisition time (smaller matrix size distributed over smaller FOV, maintaining but not reducing pixel dimensions). The interdependence of FOV, matrix size, and pixel dimensions is outlined in Table 6 and illustrated in Fig. 41.

Provided that the anatomy of interest is positioned isocentrically within the FOV, aliasing about the periphery of the image is an acceptable trade-off for the gain in spatial detail or throughput achieved by selecting a small FOV. For instance, a FOV as small as 12 cm may be suitable and desirable for pituitary imaging (Fig. 41). The wraparound artifact does not extend into the sellar region, and there is no compromise of diagnostically important image detail. Furthermore, the annoying presence of aliasing artifact about the periphery of the unreprocessed image can be eliminated by performing

TABLE 6. *Interdependence of pixel dimensions on field of view and matrix size*

FOV (cm)	Pixel dimensions (mm)	
	128 × 128 matrix	256 × 256 matrix
48 × 48	3.75 × 3.75	1.88 × 1.88
40 × 40	3.13 × 3.13	1.56 × 1.56
32 × 32	2.50 × 2.50	1.25 × 1.25
24 × 24	1.88 × 1.88	0.94 × 0.94
20 × 20	1.56 × 1.56	0.78 × 0.78
16 × 16	1.25 × 1.25	0.63 × 0.63
12 × 12	0.94 × 0.94	0.47 × 0.47
8 × 8	0.63 × 0.63	0.31 × 0.31

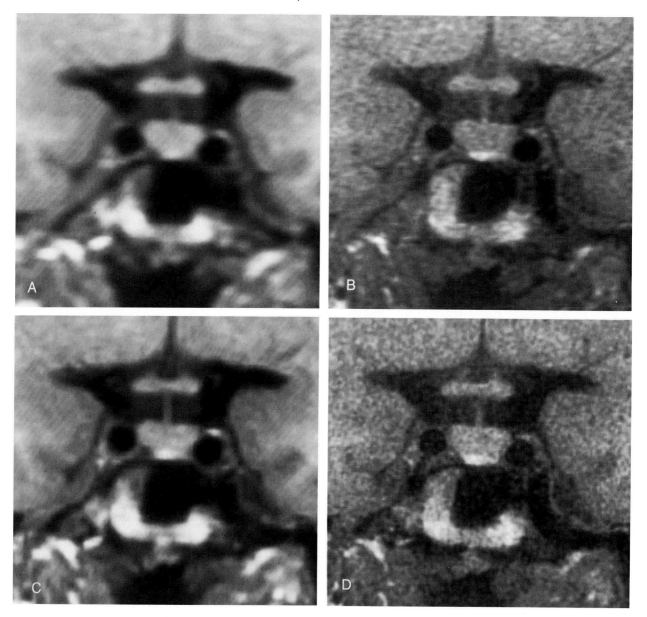

FIG. 41. Thin-section coronal images of sella using four different combinations of matrix size (128 × 128 and 256 × 256) and FOV (24 × 24 cm and 12 × 12 cm). All images were secondarily magnified to achieve similar anatomic proportions. Each pulse sequence was performed using instrument parameters: TR = 600 msec, TE = 20 msec, number of excitations (data sets) is six. **A:** Image matrix, 128 × 128 pixels; FOV, 24 × 24 cm; acquisition time, 7 min, 43 sec. **B:** Image matrix, 128 × 128 pixels; FOV, 12 cm × 12 cm; acquisition time, 7 min, 43 sec. **C:** Image matrix, 256 × 256 pixels; FOV, 24 cm × 24 cm; acquisition time, 15 min, 23 sec. **D:** Image matrix, 256 × 256 pixels; FOV, 12 cm × 12 cm; acquisition time, 15 min, 23 sec. Note improvement in spatial resolution when either progressing to a larger matrix size while maintaining FOV constant (A–C to B–D) or maintaining matrix size constant by reducing FOV (A–B or C–D). The improvement in spatial resolution is achieved in each case only with a sacrifice in SNR and, when progressing to a larger matrix size, a doubling in imaging time. Aliasing artifact "wrapped around" into either temporal lobe laterally and the centrum semiovale superiorly on the 12-cm FOV images but did not extend into the isocentrically situated region of interest and hence is excluded from these magnified images.

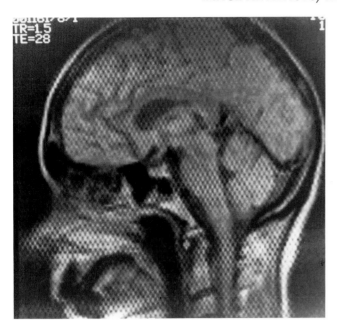

FIG. 42. Radiofrequency interference artifact. Various geometric designs such as this "herringbone pattern" are occasionally produced as a manifestation of RF interference. Isolated RF interference from an extraneous or commercial source may occasionally be depicted as a single line or band of artifact in the frequency-encoded direction.

an interpolated magnification of the region of interest prior to photography.

The ability to offset the FOV away from the geometric center of the magnet when using conventional cylindrical receiver coils extends the flexibility of high-resolution MRI. This technique enables improved delineation of "off-axis" anatomy, such as temporomandibular joints or shoulders, by displacing wraparound artifact away from the region of diagnostic importance.

The use of surface coils, especially the availability of an assortment of coils of various sizes, obviates the need for much concern about aliasing. A surface coil with an appropriately small FOV can be selected and applied directly at or at least in close proximity to the surface anatomy of interest. The limited sensitivity range of these devices can be regarded as a technical bonus that effectively suppresses the visibility and significance of aliasing artifact.

Radiofrequency Interference

The MR image can be degraded by RF noise originating from several sources including (a) "thermal" noise generated by low-level eddy currents induced by the interaction of patient anatomy with time-varying magnetic fields; (b) malfunctions of the system hardware at various levels, including gradient and transmitter coils and amplifiers; and (c) extrinsic RF noise from outside

the shielded imaging room (29). The first category represents background threshold noise, which ultimately limits the spatial resolving ability of MRI (especially for low-contrast interfaces) but is seldom discerned specifically as artifact on displayed images. The RF interference patterns produced intrinsically from system hardware components often result in easily recognized geometric patterns of image artifact, such as the herringbone pattern illustrated in Fig. 42. Stray RF energy of an isolated frequency (such as that from a communication system) incorporated by the resonance bandwidth of an MR system can result in a discrete linear or bandlike projection of artifact oriented along the frequency-encoded direction of a two-dimensional Fourier transform image.

REFERENCES

1. Brant-Zawadzki M, Davis PL, Crooks LE, et al. NMR demonstration of cerebral abnormalities: comparison with CT. *AJNR* 1983;4:117–24.
2. Alfidi RJ, Haaga JR, El Yousef SJ, et al. Preliminary experimental results in humans and animals with a superconducting whole-body, nuclear magnetic resonance scanner. *Radiology* 1982;143:175–81.
3. Doyle FH, Pennock JM, Banks LM, et al. Nuclear magnetic resonance imaging of the liver: initial experience. *AJR* 1982;138:193–200.
4. James AE, Partain CL, Holland GN, Gore JC, Rollo FD, Harms SE, Price RR. Nuclear magnetic resonance imaging: the current state. *AJR* 1982;138:201–10.
5. Bradley WG Jr., Waluch V. Blood flow: magnetic resonance imaging. *Radiology* 1985;154:443–50.
6. von Schulthess GK, Higgins CB. Magnetic Resonance. Blood flow imaging with MR: spin-phase phenomena. *Radiology* 1985;157:687–95.
7. Waluch V, Bradley WG. NMR even echo rephasing in slow laminar flow. *JCAT* 1984;8:594–8.
8. Pele NJ, Glover GH, Charles HC. Respiration artifacts in MRI. In: *Proceedings of the Society of Magnetic Resonance in Medicine, Aug 19–23, London, 1985.*
9. Haase A, et al. Rapid images and NMR movies. In: *Proceedings of the Society of Magnetic Resonance in Medicine, Aug 19–23, London, 1985.*
10. Kuhns LR, Thornbury J, Seigel R. Variation of position of the kidneys and diaphragm in patients undergoing repeated suspension of respiration. *JCAT* 1979;3:620–1.
11. Lanzer P, Botvinick EH, Schiller NB, et al. Cardiac imaging using gated magnetic resonance. *Radiology* 1983;150;121–7.
12. Hauge O, Falenburg H. Neuropsychologic reactions and other side effects after metrizamide myelography. *AJNR* 1982;3:229–32.
13. Winkler ML, Hricak H. Pelvis imaging with MR: technique for improvement. *Radiology* 1986;158:848–9.
14. Gelmer HJ. Adverse side effects of metrizamide in myelography. *Neuroradiology* 1979;18:119–23.
15. Schultz CL, Alfidi RJ, Nelson AD, Kopiwoda SY, Clampitt ME. The effect of motion on two-dimensional Fourier transformation magnetic resonance images. *Radiology* 1984;152:117–21.
16. Kelly WM, Kucharczyk W, Sze G, Davis DO, Brant-Zawadzki M. MRI of CSF Dynamics. In: *Annual Meeting of the American Society of Neuroradiology, 24th, San Diego, Jan 18–23, 1986.*
17. Brant-Zawadzki M, Kelly W, Kjos B, Newton TH, Norman D, Dillon W, Sobel D. Magnetic resonance imaging and characterization of normal and abnormal intracranial cerebrospinal fluid (CSF) spaces. Initial observations. *Neuroradiology* 1985;27:3–8.
18. Hackney DB, Gorssman RI, Zimmerman RA, Spagnoli MV,

Goldberg HI, Bilaniuk LT. Low sensitivity of magnetic resonance imaging to small changes in protein concentration in fluids. In: *Annual Meeting of the American Society of Neuroradiology, 24th San Diego, Jan 18–23, 1986.*

19. Bradley WG, Kortman KE. Use of aqueductal flow void phenomenon in the diagnosis of normal pressure hydrocephalus. In: *Annual Meeting of the American Society of Neuroradiology, 24th, San Diego, Jan 18–23, 1986.*

20. Kneeland JB, Shimakawa A, Wehrli FW. Effect of intersection spacing on MR image contrast and study time. *Radiology* 1986;158:819–22.

21. Soila KP, Viamonte M Jr, Starewicz PM. Chemical shift misregistration effect in magnetic resonance imaging. *Radiology* 1984;153:819–20.

22. Frahm J, Haase A, Hanicke W, Matthaei D, Bomsdorf H, Helzel T. Chemical shift selective MR imaging using a whole-body magnet. *Radiology* 1985;156:441–4.

23. Dixon WT. Simple proton spectroscopic imaging. *Radiology* 1984;153:189–94.

24. Menhardt W, Vollmann W, Kunz D. A new method to separate fat and water in MR imaging. In: *Annual Meeting of the Society of Magnetic Resonance in Medicine, 3rd, New York, Aug 13–17, 1984.*

25. Davis PL, Crooks L, Arakawa M, McRee R, Kaufman L, Margulis AR. Potential hazards in NMR imaging: heating effects of changing magnetic fields and RF fields on small metallic implants. *AJR* 1981;137:857–60.

26. Kelly WM, Paglen PG, Pearson JA, San Diego AG, Soloman MA. Ferromagnetism of intraocular foreign body causes unilateral blindness after MR study. *AJNR* 1986;7:243–5.

27. Finn EJ, Di Chiro G, Brooks RA, Sato S. Ferromagnetic materials in patients: detection before MR imaging. *Radiology* 1985;156:139–41.

28. New PFJ, Rosen BR, Brady TJ, Buonanno FS, Kistler JP, Burt CT, Hinshaw WS, Newhouse JH, Pohost GM, Taveras JM. Nuclear magnetic resonance. Potential hazards and artifacts of ferromagnetic and nonferromagnetic surgical and dental materials and devices in nuclear magnetic resonance imaging. *Radiology* 1983;147:139–48.

29. Schenck JF, Hart HR Jr, Foster TH, Edelstein WA, Hussain MA. High resolution magnetic resonance imaging using surface coils. In: Kressel, HY, ed. *Magnetic resonance annual 1986.* New York: Raven Press, 1986.

30. Bracewell RN. In: *The Fourier transform and its applications.* New York: McGraw Hill, 1978.

31. Goodenough D, Weaver K, Davis D, LaFalce S. Volume averaging limitations of computed tomography. *AJR* 1982;138:313–6.

CHAPTER 5

Magnetic Resonance Appearance of Flowing Blood and Cerebrospinal Fluid

William G. Bradley, Jr.

The effect of motion on the intensity of the nuclear magnetic resonance (NMR) signal has been known since the early days of analytical NMR. Hahn (1,2) was the first to describe the effects of random motion due to autodiffusion on the intensity of the spin-echo signal. When magnetic resonance (MR) imaging was first performed in the late 1970s, signal loss was noted within arteries and attributed to high flow rates (3). In the early 1980s, several causes of increased signal intensity were described, generally associated with slow flow in veins and dural sinuses (4,5). Recently, similar flow phenomena have been observed due to CSF motion within the ventricular system (6) and in the spinal subarachnoid space (7). Understanding these flow phenomena has provided the basis for the development of specialized MR imaging sequences intended to quantitate blood and CSF flow velocities (8–13). In addition, sequences have been developed (14–16) to visualize vessels without contrast ("MR angiography"). The purpose of this chapter is to describe these flow phenomena as they affect signal intensity on routine MR acquisitions.

BLOOD FLOW PHENOMENA

Flowing blood can appear bright or dark, depending on the velocity, the direction of flow, certain geometric factors (e.g., slice position within a multislice volume), and the specific MR pulse sequence used (5). When considering flow phenomena, it is useful to define the "isochromat" as a hypothetical small volume of protons that remain in phase for the duration of MR pulsing sequence (4,17). It is also useful to distinguish different types of flow. Slow flow is generally "laminar"; i.e., it can be described in terms of laminae or shells of increasing velocity as one moves in toward the center from the vessel wall (18,19). The maximum velocity occurs at the center of the vessel, and there is no flow adjacent to the vessel wall in the "boundary layer" (19). The plot of velocity versus radial position in laminar flow has a par-abolic profile (Fig. 1). The average velocity is exactly half the maximum velocity in the center of the vessel (18,19).

As the velocity increases, flow becomes "turbulent." "High velocity" and "turbulence" are not equivalent terms (18). Laminar flow can be maintained at high velocity in small-diameter tubes (Fig. 2). On the other hand, turbulence occurs at lower velocities in larger diameter tubes. Turbulence is present when fluctuating velocity components are found in both the axial and nonaxial directions (Fig. 1). The velocity profile for turbulent flow tends to be flatter than the parabolic profile seen in laminar flow (Fig. 1). In the extreme, the velocity profile is flat; i.e., there is "plug" flow. It should be noted, however, that plug flow is an idealized state in which all fluid elements move at the same velocity (19). In practice, plug flow is never achieved across the entire diameter of the vessel and is always associated with random nonaxial motion, i.e., turbulence (19).

As flow becomes turbulent, there is a transitional zone (18) between the laminar flow zone in the boundary layer at the periphery and the fully developed turbulent flow in the center of the vessel (Fig. 3). Curiously, the magnitude of the random fluctuating velocity components (i.e., the intensity of turbulence) is greatest in the buffer zone separating the turbulent core from the laminar sublayer (18,19).

As an approximation, onset of turbulence can be predicted by using the Reynolds number Re (18,19), which is a dimensionless ratio:

$$Re = \frac{Density \times velocity \times tube\ diameter}{Viscosity}$$

For Reynolds numbers less than approximately 2,100, laminar flow is generally present; for Reynolds numbers greater than 2,100, turbulent flow may be seen. The lowest velocity at which turbulence occurs is plotted as a function of vascular diameter in Fig. 2 for water and

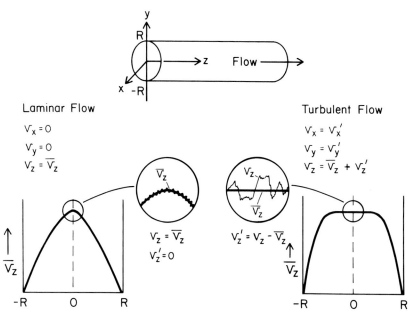

FIG. 1. Comparison of laminar and turbulent flow. For flow in a tube of radius R in the axial (z) direction, velocity components in the nonaxial direction (v_x and v_y) are zero during laminar flow. Actual velocity in the axial direction (v_z) is equal to the time-smoothed mean ($\bar{v}_z$). In turbulent flow, fluctuating velocity components are present (indicated by superscript primes, e.g., v'_x). (From ref. 18.)

blood. It should be emphasized that the concept of the Reynolds number is a gross approximation, only applying to steady flow in smooth-walled vessels that do not branch (19,20). The pulsatile flow in arteries has components of both laminar flow and turbulence and is thus sometimes described as "disturbed flow" (20). Flow past a stenosis also has a mixture of laminar and turbulent characteristics. Laminar flow is generally found in the orifice (due to the smaller diameter), whereas turbulence may be present downstream from the orifice, where the diameter again increases (18). Flow downstream from an obstruction is also associated with laminar flow within large-scale recirculation zones or "eddies" (18).

CAUSES OF SIGNAL LOSS

There are two basic causes of signal loss in MR that produce the "flow void," time-of-flight effects (5,18,21) and dephasing effects (22,23). Time-of-flight effects are simply due to isochromats not remaining within the selected slice long enough to be exposed to the 90° and 180° radiofrequency (RF) pulses required to produce a spin-echo signal. This effect has also been called "high-velocity signal loss" (5) and is illustrated in Fig. 4. Although isochromats must remain within the slice for the selective 90° and 180° pulses, they need not be within the slice at the time of the spin-echo (5). Thus, motion between the time of the last 180° pulse and the spin-echo does not reduce signal intensity (5).

Dephasing results from the differential motion of isochromats through a gradient (4,22,23). Three mag-

netic field gradients are required to produce an image. In the two-dimensional Fourier transform technique that is generally used clinically, these are described as the "slice-selected," "phase-encoding," and "frequency-encoding" (i.e., "readout") gradients. Gradients used to construct an MR image must be "symmetric" so there is no "phase buildup" along any axis in the image for stationary tissue. (Specifically, the integral of any gradient with respect to time must be zero over the period of the spin-echo acquisition.) Thus, for any positive gra-

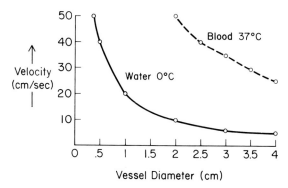

FIG. 2. Reynolds number (Re) prediction of turbulence: Re (dimensionless) = density (g/cm³) × average velocity (cm/sec) × tube diameter (cm) × viscosity (centipiose = 0.01 g/cm-sec). Laminar flow, Re < 2,100; turbulent flow, Re > 2,100. The Reynolds relationship is shown and velocity of onset of turbulence plotted for different vascular diameters for blood and water. Notice that turbulence occurs at lower velocities in larger diameter vessels and that blood, with its greater viscosity, can maintain laminar flow at higher velocities than water. (From ref. 18.)

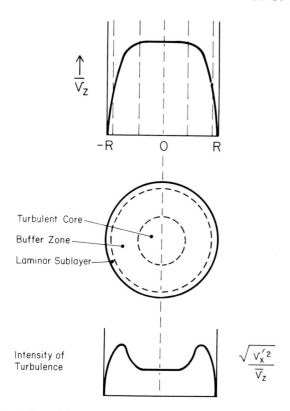

FIG. 3. Transitional flow. The flattened flow profile of the time-smooth mean velocity (v_z) is shown in lateral projection in a tube of radius R (*top*). In axial view, the three zones (turbulent core, buffer zone, and laminar sublayer) are demonstrated (*middle*). In lateral projection, the intensity of turbulence is plotted as a function of radial position. The magnitude of the fluctuating velocity component, i.e., the intensity of turbulence (*bottom*), is greatest in the buffer zone. (From ref. 18.)

The signal loss or "flow void" (21) associated with the combined effects of high velocity, turbulence, and first-echo dephasing allows blood vessels to be distinguished from the surrounding stationary tissue (3,24–26). This natural contrast is useful in the identification of normal (or occluded) vessels (Fig. 5), anteriovenous malformations (AVMs) (Fig. 6), and aneurysms (Fig. 7).

CAUSES OF INCREASED SIGNAL

Although signal loss is generally associated with flow through arteries, it should be remembered that arterial flow is pulsatile and that the signal loss is actually due to the flow that occurs during systole (20). There is relatively little flow occurring during diastole, and thus there is much less signal loss during that phase of the cardiac cycle. Vessels that are intentionally gated to the EKG and imaged during diastole have higher signal intensities based on the T1 and T2 of stagnant liquid blood (Fig. 8). Similarly, chance synchronization of the cardiac and MR cycles ("pseudogating") can lead to increased signal intensity (5). For example, if the heart rate

dient, a compensating negative gradient must be applied. To the extent that the isochromats within a voxel experience different values of the net magnetic field from moment to moment (over the interval TE from the time of the 90° pulse to the time of the echo), they will get out of phase; i.e., they will lose the coherence induced by the 90° pulse (22,23). The random motion of isochromats associated with turbulent flow results in dephasing, irreversible loss of coherence, and decreased signal intensity (18). (This is similar to the irreversible loss of coherence that results from randomly fluctuating internal magnetic fields within a tissue that cause T2 decay.) When laminar flow is present, there is a velocity gradient across the vessel and thus across each voxel spanning the vessel. Isochromats within the voxel move through the magnetic field gradients at slightly different speeds and thus lose phase coherence (22,23) and signal intensity ("first-echo dephasing"). Unlike the irreversible loss of signal intensity associated with turbulence, however, some of this signal loss can be recovered if flow continues at the same velocity through a second spin-echo acquisition (see "even-echo rephasing" below).

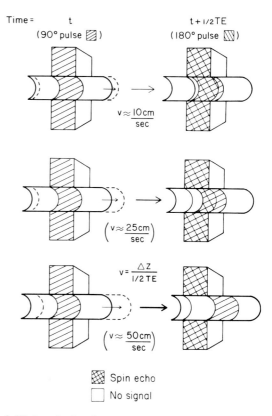

FIG. 4. High-velocity signal loss. Signal is lost from protons that are not within the slice to acquire both the 90° and 180° selective pulses. Total signal loss occurs when the velocity is such that a distance of one slice thickness Δz is traversed during the interpulse interval TE/2. (From ref. 18.)

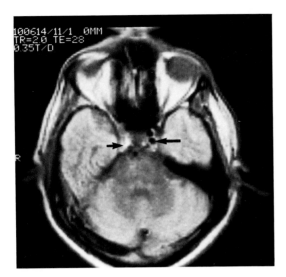

FIG. 5. Occluded right internal carotid artery. Expected "flow void" is noted in left internal carotid artery producing low intensity appearance (*arrow*). Flow void is not observed in occluded right internal carotid artery (*arrowhead*).

is 60 beats per minute (i.e., one cardiac cycle per second) and the TR is also 1 sec, then the cardiac and MR cycles may become synchronized. During a TR of 1 sec, 10 slices are acquired in numerical order on our unit. Those slices acquired during cardiac systole (approximately 30% of the cardiac cycle at this heart rate, i.e., three slices) will experience rapid flow and those acquired during diastole, no (or reduced) flow. Increased intraluminal signal can be seen when diastolic pseudogating is present (Fig. 9). (Although this is not a true cause of flow-induced increased signal, it is a cause of

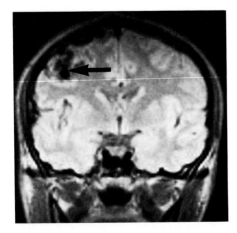

FIG. 6. Arteriovenous malformation. Signal loss is noted in rapidly flowing blood within arteriovenous malformation (*arrow*) due to time-of-flight effects, dephasing, and turbulence.

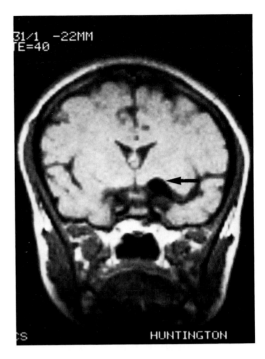

FIG. 7. Aneurysm. Signal loss in aneurysm of left middle cerebral artery (*arrow*) due to rapid flow.

increased intraluminal signal in arteries). When seen clinically, it can be distinguished from pathology (i.e., tumor or thrombus) by obtaining images through the same section intentionally gated to cardiac systole (5).

When isochromats in the blood first flow into an imaging volume, they enter with full magnetization. They are thus capable of generating a stronger signal (Fig. 10A) than the partially saturated protons in the adjacent stationary tissue, which are still recovering magnetization along the T1 relaxation curve. This entry phenomenon has been termed "flow-related enhancement" (5).

Intensity increases in the entry slice (i.e., the first slice encountered by the flowing blood) as the flow rate initially increases. Enhancement continues to a maximum value (Fig. 10B) where the partially saturated protons previously in the entry slice are totally replaced by fresh unsaturated protons in the interval TR between repetitions (5). This effect is initially seen in the center of the vessel where the velocity is greatest. The optimum effect is at an average velocity v of one slice thickness Δz per TR: $v = \Delta z/TR$ (5). Further increases beyond this optimum velocity result in some signal loss in the entry slice due to time-of-flight effects ("high-velocity signal loss") and increasing first-echo dephasing (Fig. 11). Total signal loss occurs when all the protons originally tagged by the 90° pulse leave the slice prior to the refocusing 180° pulse, i.e., at velocity $\Delta z/\frac{1}{2}TE$ (18). This is usually only observed in the center of the vessel (18), since the velocity near the vessel wall is decreased by shearing forces (19).

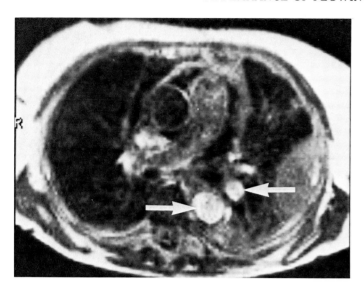

FIG. 8. Cardiac gated, diastolic image of the mediastinum. High signal intensity (*arrows*) is noted in the descending aorta and pulmonary vessels due to slow diastolic flow.

If multiple slices are acquired in a single acquisition, flow at higher velocities may introduce unsaturated (high intensity) spins into slices deeper (Fig. 12) into the imaging volume. Flow-related enhancement may then be observed (Fig. 13) on multiple slices (18). When flow-related enhancement is discussed for inner volume slices, it is important to consider the velocity of the fluid relative to the velocity at which the imaging plane moves through the imaging volume: $\Delta z/(TR/n)$, Δz being the sum of the slice thickness and the gap and TR/n being the interval at which successive slices are excited (23). Two velocity ranges can then be considered (23): those *above* the velocity at which the imaging plane moves through the imaging volume ("high-velocity flow-related enhancement") and those *below* this velocity ("low-velocity flow-related enhancement"). Isochromats demonstrating high-velocity flow-related enhancement generally have a velocity high enough to reach the slice in the interval between the 90° pulses at different levels. If n slices total are acquired during the interval TR, 90° pulses are applied at different levels at intervals TR/n. If we assume that consecutive slice excitation occurs in the direction of flow, then the velocity required (18) for an isochromat to demonstrate flow-related enhancement in slice m (counting in from the entry slice) is $m \times \Delta z/(TR/n)$, where Δz is the sum of the slice thickness and gap (if any). For slices deeper into the imaging volume, i.e., further from the entry surface, the velocities required for flow-related enhancement generally increase. As the velocity increases, there is increasing signal loss due to time-of-flight and dephasing effects (22,23). The latter cause of signal loss results from the steeper parabolic velocity profile at higher flow rates, which leads to a higher phase gradient across the voxel at the time of the echo (22,23). The higher phase gradient produces greater loss of coherence and thus greater signal loss.

Flow-related enhancement can also occur at lower velocities that have a "clever" flow pattern, avoiding exposure to 90° pulses en route to the slice. Just as flow-related enhancement occurs in the entry slice at the low velocity of $\Delta z/TR$, so flow-related enhancement can potentially occur in deeper slices at flow rates of $m\ \Delta z/TR$ (where m is the slice number, counting in from the entry surface). For slices deeper into the imaging volume, however, we must now subtract isochromats

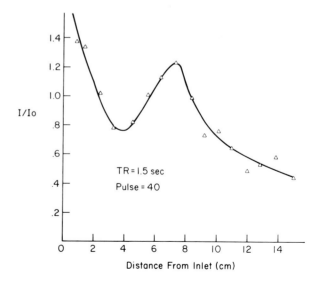

FIG. 9. Diastolic pseudogating. When there is chance synchronization of the cardiac and MR cycles (e.g., for a heart rate of 40 and a TR of 1.5 sec), several slices will be acquired during systole (showing low intraluminal signal due to rapid flow), and several slices will be acquired during diastole (showing higher signal due to slow or absent flow). The high signal intensity in the entry slices reflects flow-related enhancement. The central peak at slice 7 reflects maximal diastolic pseudogating in this flow phantom intensity plot. (From ref. 5.)

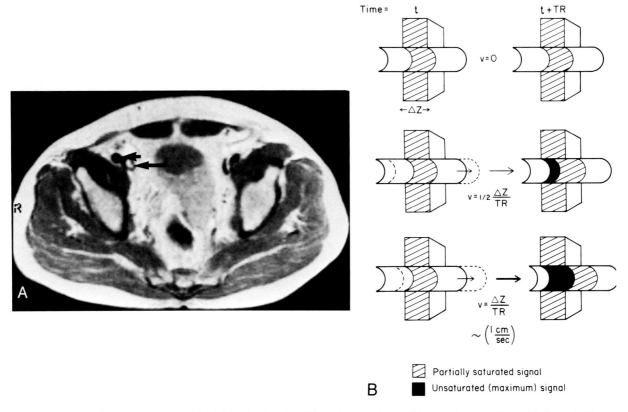

FIG. 10. Flow-related enhancement and high-velocity signal loss in a patient with carcinoma of the bladder. **A:** Increased signal in slowly flowing femoral veins (*arrow*) is due to fully magnetized protons entering first slice of multislice imaging volume. Absence of signal from the adjacent femoral arteries (*arrowhead*) reflects loss of signal due to turbulence, dephasing, and time-of-flight effects. **B:** Flow-related enhancement occurs during slow flow when unsaturated protons enter first slice with full magnetization and emit stronger signal than protons in adjacent, partially saturated, stationary tissue. Maximum effect occurs at the velocity where unsaturated protons replace the protons previously in the slice during the interval TR. (From ref. 5.)

that have been exposed to a 90° pulse prior to arriving at the deeper slice (23). Protons in gaps between slices and those at the edge of the slice that experience less than a 90° pulse (27) will also contribute to the flow-related enhancement in the deeper slice. The effect is decreased, however, for slices deeper in the imaging volume, since a higher proportion of the spins have become exposed to 90° pulses en route to the slice. If the protons at the edge of a slice experience less than 90° of rotation, a portion of the original longitudinal magnetization is retained, allowing at least partial flow-related enhancement. The degree of flow-related enhancement within a particular slice is thus due to the sum of the unsaturated and partially saturated protons that arrive at the slice with greater residual magnetization than that recovered by the surrounding (stationary) protons in the interval TR.

Flow-related enhancement in the low-velocity range tends to produce higher intensities than that at high velocity. This reflects the greater losses due to first-echo dephasing and time-of-flight effects at higher velocities.

Flow-related enhancement can also be seen for flow in the opposite direction to that of the imaging plane as it

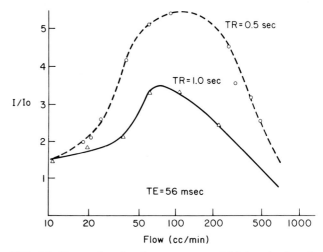

FIG. 11. Flow-related enhancement and high-velocity signal loss demonstrated in flow phantom. Intraluminal signal *I* is initially increased (relative to stationary signal I_0) due to unsaturated protons first entering volume. Effect is seen at low velocity and is accentuated at shorter TR. Signal is lost as velocity is increased due to protons leaving section prior to emitting spin echo (high-velocity signal loss). (From ref. 5.)

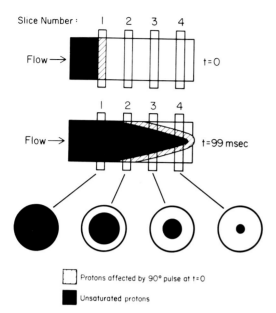

FIG. 12. Multislice flow-related enhancement. At higher velocities, the parabolic laminar profile can project several slices into the imaging volume. To demonstrate flow-related enhancement, unsaturated protons must traverse the distance from the entry surface to the inner slice during the time between 90° pulses (e.g., 100 msec). Cross-sections of the cone-shaped parabolic profile result in decreasing cross-sectional area for the central zone of unsaturated protons deeper into the imaging volume. Velocity range, 10–50 cm/sec; intensity decreased by high-velocity signal loss. (From ref. 18.)

moves through the imaging volume. In this case, only high-velocity flow-related enhancement is possible; i.e., for flow rates greater than $m \Delta z/(TR/n)$, since isochromats with slower velocities would be exposed to the preceding 90° pulse.

EVEN-ECHO REPHASING

In Fig. 14 the slow-flowing blood in the basal veins of Rosenthal has a significantly stronger signal on the second 56-msec spin echo than on the initial 28-msec echo. This is seen frequently in large veins and dural sinuses and is associated with slow laminar flow (4). The more intense intraluminal signal in the second-echo image is due to a rephasing phenomenon that occurs after each 360° of rotation following the initial 90° pulse; that is, for all even echoes in a multiple-echo train (4). Appreciation of this phenomenon requires an understanding of the phasing and dephasing that occurs during the spin-echo sequence.

Figure 15 is a schematic diagram of the Carr-Purcell-Meiboom-Gill spin-echo sequence (28). Following the 90° pulse, isochromats begin to get out of phase due to magnetic field nonuniformities. Isochromats in a slightly stronger part of the field precess at a higher frequency and tend to get ahead of those in weaker parts of the magnetic field. This results in the flaring of the magnetization vectors in the rotating reference frame shown in Fig. 15. Following a 180° rotation about the y axis, dephased isochromats are flipped so that those that led now lag. Since they remain in a slightly stronger part of the magnetic field, however, they continue to precess at the higher frequency and eventually catch up to their more slowly precessing counterparts to generate a spin echo.

The same phenomenon can be demonstrated by the spin-phase graph that was introduced by Singer (17). As shown in Fig. 16, isochromats in a stronger part of the field gain phase until the 180° pulse when phase is reversed, and they suddenly lose exactly the amount of

FIG. 13. Multislice flow-related enhancement in the right common carotid artery (TR = 1.5 sec, TE = 28 msec, nongated). Decreased intraluminal signal is noted for slices deeper into the imaging volume. (Slice 1 is lowest entry slice.) (From ref. 18.)

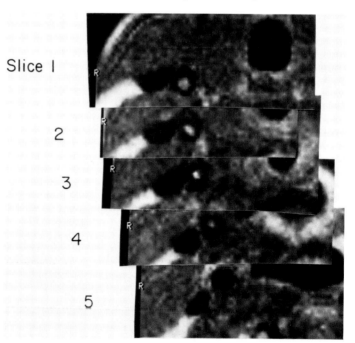

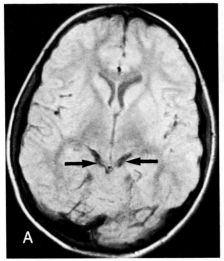 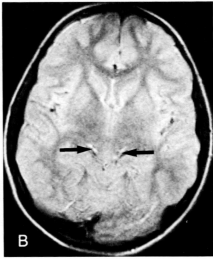

FIG. 14. Even-echo rephasing. Comparison of the first- (28 msec) echo image (A) with the second- (56 msec) echo image (B). The second-echo image has higher signal in the basal veins of Rosenthal (*arrows*) due to rephasing of isochromats in slow laminar flow.

phase they had just gained. They continue to gain or lose phase at the same rate and regain coherence with their more slowly precessing counterparts at the time of the spin echo. At this time, there is no difference in phase angle between different portions of the voxel. If the isochromats are allowed to dephase after the first spin echo, they can be rephased by a second 180° pulse, producing a second spin echo.

If blood flows into an increasing magnetic field gradient (Fig. 17), isochromats on the leading edge of the voxel start in a stronger part of the magnetic field and gain phase more rapidly than those on the lagging edge in the weaker part of the magnetic field. If there were no flow in the vessel, isochromats in different portions of the magnetic field would dephase as they do in any other nonuniform magnetic field (Fig. 18A). When there is flow into an increasing magnetic field gradient, the phase changes can no longer be represented by straight

lines but are now quadratic curves (4,5) that gain phase somewhat more rapidly (Fig. 18B).

If all isochromats were to move at the same velocity (as in plug flow), they would each increase in phase at the same rate. When laminar flow is present, a parabolic profile exists so that the protons in the center of the stream move at a higher velocity than those at the periphery (Fig. 19). Protons in the center of the stream are also on the leading edge of the voxel and therefore are in a stronger field. These isochromats gain phase at an even greater rate than those on the lagging edge. At the time of the first spin echo, coherence is not totally regained, because there is a phase difference between isochromats on the leading and lagging edges of the voxel. Following an additional 180° of rotation for the second echo, that phase difference is corrected so that coherence is reestablished (4,5).

Loss of intensity in the first echo ("first echo dephas-

FIG. 15. Carr-Purcell-Meiboom-Gill (CPMG) spin echo. In rotating reference frame. Magnetization (*solid arrow*) is rotated into transverse (*x'–y'*) plane by 90° radio-frequency (RF) pulse. Dephasing causes flaring of the magnetization because some protons precess faster and some slower than average (due to relatively stronger and weaker local magnetic field). After interpulse interval (TE/2), a 180° pulse is applied, which causes rotation about the *y'* axis, and flared magnetization vectors begin to rephase. At time (TE), rephasing is complete, and coherent spin echo is emitted. (From ref. 5.)

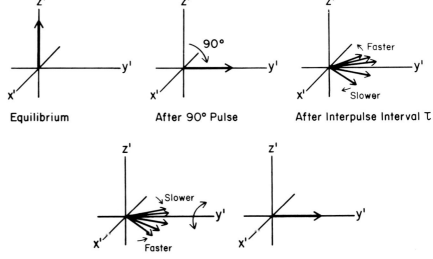

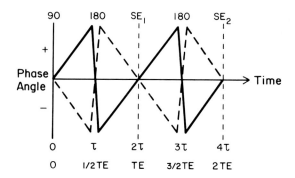

FIG. 16. Spin-phase graph. Phase is either lost or gained relative to average precessional frequency by protons in relatively weaker and stronger parts of the magnetic field. Sign of phase is reversed by each 180° pulse (at $\frac{1}{2}$TE and $\frac{3}{2}$TE). Coherence is reestablished at the time of each spin echo (SE$_1$ and SE$_2$). (From ref. 5.)

ing") can be considered analogous to partially reversible loss of coherence during a free induction decay (FID), which primarily reflects fixed-field nonuniformities in the main magnetic field. In this sense, the temporary loss of coherence at the time of the first spin echo in laminar flow might be compared with loss of coherence in an FID that is regained at the time of the spin echo (5). If the signal intensities of the first and second echoes are used to calculate a T2 value, it will be negative. This has been used as a sign of slow flow (29).

The dephasing-rephasing effect is demonstrated on the computer simulations in Figs. 20 and 21 showing plug flow and laminar flow into an increasing magnetic field gradient (5). The two simulations shown are for equal volumetric flow rates and indicate a much different phase history for laminar flow than for idealized plug flow at the time of the first spin echo. Since signal loss is due to loss of coherence, i.e., different phase angles within a voxel at the time of the spin echo, signal

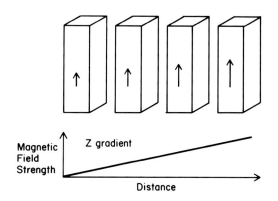

FIG. 17. Dephasing of staggered isochromats during flow. Four isochromats are shown flowing into increasing (slice-selecting) z gradient. Isochromats on leading edge of voxel are in stronger magnetic field (indicated by *longer arrow*) than isochromats on lagging edge. Isochromats on leading edge gain phase more rapidly than those behind. (From ref. 5.)

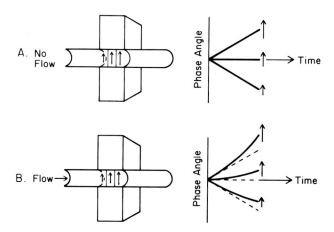

FIG. 18. Accelerated phase gain due to flow into an increasing magnetic field. When a gradient is present without flow (**A**), rephasing occurs as it would in any other nonuniform magnetic field. When blood flows into an increasing magnetic field (**B**), phase is gained more rapidly than if the blood were stationary. (From ref. 5.)

should only be lost in the laminar flow case. Although there is a positive phase angle at the time of the first echo in plug flow, all isochromats have experienced the same increase in phase, and thus they remain coherent. Zero phase angle is reestablished following 360° rotation at the time of the second spin echo for both flow situations.

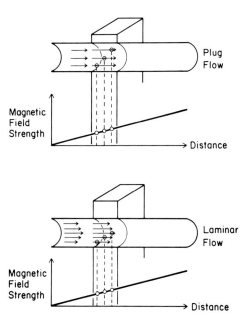

FIG. 19. Blood flow into a magnetic field gradient. In plug flow all isochromats move at the same velocity. Phase gain is related to this velocity and to position in the voxel. Isochromats on the leading edge of the voxel gain phase more rapidly than those on the lagging edge. In laminar flow, isochromats in the center of the tube move at a higher velocity than those near the periphery. Protons on the leading edge of the voxel gain phase more rapidly not only due to position in the voxel but also because they flow at a higher velocity than those at the periphery. (From ref. 5.)

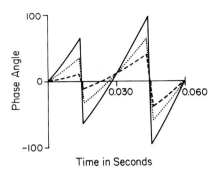

FIG. 20. Computer simulation of plug flow. Phase angle of isochromats in stronger half of field is plotted as a function of time (spin echoes occur at 0.030 and 0.060 sec). Isochromats remain in phase with positive phase angles at time of first spin echo, thus there is no less of signal (merely a phase shift relative to stationary protons). Isochromats return to zero phase shift (relative to stationary protons) on the second spin echo at 0.060 sec. (From ref. 5.)

(This analysis totally ignores the loss of coherence due to turbulence in plug flow).

The spread of the phase angles at the time of the first echo in laminar flow increases as the flow rate increases and the parabolic profile steepens, increasing the range of velocities present. Thus, the first echo becomes less intense relative to the rephased second echo as the velocity increases (Fig. 11). As the velocity continues to increase, the difference in intensity between the two echoes decreases due to high-velocity signal loss. Eventually, the intensities of the two echoes become equal as the enhancing effect of rephasing is countered by the increased signal loss due to time-of-flight effects. With further increases in velocity, the second echo becomes progressively weaker than the first, and eventually all signal is lost.

CSF Flow Phenomena

The same MR phenomena that increase or decrease the intensity of flowing blood can also alter the intensity of CSF within the ventricles and the subarachnoid space. CSF is produced at a rate of approximately 500 ml/day primarily in the choroid plexus of the lateral and third ventricles. The bulk flow of CSF results in net movement from the choroid plexus within the ventricles to the arachnoid villi. Magnetic resonance pixel intensity, however, reflects the *linear velocity* of CSF during the period of signal acquisition. This is expected to be greatest through the narrowest part of the ventricular system, i.e., through the aqueduct. CSF flow is pulsatile, due to transmitted cardiac pulsations (30). Although the motion of CSF appears to primarily reflect expansion of the choroid plexus during cardiac systole, other factors, such as generalized systolic cerebral expansion (31) and pulsation of the large arteries at the base of the brain (32), may also contribute to CSF motion. This to-and-

fro motion of CSF through the aqueduct allows ventricular reflux of radionuclide to occur during nuclear cisternography in communicating hydrocephalus, including the chronic, normal pressure form (33). The linear velocity of CSF flowing through the aqueduct depends to a much greater extent on transmitted cardiac pulsations than on the rate of production of CSF.

Causes of Signal Loss

Just as the signal of flowing blood is decreased due to first echo dephasing and time-of-flight effects, signal loss can be observed when there is motion of CSF (6,34,35). These effects are greatest where the velocity is highest, i.e., in the aqueduct (Fig. 22). Signal loss due to the random dephasing motion of turbulence may be observed in the upper portion of the fourth ventricle (6) due to a venturi effect.

The signal loss due to CSF motion is particularly prominent on heavily T2-weighted images on which the CSF is white. The effect is also increased as the slice thickness is decreased and the spatial resolution is increased due to steeper gradients and, thus, greater dephasing (6). The signal loss can be confusing, particularly in the lateral spinal subarachnoid space, where flow-related signal loss can mimic vascular malformations.

Causes of Increased Signal

Increased CSF signal can be seen in the entry slice of a multislice imaging volume when there is pulsatile, to-and-fro motion of CSF (36). This flow-related enhancement is most evident on T1-weighted, short-TR images,

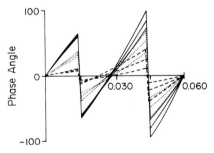

FIG. 21. Computer simulation of laminar flow. Phase angle of isochromats at different positions in voxel field are plotted as a function of time with spin echoes occurring at 0.030 and 0.060 sec. Three groups of three curves each are shown. Within each group the isochromats that gain phase most rapidly (i.e., quadratically in time) are in the center of the tube, where flow velocity is greatest. Group with *solid lines* is on leading edge of voxel in stronger part of gradient field; group with *dashed line* is on lagging edge of voxel in weaker portion of gradient field. Spread of phase angles at 0.030 sec is indicative of first echo dephasing. This loss of coherence decreases the intensity of the first echo signal. Complete rephasing occurs at the time of the second spin echo at 0.060 sec. (From ref. 5.)

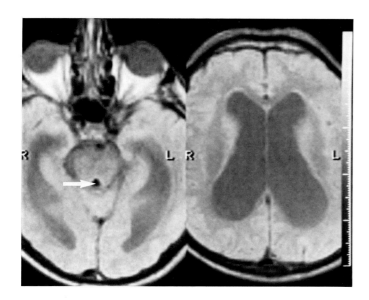

FIG. 22. Aqueductal flow void. Decreased signal is noted in aqueduct (*arrow*) relative to CSF in lateral ventricles. This reflects higher velocity of CSF through aqueduct than through lateral ventricles. This sign is accentuated in states with decreased ventricular compliance, e.g., normal pressure hydrocephalus. (From ref. 6.)

as was the case with the flowing blood. The effect is most evident at short TR, since the high-intensity "enhanced" CSF has greater contrast with the lower intensity stationary CSF. The high intensity produced within the ventricular system can be potentially confused with a high-intensity mass (Fig. 23A). When slow flow continues over the interval between the 90° pulse and a second spin-echo, even-echo rephasing can occasionally be observed as well (Fig. 23B). Subtle increase in intensity can often be observed in the basal cisterns in the lowest sections in a multislice acquisition (36).

The chance synchronization of the cardiac and MR cycles during diastole that produced increased signal during pulsatile blood flow ("diastolic pseudogating") can also increase signal during pulsatile CSF flow. Gated images of the brain may have variable CSF signal intensities, depending on the phase of the cardiac cycle. The increased signal due to chance diastolic synchronization may potentially be mistaken for a true mass (Fig. 24).

Clinical Applications of CSF Flow Phenomena

The intensity of the CSF in the aqueduct is generally less than that in the lateral ventricles due to the higher velocity back and forth through the aqueduct (Fig. 22). Although this "aqueductal flow void" can be seen in normal patients, it is much more prominent in patients with chronic communicating hydrocephalus who present with the clinical triad of dementia, gait disturbance, and incontinence. When onset of symptoms is insidious (rather than stepwise) and the ventricles are dilated out of proportion to the cortical sulci, these patients may be considered to have the syndrome of "normal pressure hydrocephalus" (NPH) (37).

To compare the aqueductal flow void sign as a possible indicator of NPH, the MR images of 60 patients were evaluated retrospectively (6). Of these, 16 were unselected, consecutive "normals" (i.e., no MR evidence of hydrocephalus or other abnormality), 11 were "nor-

FIG. 23. High-intensity CSF flow artifact. High intensity (*arrow*) in fourth ventricle on entry slice of multislice imaging volume due to to-and-fro motion of CSF and flow-related enhancement. (Overlapping acquisition containing slice at same level showed no abnormality a few minutes later.) On second echo image at same level, further intensity increase is noted due to even-echo rephasing.

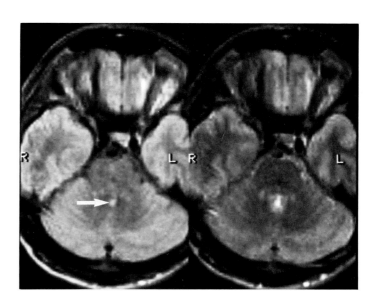

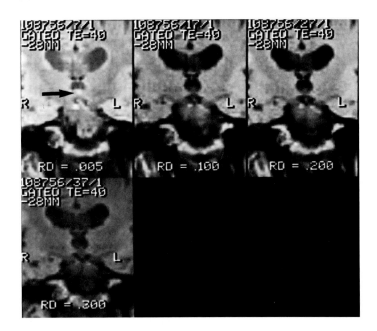

FIG. 24. Cardiac gated images through the third ventricle. Image acquired during cardiac diastole (R delay = 5 msec) has higher third ventricular CSF signal (*arrow*) compared to the images acquired in systole. This reflects slower, retrograde flow of CSF in diastole.

CSF in the aqueduct ("systolic pseudogating"), 20 had clinical NPH (i.e., chronic communicating hydrocephalus), seven had acute communicating hydrocephalus with elevated pressure, five had hydrocephalus *ex vacuo,* and one had internal obstructive hydrocephalus due to compression of the aqueduct. All patients had axial images obtained at 5 or 10 mm intervals with a TR of 2.0 sec and TE of 28 and 56 msec. The intensity of the CSF in the lateral ventricles and aqueduct was measured using a cursor-defined region of interest on both first and second echo images.

Figure 25 demonstrates the distribution of the mean pixel intensities in the aqueduct and lateral ventricles on first (TE = 28 msec) and second (TE = 56 msec) echo images at TR = 2.0 sec in normal cases and in various disease states. The data are plotted as a distribution of the means as follows: The midpoint (peak value) of the curve at half-maximum is the mean value, and the width of the curve is the standard error of the mean. The peak heights have been normalized for uniformity and thus have no physical meaning.

Figure 25 demonstrates that the intensity of the CSF in the aqueduct is lower than that in the lateral ventricle on the first echo image, even in nonselected, consecutive normal cases. The CSF intensity in the aqueduct is rela-

FIG. 25. Aqueduct/lateral ventricle CSF intensity ratios in healthy and various hydrocephalic states. The greatest relative aqueductal signal loss is noted in NPH and the least is noted in atrophy, reflecting varying degrees of ventricular compliance. Although aqueductal signal loss can also be observed in healthy individuals, this is noted less frequently and to a lesser degree than in patients with NPH. (From ref. 6.)

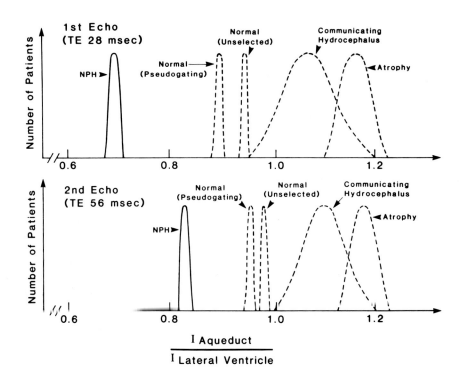

tively higher (compared to the lateral ventricle) on the second echo image. This is believed to reflect the higher linear flow velocity through the aqueduct (compared to the lateral ventricle) with first-echo dephasing and even-echo rephasing, respectively. In normal patients selected on the basis of visually apparent low-intensity CSF in the aqueduct, the measured intensity of the aqueductal CSF is significantly lower than that in the lateral ventricles. This is presumably on the basis of chance synchronization of the MR acquisition through the aqueduct and cardiac systole (i.e., "systolic pseudogating").

In patients with clinical NPH, the signal intensity in the aqueduct is decreased to an even greater extent compared to normal patients with or without obvious systolic pseudogating and compared to patients with acute communicating hydrocephalus or atrophy.

Although the actual CSF flow-time relationships have not been demonstrated experimentally in these disease states, a good deal is known about the CSF pressure-time waveform (38,39). This waveform depends on the "effective volume" of CSF in contact with the choroid plexus as well as the surface area and the elasticity of the tissues adjacent to this CSF volume. The effective volume of CSF is that volume in contact with the choroid plexus, modified by the degree of interposing resistances. Thus, the effective volume of CSF in aqueductal stenosis is that volume within the lateral ventricles, whereas the effective volume of CSF in communicating hydrocephalus is much greater, including that over the convexities. For internal obstructive hydrocephalus, the pulse pressure depends primarily on the elasticity of the periventricular tissues. For communicating forms of hydrocephalus, the pulse pressure depends on the greater surface area of the "effective CSF volume," the elasticity of the tissues adjacent to this CSF volume, and on the venting of venous blood from the intracranial cavity during the cardiac cycle. Generally, the CSF pressure rise during systole is greater and occurs earlier in hydrocephalus than in normal patients. Internal obstructive hydrocephalus and NPH have the highest pulse pressures (lowest compliance), whereas acute forms of communicating hydrocephalus have lower pulse pressures (due to somewhat decreased compliance and greater surface area) compared to normal or atrophic states (with normal compliance) (39).

On the basis of empiricism alone, the observation of decreased aqueductal signal (using these sequence parameter times) could be considered a secondary MR sign of NPH (6). This would be of significant clinical utility, since NPH remains a difficult entity to diagnose and is also one of the few potentially treatable causes of dementia (40). It is tempting, however, to speculate on the pathophysiologic mechanism responsible for this observation (Fig. 26).

The choroid plexus of the third and lateral ventricles expands during cardiac systole. Since CSF is a noncompressible fluid, there are several possible sequelae of choroid plexus expansion. The ventricles can expand by a volume equal to the expansion of the choroid plexus, a volume of CSF (equal to the volume of the expanded choroid plexus) can be vented through the aqueduct, the intraventricular pressure can rise, or a combination of these can occur.

The altered compliance of the ventricles in hydrocephalus has been discussed and modeled extensively by Hakim (37,41) and others (38,39). Compliance is decreased to the greatest extent in chronic communicating hydrocephalus (NPH), which both increases the relative outflow of CSF through the aqueduct and increases the intraventricular pressure pulsations. The pulse pressure in NPH has been likened to a "water hammer" (30) and has been shown to be up to six times that of normal patients (42). The relatively more elastic periventricular tissue in acute forms of communicating hydrocephalus and hydrocephalus *ex vacuo*, i.e., atrophy, allow greater systolic expansion of the ventricles and thus have relatively less pulsatile aqueductal CSF flow. The greater flow of CSF through the aqueduct in NPH is felt to reflect decreased periventricular elasticity.

The reason for the lack of aqueductal signal loss is uncertain in acute communicating hydrocephalus and in atrophy. Perhaps the systolic expansion of the larger

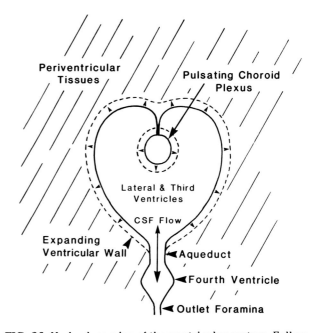

FIG. 26. Hydrodynamics of the ventricular system. Following systolic expansion of the choroid plexus, the ventricles must expand, CSF must be vented through the aqueduct, the intraventricular pressure must rise, or a combination of these events must occur. The relative compliance of the periventricular tissues and the ependymal surface area will determine the degree to which CSF pulsates through the aqueduct. There is greater aqueductal CSF flow in noncompliant states such as NPH. There is relatively less aqueductal flow in patients with normal compliance and normal-size ventricles, and there is even less aqueductal flow in patients with normal compliance and enlarged ventricles (i.e., in patients with atrophy). (From ref. 6.)

and relatively more compliant ventricles results in relatively greater dephasing within the lateral ventricles and less aqueductal CSF flow, particularly in the atrophic state. In acute communicating hydrocephalus, greater resistance to ventricular outflow (transmitted back from the obstructed arachnoid villi) may result in relatively decreased CSF motion through the aqueduct.

Although the low-intensity appearance of aqueductal CSF on these mildly T2-weighted images may be considered to be a secondary MR sign of NPH, clinical use of these phenomena will probably await the implementation of quantative CSF flow sequences. Such sequences (which display intracranial CSF motion in various phases of the cardiac cycle) are currently being developed.

ACKNOWLEDGMENT

I thank Leslee Watson, Jay Mericle, and Terry Andrues for technical assistance; Catherine Reichel Clark for artwork; and Kaye Finley for manuscript preparation.

REFERENCES

1. Hahn EL. Spin echoes. *Phys Rev* 1950;80:580–94.
2. Hahn EL. Detection of sea water motion by nuclear precession. *J Geophys Res* 1960;65:776–7.
3. Hawkes RC, Holland GN, Moore WS, Worthington BS. Nuclear magnetic resonance (NMR) tomography of the brain: a preliminary clinical assessment with demonstration of pathology. *J Comput Assist Tomogr* 1980;4:577–86.
4. Waluch V, Bradley WG. NMR even echo rephasing in slow laminar flow. *J Comput Assist Tomogr* 1984;4:594–8.
5. Bradley WG, Waluch V. Blood flow: magnetic resonance imaging. *Radiology* 1985;154:443–50.
6. Bradley WG, Kortman KE, Burgoyne B. Flowing cerebrospinal fluid in normal and hydrocephalic states: appearance on MR images. *Radiology* 1986;159:611–6.
7. Rubin J, Enzmann DR. Imaging spinal CSF pulsation by 2DFT MR: significance during clinical scanning. In: *Annual meeting of the American Society of Neuroradiology, Jan 18–23, San Diego, 1986.*
8. Wehrli FW, MacFall JR, Axel L, et al. Approaches to in-plane and out-of-plane flow imaging. *Noninvasive Med Imag* 1984;1(2):127–36.
9. Wehrli FW, Shimakawa A, MacFall JR, et al. MR imaging of venous and arterial flow by a selective saturation-recovery spin echo (SSRSE) method. *J Comput Assist Tomogr* 1985;9(3):537–45.
10. Feinberg DA, Crooks LE, Sheldon P, et al. Magnetic resonance imaging the velocity vector components of fluid flow. *Magn Reson Med* 1985;2:555–66.
11. Shimizu K, Matsuda T, Sakurai T, et al. Visualization of moving fluid: quantitative analysis of blood flow velocity using MR imaging. *Radiology* 1986;159:195–9.
12. Feinberg DA, Crooks LE, Hoenninger J III, et al. Pulsatile blood velocity in human arteries displayed by magnetic resonance imaging. *Radiology* 1984;153:177.
13. Feinberg DA. Velocity measurements of flowing CSF. In: *Annual meeting of American Society of Neuroradiology. Jan 18–23, San Diego, 1986.*
14. Valk PE, Hale JD, Kaufman L, Crooks LE, Higgins CB. MR imaging of the aorta with three-dimensional vessel reconstruction: validation by angiography. *Radiology* 1985;157:721–5.
15. Wedeen VJ, Rosen BR, Buxton R, Brady TJ. Projective MRI angiography and quantative flow-volume densitometry. *Magn Reson Med* 1986;3:226–41.
16. Miller DL, Reinig JW, Volkman DJ. Vascular imaging with MRI: inadequacy in Takayasu's arteritis compared with angiography. *AJR* 1986;146:949–54.
17. Singer JR. NMR diffusion and flow measurements and an introduction to spin phase graphing. *J Phys [E]* 1978;11:281–91.
18. Bradley WG, Waluch V, Lai K, Fernandez E, Spalter C. The appearance of rapidly flowing blood on magnetic resonance images. *AJR* 1984;143:1167–74.
19. Bird RB, Stewart WE, Lightfoot EN. *Transport phenomena.* New York: Wiley, 1960;153–8.
20. McDonald DA. *Blood flow in arteries.* Baltimore: Williams & Wilkins, 1960:20.
21. George CR, Jacobs G, MacIntyre WJ, et al. Magnetic resonance signal intensity patterns obtained from continuous and pulsatile flow models. *Radiology* 1984;151:421–7.
22. Von Schulthess GK, Higgins CB. Blood flow imaging with MR: spin-phase phenomena. *Radiology* 1985;157:687–95.
23. Valk PT, Hale JD, Crooks LE, et al. MRI of blood flow: correlation of image appearance with spin-echo phase shift and signal intensity. *AJR* 1986;146:931–9.
24. Kucharczyk W, Lemme-Pleghos L, Uske A, et al. Intracranial vascular malformations: MR and CT imaging. *Radiology* 1985;156:383–9.
25. Cohen JM, Weinreb JC, Redman HC. Arteriovenous malformations of the extremities. MR imaging. *Radiology* 1986;158:475–9.
26. Hricak H, Amparo E, Fisher MR, Crooks LE, Higgins CB. Abdominal venous system: assessment using MR. *Radiology* 1985;156:415–22.
27. Kneeland JB, Shimakawa A, Wehrli FW. Effect of intersection spacing on MR image contrast and study time. *Radiology* 1986;158:819–22.
28. Farrar TC, Becker Ed. *Pulse and Fourier transform NMR: introduction to theory and method.* New York: Academic Press, 1971.
29. Kucharczyk W, Brant-Zawadzki M, Lemme-Plaghos L, et al. MR technology: Effect of even-echo rephasing on calculated T2 values and T2 images. *Radiology* 1985;157:95–101.
30. Bering EA Jr. Choroid plexus and arterial pulsations of cerebrospinal fluid. Demonstration of the choroid plexuses as a cerebrospinal fluid pump. *Arch Neurol Psychiatry* 1955;73:165–72.
31. Laitinen L. Origin of arterial pulsation of cerebrospinal fluid. *Acta Neurol Scan* 1968;44:168–76.
32. Du Boulay G. Specialisation broadens the view. *Clin Radio* 1972;23:401–9.
33. Tator CH, Fleming JFT, Sheppard RD, et al. A radioisotopic test for communicating hydrocephalus. *J Neurosurg* 1968;28:327–40.
34. Bergstrand G, Bergstrom M, Nordell B, et al. Cardiac gated MR imaging of cerebrospinal fluid flow. *J Comput Assist Tomogr* 1985;1003–6.
35. Sherman JL, Citrin CM. Magnetic resonance demonstration of normal CSF flow. *AJNR* 1986;7:3–7.
36. Bradley WG, Kortman KE, Tsuruda JS, Bucon KA. Flow related causes of increased signal in the CSF. In: *Annual meeting of the Society of Magnetic Resonance in Medicine. Aug 18–22. Montreal, 1986.*
37. Adams RD, Fisher CM, Hakim S, Sweet WH. Symptomatic occult hydrocephalus with 'normal' cerebrospinal fluid pressure: a treatable syndrome. *N Engl J Med* 1965;273(3):117–26.
38. Di Rocco C. Hydrocephalus and cerebrospinal fluid pulses. In: Shapiro K, Marmarou A, Portnoy H, eds, *Hydrocephalus.* New York: Raven Press, 1984;231–49.
39. Foltz EI. Hydrocephalus and CSF pulsatility: clinical and laboratory studies. In: Shapiro K, Marmarou A, Portnoy H, eds, *Hydrocephalus.* New York: Raven Press, 1984;337–62.
40. Greenberg JO, Shenkin HA, Adam R. Idiopathic normal pressure hydrocephalus: a report of 73 patients. *J Neurol Neuros Psychiatry* 1977;40:336–41.
41. Hakim S, Venegas JG, Burton JD. The physics of the cranial cavity, hydrocephalus and normal pressure hydrocephalus: mechanical interpretation and mathematical model. *Surg Neurol* 1976;5:187–210.
42. Ekstedt J, Friden H. CSF hydrodynamics of the study of the adult hydrocephalus syndrome. In: Shapiro K, Marmarou A, Portnoy H, eds, *Hydrocephalus.* New York: Raven Press, 1984;363–82.

CHAPTER 6

Paramagnetic Contrast Media for Magnetic Resonance Imaging of the Central Nervous System

Michael T. McNamara

Presently, a variety of radiofrequency (RF) and magnetic field gradient pulse sequences is used to manipulate magnetic resonance (MR) image contrast. Such manipulation may be performed by altering the RF pulse sequence repetition time (TR), the spin–echo delay time (TE), the inversion-delay time (TI), and the flip angle. The detection and characterization of a lesion or structure may thus be optimized. Although such contrast manipulation is noninvasive, magnetic resonance imaging (MRI) still suffers somewhat from lack of specificity. Also, the use of multiple imaging sequences to locate and characterize a lesion may prolong the imaging time and, thus, might place an economic burden on the system. Paramagnetic pharmaceuticals offer promise in this regard. They shorten tissue relaxation times, thus permitting the use of shorter imaging parameters, and in some circumstances, may obviate additional and more time-consuming pulse sequences. Paramagnetics could expand the sensitivity and specificity of MRI and provide functional information with regard to tissue perfusion, tissue viability, and blood–brain barrier integrity.

The use of paramagnetic compounds is not new to MR. As early as 1946, Block (1) used $Fe(No_3)_3$ to shorten relaxation times of water protons. The use of paramagnetic ions *in vivo* was proposed in (1976) by Lauterbur et al. (2) who injected manganous salt solutions in order to provide information about myocardial perfusion. Since that time there have been a variety of paramagnetic pharmaceuticals that have been utilized for MRI. They include simple molecular oxygen, paramagnetic ions, in both chelated and unchelated form, and nitroxide spin labels (3). Due to a heightened awareness of the need for tissue-specific information, paramagnetic labeled monoclonal antibodies for tumor enhancement have also been proposed (4). Thus far, the lanthanide series complexes have demonstrated the most ideal combination of strong relaxivity and clinical

safety to warrant clinical investigation. Manganese is also strongly paramagnetic but in ionic form is limited by acute toxicity, prolonged body retention, and a small margin of safety between the effective dose and toxic dose.

THEORETICAL BASIS

Unlike conventional radiographic contrast agents that are directly visualized, paramagnetic contrast agents produce local alterations in magnetic environments that directly influence the MR signal intensity obtained from protons. Thus, it is the effect of enhancement of proton relaxation (PRE) that appears on MR images; the paramagnetic contrast media themselves are not directly visualized.

Paramagnetic substances are defined as those that are attracted to and align with an external magnetic field but resume a random orientation when the external field is removed. They are all characterized by the presence of at least one unpaired electron. Under the influence of an external magnetic field, paramagnetic compounds create local magnetic fields that enhance relaxation of protons within local spheres of influence (the local environment that is affected) surrounding each paramagnetic molecule. Proton relaxation enhancement is the process whereby the relaxation times, T1 and T2, are shortened, with resultant alterations of MR signal intensity. For spin-echo pulse sequences, the expression for MR signal intensity is related to T1 and T2 as follows:

$$I = N(\text{H})f(v)e^{-\text{TE/T2}}(1 - e^{-\text{TR/T1}})$$

where $N(\text{H})$ is the local hydrogen density; TR is the repetition time, measured in seconds; TE is the echo delay, measured in milliseconds; $f(v)$ is a function of both the speed with which the hydrogen nuclei move through the region being imaged and of the fraction of the total number of nuclei that are moving. From this expression, it is apparent that an increase in spin-echo intensity can be produced by T1 shortening, T2 prolongation, or by an increase in spin density. Since PRE produces shortening of both T1 and T2, paramagnetic agents will produce potentially opposing effects on spin-echo signal intensity. In order to produce an increase in MRI signal intensity, the T1 shortening effect must predominate over the intensity-decreasing effect of T2 shortening. In general, pharmacologic doses presently used produce such predominant T1 shortening and thus cause an increase in MR spin-echo signal intensity.

The most commonly used paramagnetic substances in MRI are paramagnetic ions. The transition metal and lanthanide series elements are paramagnetic substances that are characterized by unpaired electrons in the 3d and 4f orbitals, or subshells, respectively. The paramagnetic strength is related to the number of unpaired electrons. This strength is expressed in terms of Bohr magnetons (μ_B), a measure of the magnetic moment of the substance. Thus, the strongest of the transition metal and lanthanide series elements are manganese (5.9 μ_B), with five unpaired electrons, one in each of the five 3d subshells; and gadolinium (8.0 μ_B), with seven unpaired electrons, one in each of the seven 4f subshells, respectively. Other paramagnetic elements include cobalt, iron, copper, nickel, and chromium.

As discussed in Chapter 1, populations of hydrogen protons within a stationary magnetic field may exist in one of two discrete energy levels. These are the low energy level, in which the proton is parallel to the magnetic field, and the high energy level, in which the proton spin is antiparallel to or aligned against the field. Application of RF field to the system at the resonance frequency produces a net upward transition from the lower energy level to the higher energy level, producing a nonequilibrium situation. In order for a nuclear magnetic resonance (NMR) signal to persist, there must be replenishment of the number of nuclei in the lower energy state. This replenishment results from transitions that cause the perturbed system (which resulted from RF application) to return to the equilibrium spin (proton) distribution. These transitions are called relaxation processes. There are two types of relaxation processes: spin-lattice (longitudinal) and spin-spin (transverse) relaxation. Spin-lattice relaxation is designated as T1. Spin-spin relaxation is characterized by T2. These relaxation processes result in one sense from random magnetic or electric fields and their impact on the spinning proton dipole. These random fields may result from magnetic moments of other nuclei, such as nearby protons, or from magnetic moments of unpaired electrons. In the clinical situation in which protons are being imaged,

direct interaction between nearby protons, known as dipole-dipole relaxation (R_{DD}), is the dominant mechanism for relaxation. For two protons P_1 and P_2 separated by distance d, the energy of this process is characterized by

$$R_{DD} = (u_1 \times u_2)/d^3$$

where u_1 and u_2 are the magnetic moments of the protons. It is evident that the strength of this relaxation interaction decreases significantly as the distance separating them increases. Dipole-dipole relaxation results from interactions between protons in the same molecule (intramolecular) and between protons or adjacent molecules (intermolecular). In pure water systems, the intramolecular interactions predominate over the intermolecular interactions.

Relaxation may also be mediated by interactions between proton nuclei and nearby electrons. This is known as scalar relaxation. As mentioned above, it is not as important as the stronger dipole-dipole relaxation mechanism.

Relaxation processes that are mediated by paramagnetic substances are particularly more influential than dipole-dipole or scalar relaxation. Paramagnetic substances create their effect because of their possession of one or more unpaired electrons. This results in uncanceled electron spins, which produce a net magnetic moment. Since both nuclei and electrons may have net magnetic moments, they both may technically be classified as paramagnetic; however, the magnetic moment of an electron is 657 times stronger than the magnetic moment of a proton. Since the relaxation mechanism is related to the square of the magnitude of the involved magnetic moments, an unpaired electron has a relaxation mechanism that is approximately 500,000 (657^2) times more potent than the dipole-dipole interaction of a proton. The nuclei that are commonly imaged (hydrogen, sodium, fluorine, phosphorus) are dipoles, but they are relatively weak compared to paramagnetic substances because the magnetic moment of an unpaired electron is so much stronger than the magnetic moments of nuclei. Although the dipole moments of nuclei give rise to a dipole field that causes both nuclear relaxation and chemical shifts, the electron dipole moments result in much greater relaxation and chemical shifts of nuclei compared to nuclear dipoles. In summary, even though nuclear relaxation is usually dominated by dipole-dipole relaxation and to a lesser extent by scalar relaxation, which is an electron-mediated process, the presence of paramagnetic species in sufficient quantity will easily provide the predominant mechanism for relaxation.

In a system with paramagnetic agents, there are also two types of electron-nucleus interactions that contribute to T1 and T2 relaxation. These are dipole-dipole coupling and scalar coupling. Dipole-dipole coupling depends on the electron–nucleus distance and decreases inversely proportional to the sixth power of this distance (Eq. 1, below). Scalar coupling requires the presence of a finite density of elctron spins in immediate proximity (first coordination sphere) to the proton undergoing relaxation. There will be no scalar contribution to relaxation for protons that are not within the first sphere of coordination of the paramagnetic ion (i.e., the electron spin).

The paramagnetic species creates randomly fluctuating electromagnetic fields because of the inherent motion (tumbling) of its large magnetic moment. When the frequency components of these rapidly changing magnetic fields match the precessional frequency of the local protons, there is a resultant induction between energy spin states (that is, between parallel and antiparallel spin states), which shortens T1. In addition, the strong magnetic moment of the paramagnetic species creates more widely fluctuating magnetic fields that augment the loss of phase coherence of the proton spins, resulting in T2 shortening. In summary, paramagnetics produce shortening of both T1 and T2. Solomon (5) and Bloembergen (6) derived equations for the paramagnetic contribution to T1 and T2 relaxation times of a nucleus with spin ½ that have come to be known as the Solomon-Bloembergen equations:

$$\frac{1}{T_{1M}} = \frac{2}{15} \frac{S(S+1)\gamma^2 g^2 \beta^2}{r^6}$$

$$\times \left(\frac{3\tau_c}{1 + \omega_I^2 \tau_c^2} + \frac{7\tau_c}{1 + \omega_s^2 \tau_c^2} \right)$$

$$+ \frac{2}{3} \frac{S(S+1)A^2}{\hbar^2} \left(\frac{\tau_e}{1 + \omega_s^2 \tau_e^2} \right) \quad [1]$$

$$\frac{1}{T_{2M}} = \frac{1}{15} \frac{S(S+1)\gamma^2 g^2 \beta^2}{r^6}$$

$$\times \left(4\tau_c + \frac{3\tau_c}{1 + \omega_I^2 \tau_c^2} + \frac{13\tau_c}{1 + \omega_s^2 \tau_c^2} \right)$$

$$+ \frac{1}{3} \frac{S(S+1)A^2}{\hbar^2} \left(\tau_e + \frac{\tau_e}{1 + \omega_s^2 \tau_e^2} \right) \quad [2]$$

where S is the electron spin quantum number; g is the electronic g factor; β is the Bohr magneton; ω_I and ω_s ($=657 \omega_I$) are the Larmor angular precession frequencies for the nuclear spins and electron spins, respectively, r is the ion-nucleus distance; A is the hyperfine coupling constant; and τ_c and τ_e are the correlation times for the dipolar and scalar interactions, respectively. In both Eqs. 1 and 2, the first term represents the dipolar contribution to relaxation, and the second term defines the scalar component of relaxation.

Discussion of the correlation time τ_c in Eqs. 1 and 2 requires a knowledge of the nature of relaxation times. Again, classical description of relaxation in liquids says that relaxation is primarily governed by dipole-dipole interactions. Since clinical MRI is primarily concerned with protons in tissues that are composed primarily of water, this model is appropriate. To reiterate, the time required for relaxation of a system of protons is related to the probability for transition from the high-energy (antiparallel) nuclear spin state to the low-energy (parallel) spin level.

With respect to nuclear magnetization, the correlation time τ_c is an expression that relates the length of time that a nuclear magnetization is maintained in a given orientation with respect to the field causing relaxation. Stated otherwise, τ_c is the rate of fluctuations of magnetic fields that is produced by dipoles such as protons and paramagnetic species. These field fluctuations are caused by molecular motion, due to rotational, translational, and chemical exchange motion, or by fluctuation of the electron spin moment. The correlation time τ_c may be expressed in terms of multiple components as

$$1/\tau_c = 1/\tau_r + 1/\tau_s + 1/\tau_m$$

$$1/\tau_e = 1/\tau_s + 1/\tau_m$$

where τ_r is the rotational correlation time; τ_s is the electron spin relaxation time; and τ_m is the mean lifetime of a nucleus within the sphere of influence of a paramagnetic ion. The important points to glean from these expressions are that (a) the correlation time with lowest value will predominate over the contribution of others; (b) as the motions of nuclei decrease in speed, the correlation time gets larger; and (c) ions bound to macromolecules produce larger values of τ_r due to slowing of rotational motion, allowing larger contribution of τ_s and τ_m to relaxation. In terms of paramagnetic effects on relaxation, slowing of the rotational motion of the paramagnetic ion results in increased T1 shortening and increase in spin-echo imaging intensity. Such may be the case with binding of paramagnetic compounds to macromolecules, such as plasma proteins.

Finally, it is also important to consider the dipole-dipole term of the Solomon-Blombergen equations to note that the strength of this interaction between the paramagnetic ion and the nucleus is inversely proportional to the sixth power of the distance between them. In practical terms, this places some limitations on the size of the carrier molecule or ligand for a paramagnetic ion. It may be that an organ-specific paramagnetic contrast agent, such as a macromolecular protein-paramagnetic structure for perfusion assessment or a paramagnetically labeled monoclonal antibody, would produce less proton relaxation enhancement because of this limitation. Superimposed on this space limitation is the fact that PRE is proportional to the number of water molecules that are directly coordinated with the paramagnetic ion. The presence of a ligand or protein to which the ion is bound diminishes the relaxing ability of the ion because of displacement of water from the solution sphere. Because of the serious toxicity of many paramagnetic species, they must be chelated in order to facilitate excretion and diminished toxicity, and it is thus inevitable that the effectiveness of relaxation will diminish compared to that of the free ion.

The relaxation constants T1 and T2 may be expressed in terms of relaxation rates 1/T1 and 1/T2, respectively. With this expression it became easier to assess the contribution of paramagnetic ions to proton relaxation as follows:

$$1/T_{obs} = 1/T_d + 1/T_p$$

where $1/T_{obs}$ is the observed or measured relaxation rate; $1/T_d$ is the inherent tissue diamagnetic contribution to relaxation rate; and $1/T_p$ is the paramagnetic contribution to proton relaxation. The above expression is true for both T1 and T2 relaxation.

The magnitude of PRE is concentration dependent. As concentration increases, the magnitude of T1 and T2 relaxation rate enhancement (i.e., T1 and T2 shortening) increases. Clinically, approximately 0.1 to 1.0 mM concentrations of paramagnetic ions are required to produce visible alteration to signal intensity. With the heightened use of higher field strength units, it is noteworthy that paramagnetic substances exhibit field dependence and are more effective at low field strengths (8).

GADOLINIUM-DTPA

Gadolinium is a rare-earth series element that cannot be administered in ionic form because of serious toxicity. Acute toxicity includes hypotension, cardiovascular collapse, anticoagulation, and on a cellular level, includes fatty degeneration of hepatocytes, hepatic necrosis, and prolonged retention in the reticuloendothelial system (9). For this reason, gadolinium is chelated to facilitate excretion and to prevent binding to other chelates. The most promising chelate thus far has been diethylenetriaminepentaacetic acid (DTPA) because its formation constant, which is a measure of the strength of the affinity that a ligand has for a particular ion species (Gd-DTPA), is extremely high, approximately 10^{23}. The formation constant for Gd–ethylenediaminetetraacetic (EDTA), another chelate, is only 10^{17} and is thus less ideal than Gd-DTPA. Even though chelation occupies eight of the nine or ten coordination sites of gadolinium, access of local protons to gadolinium is sufficient for the complex to remain strongly paramagnetic.

It is well tolerated in biologic systems, with an LD_{50} of approximately 10 mmol/kg (11). Gadolinium-DTPA is excreted primarily by glomerular filtration, with a half-life of approximately 20 min (12). By 7 days after intravenous administration of Gd-DTPA, 90% of the dose has been recovered in the urine, 7% in feces, and less than 0.3% remains in the body in the liver (0.08%) and kidneys (0.1%). To facilitate water solubility, *N*-methylglucamine is added to Gd-DTPA. Presently, a dose of 0.1 mmol/kg is being administered to humans, which is 1/100 of the LD_{50} of Gd-DTPA.

Investigators have demonstrated utility for Gd–DTPA as an MRI contrast agent in numerous experimental models (11,13). It has proven useful for enhancement of renal function (11), myocardial perfusion (13), myocardial infarction (14), inflammatory lesions (11), abnormalities of the blood-brain barrier (BBB) (15), and tumor enhancement (16).

GADOLINIUM-DTPA IN THE CENTRAL NERVOUS SYSTEM

Magnetic resonance imaging of the central nervous system (CNS) has undoubtedly demonstrated excellent sensitivity for the detection of a variety of lesions (17). The need for contrast agents in MRI of the CNS stems from the somewhat limited specificity of MRI in differentiating abnormalities that increase the water content of the tissue and may or may not disrupt the BBB. Also, some CNS lesions are isointense relative to normal brain tissue on a limited number of pulse sequences.

Brasch and co-workers (3) used a prototype nitroxide spin label (NSL) called TES to enhance experimental lesions involving the BBB. NSLs are a group of strongly paramagnetic organic compounds that are characterized by a single unpaired electron. They are chemically stable over a broad range of pH and temperature and are chemically versatile. A potential drawback is that they are reduced to a nonparamagnetic species by ascorbic acid. In that study, dogs with experimentally induced cerebritis (streptococcal abscess) or radiation damage were imaged with MR before and after intravenous administration of 0.9 g/kg TES. TES produced significant T1 shortening and increased spin–echo signal intensity in all of the lesions studied. Grossman (18) studied enhancement of experimental brain abscess in a primate model and produced visible enhancement of the lesions with Gd-DTPA. Brasch (11) also demonstrated dramatic enhancement of radiation cerebritis using 0.5 mmol/kg Gd-DTPA in a canine model. These early experiments verified the use of Gd-DTPA to depict an active disruption of the BBB.

Preliminary investigation also demonstrated that Gd-DTPA may be useful for obtaining temporal physiological information about acute cerebral ischemia (16). We

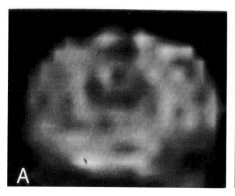 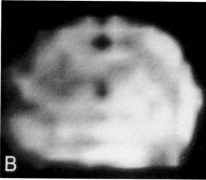 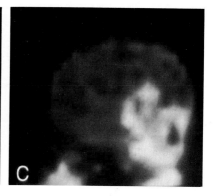

FIG. 1. Acute (24 hr) experimental infarct in a cat brain. **A:** TR = 500; TE = 28 msec (pre-contrast). **B:** TR = 2,000; TE = 56 msec. **C:** TR = 500; TE = 28 msec with Gd-DTPA (post-contrast). Note high intensity of left parietal temporal cortex seen on the T2-weighted image (**B**). Image 10 min postinjection of 0.2 mmol/kg Gd-DTPA demonstrates significant enhancement of left cerebral cortex and deep white matter on the T1-weighted image (**C**; compare to **A**) due to T1 shortening in region of BBB damage.

have administered 0.25 mmol/kg Gd-DTPA to cats that underwent middle cerebral arterial occlusion for variable periods of time. No enhancement occurred in infarcts that were less than 2 hr old. Infarcts aged 16 to 24 hr enhanced rapidly due to BBB breakdown, and infarcts aged 72 to 168 hr were characterized by delayed enhancement, presumably due to more pronounced vasogenic edema and diminished circulation (Fig. 1).

Carr et al. (19) reported their initial experience with 0.1 mmol/kg Gd-DTPA as an MRI contrast agent in 20 patients with cerebral tumors (12 patients), hepatic neoplasms (six patients), transitional cell carcinoma of the bladder (one patient), and hepatic cysts (one patient). Contrast enhancement was apparent in all of the neoplastic lesions. The CNS tumors demonstrated ring enhancement (seven patients), central enhancement (three patients), and patchy enhancement (two patients). All 12 of the tumors were identified with computed tomography (CT). In two cases, additional lesions were seen with MR that were not seen on CT; in one of these, small centrally enhanced lesions were seen bilaterally, and an additional cerebellar lesion was seen. Comparing the two modalities subjectively, the authors noted greater MR enhancement compared to CT in eight cases, equal enhancement in three cases, and less MRI enhancement in one case. The extent of tumors as evidenced by enhancement was greater on MRI in five cases, equal in three cases, and greater on CT in one case. In another report by Carr et al. (20) contrast enhancement of cerebral neoplasms was produced in 12 patients studied.

Clinical trials have been conducted at four medical institutions in the United States to assess the effects of Gd-DTPA on MR images of patients with suspected brain tumors (12,21). In more than 60 lesions in 27 patients by MRI in our institution, Gd-DTPA produced

definite enhancement in 33 (54%); however, on T2-weighted images acquired prior to contrast administration, 31 of the 33 enhancing lesions were readily identified. Therefore, routine MRI (T2 weighted) identified lesions both without and with an active breach of the BBB; however, Gd-DTPA-enhanced MRI (T1 weighted) showed only the lesions with an active BBB break.

The two lesions that were rendered visible by Gd-DTPA were small punctate metastatic foci in two patients that had multiple other intracranial metastases that were visible on precontrast T2-weighted images.

Overall, Gd-DTPA improved the ease of identification of eight lesions, which included the two metastases (Fig. 2) described above and six meningiomas (Fig. 3). Of note was the finding of disappearance (two lesions) or diminished visibility (two lesions) of lesions on post-Gd-DTPA T2-weighted images compared to precontrast T2-weighted images. This was in a patient with multiple sclerosis and was due to T2 shortening, which outweighed the T1 effect (Fig. 4).

The role of paramagnetic contrast agents such as Gd-DTPA has yet to be defined in MRI of the brain. Since most lesions induce an increase in the water content, they and the surrounding edema are easily detected on T2-weighted images unless the lesion is very small and the study suboptimal. However, a Gd-DTPA T1-weighted study will likely be utilized to help characterize the lesions identified on T2-weighted images. Thus, many patients with obvious pathology on routine MRI may undergo Gd-DTPA-enhanced studies; however, it must be remembered that not all lesions are enhanced by Gd-DTPA. Visualized enhancement of a lesion indicates a viable blood supply and an abnormal BBB. Thus, active breakdown of the BBB can be inferred when enhancement occurs. This helps to distinguish lesions that are recent and progressive and those that have an active

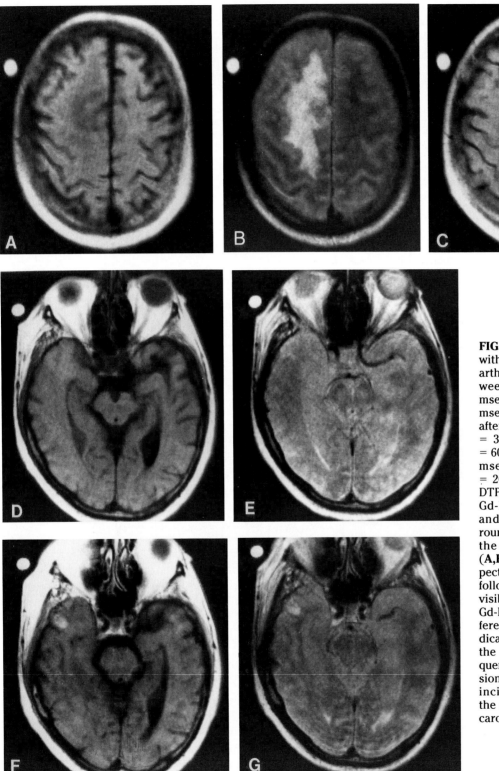

FIG. 2. Sixty-two-year-old man with left-arm weakness and dysarthria that progressed during 3 weeks. **A:** TR = 500; TE = 30 msec. **B:** TR = 2,000; TE = 60 msec. **C:** TR = 500; TE = 30 msec after Gd-DTPA. **D:** TR = 500; TE = 30 msec. **E:** TR = 2,000; TE = 60 msec. **F:** TR = 500; TE = 30 msec after Gd-DTPA. **G:** TR = 200; TE = 60 msec after Gd-DTPA. The lesion enhances with Gd-DTPA (**C**). Its localization and differentiation from surrounding edema are possible on the pre-Gd-DTPA sequences (**A,B**). Primary tumor was suspected. The temporal focus seen following Gd-DTPA (**F,G**) is not visible on the sequences before Gd-DTPA (**D,E**). Note slight differences of slice orientation indicating patient motion between the pre- and post-Gd-DTPA sequences. Biopsy of the large lesion found adenosarcoma. Note, incidentally, enhancement of the cavernous sinus but not the carotid arteries.

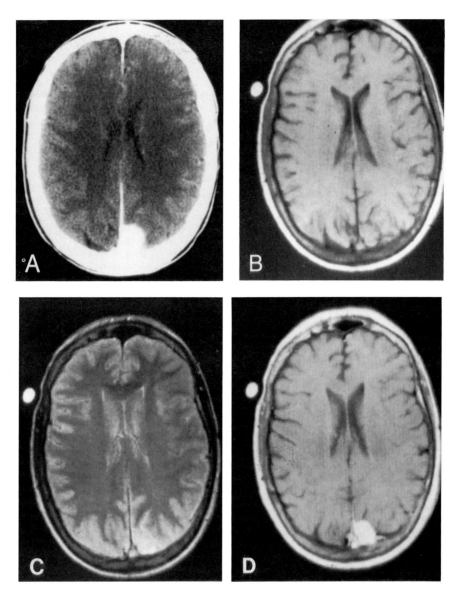

FIG. 3. Elderly woman studied for retinal ischemia. Incidental meningioma found on CT. **A:** Post contrast CT scan showing an en-plaque meningioma of the left occipital convexity with calvarial thickening. **B:** TR = 500; TE = 30 msec. **C:** TR = 2,000; TE = 60 msec. **D:** TR = 500; TE = 30 msec after Gd-DTPA. The nonenhanced images barely show the ill-defined meningioma, which is isointense to gray matter on the T1-weighted images and slightly hyperintense on the T2-weighted image (**B,C**). Obvious enhancement of the lesion is seen with Gd-DTPA. Note partial invasion of the dura around the sagittal sinus (**D**).

blood supply. This distinction may be especially important in elderly patients who often have high-intensity white-matter foci on T2-weighted images and in whom presence of a more active and serious process, such as metastases or stroke, is difficult to ascertain. The pattern of enhancement, albeit nonspecific, may help in localizing the focus of BBB breakdown within the lesion or surrounding edema and can also allow identification of liquifaction, necrosis, or cyst formation within a tumor.

Lack of enhancement in an active lesion may be due to lack of perfusion to the abnormality, insufficient BBB breakdown (Fig. 5), predominant T2 effect canceling the effect of T1 shortening or insufficient T1 shortening to overcome the initially prolonged T1 due to intrinsically long tumor relaxation characteristics and due to local edema.

Recently investigators have demonstrated that Gd-DTPA may also be useful in improving delineation of

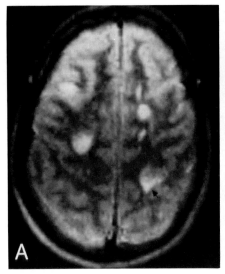

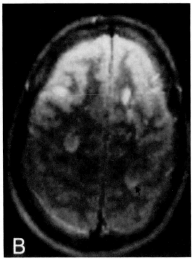

FIG. 4. Thirty-seven-year-old man with history of seminoma 4 years ago, recent decline in mental status, and focal neurologic exam. **A:** TR = 2,000; TE = 60 msec. **B:** TR = 2,000; TE = 60 msec after Gd-DTPA. Multiple foci of high intensity are consistent with the diagnosis of multiple sclerosis (**A;** *arrows*). Note that several of the lesions seen on the T2-weighted study fade or disappear after administration of Gd-DTPA (**B;** *arrows*).

FIG. 5. Forty-three-year-old man with AIDS and altered mental status. **A:** CT with contrast. Large low-density lesion in right hemisphere with central ring enhancement. **B:** TR = 500; TE = 30 msec. **C:** TR = 2,000; TE = 60 msec. **D:** TR = 500; TE = 30 msec following Gd-DTPA. The low-intensity lesion on the T1-weighted image (**B**) shows persistent low intensity within a larger region of high intensity on the T2-weighted image (**C**). Ring enhancement is produced by Gd-DTPA (**D**), analogous to the CT scan, both suggesting abscess in this region. A left hemispheric lesion is seen on the T2-weighted image (**C**) that was not seen in CT or on T1-weighted images before or after Gd-DTPA. Biopsy of the ring lesion revealed lymphoma on the right; toxoplasmosis was proven on the left.

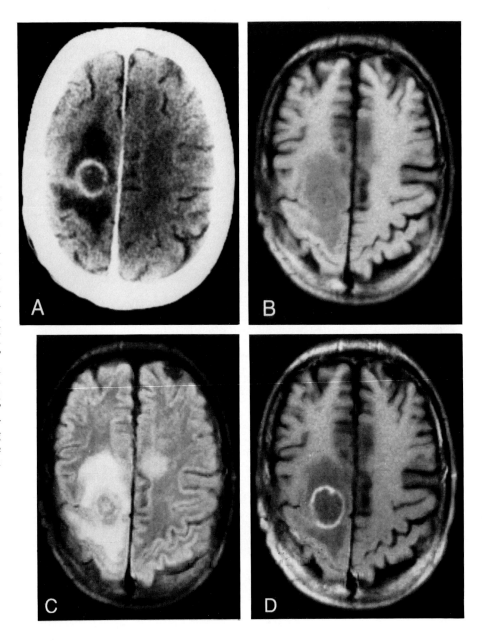

intraspinal tumors. Treisch et al. examined 9 patients with intramedullary spinal tumors, before and after intravenous injection of 0.1 mmol/kg of Gd-DTPA (22). Enhancement was noted in 8 of the 9 tumors and, compared to the precontrast T2-weighted images, improved tumor delineation was achieved in 5 patients, particularly in 2 patients with recurrent ependymomas adjacent to postsurgical scar tissue. Yoshikawa et al. found higher contrast between tumor and normal cord or brain stem tissue on post-Gd-DTPA T1-weighted images compared to precontrast T2-weighted images in 9 of 11 patients with intramedullary tumors (23). In both studies the extent of the lesions were better seen on MR images compared to CT, particularly following administration of Gd-DTPA. Thus, early results indicate that while nonenhanced T2-weighted MR images are sensitive for detecting intraspinal lesions, Gd-DTPA may be useful for improving the delineation of intramedullary tumors from normal tissue or from scar tissue with the potential added benefit of decreasing the examination time.

In summary, it appears that Gd-DTPA may produce contrast separation of tumors and other lesions from adjacent brain and spine tissues on T1-weighted images; however, the applicability of the preliminary findings to routine clinical MR is still premature. It may be that Gd-DTPA will be useful to define better the extent of BBB damage and also to identify lesions that are isointense on routine imaging sequences such as meningiomas. Our experience suggests that T2-weighted sequences will still be necessary to optimize sensitivity to detection of disease because they identify many more lesions that Gd-DTPA-enhanced T1-weighted images. Gd-DTPA may allow characterization of lesions that are first detected with T2-weighted sequences.

REFERENCES

1. Bloch F, Hansen W, Packard M. The nuclear induction experiment. *Physiol Rev* 1946;70:474.
2. Lauterbur PC, Mendoca-Dias M, Ruden AM. Segmentation of tissue water proton spin–lattice relaxation rates by the *in vivo* addition of paramagnetic ions. *In:* Dutton PO, Leigh JS, Scarpa A, eds. *Frontiers of biological energetics.* New York:Academic Press, 1978.
3. Brasch RC, Nitecki DE, Brant-Zawadzki M, et al. Brain nuclear magnetic resonance imaging enhanced by a paramagnetic contrast agent: preliminary report. *AJNR* 1983;4:1035–9.
4. McNamara MT, Ehman RL, Quay SC, et al. Alterations of MR tumor relaxation times using paramagnetic labelled monoclonal antibody [Abstr.]. 70th Scientific Assembly of the Radiological

Society of North America, Chicago, 1984. Easton, Pa.: Radiological Society of North America, p. 292.
5. Solomon I. Relaxation processes in a system of two spins. *Phys Rev* 1955;99:559.
6. Bloembergen N: Proton relaxation times in paramagnetic solutions. *J Chem Phys* 1957;27:572.
7. Reference deleted in proof.
8. Koenig SH, Brown RD III. Solvent nuclear magnetic relaxation dispersion (NMRD) in solutions of paramagnetic proteins: a critical analysis by example. In: Bertini I, and Drago RS, eds. *ESR and NMR of paramagnetic species in biological and related systems.* 89–115, 1979.
9. Arvela P: Toxicity of rare earths. *Prog Pharmacol* 1979;2:71–114.
10. Weinmann HJ, Brasch RC, Press WR, Wesbey GE. Characteristics of gadolinium-DTPA complex: a potential NMR contrast agent. *AJR* 1984;142:619–24.
11. Brasch RC, Weinmann HJ, Wesbey GE. Contrast-enhanced NMR imaging: animal studies using gadolinium-DTPA complex. *AJR* 1984;142:625–30.
12. Brant-Zawadzki M, Berry I, Osaki L, Brasch RC, Murovic J, Norman D. Gd-DTPA in clinical MR imaging of the brain—I: intraaxial lesions. *AJNR (in press).*
13. McNamara MT, Higgins CB, Ehman RL, Revel D, Sievers R, Brasch RC. MRI of acute myocardial ischemia: magnetic resonance contrast enhancement with gadolinium-DTPA. *Radiology* 1984;153:157–63.
14. Wesbey GE, McNamara MT, Higgins CB, et al. Effect of gadolinium-DTPA on the magnetic relaxation times of normal and infarcted myocardium. *Radiology* 1984;153:164–7.
15. McNamara MT, Brant-Zawadzki M, Berry I, Pereira B, Weinstein P, Derugin N, Moore S, Kucharczyk W, Brasch RC. Acute experimental cerebral ischemia: MRI enhancement using Gd-DTPA. *Radiology* 158:149–55.
16. McNamara MT, Epstein A, Williams B et al. Nonspecific tumor enhancement using paramagnetic contrast media [Abstr.]. 70th Scientific Assembly of the Radiological Society of North America, Chicago, 1984, p. 145.
17. Brant-Zawadzki M, Norman D, Newton TH, et al. Magnetic resonance imaging of the brain: the optimal screening technique: *Radiology* 1984;152:71–7.
18. Grossman RI, Wolf G, Biery D, et al. Gadolinium-enhanced nuclear magnetic resonance images of experimental brain abscess. *JCAT* 1984;8(2):204–7.
19. Carr DH, Brown J, Bydder GM, et al. Gadolinium-DTPA as a contrast agent of MRI: initial clinical experience in 20 patients. *AJR* 1984;143:215–24.
20. Carr DH, Brown J, Bydder GM, et al. Intravenous chelated gadolinium as a contrast agent in NMR imaging of cerebral tumors. *Lancet* 1984;1:484–6.
21. Berry I, Brant-Zawadzki M, Osaki L, Brasch RC, Holland B, Rosenblum S, McMurdo K, Norman D, Newton TH. Gadolinium-DTPA enhancement of intracranial lesions: quantitative aspects. Presented at Radiological Society of North America, Chicago, November 1985 *(in press).*
22. Treisch J, Claussen C, Massih M, Kornmesser W, Felix R. Intraspinal tumors in plain and Gd-DTPA-enhanced magnetic resonance imaging [Abstr.]. Book of Abstracts, Fifth Annual Meeting of the Society of Magnetic Resonance in Medicine, pp. 813–4. Montreal, Canada, August 19–22, 1986.
23. Yoshikawa K, Aoki K, Momose T, Okada Y, Minami M, Itoh M, Nishikawa J, Iio M. Gd-DTPA as contrast agent in MR imaging of spinal intramedullary tumors [Abstr.]. Book of Abstracts, Fifth Annual Meeting of the Society of Magnetic Resonance in Medicine, pp. 545–6. Montreal, Canada, August 19–22, 1986.

CHAPTER 7

Magnetic Resonance Spectroscopy: Principles and Potential Applications

Michael E. Moseley, Isabelle Berry, Wil M. Chew,
Michael Brant-Zawadzki, and Thomas L. James

Magnetic resonance imaging (MRI) has firmly established itself as a valuable clinical and research tool for the examination of the central nervous system. As discussed in Chapters 1 and 2, MRI functions by providing proton maps of the brain of submillimeter spatial resolution in two and three dimensions, does so non-invasively, and is without harmful radiation effects. The images are produced by purposeful alteration of the static external magnetic field (B_0), which bestows a distinct resonant frequency on the protons of the region sampled. This distinct frequency indicates the specific location of the protons within the three-dimensional space in which B_0 is modified. The intensity of the signal reflects the density of protons and limited aspects of their biochemical milieu. The potential importance of magnetic resonance spectroscopy (MRS) and its future clinical utility are related to its promise to provide spatial maps in which each imaging pixel (or voxel) can be opened to reveal a dossier of the biochemical processes taking place at a molecular level within that region in real time. MRS can, in short, provide the clinician with a rapid, multifaceted, noninvasive biochemical analysis within a region of interest.

The use of MRS to study *in vivo* processes is only as old as MRI technology and has developed at a similarly fast pace. Based on the initial observations that MRS could detect and follow phosphorus-31 (^{31}P) signals from metabolites in solution, studies of intact cell preparations allowed monitoring of important cellular events: metal ion binding, compartmentation, phosphoryl transfer kinetics, changes in metabolite concentrations as a function of time, and the rapid alterations of intra- and extracellular pH in a variety of normal and pathological states. Within the last 5 years, similar studies using carbon-13 (^{13}C), proton (^{1}H), and sodium-23 (^{23}Na) MRS have been done in intact live animals, by placing special magnetic resonance radiofrequency (RF) coils ("surface coils") directly over the region of interest. Recently, several books and numerous review articles have appeared which describe MRS at length and chronicle the evolution of this technique (1,2). Within the last year, the feasibility of using MRS in humans has been demonstrated with surface coils, and ^{31}P, ^{1}H, and ^{13}C spectra have been obtained. The human applications of MRS have come about through the evolution of magnet technology. As the magnetic field strengths and the available bore space have increased, a major effort to improve the homogeneity of the magnetic field has been made, since MRS requires a magnetic field at least five times higher and 50 times more uniform than that needed for routine MRI. Larger, 100 cm bores in clinical magnets with fields of 1.5 to 2.2 tesla (T) suitable for MRS are now being delivered, and allow MRI and MRS studies to be feasible on the same patient at the same time. As the MRI and MRS techniques develop, their distinctions will begin to blur and may eventually disappear; true "biochemical metabolite imaging" and "volume-defined spectroscopy" are the goals we expect to be realized in the clinical area.

BASIC PRINCIPLES

Foundations of nuclear magnetic resonance (NMR) have been set down in the last three decades. Clinical feasibility of NMR has led to the use of the terms MRI, for imaging, and MRS, which is the implied use of NMR for *in vivo* spectroscopy. This terminology emphasizes the fundamental similarity of the two methods: the basic ideas of MRS are essentially those of NMR and an in-depth treatment of NMR in general, and in biochemistry in particular, has been published (3)

In essence, MRI is a sophisticated refinement of MRS with one major difference between the two. In MRI, the

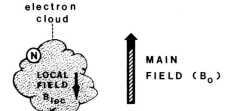

FIG. 1. Depiction of how the local electron distributions in a molecule produce a local field ($\mathbf{B}_{loc}$) which alters the main magnetic field ($\mathbf{B}_0$), yielding an effective field ($\mathbf{B}_{eff}$) "felt" by the nucleus in question (N).

$$B_{eff} = B_0 - B_{loc}$$

operator knowingly changes the homogeneity of the external magnetic field in a relatively gross but predetermined pattern in order to effect a change in the resonant frequency of the nuclei being sampled, that change providing spatial localization of the particular nucleus. In MRS, a very homogenous field, $\mathbf{B}_0$, is created in a region of interest. Any deviation from the expected resonant frequency for a nucleus must reflect microenvironmental field gradients induced by the chemistry of the tissue (Fig. 1). These subtle gradients are created by the grouping of electrons (electron cloud) around various nuclei in the molecule within which the target nucleus resides. This nucleus then "sees" and resonates in response to this local, slightly altered magnetic field (effective $\mathbf{B}$ or $\mathbf{B}_e$) when compared to the $\mathbf{B}_0$ set up by the instrument. By measuring this change in resonant frequency we can determine the type of molecule in which the nucleus is bound, and even the various positions of the given nucleus within the *same* molecule, because the electron clouds will vary from place to place (Fig. 2).

A nucleus of phosphorus, hydrogen, or carbon, for example, will absorb RF energy and "resonate" when placed in a magnetic field of strength $\mathbf{B}_0$ and irradiated with a certain RF:

$$\nu = \delta \mathbf{B}_e / 2\pi \qquad [1]$$

where δ is the gyromagnetic ratio inherent for the nucleus being studied, and $\mathbf{B}_e$ is the "effective" or resulting magnetic field strength. For MRI, consider two tubes of water in a field $\mathbf{B}_0$ modified by the purposeful introduction of a magnetic field gradient of strength $\Delta \mathbf{B}_0$. The values of $\mathbf{B}_e$ which determine hydrogen resonance in the two tubes will be $\mathbf{B}_0 + \Delta \mathbf{B}_0$ and $\mathbf{B}_0 - \Delta \mathbf{B}_0$ for the tubes in

the stronger and weaker fields, respectively. Thus two "resonances" will be observed, and the location of each tube along the predetermined gradient is easily determined, allowing localization. In MRI the created $\mathbf{B}_0$ differences are of the order of 10^{-4} T. In MRS, however, these differences are much smaller (hence the much greater need for homogenous fields!) and, as discussed above, created by the inherent atomic environment surrounding the nucleus.

For MRS, consider the three phosphorus nuclei in a molecule (or molecules) of ATP within a homogenous ($\mathbf{B}_0$) region of interest. Since each nucleus is in a slightly different molecular environment, the $\mathbf{B}_e$ values for each nucleus will be slightly different and three separate resonant frequencies will be observed from the region studied, based on Eq. 1. The frequency differences between the resonances can be accurately measured in an NMR or MRS spectrometer and are termed "chemical shifts" relative to some external or internal reference of the phosphorus nucleus. Having a reference is a practical way of being more accurate, and of measuring differences in resonant frequencies instead of absolute values. (Differences are in the range of hertz, whereas frequencies are in the range of megahertz.) These differences in frequencies are dependent on the spectrometer field; relating the measurement to the basic frequency of the spectrometer for that nucleus allows us to compare data from different spectrometers. Inherent chemical shifts for the same nuclei in different locations can be denoted in a dimensionless ratio of "parts per million" (ppm) according to the equation

$$\gamma = \frac{(\nu_R - \nu_S) \times 10^6}{\nu_I} \qquad [2]$$

FIG. 2. Electron "clouds" give rise to small changes in the magnetic field in the region of the molecule. These small changes result in separate resonances for each hydrogen nucleus which depend on location within the molecule.

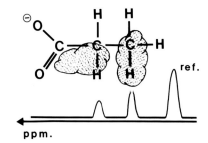

where ν_S, ν_R and ν_I are the sample frequency, the reference frequency, and the normal instrument frequency, respectively, for the nuclear species being studied. Because the field strength of the instrument (B_0) determines ν_I, using Eq. 2 to determine chemical shift in terms of parts per million allows comparison of results at different field strengths, since the units of frequency cancel out.

THE ^{31}P SPECTRUM

The general characteristics of a hypothetical ^{31}P spectrum are shown in Fig. 3. The different resonant frequencies of the various ^{31}P nuclei are shown as chemical shifts relative to the internal reference (at 0 ppm) of phosphocreatine (PCr, peak C) distributed along the horizontal axis. The spectrum shown is typical of ^{31}P spectra *in vivo* and is comprised of the separate resonant signals from several molecules. From left to right in Fig. 3, separate signals are recorded from simple sugar phosphates (fructose-6-phosphate), for example, (peaks A), inorganic or "waste" phosphates (peak B), phosphocreatine (peak C), and the three different ^{31}P nuclei in adenosine triphosphate (ATP). The "peak area," as shown in Fig. 3, is directly proportional to the number of nuclei contributing to the signal. Thus, if the number of phosphocreatine ^{31}P nuclei in the sample is known, the relative peak areas can be used to derive absolute concentrations of the metabolites in the sample being observed.

The splitting evident in several of the peaks is a consequence of "spin–spin coupling." In addition to the local fields caused by its surrounding electrons, a nucleus also experiences even smaller, local fields produced by the presence of other nuclei in the vicinity. The mutual interaction between nuclei is called spin–spin coupling, and leads to the splitting of each population into subsets of slightly different resonant frequencies. In contrast to the chemical shift, the spin–spin coupling is not a function of the applied field and reflects only the

extent of the influence of a nearby nucleus. This is mainly expressed through the chemical bonds: therefore, the spin–spin coupling can be used to derive important information about the conformation of the molecules. For *in vivo* spectra, the peaks are often quite broad and this splitting is not observed.

Another important consideration in MRS is the "linewidth" ($W_{1/2}$) of the metabolite signal. The linewidth is a measure of the spin–spin relaxation time (T_2). As in MRI, some magnetic field inhomogeneity inherent in the instrument is inescapable and affects T_2. This increases the linewidth of the signal peaks. Thus, for MRS it is essential that the field be as homogeneous as possible in order to (1) decrease the linewidth to its inherent T_2 dependence and thus (2) better resolve the signal peaks in the spectrum. It is for this reason of improving the field homogeneity for best resolution that MRS magnets are equipped with "shim" coils (similar to gradient coils) which can modify the main static field B_0 to its maximum homogeneity in the region of the sample.

In MRS, as in MRI, perhaps the most important consideration is that of the signal-to-noise ratio. From Fig. 3, the signal-to-noise ratio (S/N), can be seen to be defined as the "amplitude" of the signal to that of the noise in the base line. The S/N can be improved by (1) increasing the field strength of the magnet, (2) improving or maximizing RF coil characteristics (usually by decreasing the noise picked up throughout the system), and (3) signal averaging of many identical transients (excitations) where S/N increases by $\sqrt{N}$, with N being the number of transients collected in an experiment.

ACQUIRING A SPECTRUM

A typical protocol for acquiring an *in vivo* chemical shift spectrum (as in Fig. 3) would consist of first exciting the sample with a short (10–100 μsec) pulse of RF power (100–1,000 W) through a surface coil, then turning off the RF transmitter and receiving the resulting RF

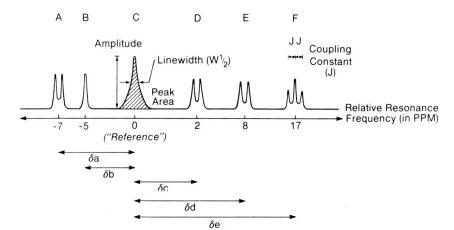

FIG. 3. Hypothetical ^{31}P spectrum showing approximate resonance frequencies of ^{31}P nuclei (in parts per million from phosphocreatine reference, see text). From left to right (peaks A–F), resonances arise from (a) sugar phosphates (SP), (b) inorganic phosphates (Pi), (c) phosphocreatine (PCr), (d) γ-adenosine triphosphate (γ-ATP), (e) α-ATP, (f) β-ATP.

signal from the sample. This signal is the so-called "free induction decay" (FID). The procedure of RF excitation and reception can be repeated *N* times, letting the computer sum the individual FIDs. Fourier transformation of the averaged sum of the FIDs yields the characteristic frequency versus amplitude spectrum (Fig. 3). To acquire a ^{31}P spectrum *in vivo,* the time required varies from 0.5 to 20 min, depending on the S/N desired, the sizes of the sample and the coil, and the magnetic field strength.

IMPORTANT NUCLEI FOR MRS

Table 1 lists those nuclei most useful for MRS experiments in order of decreasing relative sensitivity. The relative sensitivity of an isotope for NMR is the product of its natural abundance and its ability to resonate. It dictates the intensity of the signal produced when submitted to the NMR equipment. The overwhelming popularity of proton NMR is clear from its sensitivity. Though protons of water are by far the most easily observed *in vivo,* which is ideal for proton MRI, their signal overwhelms that from protons in other molecules and presents problems for the observation of other proton-bearing species such as lactate. One must also consider the density of the nuclei *in vivo;* for example, fluorine is rarely found in large concentrations *in vivo,* but is extremely useful as a MRS "tag" for tracer studies, using perfluorinated blood substitutes or fluorinated sugars, for example. Table 1 also explains why multinuclear imaging (^{31}P imaging, for example) has not become widely used. However, the biochemical information obtainable from the less sensitive nuclei, such as ^{31}P, makes the extra effort to observe them with magnetic resonance worthwhile.

^{31}P MRS

Despite the high sensitivity of protons relative to ^{31}P nuclei, most MRS studies have focused on phosphorus, in that a number of metabolites are present *in vivo* in the

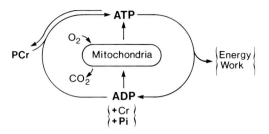

FIG. 4. ATP is a molecule which is a carrier of energy within the cell. By splitting off the last phosphate the cell can release energy for useful work, yielding ADP and inorganic phosphates. A supply of oxygen and glucose catabolites is needed in the mitochondria so that the electron transport chain can generate the high energy intermediates needed to restore ATP from ADP +Pi. In some organs, in emergency situations, e.g., lack of oxygen, ADP can be coupled with a high energy phosphate group donated by phosphocreatine (a high energy phosphate storehouse) to restore some ATP.

millimolar concentration range needed for convenient observation via MRS. Several of these metabolites are described in Fig. 3, and give sharp signals of narrow linewidths sufficient for adequate spectral resolution. The metabolites observed in a ^{31}P spectrum present an almost ideal picture or "dossier" of the real-time processes of energy metabolism taking place *in vivo.* Further, the relative ratios of the metabolites can be used as "fingerprints" for identifying different organs, tissues, disease states, and even aging. The interested reader is again referred to the literature (1,2,4–6) for further detail. Figure 4 quickly gives an idea of the roles played in cellular function by the metabolites amenable to examination using MRS. The ^{31}P spectrum, in effect, "freezes" the biochemical equilibrium in time.

Other useful information can be gleaned from the ^{31}P *in vivo* spectrum. From Fig. 3, the chemical shift of the inorganic phosphate peak changes with pH (up to 2.3 ppm), as this molecular species gives up or takes on an extra proton, thus changing the local magnetic field (and hence, resonant frequency) for the phosphorus nuclei. The chemical shift difference between the inorganic phosphate peak and the "reference" phosphocreatine peak (which does not change position) can be used to determine the pH. If the pH in the cell decreases, inorganic phosphates take on a proton, and the phosphorus nuclei resonate more closely in frequency to those of PCr.

The shift in the inorganic phosphate peak with pH allows for compartmentation studies, too. Biologic compartments are entities separated by semipermeable membranes. This definition includes macroscopic compartments (e.g., CSF spaces) as compared to intravascular space, as well as extracellular space as opposed to intracellular space. The distinction between extra- and intracellular molecules, difficult to assess by direct mea-

TABLE 1. *Properties of selected nuclei studied by MRS*

Nucleus	Natural abundance (%)	Relative sensitivity for same number of nuclei at constant field strength (% relative to ^{1}H)
^{1}H	99.98	100.0
^{19}F	100.00	83.3
^{23}Na	100.00	9.25
^{31}P	100.00	6.63
^{13}C	1.108	1.59
^{15}N	0.365	0.104
^{39}K	93.1	0.051

Reproduced from James (3).

surements, can benefit from NMR because intracellular and extracellular subsets of the same component do not have the same resonant frequency (7).

Further, the chemical shift of the β-ATP nuclei (peak F in Fig. 3) can vary, depending on metal ion binding. Finally, the rates of bioenergetic reactions *in vivo* can be measured noninvasively by the use of ^{31}P phosphoryl transfer experiments in which one peak in the ^{31}P spectrum is selectively excited, after which changes in the other peaks are monitored (8). From these changes, as well as knowledge of the spin–lattice relaxation time (T_1) of the nuclei involved, the unidirectional rate constants for the forward or reverse phosphoryl transfer reaction can be determined. In this manner, sophisticated studies of enzyme kinetics and their abnormalities can be obtained.

Given the wealth of information regarding biochemical processes which MRS may elucidate, the efforts aimed at developing this technology for clinical use become understandable. The actual value of clinical MRS must now be determined pragmatically.

MRS AND BRAIN INJURY

As was the case with MRI, much of the initial study of the application of ^{31}P MRS has been done on the brain. As the magnet technology has matured, homogeneous magnets of wider bore have become available for large animal and human brain research (9,10). Indeed, manufacturers now offer magnets of 33 to 100 cm bore with fields from 2.0 to 4.7 T in complete systems that provide MRI and MRS capabilities within the same system. Using a magnet with a 33 cm bore, we are investigating hemispheric brain injury models in larger animals at 2.0 T, in which proton MRI is correlated with ^{31}P and proton MRS. To do this, two surface coils are placed side by side over each hemisphere in the brain of the cat, for example (Fig. 5); each coil is tunable to ^{31}P and proton frequencies (35 and 86 MHz, respectively). When

placed over the brain hemisphere, the surface coil "sees" tissue under the coil to a depth of approximately one radius (1.5 cm). The RF pulses are applied in sequences to minimize the response from tissues just below the coil, termed "depth pulse sequences" (11). This helps to localize the signal received by the coil to a region within the brain.

Figure 6 depicts the changes in brain ^{31}P metabolism occurring over a period of 12 hr following a middle cerebral artery occlusion (MCAO) of the right hemisphere. The bottommost spectra from the left and right hemispheres (Fig. 6A), taken before occlusion, show normal metabolism. Brain spectra from larger animals and humans contain a peak (Fig. 6A, third peak from the left) which is a result of the presence of phosphodiesters in the brain. One hour after occlusion, several changes are noted: (1) the "storehouse" of phosphate groups for energy metabolism, PCr, has begun to disappear; (2) the inorganic phosphate signal has shifted toward PCr, denoting a decrease in intracellular pH; (3) there is a simultaneous increase in inorganic phosphate concentration. These changes are the hallmarks which indicate the depletion of substances needed for energy metabolism and are a harbinger of cellular injury. After this time, the ATP resonances will disappear as the mitochondria shut down, and PCr is depleted as the cells begin to die. At this point, the animal shows definite deficits in neurologic functions. If the injury can be quickly reversed, the animal can sometimes recover. After 12 hr, the right hemisphere shows only inorganic phosphate; it is essentially dead and will not recover fully. The left, unoccluded hemisphere appears to be normal throughout the occlusion.

OTHER NUCLEI IN BRAIN MRS

The biochemical information given in Figs. 3, 4, and 6 explains the popularity and utility of ^{31}P MRS. In addition, ^{1}H and ^{13}C MRS are also finding use in studies

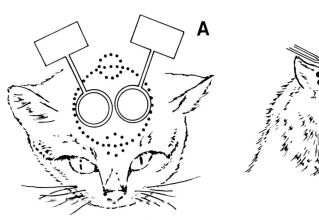

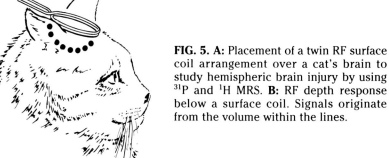

FIG. 5. A: Placement of a twin RF surface coil arrangement over a cat's brain to study hemispheric brain injury by using ^{31}P and ^{1}H MRS. **B:** RF depth response below a surface coil. Signals originate from the volume within the lines.

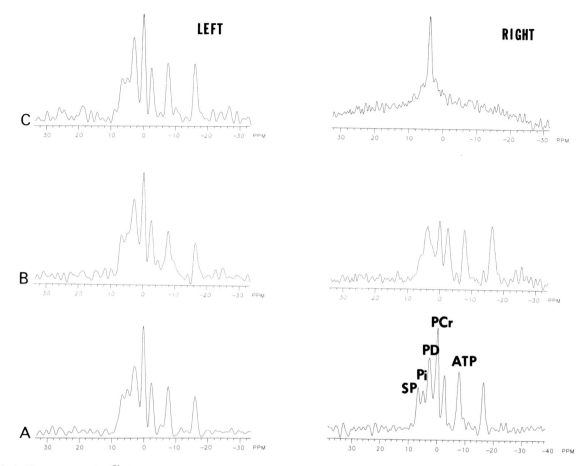

FIG. 6. A: Phosphorus-31 (^{31}P) spectra (34.6 MHz) from left and right hemispheres of a cat's brain using coil arrangement in Fig. 3. Spectra are taken prior to MCAO. Each spectrum results from signal averaging of 128 free induction decays with a pulse repetition rate of 2.5 sec. The peaks are **left** to **right**: sugar phosphates (SP), inorganic phosphates (PI), phosphodiesters (PD), phosphocreatine (PCr), and γ-, α- and β-ATP. **B:** Left and right hemispheric spectra 1 hr following occlusion. **C:** Left and right spectra 12 hr after occlusion. The right, injured hemisphere is essentially dead.

of brain metabolism and brain injury. Carbon is present in the brain in sufficient concentration, but the relative insensitivity of the ^{13}C nucleus (Table 1) at 1% isotope abundance makes observation difficult. Nonetheless, ^{13}C MRS has been demonstrated. Figure 7 shows a ^{13}C spectrum of a rat brain at a field strength B_0 of 5.6 T. The methylene (–CH$_2$–) signal from brain lipids and proteins is the most observable. Future studies could be based on various enriched ^{13}C tracers introduced into the carbohydrate substances of the brain. In this manner, alterations of carbohydrate metabolism could help elucidate various mechanisms of disease processes within this organ.

Proton spectra are dominated by an immense water peak which is 10,000 times stronger than proton signals from other observable proton-containing metabolites, such as lactate, *N*-acetylaspartate, and glutamate. The sheer size of the water peak "drowns" out the other peaks, reducing their amplitudes to the level of noise. Techniques are available to "suppress" the water signal, revealing the other signals with sufficient signal-to-noise ratio. Further, by employing RF coils that can excite and

observe ^{31}P and protons, both types of nuclei can be used to study brain injury from complementing spectra. Such a method is used in animal models to monitor ^{31}P

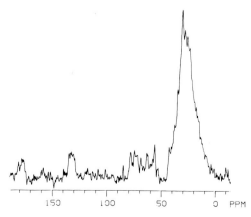

FIG. 7. Carbon-13 (^{13}C) MRS spectrum of *in vivo* rat brain at 5.6 T, after infusion of universally ^{13}C-labeled glucose (20 atom%). Spectrum is comprised of 1,000 scans (total time = 13.4 min). Large peak at 30 ppm is that of (–CH$_2$–)$_n$ lipid carbon nuclei.

NORMAL LEFT SIDE

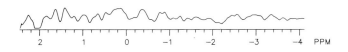

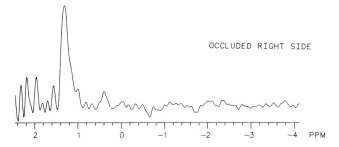

OCCLUDED RIGHT SIDE

FIG. 8. Proton MRS at 2.0 T with dual surface coil design (Fig. 5) showing lactate (at 1.3 ppm) accumulation in brain 12 hr after MCAO (obtained simultaneously with the ^{31}P results in Fig. 6). Normal brain tissue contains no observable lactate, whereas injured or recently dead tissue shows lactate accumulation.

and protons at the same time. Figure 8 shows lactate accumulation in the two hemispheres in the same animal whose ^{31}P spectrum was shown in Fig. 6, about 12 hr after the original MCAO. The injured hemisphere shows lactate accumulation, as evidenced by the presence of a peak observable at 1.3 ppm, whereas the normal contralateral side shows no observable lactate concentrations.

PRESENT STATUS AND FUTURE OF MRS

At present, MRI can produce *in vivo* [1]H (water proton!), ^{19}F and [23]Na images, because of the relative sensitivity and presence of a dominant single-frequency peak. A desirable technique for the future would be ^{31}P MRI, despite its low sensitivity and the presence of several ^{31}P peaks. Although it is possible to produce a ^{31}P image by exciting only one ^{31}P species using its specific resonance frequency in the spectrum, the low S/N would require many acquisitions to produce the image. At this point, it is conceivable that future techniques will allow this problem to be overcome for clinical use. If so, a metabolic map could be obtained, for example, of the biochemical evolution of inorganic phosphate in injured brain regions. Images could then be obtained of other metabolites in the same fashion, by using either ^{31}P nuclei associated with ATP or protons associated with lactate.

Such multinuclear metabolic or functional imaging techniques require the initial use of field gradients which can slice or select out a defined region in one dimension, so that MRS spectra may be obtained from such a localized sample (12). This has already been advanced to a stage at which we can define three-dimensional cubes (voxels) in phantoms (13). Future refinement will allow MRS to be done in a well-defined volume in humans using the new generation of high-field imaging spectrometers.

Finally, the two approaches can be combined to produce a three- or four-dimensional data array in which two or three dimensions of the data matrix will define the spatial image as in MRI currently. The final dimension would then be a one-dimensional chemical shift spectrum of a desired nucleus.

Whichever technique develops further with time, it is clear that the future of MRI and MRS will involve their convergence, which will blur the distinction between them and thus produce clinical tools of unprecedented and enormous utility.

REFERENCES

1. James TL, Margulis AR, eds. *Biomedical magnetic resonance.* San Francisco: Radiology Research and Education Foundation, 1984.
2. Gadian DG. *Nuclear magnetic resonance and its applications to living sysems.* Oxford: Oxford University Press, 1982.
3. James TL. *Nuclear magnetic resonance in biochemistry.* New York: Academic Press, 1975.
4. Shaw D. *In vivo* chemistry with NMR. In: Kaufman L, Crooks L, Margulis AR, eds. *Nuclear magnetic resonance imaging in medicine,* New York: Igaku-Shoin, 1982:147–85.
5. Shulman RG. NMR spectroscopy of living cells. *Sci Am* 1983;248:86–97.
6. Burt CB, Koutcher JA. Multinuclear NMR studies of naturally occurring nuclei. *J Nucl Med* 1984;25:237–48.
7. Seeley PJ, Busby SJW, Gadian DG. A new approach to metabolite compartmentation in muscle. *Biochem Soc Trans* 1976;4:62–6.
8. Koretsky AP, Weiner MW. Phosphorus-31 nuclear magnetic resonance magnetization transfer measurement of exchange reactions *in vivo.* In: James TL, Margulis AR, eds. *Biomedical magnetic resonance,* San Francisco: Radiology Research and Education Foundation, 1984:209–31.
9. Hilberman M, Subramanian VH, Haselgrove J, et al. *In vivo* time-resolved brain phosphorus nuclear magnetic resonance. *J Cerebral Blood Flow Metab* 1984;4:334–42.
10. Brindle KM, Smith MB, Rajngopalan B, et al. Spectral editing in P-31 NMR spectra of the human brain. *J Magn Reson* 1985;61:559–63.
11. Bendall MR. Surface coils and depth resolution using the spatial variation of the radiofrequency field. In: James TL, Margulis AR, eds. *Biomedical magnetic resonance,* San Francisco: Radiology Research and Education Foundation, 1984:99–127.
12. Bottomley P, Foster T, Darrow R. Depth-resolved surface coil spectroscopy (DRESS) for *in vivo* H-1, P-31 and C-13 NMR. *J Magn Reson* 1984;59:338–42.
13. Muller S, Aue WP, Seelig J. NMR imaging and volume selective spectroscopy with a single surface coil. *J Magn Reson* 1985;63:530–43.

CHAPTER 8

Functional Neuroanatomy by Magnetic Resonance Imaging

Jack DeGroot

CONTROL OF MOTOR FUNCTION

Pyramidal System (Corticospinal and Corticobulbar Tract)

The pyramidal or voluntary motor system begins in the frontoparietal region of the cerebral cortex around the central sulcus. The precentral gyrus (cortical area 4), the premotor gyrus (area 6), and the postcentral gyrus (areas 3, 1, and 2), all contribute to the formation of the descending corticospinal and corticobulbar systems.

There is an orderly organization of the cortical areas from which these tracts arise: Leg muscles are represented at the top of the hemisphere, head muscles near the lateral fissure, and other body regions are represented in between. This representation is maintained throughout, from motor cortex to the white matter of the corona radiata, internal capsule (posterior limb), cerebral peduncle, pons, and medulla into the spinal cord for the corticospinal (pyramidal) tract (Figs. 1–19, bold arrows). The corticobulbar fibers from the cortical face region end in the motor nuclei of the brainstem, which give rise to the motor components of cranial nerves.

Most fibers of the corticospinal tract cross just before descending into the lateral column of the spinal cord; the remaining fibers stay on the same side until they reach the segment of destination, where they then decussate. Secondary fibers of the motor system arise in the spinal cord gray matter as peripheral (motor) nerves to supply the muscles of the extremities and the body. Lesions limited to the corticospinal tract itself may lead to a flaccid paralysis with reduced deep tendon reflexes. However, spinal cord lesions of the corticospinal tract usually involve, in addition, other descending tracts that modify gross motor function automatically (rubrospinal, reticulospinal); the result then is a spastic paralysis with increased and abnormal reflexes ("upper motor neuron lesion"). Interruption of the peripheral motor fibers leads to flaccid paralysis with reduced or absent reflexes ("lower motor neuron lesion").

Basal Ganglia (Extrapyramidal System)

The basal ganglia are deep gray-matter nuclei that are interconnected with extensive cortical regions as well as parts of the thalamus. This system of so-called extrapyramidal fiber tracts and gray-matter areas exerts an influence on the motor cells of the spinal cord that is not under volitional control, in contrast to the corticospinal system.

A list of the major components includes the caudate nucleus (C), putamen (P; together with the caudate nucleus referred to as striatum), the globus pallidus (G), the claustrum and the subthalamic nucleus (not shown), the red nucleus (R), and the substantia nigra (S); the putamen and globus pallidus are sometimes referred to as the lentiform nucleus (Figs. 2–6 and 12–17).

There are extensive interconnections among many individual components of this system; one pathway is from the cerebral cortex to the caudate nucleus, from where connections travel to the putamen and the globus pallidus. Some fibers then loop back to the thalamus (T) and hence feed back to the cerebral cortex, whereas others descend to the subthalamic and red nuclei as well as the substantia nigra. From here, descending pathways reach the motor cells of the anterior spinal cord. There is a cerebellar outflow that similarly reaches the red nucleus and the ventral thalamus, so that the extrapyramidal system is also influenced by cerebellar function.

Lesions in individual nuclei of the basal ganglia system may interrupt one or more of these pathways, thus leading to forms of motion disorder (dyskinesis). Athetosis may be caused by lesions in several areas; the cau-

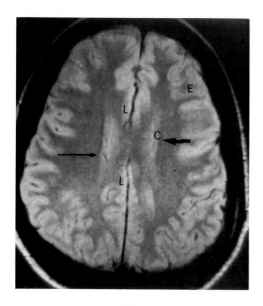

FIG. 1

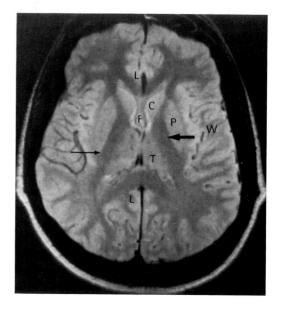

FIG. 3

date nucleus is related to chorea, the subthalamic nucleus to ballismus, the substantia nigra to parkinsonism.

Cerebellum

The cerebellum is involved in the coordination of primitive movements concerned with maintenance of position (archicerebellum); fine movements, especially in the extremities (neocerebellum); and propulsive, automatic movements, such as walking, running, or swimming (paleocerebellum). The cerebellar cortex can thus be divided in the flocculus and nodule of the vermis, which are the "oldest" part, whereas the anterior

lobe and posterior vermis are considered to be paleocerebellar cortex. The neocerebellar cortex extends over all other cerebellar regions (Figs. 6–11 and 19).

These various functions of the cerebellum are reflected by their incoming signals; the vestibular nerve and nuclei (via the inferior cerebellar peduncle) project to the archicerebellum. Extensive cerebral cortical regions in the frontoparietal and temporal lobes project to the pontine nuclei, from where fibers cross via the large middle cerebellar peduncles (M) to the neocerebellar cortex. The spinal cord and lower brainstem influence the paleocerebellum via the inferior cerebellar peduncle (I). The outflow from the cerebellum is mainly by way of

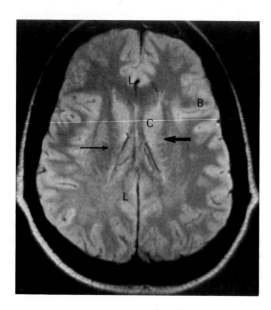

FIG. 2

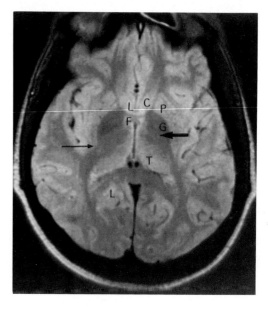

FIG. 4

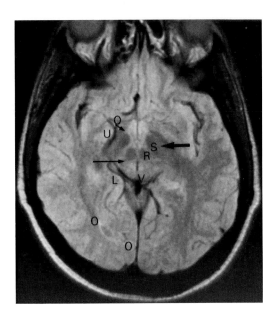

FIG. 5

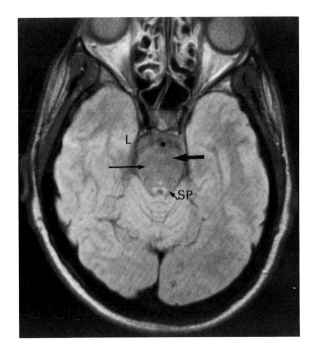

FIG. 7

the dentate nucleus and the superior cerebellar peduncles (SP), ending in the contralateral red nuclei (R) and ventral thalamus (T). From these relay stations, fibers descend to the contralateral spinal cord, or go back to the cerebral cortex and extrapyramidal system.

Neocerebellar lesions result in loss of fine coordination of muscle movements: repetitive opposite movements can no longer be executed quickly or correctly (adiodochokinesis); target-directed movements are performed poorly (dysmetria, and intention tremor); and there is general hypotonia of the muscles. Disturbances

of position and truncal ataxia, resembling drunkenness, result from lesions in the archicerebellum or the paleocerebellum or their afferent pathways.

Control of Eye Movements

Whereas each eye muscle is innervated by a single cranial nerve, the coordination of movements of both

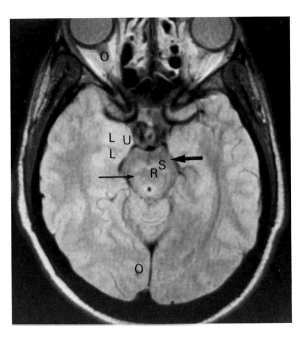

FIG. 6

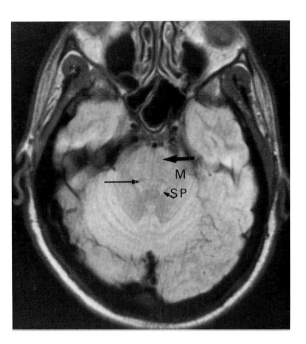

FIG. 8

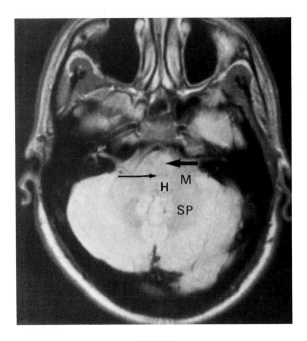

FIG. 9

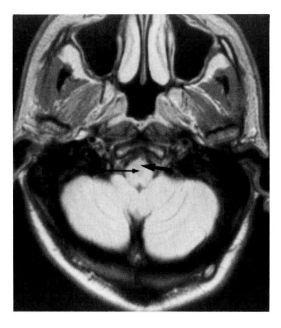

FIG. 11

eyes together (conjugate gaze) is more complex. A cerebral cortical eye field (area 8, E) is located in the middle frontal gyrus; this area coordinates movements of both eyes together (Figs. 1 and 13). Cortical areas in the occipital lobes (area 17) not only are the terminal projection area for visual stimuli from the retinae, but are involved with the smooth pursuit of moving objects in the visual fields. Both cortical regions connect to the so-called pretectal region, the superior colliculi, and other midbrain areas. Lesions in this pretectal area may

impair the conjugate vertical gaze movements (Parinaud syndrome; V in Figs. 5 and 18).

The nuclei of the oculomotor (III) and the trochlear (IV) lie in the midbrain, the abducens nuclei (VI) in the pontine tegmentum just under the fourth ventricle. These nuclei, as well as the vestibular complex, are interconnected on each side by the medial longitudinal fasciculus (MLF). A conjugate lateral gaze center is located in the paramedian pontine reticular formation. Lesions in this region disrupt contralateral lateral (horizontal) gaze movements, whereas interruption of the MLF alone (e.g., by a multiple sclerosis plaque) leads to a so-called internuclear ophthalmoplegia, in which lateral gaze movements are disrupted while abduction is still possible (H in Figs. 9 and 19).

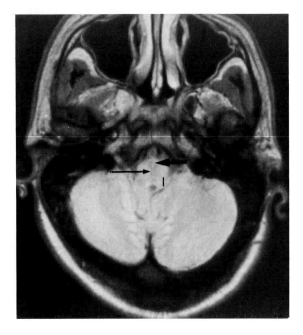

FIG. 10

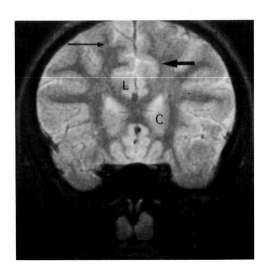

FIG. 12

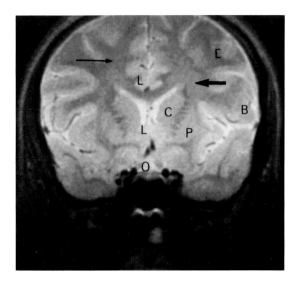

FIG. 13

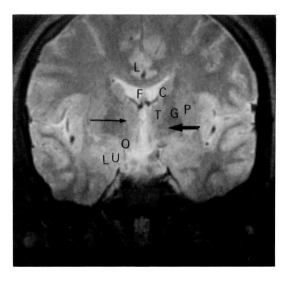

FIG. 15

The size of the pupil is controlled by the interaction between the dilator muscle fibers (sympathetic innervation) and the constrictor muscle (parasympathetic by way of the oculomotor nerve). Interruption of the sympathetic innervation of one eye, e.g., in Horner's syndrome, leads to a small, constricted pupil (miosis). Interruption of the oculomotor nerve fibers (e.g., by compression due to uncal herniation) results in a wide pupil (mydriasis).

SENSORY SYSTEMS

General Sensory Systems (from the Body)

Impulses of fine and discriminative touch, as well as proprioception or position sense, from the peripheral sense organs in the skin and tendons are conveyed by the dorsal column or lemniscal system to the sensory cortex (Figs. 1–19, thin arrows). This system courses in the dorsal columns of the spinal cord, then in the contralateral brainstem, to the posterior thalamus (T). The pathway then projects by way of the posterior internal capsule to the postcentral gyrus of the parietal lobe, so that the lower body is represented at the top of the hemisphere, and the upper extremity at the middle of the postcentral gyrus. The sensation in the face is conveyed by the trigeminal system (see below). Discrete lesions in the so-called dorsal column system may result in loss of position and tactile sense in well-defined areas of the body.

A second sensory or spinothalamic system relays impulses of sharp pain, temperature (hot or cold), and gross mechanical distortion from the periphery to the thalamus and cerebral cortex. This system courses from

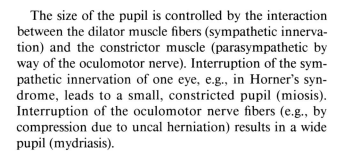

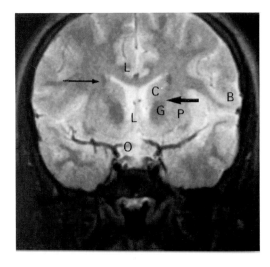

FIG. 14

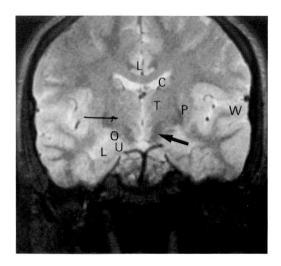

FIG. 16

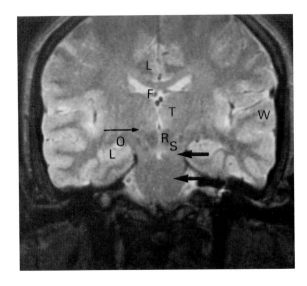

FIG. 17

the spinal cord through the brainstem, to end in the posterior thalamus (T), hence its name. Collateral fibers are given off in the spinal cord as well as in the brainstem, to form a polysynaptic spinoreticular tract, which ascends to another area in the thalamus. The latter, ill-defined, fiber system is involved in the sensation of dull, chronic pain.

The spinothalamic system then projects from the posterior thalamus (T) by way of the posterior internal capsule to the postcentral gyrus of the parietal lobe and adjacent gyri. The lower extremity is represented at the top of the hemisphere. The upper extremity and neck are localized lower in the postcentral gyrus. Discrete lesions in the spinothalamic systems may result in the loss of sharp pain and temperature sensation.

Trigeminal System (Sensory from the Face)

Sensation in one half of the face (touch, pain, temperature) is relayed to the cerebral cortex chiefly by way of

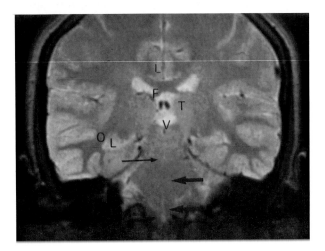

FIG. 18

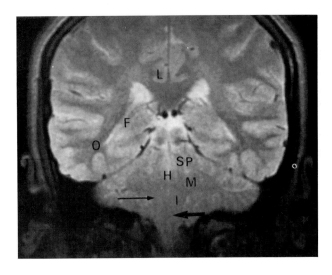

FIG. 19

the sensory fibers of the fifth nerve (trigeminus). These fibers synapse in the pons for touch, or in the lower part of the brainstem for pain and temperature. Secondary fibers of the trigeminal system then ascend in the contralateral half of the brainstem, to end in the posteromedial part of the thalamus (T). From there, thalamocortical fibers course by way of the posterior internal capsule to the lower portion of the postcentral gyrus, where the face is represented. Discrete lesions in the trigeminal system (e.g., caused by multiple sclerosis plaques) may lead to well-defined areas of sensory loss in the face. Irritation (of parts) of the system may result in painful sensation ("tic douloureux") of the face, usually restricted to the area innervated by one division of the fifth nerve.

OPTIC SYSTEM

Retina cells give rise to the optic nerves (O), which partially cross in the optic chiasma to become the optic tracts (O; Figs. 5, 6, 13–16). These tracts, containing visual impulses from a retinal half of each globe, end in the lateral geniculate bodies of the thalamus. The final portion of the pathway is by way of the optic or geniculocalcarine radiation, which terminates in the visual cortex (O, area 17) above and below the calcarine fissure in the occipital lobes (Figs. 5–7, 18, 19). Because of the image reversal by the lens, the portions of the visual fields represent portions of the opposite retinas: e.g., upper visual fields = lower halves, right visual fields = left halves of the retinas. The lower part of optic radiation loops around the inferior horn of the lateral ventricle, far forward into the temporal lobe. This "Meyer's" loop, carrying impulses from the lower half of both retinas, may be interrupted by a large temporal lobe lesion, resulting in a contralateral upper quadrantopia. A lesion of an entire geniculate body, or transection of an optic tract, may lead to contralateral homonymous hemianopia. Total destruction of the visual cortex of one side, e.g., with posterior cerebral artery occlusion, may result in a similar visual deficit, usually with some sparing of the area of sharp vision. A lesion in the middle of the chiasm, such as may occur with a pituitary tumor with suprasellar extension, may cause a (partial or complete) bitemporal hemianopia, since fibers from the nasal half of each retina are interrupted in this location. Some of the fibers (or their collateral processes) in the optic tract terminate in the pretectal region, between the thalamus and midbrain. From this ill-defined area connections course to both third nuclei, as part of the circuit for the pupillary light reflex.

Olfaction: Limbic System

Olfaction, the sense of smell, is a primitive and simple system that projects from the olfactory bulbs to a projection area in the temporal lobe near the uncus (U; Figs. 5, 6, 16, 17). Olfactory stimuli may produce reflexes controlled by hypothalamic and other areas. Structures lying deep in the medial temporal lobe were once thought to be olfactory centers, but in recent decades the functions of the hippocampus, amygdala, parahippocampal gyrus, cingulate gyrus, and other so-called limbic system components (L) have been elucidated. The limbic system has a complex, primitive influence on a variety of noncognitive functions (Figs. 1–7 and 12–19). Autonomic system functions are subject to the control of certain limbic system areas; hypothalamic and pituitary function is likewise influenced by the limbic system. Certain patterns of primitive behavior, or drives, e.g., feeding, drinking, propagation, aggression, are subject to limbic-hypothalamic influence. The hippocampus and its outflow fibers in the fornix (F) play a role in the consolidation and retention of recent memory.

Central Control of Speech

Several regions in the dominant hemisphere have traditionally been associated with aspects of speech. The so-called sensory speech area (W, of Wernicke), located in the superior temporal gyrus region, is involved in the understanding of spoken words and sentences (Figs. 3, 16, 17). A lesion in this area leads to sensory aphasia. The so-called motor speech area (B, of Broca), located in the lower precentral gyrus area, is associated with the formation of audible speech (Figs. 2, 13, 14). Lesions in this area may lead to inability to formulate intelligible speech. Lesions in the angular gyrus behind the lateral fissure have been associated with so-called anomia—the inability to identify and name objects and persons. A subcortical fiber (arcuate) system, interconnecting all speech areas, appears to result in so-called global aphasia, when destroyed. Although there is considerable clinical evidence that destruction of all these traditional areas leads to forms of aphasia, recent work may modify these concepts.

ABBREVIATIONS USED IN ILLUSTRATIONS

B   Motor speech area (of Broca)
C   Caudate nucleus
E   Cortical eye field
F   Fornix
G   Globus pallidus
H   Lateral (horizontal) gaze center
I   Inferior cerebellar peduncle
L   Limbic system components
M   Middle cerebellar peduncle
O   Optic system
P   Putamen
R   Red nucleus
S   Substantia nigra
SP Superior cerebellar peduncle
T   Thalamus
U   Uncus
V   Vertical gaze center
W   Sensory speech area (Wernicke)

Note: In Figures 1 to 19, structures are labeled on one side only; *thick arrows* on right half of figures indicate motor system; *thin arrows* on left half of figures indicate general sensory system. Figures 1 to 11 are (trans)axial MR images (T2 weighted); Figs. 12 to 19 are coronal magnetic resonance images (T2 weighted).

CHAPTER 9

Degenerative Brain Disorders and Brain Iron

Burton P. Drayer

High-field-strength [e.g., 1.5 tesla (T)] magnetic resonance imaging (MRI) provides a sensitive, *in vivo* method for mapping the normal and pathological distribution of iron in the brain with excellent anatomic specificity (1,2). In all adult individuals studied using a multislice, spin-echo (SE) pulse sequence for T2-weighted (e.g., TR = 2,500 msec and TE = 80 msec) imaging, a prominent decreased signal intensity (decreased T2) was noted in the globus pallidus, red nucleus, reticular substantia nigra, and dentate nucleus of the cerebellum (1,2). The normal decreased signal intensity on SE 2,500/80 images correlates directly with previous autopsy studies (3) on 98 normal brains of age 13 to 100 years that describe a preferential accumulation of brain iron in the globus pallidus (21 mg Fe/100 g), red nucleus (19 mg Fe/100 g), reticular substantia nigra (18 mg Fe/100 g), putamen (13 mg Fe/100 g), caudate nucleus (9 mg Fe/100 g), and thalamus (5 mg Fe/100 g). Our own studies using both high-field MRI *in vivo* and Perls staining for ferric iron on autopsy brains confirm this iron accumulation (2).

MRI FINDINGS

There is no significant brain iron noted at birth on either MRI or Perls staining (2,4). There is a progressive increase in nonheme iron through childhood until adult levels are reached at about 15 to 20 years of age (2,3,5). Although the globus pallidum iron remains fairly con-

TABLE 1. *Brain iron and neurological diseases*

Disease	Localization of Fe excess	Ref.
Normal distribution		
Infancy	Fe absent	2, 4
Adult (Fig. 1)	GP/SN reticulata/red nucleus/dentate nucleus	2, 3
Aging	Adult + putamen	2, 3
Neurodegenerative		
Parkinson's disease (Figs. 2 and 3)	Putamen/SN compacta	14
Parkinson's plus syndrome (Fig. 4)	Putamen/SN compacta	13
Hallevorden-Spatz	GP/SN reticulata	17
Huntington's chorea	Caudate/putamen	17
Motor neuron disease (Fig. 5)	Putamen	16
Alzheimer's disease (Fig. 6)	Cerebral cortex	1, 15
Demyelinating: multiple sclerosis[b] (Fig. 7)	Thalamus/putamen	11, 12
Neoplasm/radiation		
Radionecrosis	Endothelial and glial cells	5
Glioma	Transferrin receptors?	1
Hemorrhage		
Intracerebral hematoma	Rim macrophages	9
Vascular malformation (Fig. 8)	Malformation + rim	9, 10
Hemorrhagic infarction (Fig. 9)	Gyral/basal ganglia	10

[a] Greatest abnormal iron accumulation in Parkinson's disease with poor drug response.
[b] Decreased signal intensity (probably due to iron effect) in moderate and severe disease.

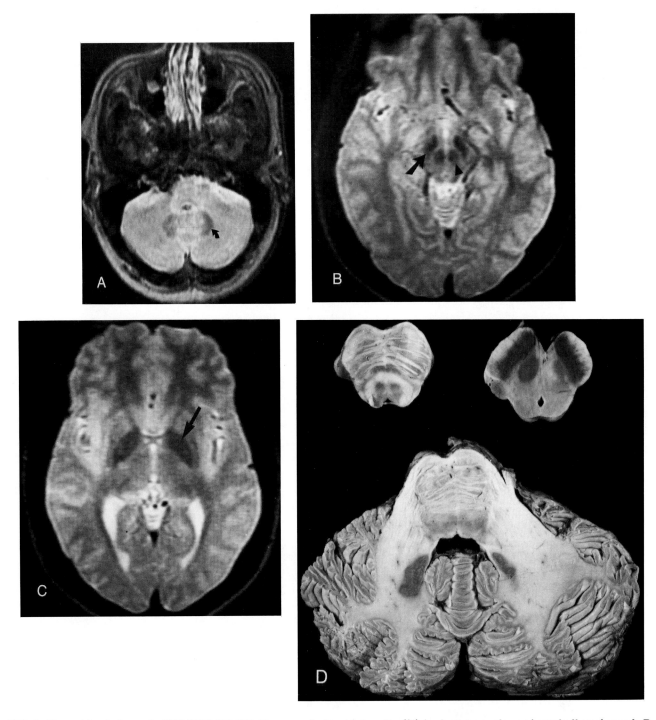

FIG. 1. Normal brain iron. **A:** MRI (SE 2,500/80): Decreased signal intensity (SI) in dentate nucleus of cerebellum (*arrow*). **B:** MRI (SE 2,500/80): Decreased SI in red nucleus (*arrowhead*) and pars reticulata of substantia nigra (*arrow*). **C:** MRI (SE 2,500/80): Decreased SI in globus pallidum (*arrow*). **D:** Perls staining (44-year-old): Increased iron in dentate nucleus, red nucleus, and substantia nigra. **E:** Perls staining (44-year-old): Increased iron in globus pallidum versus putamen or thalamus. **F:** Perls staining (84-year-old): Caudate and putamen iron now equal the concentration in the globus pallidum consistent with normal senility.

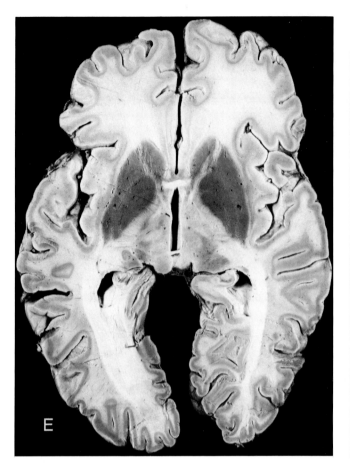
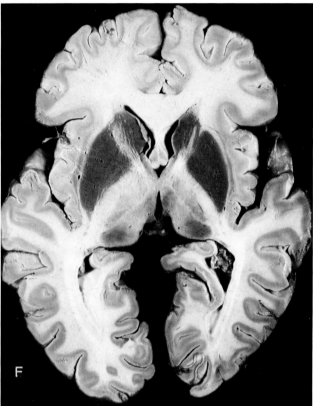

FIG. 1. (continued)

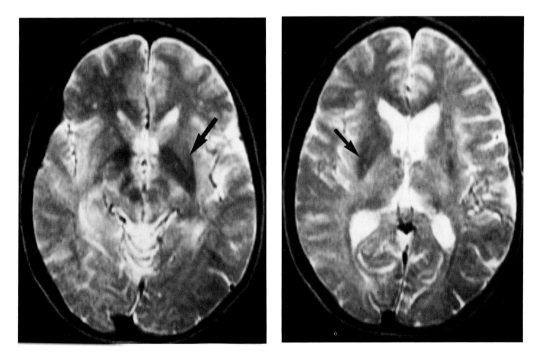

FIG. 2. Parkinson's disease. Abnormally decreased SI (SE 2,500/80) putamen (*arrows*) so that it almost equals that in the globus pallidum, most likely due to excessive iron accumulation in putamen.

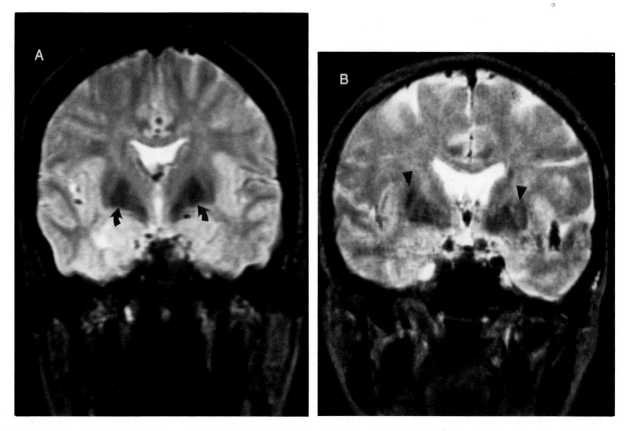

FIG. 3. Parkinson's disease versus normal, age-matched control. **A:** Normal. Coronal MRI exhibits prominent decreased SI (SE 2,500/80) in globus pallidum (*arrows*), compared to putamen due to the normally higher iron concentration in the globus pallidum. **B:** Parkinson's disease. The decreased SI (SE 2,500/80) in the putamen (*arrowheads*) is almost as prominent as in the globus pallidum.

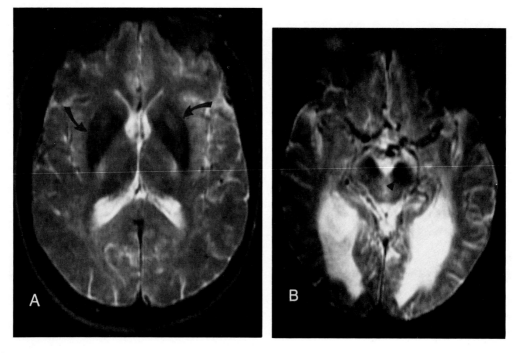

FIG. 4. Parkinson's plus. Abnormally decreased SE (SE 2,000/100) in putamen (*arrows*) and pars compacta of substantia nigra (*arrowheads*), suggesting increased iron deposition.

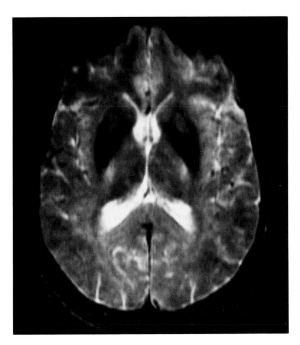

FIG. 5. Motor neuron disease. Abnormally decreased SI (SE 2,000/100) in putamen similar to that seen with Parkinson's disease.

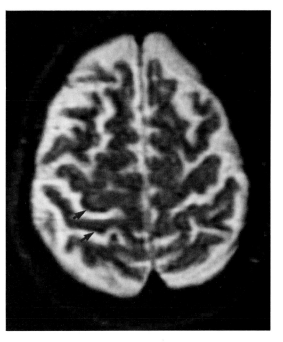

FIG. 6. Alzheimer's disease. Dilated cortical sulci with adjacent gyral decreased SI (SE 2,500/80) most prominent in the right parietal region (*arrows*), consistent with increased iron distribution.

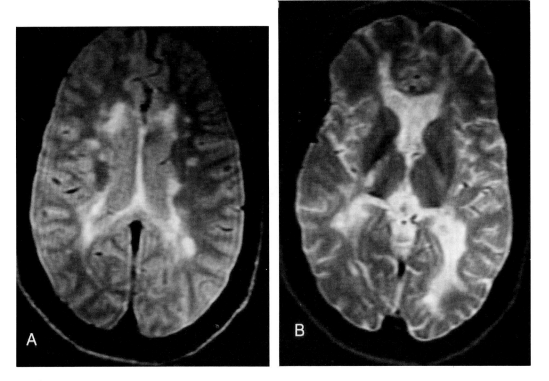

FIG. 7. Multiple sclerosis. **A:** Multiple areas of increased SI (SE 2,500/40) in a prominently periventricular location consistent with multiple sclerosis. **B:** Abnormally decreased SI (SE 2,500/80) in the putamen, caudate nucleus, and thalamus, suggesting an increased accumulation of iron or other trace metal in these gray-matter structures in association with white-matter disease (multiple sclerosis).

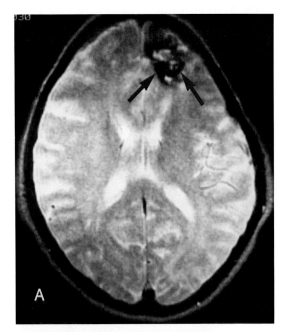

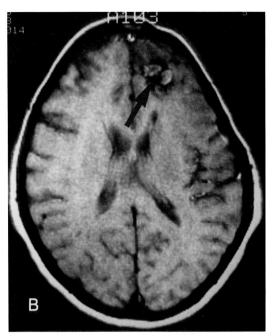

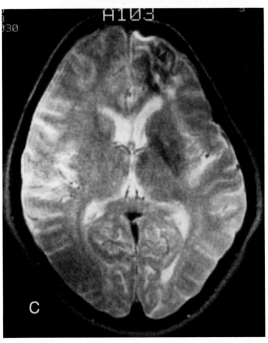

FIG. 8. Cavernous angioma. **A:** Abnormally decreased SI (SE 2,500/80) consistent with hemosiderin-stained macrophages in a cavernous angioma with prior hemorrhage (*arrows*). Intermixed increased SI is also typical of cavernous angioma. **B:** The decreased SI in the cavernous angioma is less prominent on this more T1-weighted image (SE 600/25), since the hemosiderin effect dominantly effects T2. **C:** Hemosiderin-stained cortex (*arrowhead*) secondary to prior surgery clearly defined as decreased SI on T2-weighted (SE 2,500/80) image.

stant with aging, the striatal iron concentrations continue to slowly increase so that putaminal iron may approach globus pallidal concentration by the eighth decade (2,3).

The mechanism of brain iron accumulation is unknown. Iron-transferrin from the bloodstream does not readily cross an intact blood-brain barrier (6). Transferrin receptors on brain capillary endothelial cells are not highest in concentration at sites of iron accumulation. Similar preferential iron distribution has been noted in studies of various animals, including the baboon, dog,

and rat (6). Iron is an important cofactor in oxidative phosphorylation, dopamine synthesis and turnover, and hydroxyl free radical formation (5,7). Brain iron is predominantly intracellular, with largest concentrations in oligodendroglia and astrocytes in the form of ferritin (6).

There are a variety of brain disorders in which neuropathological evidence has suggested an abnormal accumulation or distribution of iron as ferritin or hemosiderin. We have studied more than 200 patients with iron-deposition disorders, and the findings are summarized in Table 1.

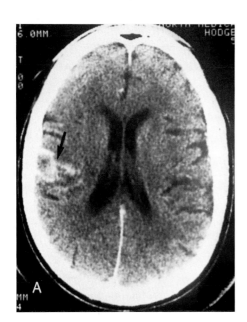
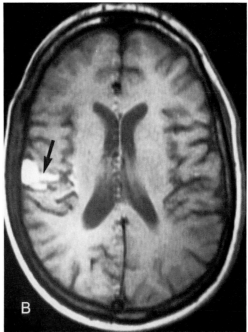
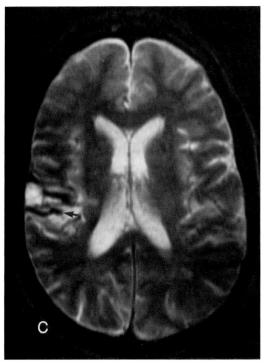

FIG. 9. Hemorrhagic infarction (10 days). **A:** Abnormal gyral enhancement on intravenously enhanced computerized tomography. **B:** Increased SI in a gyral pattern on a T1-weighted (SE 600/25) image due to methemoglobin. **C:** Decreased SI (*arrows*) in a gyral pattern on T2-weighted (SE 2,500/80) image due to hemosiderin-laden macrophages.

DISCUSSION

A knowledge of brain iron distribution is critical to the interpretation of high-field-strength MR images. It is of interest that this striking T2 relaxation time decrease in basal ganglia structures is not associated with similar declines in the T1 relaxation time. This is therefore not a typical paramagnetic effect; rather, it is related to local field heterogeneity, magnetic susceptibility, and diffu-

sion effects caused by ferritin or hemosiderin and proportionally related to the magnetic field strength (2,8–10). The ability to map accurately *in vivo* the distribution of brain iron should result in exciting new strategies for both diagnosing and understanding better the disease process and response to therapeutic interventions. Of additional importance, brain iron may provide an important marker of brain development and peroxidation reactions associated with aging.

REFERENCES

1. Drayer BP. Neurometabolic applications of magnetic resonance In: *Syllabus: American college of radiology categorical course on magnetic resonance.* Maryland: Bethesda, 1985:185–211.
2. Drayer BP, Burger P, Darwin R, et al. Magnetic resonance imaging of brain iron. *AJNR* 1986;7:373–80.
3. Hallgren B, Sourander P. The effect of age on the non-haemin iron in the human brain. *J Neurochem* 1958;3:41–51.
4. Diezel PB. Iron in the brain: a chemical and histochemical examination. In: Waelsch H, ed. *Biochemistry of the developing nervous system.* New York: Academic Press, 1955:145–52.
5. Seitelberger F. Pigmentary disorders. In: Minckler J, ed. *Pathology of the nervous system.* New York: Blakiston (McGraw-Hill), 1972:1324–38.
6. Hill JM, Switzer RC III. The regional distribution and cellular localization of iron in the rat brain. *Neuroscience* 1984;11:595–603.
7. Halliwell B, Gutteridge JMC. Oxygen radicals and the nervous system. *TINS* 1985;8:22–6.
8. Brittenham GM, Farrell DE, Harris JW. Magnetic susceptibility measurements of human iron stores. *N Engl J Med* 1982;307:1671–5.
9. Gomori JM, Grossman RI, Goldberg HI, et al. Intracranial hematomas: imaging by high-field MR. *Radiology* 1985;157:87–93.
10. Voorhees D, Drayer B, Djang W, et al. High field MR imaging of acute and chronic hemorrhage. *AJNR* 1986;7:A536.
11. Craelius W, Migdal MW, Luessenhop CP, et al. Iron deposits surrounding multiple sclerosis plaques. *Arch Pathol Lab Med* 1982;106:397–9.
12. Drayer BP, Hurwitz B, Heinz ER, et al. High field MR imaging and multiple sclerosis: decreased thalamic T_2 relaxation time. *AJNR* 1986;7:A556.
13. Drayer BP, Olanow CW, Burger P, et al. Parkinson plus syndrome: Diagnosis using high field MR imaging of brain iron. *Radiology* 1986;159:493–8.
14. Earle KM. Studies on Parkinson's disease including x-ray, fluorescent spectroscopy of formalin-fixed brain tissue. *J Neuropathol Exp Neurol* 1968;27:1–14.
15. Hallgren B, Sourander P. The non-haemin iron in the cerebral cortex in Alzheimer's disease. *J Neurochem* 1960;5:307–10.
16. Klintworth GK. Huntington's chorea—morphologic contributions of a century. In: Barbeau A, Chase TN, Paulson GW, eds. *Advances in neurology.* New York: Raven Press, 1973:353–68.
17. Park BE, Netsky MG, Betsill WL. Pathogenesis of pigment and spheroid formation in Hallervorden-Spatz syndrome and related disorders. *Neurology* 1975;25:1172–8.

CHAPTER 10

Common Congenital Malformations of the Brain

T. P. Naidich and R. A. Zimmerman

In nearly all cases, congenital malformations are characterized most easily by their anatomic features and are best imaged with T1-weighted short TR/short TE pulse sequences. T2-weighted, long TR/long TE images are used primarily for the phakomatoses that are commonly associated with brain tumors. This chapter reviews the features of the most common congenital malformations and illustrates their typical magnetic resonance imaging (MRI) appearance (Table 1).

DISORDERS OF NEURAL TUBE CLOSURE

Encephaloceles, myelomeningoceles, and anencephaly are a related group of disorders that occur with increased frequency in the same extended families.

Encephaloceles

Encephaloceles are congenital malformations in which the meninges and brain protrude outside the cranial cavity via a defect in the bone or soft tissue (1).

Cranial meningoceles are extremely rare protrusions of the meninges alone, without protrusion of brain.

The incidence of encephalocele is approximately 1 to 3 for every 10,000 births (2). In Europe and North America, encephaloceles are most commonly occipital (71%), then parietal (10%), frontal (9%), nasal (9%), and nasopharyngeal (1%) (2). In Southeast Asia, nasofrontal encephaloceles are most common. Most cases of encephalocele appear sporadically. Occipital encephaloceles affect females predominantly. Encephaloceles at other sites are more frequent in males.

Clinically, the patients usually exhibit a midline skin-covered sac that protrudes from a microcephalic calvarium. Lateral encephaloceles are uncommon and suggest constriction of the fetal head by amnionic bands *in utero*. Symptoms are usually mild and depend on the volume of brain protruding and the location of the protrusions. Low occipital encephaloceles are associated with reduced motor coordination, high occipital encephaloceles with visual disturbances, and parietal encephaloceles with sensory and speech disturbances. Sphenoethmoidal encephaloceles form a distinct group

TABLE 1. *Congenital malformations of the brain categorized into broad groups of conditions with related features*

Category	Specific condition
Disorders of neural tube closure	Encephalocele
	Chiari II malformation and myelomeningocele
Disorders of cerebral hemispheric organization	Dysgenesis of the corpus callosum
	Interhemispheric lipoma
	Holoprosencephaly
Dysplasias of the cerebral cortex	Agyria/pachygyria
	Polymicrogyria
	Cortical heterotopias
Dysplasias of cerebellar hemispheric organization	Cystic malformations of the posterior fossa
	Cerebellar hypoplasia
	Chiari I malformation
Dyshistiogeneses (phakomatoses)	Neurofibromatosis
	Tuberous sclerosis
	Sturge-Weber syndrome

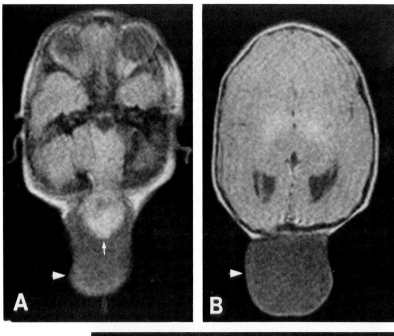

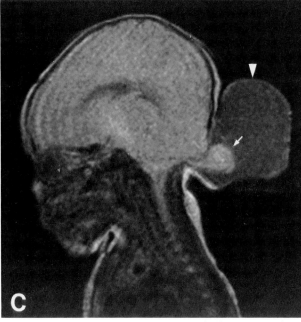

FIG. 1. Occipital encephalocele; 3-day-old girl. A portion of brain (*white arrows*) connected to the cerebellum protrudes through a midline cranial defect into a large skin-covered, CSF-filled sac (*white arrowheads*). **A, B:** Axial sections; TR 1,000 msec; TE 30 msec. **C:** Sagittal section; TR 1,000 msec; TE 30 msec.

in which nearly two-thirds of patients have midline clefts of the upper lip and/or nose; 40% have optic nerve dysplasias such as papillary-peripapillary colobomas, and 40% have dysgenesis of the corpus callosum.

In patients with encephalocele (Figs. 1–3), MRI typically displays the following:

1. microcephaly with cranium bifidum;
2. external sac with continuity of the subcutaneous fat of the scalp into the wall of the sac;
3. protrusion of CSF and variable amounts of brain through the cranium bifidum into the sac;
4. variable extension of ventricles, blood vessels, choroid plexi, and dural partitions into the sac with the brain; and

5. islands of disorganized neuroglial tissue along the walls of the sac.

Myelomeningocele and the Chiari II Malformation

Myelomeningocele is a form of spina bifida in which the neural tissue of the cord is exposed to the environment through a midline defect in the skin, soft tissue, and bone of the back. Myelomeningocele is always associated with diverse anomalies of the brain, including the Chiari II deformity (3).

In North America, the incidence of myelomeningocele and the Chiari II malformation is approximately 2

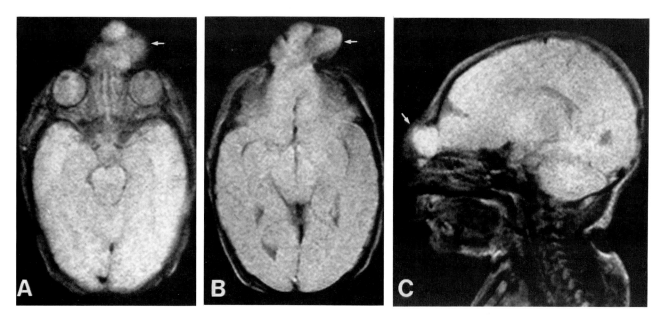

FIG. 2. Frontonasal encephalocele; 2-day-old girl. Portions of both frontal lobes form a lobulated midline mass (*white arrows*) that protrudes anteriorly above the cartilaginous portion of the nose and between the orbits, causing hypertelorism. **A, B:** Axial sections; TR 2,000 msec; TE 50 msec. **C:** Sagittal section; TR 2,000 msec; TE 50 msec.

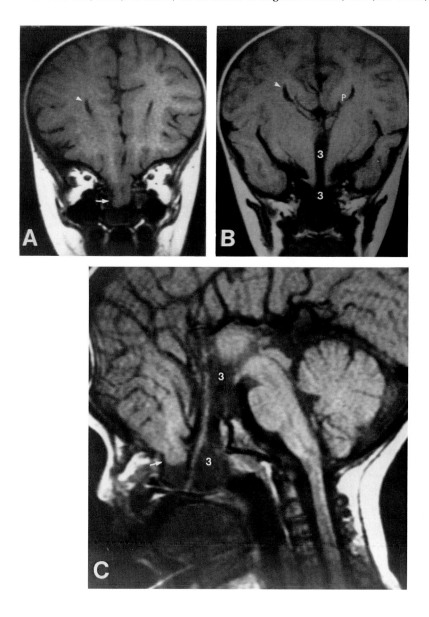

FIG. 3. Sphenoethmoidal encephalocele with callosal agenesis; 4-day-old boy. The inferior medial portions (*white arrows*) of both hemispheres and the anterior portion of the third ventricle (3) protrude inferiorly through a midline defect in the sphenoid and ethmoid bones. No corpus callosum is seen in coronal or sagittal sections. The interhemispheric fissure appears to be continuous with the third ventricle. The frontal horns (*white arrow heads*) are widely separated, concave medially and pointed superiorly. The collateral bundle of Probst (P) along the medial wall of the lateral ventricle is pathognomonic of callosal agenesis. **A, B:** Coronal sections; TR 800 msec; TE 25 msec. **C:** Sagittal section; TR 600 msec; TE 25 msec.

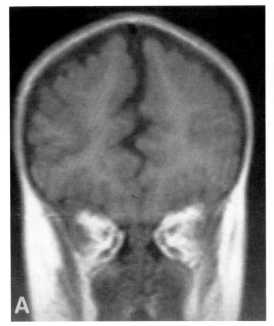

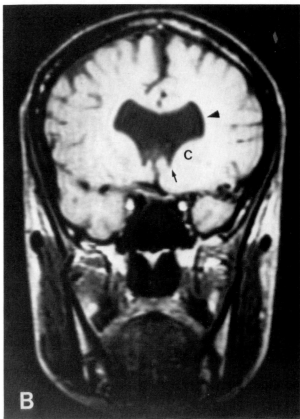

FIG. 4. Intracranial anomalies with myelomeningocele. Coronal sections in three patients. **A:** 15-month-old girl; TR 530 msec; TE 30 msec. **B:** 24-year-old woman; "partial saturation"; TR 1,500 msec. **C:** 19-month-old girl; TR 750 msec; TE 30 msec. Abnormalities commonly observed with myelomeningocele include (**A**) a "zig-zag" interhemispheric fissure with interdigitations of the medial gyri; (**B**) frontal horns with "squared-off" lateral angles (*black arrowhead*), prominent caudate impressions (C), and inferior medial points (*black arrow*); and (**C**) hypoplasia of the tentorium (*black arrowheads*) with small posterior fossa, low position of the dural venous sinuses (*white arrows*), wide incisura (*between the black arrows*), and upward growth of the cerebellum (Ce), so that it towers above the incisura in the supratentorial space and compresses the atria and the adjacent brain.

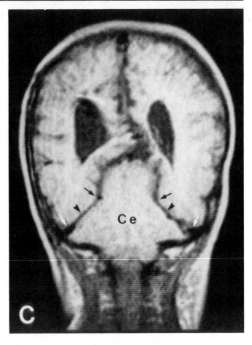

to 3 for every 1,000 births (2). Most cases are sporadic, but there is increased risk of the malformation in families with a history of neural tube defects. Females are affected about twice as often as males.

Clinical symptomatology is usually dominated by sensory motor deficits of the lower extremities. Hydrocephalus with macrocephaly and raised intracranial pressure requires shunting in 90% of patients. In 90% of patients, IQ is normal or near normal, unless there has been shunt infection. Ten percent will require custodial care.

In patients with myelomeningocele and Chiari II malformation (Figs. 4–6), MRI typically displays the following (4):

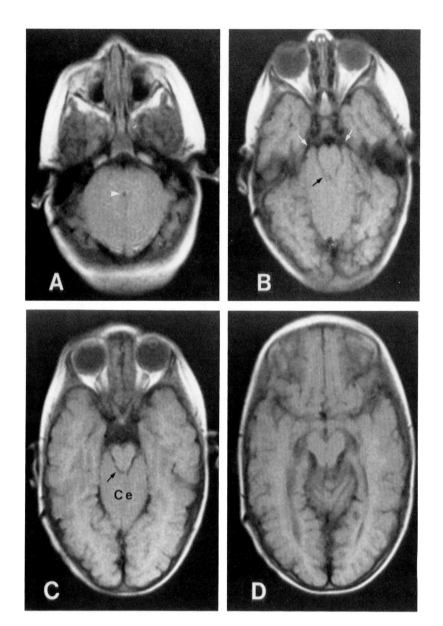

FIG. 5. Intracranial anomalies with myelomeningocele; 19-month-old girl (TR 750 msec, TE 30 msec). Serial axial MRI through the posterior fossa demonstrate nearly complete obliteration of the subarachnoid cisterns, small tubular fourth ventricle (*white arrowhead in* **A**), beaking of the tectum (*black arrows in* **B** *and* **C**), typical high position and "heart" or "bullet" shape of the upper cerebellum (Ce), and anterior extension (*white arrows*) of the cerebellum around the brainstem.

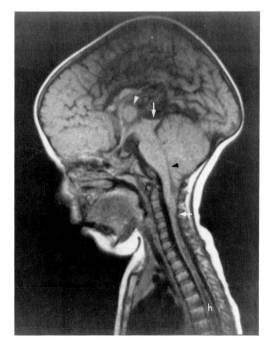

FIG. 6. Chiari II malformation. Same patient as Fig. 5; TR 750 msec; TE 30 msec. Midline sagittal image displays the large massa intermedia (*white arrowhead*), sharply beaked tectum (*white arrow*) of midbrain, elongation of the brainstem so that the caudal tip of medulla buckles behind the cervical cord to form a kink and a spur (*crossed white arrow*) at C4, elongated tubular fourth ventricle (*black arrowhead*) with dilated intracanalicular portion, associated hydromyelia (h), and growth of the cerebellum upward through the incisura behind the tectum and downward through foramen magnum behind the medulla.

1. macrocephaly with dilated (or shunted) lateral ventricles and thin cerebral mantle;

2. modest frontal horns with "squared-off" lateral angles, prominent caudate impressions, and inferior "points" (in the coronal plane);

3. large atria;

4. modest third ventricle with prominent suprapineal recess and large massa intermedia;

5. long tubular fourth ventricle that extends below foramen magnum;

6. hypoplastic falx with interdigitating medial gyri and zig-zag interhemispheric fissure;

7. hypoplastic tentorium with wide incisura and short, straight sinus;

8. low insertion of the tentorium near the foramen magnum with consequently large supratentorial space, small posterior fossa, and prominent plexus of dural venous sinuses surrounding the foramen magnum;

9. fusion of the four colliculi into a conical mass designated the tectal beak;

10. unusual, characteristic craniocaudal elongation of the cerebellum, such that the upper margin bulges superiorly through the incisura, whereas the lower margin bulges inferiorly through the foramen magnum;

11. forward growth of the cerebellum lateral and anterior to the brainstem;

12. large foramen magnum and small C1 ring with constriction of neural structures at C1; and

13. the Chiari II malformation.

The Chiari II malformation per se (Fig. 6) consists of the following (3):

1. downward displacement of the spinal cord, so that the upper cervical nerve roots ascend to their exit foramina;

2. marked elongation of the brainstem, so that the medulla extends into the cervical canal and (often) buckles backward behind the cord to form a kink and a spur at the cervicomedullary junction;

3. dysplasia and caudal elongation of the cerebellum, so that it protrudes through the foramen magnum to "rest" on the upper border of the C1 arch;

4. protrusion of a narrow tongue or "peg" of cerebellar tissue further caudally through the C1 ring behind the medulla to C2 to C4, rarely to the upper thoracic region; and

5. variable dilatation of the intracervical portion of the fourth ventricle, sometimes forming a teardrop diverticulum that protrudes caudal to the medulla behind the upper cord.

Myelomeningocele and Chiari II malformation are associated with hydromyelia in 20% to 70% of cases. Experience to date (4) suggests that hydromyelia is found most frequently in patients with dilatation of the intracervical portion of the fourth ventricle (Fig. 6).

DISORDERS OF CEREBRAL HEMISPHERIC ORGANIZATION

Agenesis of the Corpus Callosum

This signifies a constellation of anatomic deformities that includes partial and complete agenesis of the corpus callosum (5,6). The incidence of callosal agenesis is not known; however, it has been observed in 0.7% of pneumoencephalograms and approximately 2.3% of patients with developmental delay. Most cases are sporadic. Males and females are affected equally.

Isolated agenesis may be completely asymptomatic, although sophisticated testing may document that learning and memory are not shared between the hemispheres (cerebral disconnection syndrome). Most patients seen by physicians present before age 3 years with developmental delay (70%) and seizures (60%).

Associated conditions, such as trisomy 13–15, trisomy 18, Dandy-Walker malformation, and Aicardi syndrome, account for many of the other clinical features found in these patients. In patients with agenesis of the corpus callosum (Figs. 3 and 7), MRI frequently displays the following:

1. absence of all or a portion of the corpus callosum;

2. absence of some or all of the hippocampal, posterior, and anterior commissures;

3. small size, wide separation, and concave medial borders of the frontal horns with sharply angled lateral peaks;

4. lateral elongation of the foramina of Monro;

5. large size and high position of the third ventricle;

6. large, rounded atria secondary to absence of the splenium and hypoplasia of the forceps major;

7. diverging medial walls of the lateral ventricle, so that they form an angle that is open anteriorly;

8. radial array of sulci along the medial wall of the hemispheres such that the parieto-occipital and calcarine sulci fail to converge and the medial sulci orient themselves perpendicular to the narrow inferior margin of the hemisphere;

9. abnormal, sagittally oriented collateral callosal bundles (bundles of Probst) that form the medial walls of the bodies and frontal horns of the lateral ventricles;

10. abnormal formation of the cerebral cortex with agyria, pachygyria, polymicrogyria, and heterotopic gray matter;

11. hypoplasia of the hippocampal formation with patulous temporal horns (7);

12. fully communicating or multiply loculated interhemispheric cyst(s) that may act as a mass to displace and compress the adjacent hemispheres; and

13. lateral separation of the pericallosal arteries and internal cerebral veins by the high third ventricle and cyst, loss of the sweep of the pericallosal artery about the

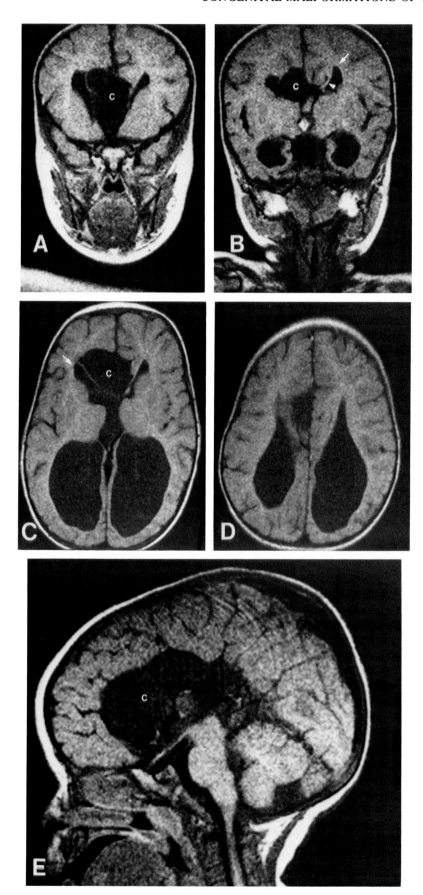

FIG. 7. Agenesis of the corpus callosum with interhemispheric cyst; 8-month-old girl. The frontal horns (*white arrows*) are small, superiorly pointed, and widely separated with concave medial borders. Probst's bundle (*white arrowhead in* **B**) is defined by the CSF within the ventricle laterally and a sulcus medially. The interhemispheric cyst (C) further separates the frontal horns. The atria and temporal horns are prominent. In **D**, the medial walls of the two lateral ventricles form an angle that is open anteriorly. In **E**, the gyri of the medial surface radiate toward the interhemispheric fissure; no corpus callosum is seen. **A, B:** Coronal MRI; TR 750 msec; TE 30 msec. **C, D:** Axial MRI; TR 750 msec; TE 30 msec. **E:** Sagittal MRI; TR 750 msec; TE 30 msec (see also Fig. 3).

genu of corpus callosum, loss of the sweep of the internal cerebral vein–vein of Galen complex about the splenium, and increased incidence of azygous anterior cerebral artery.

Lipoma of the Corpus Callosum

Lipomas of the corpus callosum are interhemispheric collections of primative and mature fat that lie in or near to the corpus callosum. They are best classed with the midline dysraphias (8–11).

The incidence of all intracranial lipomas at autopsy is approximately 0.8 per 1,000. The majority of intracranial lipomas affect the interhemispheric fissure near to the corpus callosum. Other common sites include the quadrigeminal plate, tuber cinereum, and cerebellopontine angle. No hereditary factors are known. Males and females are affected equally.

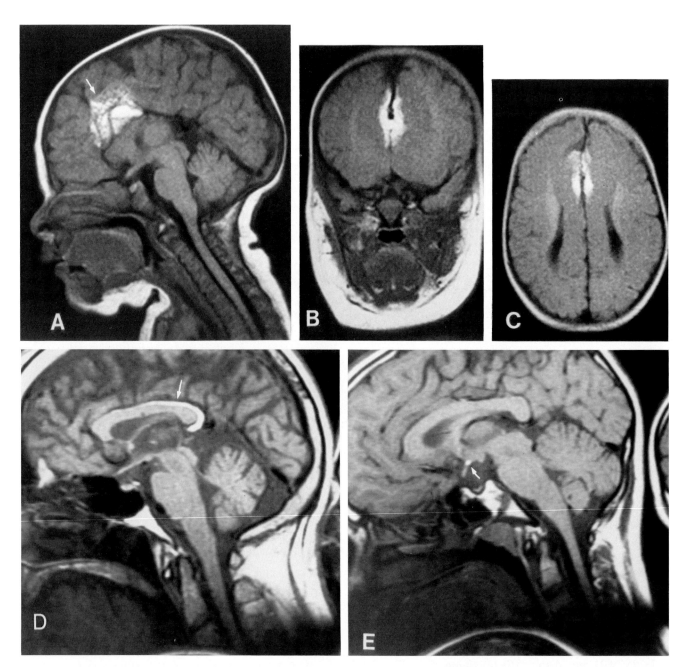

FIG. 8. Interhemispheric lipomas. **A–C:** Lipoma near the genu of the corpus callosum; 2-month-old boy: (**A**) sagittal, (**B**) coronal, (**C**) axial MRI (TR 750 msec, TE 30 msec). **D:** Lipoma curving posteriorly with the splenium, 52-year-old man; sagittal MRI (TR 600 msec, TE 30 msec). **E:** Hypothalamic lipoma; 15-year-old boy; sagittal MRI (TR 600 msec, TE 25 msec). Intracranial lipomas (*white arrows*) appear as well-defined regions of high signal intensity. Vessels that traverse the lipoma appear as curvilinear and dot-like signal voids in the high-intensity fat.

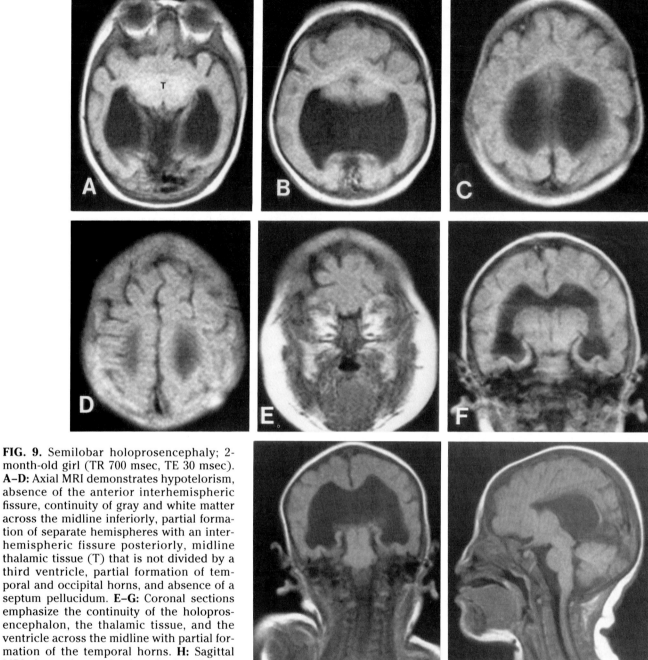

FIG. 9. Semilobar holoprosencephaly; 2-month-old girl (TR 700 msec, TE 30 msec). **A–D:** Axial MRI demonstrates hypotelorism, absence of the anterior interhemispheric fissure, continuity of gray and white matter across the midline inferiorly, partial formation of separate hemispheres with an interhemispheric fissure posteriorly, midline thalamic tissue (T) that is not divided by a third ventricle, partial formation of temporal and occipital horns, and absence of a septum pellucidum. **E–G:** Coronal sections emphasize the continuity of the holoprosencephalon, the thalamic tissue, and the ventricle across the midline with partial formation of the temporal horns. **H:** Sagittal MRI shows the predominantly dorsal location of the ventricular system.

Lipomas of the corpus callosum may be asymptomatic (10%) or may be associated with seizures (56%), mental "disturbance" (40%), paralysis (17%), and headache (16%). In patients with interhemispheric lipomas (Fig. 8), MRI may display the following:

1. a midline, nearly symmetrical mass of fat that occupies a focal zone of the interhemispheric fissure, usually near the genu of corpus callosum;

2. variable extension around the splenium, through the choroidal fissure to the choroid plexus, along cerebral clefts, and through a cranium bifidum;

3. concurrent callosal dysgenesis (37–50%);

4. concurrent subcutaneous lipoma (11%);

5. encasement of the medial interhemispheric arteries with fusiform dilatation of these vessels and increased incidence of azygous and bihemispheric anterior cerebral arteries; and

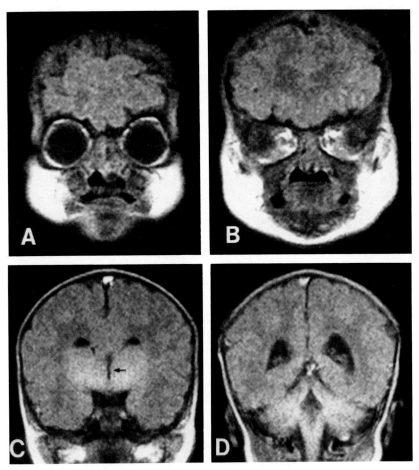

FIG. 10. Semilobar holoprosencephaly; 1-week-old boy (TR 600 msec, TE 30 msec). Coronal sections document absence of the anterior interhemispheric fissure (**A, B**); continuity of the gray and white matter across the midline anteriorly (**A–C**); partial formation of cerebral hemispheres with an interhemispheric fissure posteriorly (**C, D**); and relatively normal posterior portions of the lateral ventricles. In this patient, a midline third ventricle (*arrow*) separates the two thalami.

6. shell-like peripheral calcification or dense bone within the lipoma.

Holoprosencephaly

Holoprosencephaly is the name given to a spectrum of cerebral malformations characterized by micrencephaly (small brain), hypotelorism, and failure to form separate left and right cerebral hemispheres or thalami (12,13). From most to least severe, three points along the spectrum are designated alobar, semilobar, and lobar holoprosencephaly. The severe alobar holoprosencephaly exhibits no interhemispheric fissure, no falx, completely uncleft holoprosencephalon and basal ganglia, and a single horseshoe-shaped supratentorial ventricle. The intermediate semilobar holoprosencephaly shows partial development of the posterior interhemispheric fissure and falx, partial separation of occipito-temporal lobes, and beginning differentation of the monoventricle into temporo-occipital horns. A rudimentary third ventricle may be present. The mildest lobar form has a nearly complete interhemispheric fissure and falx, nearly normal formation of cerebral hemispheres and thalami, and nearly normal ventricles. However, the two frontal lobes remain fused across the midline at the depth of the anterior interhemispheric fissure; the frontal horns lie close together, and the septum pellucidum is absent, permitting free communication from side to side. Septo-optic dysplasia may be regarded as a mild form of lobar holoprosencephaly.

The incidence of holoprosencephaly is estimated at 1 per 16,000 births (14). Most cases are sporadic, but autosomal dominant and autosomal recessive forms exist. Males and females are affected equally.

Clinically, most patients with alobar and semilobar holoprosencephaly are detected at birth by their characteristic facies: microcephaly, hypotelorism, and one of cyclopia, ethmocephaly, cebocephaly, or absent premaxillary segment. The mild lobar holoprosencephaly may have (nearly) normal facies. Trisomy 13–15, trisomy 18, 18p⁻, and 13q⁻ syndromes are known associations that suggest possible presence of holoprosencephaly. Many patients manifest poikilothermia, spasticity, apneic spells, motor retardation, and mental retardation. Life expectancy is limited in the more severe forms.

In patients with holoprosencephaly, MRI frequently displays micrencephaly, hypotelorism, direct continuity of gray and white matter across the midline, and a single supratentorial ventricle. A large dorsal cyst may occupy

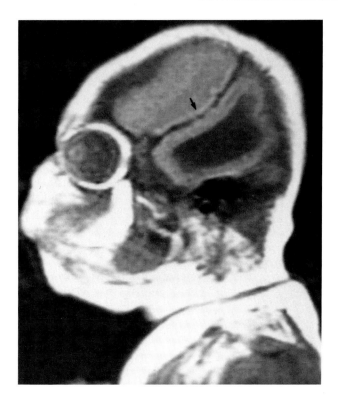

FIG. 11. Agyria; 2-day-old boy with microcephaly (TR 600 msec, TE 25 msec). Sagittal MRI demonstrates the sylvian groove (*arrow*), a smooth frontoparietal cortical surface, and absence of any opercula.

The midline, displace the holoprosencephalon anteriorly, and expand sufficiently to cause macrocephaly. The holoprosencephaly may be designated alobar (severe) holoprosencephaly when MRI demonstrates

1. complete absence of the interhemispheric fissure and falx;
2. a single unlobed, often shield-shaped holoprosencephalon;
3. absence of corpus callosum;
4. a horseshoe-shaped supratentorial monoventricle;
5. absence of the third ventricle;
6. absence of the superior sagittal, inferior sagittal, and straight sinuses with absent internal cerebral veins; and
7. increased incidence of azygous anterior cerebral arteries with hypoplastic middle cerebral arteries.

The holoprosencephaly may be designated semilobar (Figs. 9 and 10) if the MRI displays

1. partial formation of the posterior interhemispheric fissure, falx, and associated dural sinuses;
2. rudimentary, if any, corpus callosum;
3. partial differentiation of the ventricle into temporo-occipital horns;
4. a rudimentary third ventricle; and
5. variable, minimal development of the deep veins.

The holoprosencephaly may be designated lobar if MRI displays

1. a nearly complete interhemispheric fissure and falx that may be shallow anteriorly;
2. partial fusion of the two frontal lobes with direct continuity of gray and white matter across the midline, under the shallow interhemispheric fissure, in a restricted inferior frontal region;
3. well-formed occipital and temporal horns with narrow bodies of the lateral ventricles; and
4. "squared-off," fused frontal horns with absent septum pellucidum.

DYSPLASIAS OF THE CEREBRAL CORTEX

Agyria, pachygyria, polymicrogyria, and cortical heterotopias are a related group of anomalies believed to result from disordered migration of neuroblasts between the subependymal germinal matrix and the brain surface, with consequent abnormal thickness, abnormal folding, and disorganization of the cortex (15,16). Agyria (synonym: lissencephaly) signifies a smooth brain with complete absence of gyri. Pachygyria indicates a reduced number of coarse, broad, shallow gyri with less than normal folding. These differ only in de-

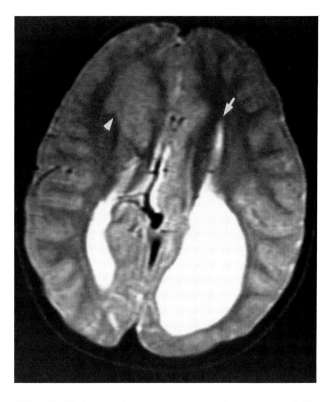

FIG. 12. Heterotopic gray matter and agenesis of the corpus callosum; 3-year-old boy (TR 2500 msec, TE 80 msec). Axial MRI demonstrates a large irregular zone of gray matter (*white arrowhead*) within the frontal white matter. Small, pointed, laterally separated frontal horns (*white arrow*), and large atria identify callosal agenesis.

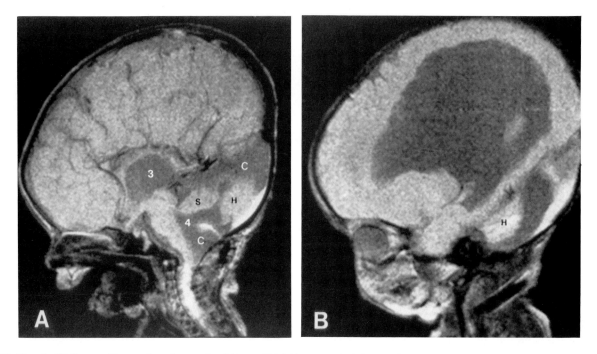

FIG. 13. Dandy-Walker malformation; 1-month-old boy (TR 2000 msec, TE 50 msec). **A:** Midline sagittal section demonstrates a dilated third ventricle (3), preserved superior vermis (S), absence of the inferior vermis, continuity between the large fourth ventricle (4) and the very large posterior fossa cyst (C), and a portion of the cerebellar hemisphere (H) that projects into the section from the side. **B:** Paramedian sagittal section demonstrates the massive dilatation of the lateral ventricle, the cerebellar hemisphere (H), and the posterior fossa cyst.

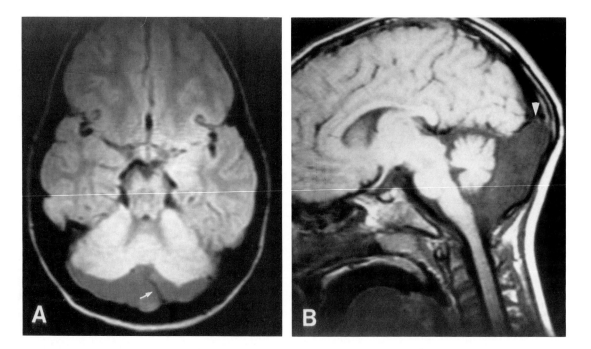

FIG. 14. Retrocerebellar arachnoid pouch; 5-year-old boy (TR 800 msec, TE 20 msec). Axial (**A**) and sagittal (**B**) MRI demonstrates an intact cerebellum and vermis that are displaced forward by a large CSF space. The space appears to be continuous with the cisterna magna, is indented by a falx cerebelli (*white arrow*), and has a superior diverticulum (*white arrowhead*) at or above the torcular.

gree and can be found in different areas of the same hemisphere.

Polymicrogyria signifies a brain with too many gyri of abnormally small size. Polymicrogyria may be mistaken for pachygyria on gross inspection, because the multiple small gyri have fused surfaces and are not exteriorized by sulci. Cortical heterotopias are islands of gray matter that may form at any point along the route of neuroblast migration, along or in association with other dysplasias of the cortex.

Agyria and pachygyria are rare disorders. Most cases are sporadic. Autosomal recessive inheritance has been found in several syndromes featuring lissencephaly (17).

The clinical features roughly parallel the degree of morphologic derangement. Patients with agyria manifest microcephaly, decerebration, lack of awareness of the environment, and severe mental retardation. Nearly all develop seizures before age 1 year and most die by age 2 years. Patients with pachygyria live longer but are severely retarded and frequently have seizures. Patients with small "patches" of polymicrogyria may be asymptomatic, but those with extensive regions are usually retarded with neurological deficits. Cortical heterotopias are associated with mental retardation and seizures less consistently than are agyria/pachygyria.

In patients with cortical dysplasia (Figs. 11 and 12), MRI usually displays

1. micrencephaly with an abnormally smooth brain surface;

2. shallow, oblique sylvian grooves with exposed insulae and absent opercula;

3. superficial position of the middle cerebral artery with absence of the sylvian triangle and sylvian point;

4. increased thickness of the cortex;

5. reduced thickness of the white matter, with hypoplastic centrum semiovale, loss of the peripheral digitations, and small corpus callosum, cerebral peduncles, and long tracts of the brainstem;

6. absence of claustrum and extreme capsules with relatively normal lentiform nuclei;

7. hypoplastic or absent olivary and pyramidal eminences of the medulla;

8. enlarged ventricle, perhaps with nodular walls from heterotopic subependymal gray matter; and

9. single or multiple isolated or concurrent islands of gray matter (1 mm–2 cm in diameter), usually near the corners of the lateral ventricles or the ventrolateral aspects of the temporal horns.

DYSPLASIAS OF CEREBELLAR HEMISPHERIC ORGANIZATION

Cystic Malformations of the Posterior Fossa

The Dandy-Walker malformation, the Dandy-Walker variant, and the retrocerebellar arachnoid pouch are a related group of malformations with the common feature of a large CSF space situated posterior to the cerebellum.

True Dandy-Walker malformation is characterized by (partial) absence of the vermis, absence of the foramen of Magendie, marked dilatation of the fourth ventricle to form a cyst that balloons behind the cerebellum, and absence of communication between the fourth ventricular cyst and the perimedullary cistern (18). The Dandy-Walker variant differs in that the fourth ventricle is smaller and better formed; the retrocerebellar cyst is smaller; and the foramen of Magendie is patent, permitting free communication between the fourth ventricular cyst and the basal cistern. The variant is believed to be far more common than the true Dandy-Walker malformation (18).

The retrocerebellar arachnoid pouch (synonym: Blake's pouch cyst) is characterized by an intact vermis, evagination of the tela choroidea of the fourth ventricle above and behind the intact vermis to form a pouch, and full communication between the fourth ventricle and the subarachnoid space (18). It is believed that the retrocerebellar arachnoid pouch is the origin of many cases of "mega cisterna magna" (19).

The incidence of Dandy-Walker malformation and its variant is not established. The condition appears to account for 2% to 4% of patients with hydrocephalus. Most cases are sporadic. Males and females are affected approximately equally.

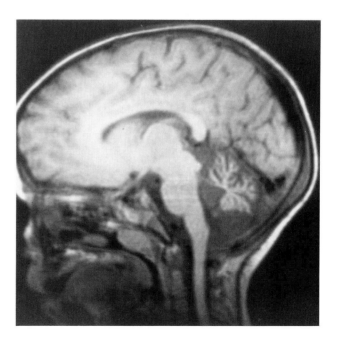

FIG. 15. Vermian-cerebellar hypoplasia; 3-year-old boy (TR 800 msec, TE 20 msec). Midline sagittal MRI demonstrates reduced size of the vermis with prominent fissures and prominent surrounding cisterns.

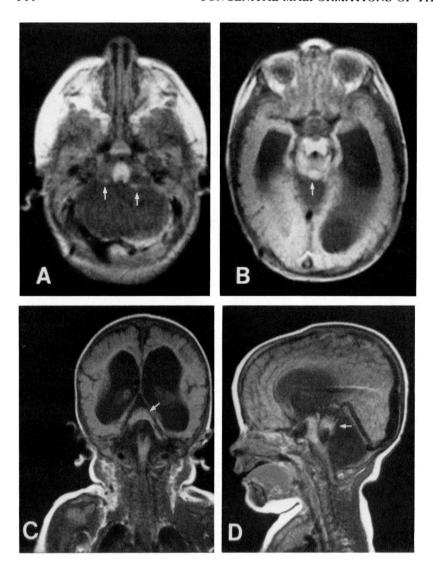

FIG. 16. Marked cerebellar hypoplasia; 8-month-old boy (TR 500 msec, TE 30 msec). Axial (**A**, **B**), coronal (**C**), and sagittal (**D**) MRI demonstrates near-total absence of cerebellum with a tiny residual portion (*white arrows*) of anterior cerebellum, a tiny brainstem, and a large CSF space where the cerebellum ought to be.

Dandy-Walker malformation and variant usually present with macrocephaly, hydrocephalus, and elevated intracranial pressure. Mental retardation is common even after successful shunting, perhaps because of the high incidence of associated cerebral anomalies, including dysgenesis of the corpus callosum (15–25%), holoprosencephaly (10–25%), and dysplasia of the cerebral and cerebellar cortices (20–25%) (18–20).

In patients with Dandy-Walker malformation (and variant) (Fig. 13), MRI usually displays

1. macrocephaly with hydrocephalus;
2. expansion of the posterior fossa with scaphocephaly and pressure erosion (scalloping) of the petrous pyramids;
3. high insertion of the tentorium above the lambda ("torcular-lambdoid inversion") with wide, more vertically oriented incisura;
4. absent inferior vermis;
5. variably persistent superior vermis that is displaced

superiorly and anteriorly into the incisura by the dilated fourth ventricle and cyst behind it;

6. hypoplastic cerebellar hemispheres;
7. ballooning of the fourth ventricle into a retrocerebellar cyst that displaces the cerebellar hemispheres anterolaterally against the petrous pyramids;
8. absence of any midline or paramedian retrocerebellar septae (true Dandy-Walker cyst); and
9. presence of midline or paired paramedian retrocerebellar septae (Dandy-Walker variant).

In patients with a retrocerebellar arachnoid pouch (Fig. 14), MRI displays

1. an enlarged CSF space above and behind an intact cerebellum and vermis;
2. frequent apparent separation of that space into supracerebellar and retrocerebellar compartments by a transverse meningeal fold;
3. frequent falx cerebelli (two-thirds of cases), which may be bifid with one fold to each side of the midline;

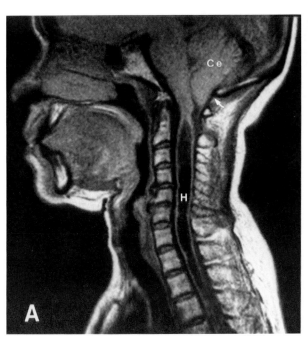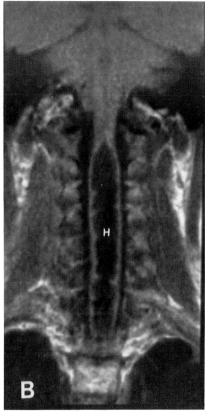

FIG. 17. Chiari I malformation with hydromyelia; 61-year-old man (TR 700 msec, TE 30 msec). **A:** The inferior portion of the cerebellum (Ce) is prolonged caudally to the posterior lip (*white arrow*) of the foramen magnum. **B:** Severe hydromyelia (H) distends the spinal cord and thins its walls, leaving "haustra-like" bands that project into the cavity. Even with severe hydromyelia, the spinal cord typically remains narrow at C1.

4. occasional high position of the tentorium (12%); and

5. dehiscence of the tentorium in the midline posteriorly (25%), with superior extension of the cyst through a hiatus into the intradural compartment between the leaves of the falx cerebri.

Cerebellar Hypoplasia

Cerebellar hypoplasia is a failure of full development of the vermis and/or the cerebellar hemispheres (15). Vermian hypoplasia may be an isolated anomaly or form part of the Dandy-Walker malformation. Cerebellar hemispheric hypoplasia may be unilateral or bilateral, modest or severe. Mild symmetrical cerebellar hypoplasia is common in trisomy 21 (Down syndrome). Severe symmetrical cerebellar hypoplasia may leave only a small remnant of the anterior lobe surrounded by freely communicating basal cisterns.

In these patients (Figs. 15 and 16), MRI displays

1. a small symmetrical remnant of vermis and anterior lobe;

2. a large retrocerebellar CSF space that does not appear to be under tension;

3. severely hypoplastic or absent cerebellar peduncles; and

4. small size of brainstem, especially the pons.

Chiari I Malformation

The Chiari I malformation is a complex anomaly characterized in part by caudal elongation of the cerebellar tonsil into the cervical spinal canal. The brainstem may be elongated mildly (21–22). The Chiari I malformation has no relationship to the Chiari II malformation and is not associated with myelomeningocele.

Patients with Chiari I malformation typically manifest one of three syndromes: (a) foramen magnum compression (22%) with ataxia, corticospinal and sensory deficits, cerebellar signs, and lower cranial nerve deficits; (b) central cord syndrome (65%) with combined, dissociated sensory loss; or (c) cerebellar syndrome (11%) with truncal ataxia, nystagmus, and limb ataxia. Pain is common (69%), particularly headache (34%) and cervi-

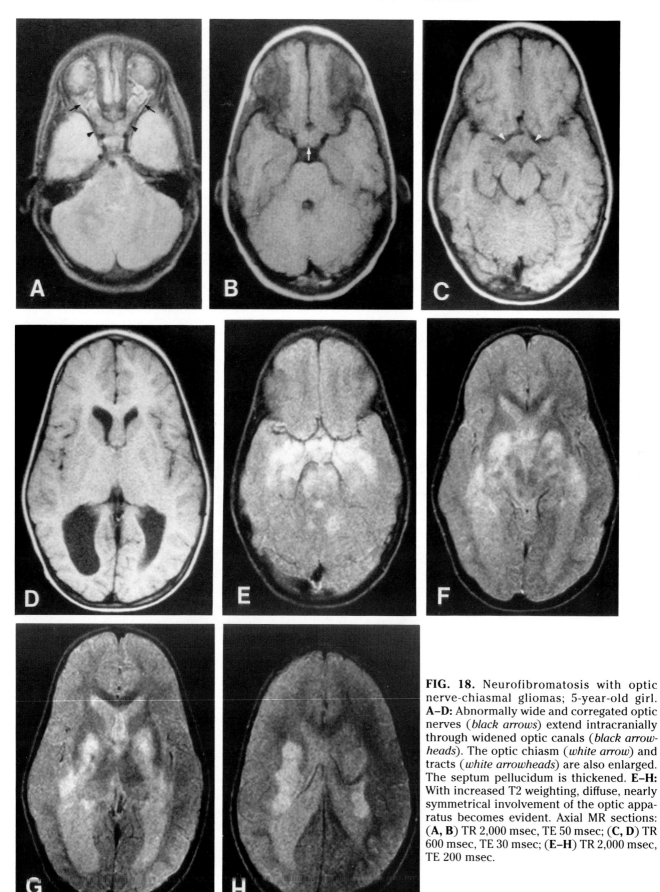

FIG. 18. Neurofibromatosis with optic nerve-chiasmal gliomas; 5-year-old girl. **A–D:** Abnormally wide and corregated optic nerves (*black arrows*) extend intracranially through widened optic canals (*black arrowheads*). The optic chiasm (*white arrow*) and tracts (*white arrowheads*) are also enlarged. The septum pellucidum is thickened. **E–H:** With increased T2 weighting, diffuse, nearly symmetrical involvement of the optic apparatus becomes evident. Axial MR sections: (**A, B**) TR 2,000 msec, TE 50 msec; (**C, D**) TR 600 msec, TE 30 msec; (**E–H**) TR 2,000 msec, TE 200 msec.

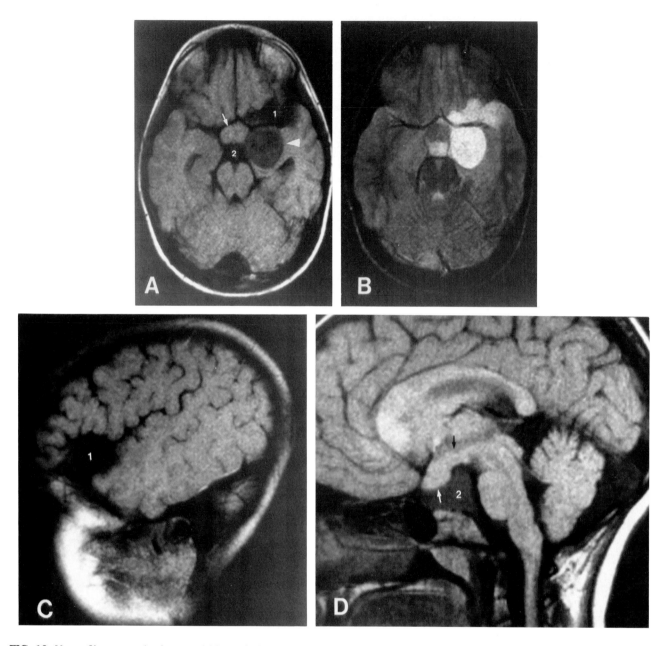

FIG. 19. Neurofibromatosis; 8-year-old boy. **A, B:** Axial MRI demonstrates an enlarged optic chiasm (*white arrow*), a round, well-defined cystic medial temporal astrocytoma (*white arrowhead*) that displaces the temporal horn, and two separate arachnoid cysts (1,2). The signal intensity of the arachnoid and tumor cysts increases with T2 weighting. **C:** The lateral arachnoid cyst (1) opens the sylvian fissure, separating the frontal and temporal lobes. **D:** Midline MRI demonstrates extension of the chiasmal lesion (*white arrow*) into the hypothalamus (*black arrow*), thickening and increased signal intensity in the corpus callosum, and the suprasellar arachnoid cyst (2). Axial section: (**A**) TR 750 msec, TE 30 msec; (**B**) TR 2,000 msec, TE 100 msec. Sagittal section: (**C**) TR 750 msec, TE 30 msec; (**D**) TR 750 msec, TE 30 msec.

cal pain (13%). Weakness (56%) and unsteadiness, with loss of balance (40%), are also frequent symptoms.

In patients with Chiari I malformation (Fig. 17), MRI displays

1. malformed craniovertebral junction with basilar impression (23–50%), assimilation of C1 to the occiput (1–10%), partial fusions of C2 and C3 (18%), Klippel-Feil deformity (5%), cervical spina bifida occulta (5–7%), and widening of the cervical spinal canal from hydromyelia (18%);

2. caudal elongation of the tonsils through foramen magnum (4%) as far as C1 (62%), C2 (25%), and C3 (3%), occasionally lower; the tonsils may be asymmetric in size and position;

3. extremely small cisterna magna, often with fibrous adhesions, matting dura, arachnoid, tonsils, and spinal cord together (41%);

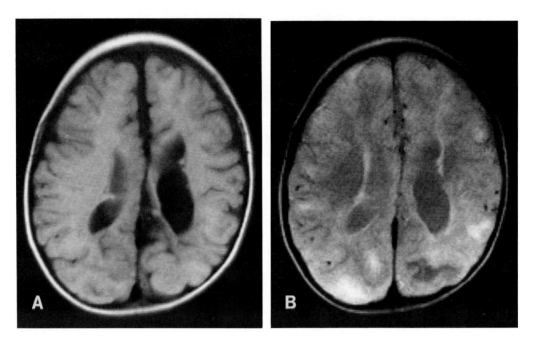

FIG. 20. Tuberous sclerosis; 2-year-old child. Axial MR demonstrates dilated lateral ventricles; multiple small subependymal tubers which increase in signal intensity in **B;** multiple cortical and subcortical tubers; and cerebral atrophy. **A:** TR 600 msec, TE 20 msec. **B:** TR 1,000 msec, TE 30 msec.

4. hydromyelia of the cervical cord (sometimes the entire cord) in 20% to 73% of cases; and

5. hydrocephalus (0–20–44%) of cases.

THE PHAKOMATOSES: NEUROCUTANEOUS SYNDROMES

The phakomatoses are hereditary developmental anomalies characterized by disordered histiogenesis with abnormal cell proliferation in the nervous system and skin. The most common of these are von Recklinghausen's neurofibromatosis, Bourneville's tuberous sclerosis, and Sturge-Weber's encephalotrigeminal angiomatosis (23).

Neurofibromatosis

Neurofibromatosis is a dyshistiogenesis of neuroectodermal and mesodermal tissue in which the neuroectodermal Schwann cell is the neoplastic element and in

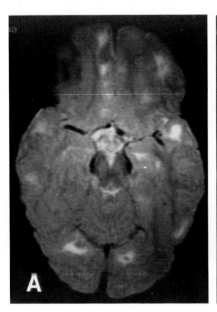
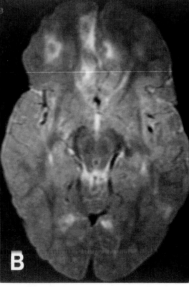

FIG. 21. Tuberous sclerosis; 2-year-old boy (TR 2,500 msec, TE 80 msec). Axial MRI demonstrates diffuse, bilateral, asymmetrical cortical and subcortical lesions with central low signal and irregular ring-like borders of high signal.

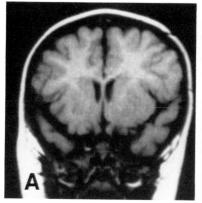 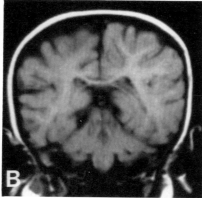 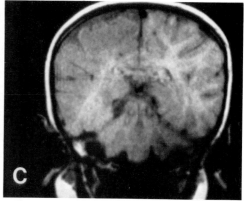

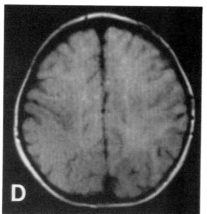 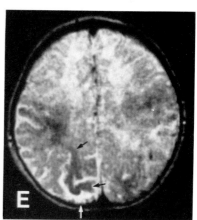

FIG. 22. Sturge-Weber syndrome; 6-month-old girl with facial port-wine stain. **A–C:** Coronal MRI demonstrates atrophy of the cerebral hemisphere on the side of the port-wine stain, expansion of the overlying cisterns, and poor myelination of the white matter. **D, E:** Axial MRI demonstrates decreasing signal intensity of the cortex (*arrows*) with increasing T2 weighting, consistent with the paramagnetic effect of iron deposited in the cortex. CSF within the dilated subarachnoid cisterns (*white arrow*) shows increased signal intensity with T2 weighting. (**A, B**) TR 1,000 msec, TE 30 msec; (**C**) TR 1,000 msec, TE 67 msec; (**D**) TR 2,000 msec, TE 67 msec; (**E**) TR 2,000 msec, TE 90 msec.

which this cell is surrounded by a widely variable degree of reactive mesenchymal hyperplasia (24). The incidence of neurofibromatosis is estimated at 1 in 2,500 to 1 in 3,300 births. It is an autosomal dominant trait with nearly 100% penetrance, variable expressivity, and a high spontaneous mutation rate. Approximately 45% to 71% of cases appear as spontaneous mutations in normal families.

Cutaneous signs of neurofibromatosis include café-au-lait spots, axillary freckles (33%), and subcutaneous nodules. These are less common in children and in patients with the central nervous system form of the disease (central neurofibromatosis). Mental retardation is observed in 10% to 30% of patients (14).

In patients with neurofibromatosis (Figs. 18 and 19), MRI commonly displays

1. cranial nerve schwannomas, especially acoustic neuromas; these appear at an earlier age than isolated acoustic neuromas and are often bilateral;
2. meningiomas, especially multiple meningiomatosis;
3. optochiasmal gliomas. These are the most common tumor in neurofibromatosis and are found in 10% of children with the disease; the tumor may affect one or both eyes, the chiasm alone, or the entire length of the visual apparatus;

4. brainstem and supratentorial gliomas;
5. arachnoid cysts;
6. sphenoid dysplasia with hypoplastic sphenoid wings, enlarged superior orbital fissure, and protrusion of the temporal lobe onto the orbit to cause pulsating exophthalmos; and
7. vascular dysplasia with multiple infarctions and even moya-moya.

Tuberous Sclerosis

Tuberous sclerosis is a dyshistiogenesis characterized, in part, by overgrowth of astrocytes. The incidence of tuberous sclerosis is approximately 1 per 1,000 births (14). It is believed to be hereditary, but the mode of transmission is not clear. Some cases may be autosomal dominant disease. Perhaps 70% to 80% appear as spontaneous mutations (17).

Clinically, tuberous sclerosis is characterized by the clinical triad of adenoma sebaceum (30–85% of cases), mental retardation (50–80%), and seizures (80%). Hypopigmented nevi (83%), shagreen patches, subungual fibromas, rhabdomyomas and sarcomas of the heart and angiomyolipomas of the kidney (80%), all suggest the diagnosis of tuberous sclerosis (25).

In patients with tuberous sclerosis (Figs. 20 and 21), MRI displays

1. cortical, subcortical, white matter, and subependymal tubers;
2. cortical heterotopias;
3. myelination defects;
4. septal, parenchymal, and diffuse tumors, especially giant-cell astrocytoma (10%);
5. hydrocephalus from obstruction of CSF flow by tumor or tuber; and
6. cerebral infarction from cerebrovascular disease.

Sturge-Weber Syndrome

Encephalotrigeminal angiomatosis is characterized by angiomatosis of the face and leptomeninges with atrophy of the subjacent cerebral hemispheres and intracortical calcification (26,27). The disease is usually unilateral but may be bilateral (15%).

The incidence of Sturge-Weber syndrome is 1 per 1,000 patients in mental institutions. It appears sporadically with no known pattern of inheritance. Estimates of the ratio of males to females with the syndrome vary widely (28).

Patients with Sturge-Weber syndrome typically exhibit a port-wine stain over the face, usually in a distribution comparable to the innervation of the superior division of the trigeminal nerve. Epilepsy is seen in more than two-thirds of cases. Mental retardation, buphthalmos or glaucoma, hemiplegia, and homonymous hemianopsia are common.

In patients with Sturge-Weber syndrome (Fig. 22), MRI displays

1. atrophy of one hemisphere, especially in the occipital and temporal lobes, with shrunken calcified gyri and enlarged sulci;
2. superficial leptomeningeal angiomas; and
3. nonfunctional or absent cortical veins with patent deep veins.

CONCLUSION

Magnetic resonance imaging is the modality of choice to display and differentiate among the diverse congenital anomalies. It shows gray and white matter well. It images the same structures in three orthogonal planes without loss of resolution. It can be repeated serially, without endangering the patient, to evaluate the evolution of the dysplasia over time. With MRI, neuroradiology becomes gross pathology, *in vivo,* when knowledge of the pathology may still be helpful to the patient.

REFERENCES

1. Diebler C, Dulac O. Cephaloceles: Clinical and neuroradiological appearance. Associated cerebral malformations. *Neuroradiology* 1983;25:199–216.
2. Friede RL. *Developmental Neuropathology* New York, Wien:Springer-Verlag, 1975.
3. Naidich TP, McLone DG, Fulling KH. The Chiari II malformation: Part IV. The hindbrain deformity. *Neuroradiology* 1983;25:179–197.
4. Naidich TP, Maravilla K, McLone DG. The Chiari II malformation. *Proceedings of the Second Symposium on Spina Bifida.* Ed. McLaurin R and McLone D. New York; Grune and Stratten, 1986 (*in press*).
5. Grogono JL. Children with agenesis of the corpus callosum. *Dev Med Child Neurol* 1968;10:613–6.
6. Kendall BE. Dysgenesis of the corpus callosum. *Neuroradiology* 1983;25:239–56.
7. Atlas S, Zimmerman RA, Bilaniuk LV, Hackney DB, Goldberg HI, Grossman RI. Developmental anomalies of the corpus callosum and limbic system. *24th Ann Meet Am Soc Neuroradiol, San Diego, Jan 18–23, 1986.*
8. Faerber EN, Wolpert SM. The value of computed tomography in the diagnosis of intracranial lipomata. *JCAT* 1978;2:297–9.
9. Suemitsu T, Nakajima S-I, Kuwajima K, Nihei K, Kamoshita S. Lipoma of the corpus callosum: report of a case and review of the literature. *Childs's Brain* 1979;5:476–83.
10. Wolpert SM, Carter BL, Ferris EJ. Lipomas of the corpus callosum. An angiographic analysis. *AJR* 1972;115:92–9.
11. Zee C-S, McComb JG, Segall HD, Tsai FY, Stanley P. Lipomas of the corpus callosum associated with frontal dysraphism. *JCAT* 1981;5:201–5.
12. Fitz CR. Holoprosencephaly and related entities. *Neuroradiology* 1983;25:225–38.
13. Manelfe C, Sevely A. Neuroradiological study of holoprosencephalies. *J Neuroradiol* 1982;9:15–45.
14. Goodman RM, Gorlin RJ. *Atlas of The Face in Genetic Disorders,* 2nd ed. St. Louis: The C.V. Mosby Co., 1977.
15. Urich H. Malformations of the nervous system, perinatal damage and related conditions in ealy life. In: Blackwood W, Corsellis J., eds. *Greenfield's Neuropathology,* 3rd ed. Chicago: Year Book Medical Publishers, Inc., pp 361–469, 1976.
16. Zimmerman RA, Bilaniuk LT, Grossman RI. Computed tomography in migratory disorders of human brain development. *Neuroradiology* 1983;25:257–63.
17. Mori K. *Anomalies of the Central Nervous System. Neuroradiology and Neurosurgery.* New York:Thieme-Stratton Inc., 1985.
18. Raybaud C. Cystic malformations of the posterior fossa: Abnormalities associated with the development of the roof of the fourth ventricle and adjacent meningeal structures. *J Neuroradiol* 1982;9:103–33.
19. Archer CR, Darwish H, Smith Jr. K. Enlarged cisternae magnae and posterior fossa cyst simulating Dandy-Walker syndrome on computed tomography. *Radiology* 1978;127:681–6.
20. Sawaya R, McLaurin RL. Dandy-Walker syndrome. Clinical analysis of 23 cases. *J Neurosurg* 1981;55:89–98.
21. Naidich TP. The craniovertebral junction: Chiari malformations I and II. in CT'82. *Internationales Computertomographie Symposium, Seefeld/Tirol, 28–30 Jan 1982.* Konstanz: Schnetztor-Verlag, pp 78–84, 1982.
22. Paul KS, Lye RH, Strang FA, Dutton J. Arnold-Chiari malformation. Review of 71 cases. *J Neurosurg.* 1983;58:183–7.
23. Gardeur D, Palmieri A, Mashaly R. Cranial computed tomography in the phakomatoses. *Neuroradiology* 1983;25:293–304.
24. Casselman ES, Miller WT, Lin SR, Mandell GA. Von Recklinghausen's disease: Incidence of roentgenographic findings with a clinical review of the literature. *CRC Crit Rev Diagn Imaging* 1977;9:387–419.
25. Kinglsey DPE, Kendall BE, Fitz CR. Tuberous sclerosis: a clinicoradiological evaluation of 110 cases with particular reference to atypical presentation. *Neuroradiology* 1986;28:38–46.
26. Bentson JR, Wilson GH, Newton TH. Cerebral venous drainage pattern of the Sturge-Weber Syndrome. *Radiology* 1971;101:111–8.
27. Probst FP. Vascular morphology and angiographic flow patterns in Sturge-Weber angiomatosis: facts, thoughts and suggestions. *Neuroradiology* 1980;20:73–8.
28. Warkany J. *Congenital Malformations, Notes and Comments.* Chicago:Year Book Medical Publishers, Inc. 1971.

CHAPTER 11

Brain Tumors

Michael Brant-Zawadzki and William Kelly

The detection of intracranial neoplasms poses a challenge for all diagnostic imaging modalities, including magnetic resonance imaging (MRI). The clinical presentation of patients harboring such neoplasms varies from subtle or nonspecific symptoms, such as headache, nausea, and subjective mental status changes (seen in up to 50% of patients with tumors in the early stages of growth), to more ominous signs, such as seizure onset, focal weakness, loss of verbal fluency, and altered visual or other sensory function.

The major advantage of MRI in this context is its unprecedented sensitivity. Clinical experience has documented the unquestionable superiority of MRI over computed tomography (CT) in detecting the tissue changes resulting from intracranial neoplasms when the two techniques are compared (1–7). This superiority results not only from optimal anatomic delineation in multiple planes of altered morphology, but especially from the clearly improved capability to detect altered tissue constituents even before any morphologic change is detected (Fig. 1). Once such an abnormality is detected, the diagnostician can begin to formulate a differential diagnosis. This process requires an understanding of the underlying principles of the imaging technique (as explained elsewhere in this volume) and a working knowledge of the clinical context as well as disease pathophysiology. The ability to characterize tumors and provide tissue specificity is as limited with MRI as it is with any imaging modality used in a vacuum. The proper role of MRI in the diagnostic algorithm will best be appreciated if both its major advantages as well as its limitations are kept in mind.

GENERAL TECHNICAL CONSIDERATIONS

Imaging of brain tumors with MRI depends not only on pathologic factors, but predictably, on technical ones as well. The location as well as the histology of the tumor influences its MRI appearance. Extraaxial lesions do not have a blood-brain barrier (BBB). They lie adjacent to bony and CSF spaces, are more likely to contain calcium, and may be found in intricate anatomic locations, such as the internal auditory canal, cavernous sinus, or foramen magnum. Therefore, their MRI identification requires not only an understanding of the signal intensity relationships of their intrinsic constituents to their surroundings on various pulse sequences but also more specific attention to the selection of slice orientation, thickness, and perhaps, paramagnetic contrast agents.

Intraaxial tumors are in general less challenging to delineate from an anatomic point of view, since they occur in the brain substance, but the variety of their morphology and constituents provide diagnostic comlexity nonetheless. Metastatic as well as primary brain tumors may produce a wide variety of nonspecific MRI changes, and knowledge of clinical presentation and pathophysiology of neoplastic processes are still the cornerstones of concise differential diagnosis.

The radiologist rarely knows in advance that the patient first referred for a diagnostic evaluation harbors a neoplasm. The clinical indication for MRI may be a first seizure, a focal neurologic sign or symptom of recent onset, a diffuse change in mental status, or a combination of these or other relatively nonspecific findings. A screening MRI sequence needs to be chosen that optimizes sensitivity to the widest possible spectrum of disease, including tumors. The long TR sequence (2,000 msec) with an early and a late echo is optimal in the vast majority of cases when no specifically localizing clues are present (8). That the axial plane is used in most instances is purely due to tradition; but the coronal plane offers advantages when evaluating lesions of the upper convexities, base of the skull or sella, or when a temporal lobe abnormality is suspected. The sagittal plane evaluates the region of the pineal gland and cerebral aqueduct to best advantage. Section thickness of 5 to 10 mm generally covers the entire brain (depending

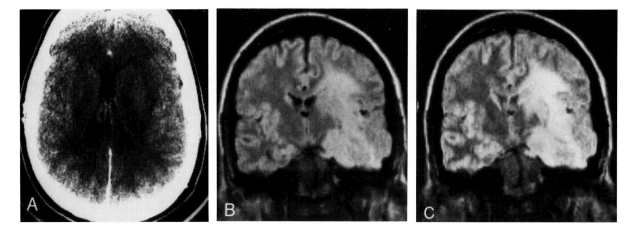

FIG. 1. Middle-aged man with recent seizure, subtle right hemiparesis. **A:** CT scan with contrast. **B:** TR 1,500, TE 28 msec. **C:** TR 1,500, TE 56 msec. The CT shows a mild shift of midline, left to right. The MRI documents a diffuse, infiltrating lesion, best seen on the second echo as a high signal intensity involving the parietal and temporal white matter (**C**). Biopsy verified an anaplastic astrocytoma.

on the interslice gap) and suffices for screening purposes. A 256 × 256 image matrix offers optimal resolution.

Once a lesion is identified within the screening sequence, a short TR sequence helps to characterize the T1 relaxation parameters of the abnormality. It should be performed in the same plane as the long TR study, but its relative speed permits additional planes to be easily obtained, if desired. Occasionally, the short TR sequence suffices for diagnostic needs, and the long TR sequence can be obviated. For instance, when the study requested is that of the pituitary gland in order to look for an adenoma, the short TR sequence is often the only one needed (see below). Thin sections are required in such cases, however. The combination of short TR and thin (2–3 mm) sections may necessitate more excitations (averages) for better signal-to-noise ratio in the resulting images. Imposing the available matrix into a limited field of view when the region of interest is small minimizes pixel size and maximizes spacial resolution, but again, the price is more noise.

Paramagnetic contrast agents [gadolinium–diethylenetriamine pentaacetic acid (DTPA)] are currently in clinical trials and will allow improved characterization of tumors. The effectiveness of such agents depends on intact perfusion of the lesion and absence or alteration of the BBB. Therefore, enhancement indicates that both phenomena are occurring. Screening technique, however, need not include the use of such agents in most cases (9).

The above discussion of technical considerations is, be design, of a general nature. More specific technical points shall be considered in the subsequent discussion of individual lesions when applicable.

GENERAL PATHOLOGICAL CONSIDERATIONS

Proton MRI signal characteristics of neoplasms are based predominantly on tumor water content, especially that of the extracellular space. The occasional presence of other substances, such as calcium, fat, hemorrhage, paramagnetic substances (e.g., melanin), will modify the predominant water signal. Cyst formation and other aspects of the morphology may help in formulating the differential diagnosis.

Edema

Metastases and many anaplastic primary brain tumors are often surrounded by edema of the brain's interstitium. The volume of water that accumulates often dictates the degree of mass effect and the accompanying neurologic deficit. The pathophysiologic mechanisms responsible for the appearance of edema are twofold. The neovascularity associated with malignant neoplasms is more permeable than the vascularity of the normal brain; that is, the normal BBB is incomplete or absent. The tight junctions between the endothelial cells of normal brain capillaries are not present in these abnormal vessels. These junctions, together with the capillary basement membrane, the foot processes of the nearby glial cells, and the various active transport mechanisms of the endothelial cells, form the normal BBB. When the BBB is damaged or absent, water leaks out of the capillaries, as do various plasma proteins (and any exogenously administered contrast agents). Progres-

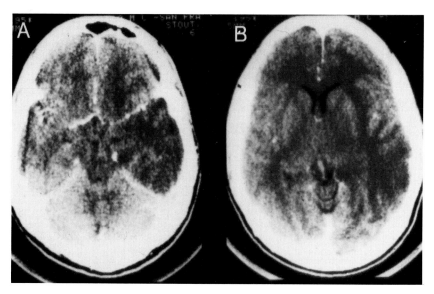

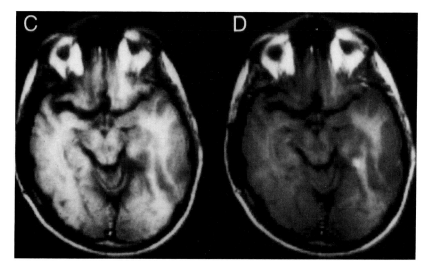

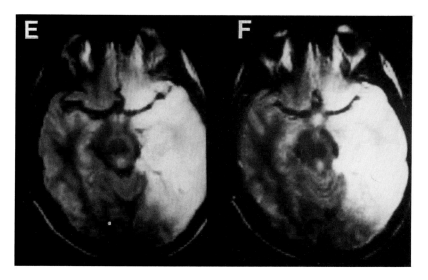

FIG. 2. Young adult man with recent personality change. **A,B:** CT with contrast, two sections. **C,D:** TR 500, TE 30 msec before and after GD-DTPA, respectively. **E,F:** TR 2,000, TE 60 msec before and after GD-DTPA, respectively. The CT shows a mass effect on the middle cerebral artery, which is enhanced by the iodinated contrast agent. Low density throughout the white matter of the posterior temporal region is seen. The short TR sequences show no definite evidence of enhancement in the tumor. The long TR sequences verified diffuse involvement of the entire temporal lobe by the lesion, as evidenced by the hyperintensity. Note that the vascular structures on both sequences without and with the paramagnetic contrast agent are seen as structures with signal void. This case emphasizes that water is more easily passed through a disrupted BBB than larger molecules such as contrast agents.

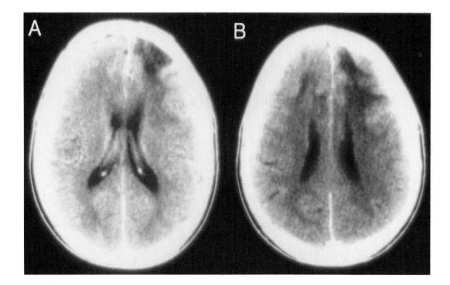

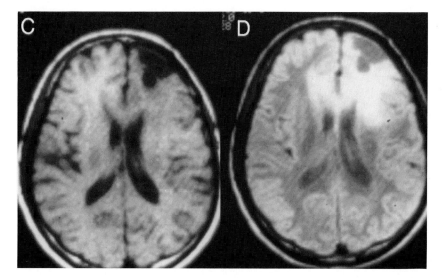

FIG. 3. Middle-aged woman, new frontal lobe signs 2 years after resection of a left frontal lobe astrocytoma. **A,B:** CT scans with contrast, two adjacent sections. **C:** TR 500, TE 30 msec. **D:** TR 2,000, TE 30 msec. The CT scan shows the site of previous frontal lobe surgery (**A**), as well as low density in both frontal lobes on the higher cut (**B**). MRI verifies the fluid-filled site of resection, surrounded by high signal intensity in the ipsilateral, as well as contralateral, lobe. There is contiguity of the abnormal tissue across the corpus callosum. Astrocytoma was found in both regions, with associated radiation necrosis on the original side. The involvement of the corpus callosum is most consistent with tumor spread, rather than simply vasogenic edema (see text).

sively more water leaks out due to the osmotic gradient and the hydrostatic forces of the blood pressure that continues to pump water out of the abnormal capillaries. The extracellular spaces of the gray matter are 10 to 20 nm across, compared to 80 nm or more in the white matter. The passage of macromolecules is permissible at a breadth of 20 nm and is hence facilitated in white matter (10). Therefore, this so-called vasogenic edema of tumors is seen predominantly in the white matter, since it is facilitated by the migration of macromolecules through the extracellular space.

More benign tumors, such as meningiomas, may cause vasogenic edema by compromising the integrity of the endothelium of the normal brain vasculature at the margins of the tumor–brain interface, because of pressure or direct invasion. A surprising amount of edema may accompany even small meningiomas for reasons that are poorly understood.

The abnormally high MRI signal produced by the vasogenic edema may make it difficult to identify the nidus of tumor within the edema that has caused it. Both the tumor's extracellular space and that of the affected white matter may have increased water content. Computed tomography may also have some difficulty providing the answer. For example, even anaplastic astrocytomas may have insufficient vascular permeability to allow leakage of contrast, although water content is raised (Fig. 2). In such instances, MRI is better able than CT to depict the abnormal tissue's presence and its extent, although neither modality can definitely separate tumor margins from edematous brain.

The practical needs in imaging tumors are to provide

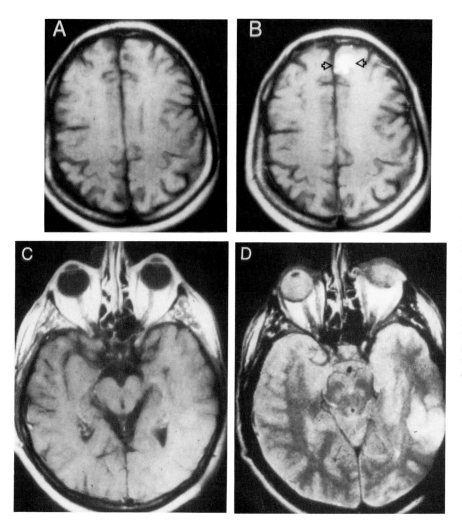

FIG. 4. Multifocal glioma. Middle-aged man with recent onset of seizures; no other symptoms. **A,B:** TR 500, TE 30 msec; before and after GD-DTPA, respectively. **C:** TR 500, TE 30 msec; after GD-DTPA. **D:** TR 2,000, TE 60 msec; before GD-DTPA. A left frontal lobe lesion is seen after GD-DTPA on the short TR sequence (*arrows;* **B**). This was also visualized on the long TR sequence prior to contrast agent administration as a focus of high signal intensity. The temporal focus did not enhance on the post-GD-DTPA study (**C**), but was well visualized on the long TR sequence despite lack of enhancement (**D**).

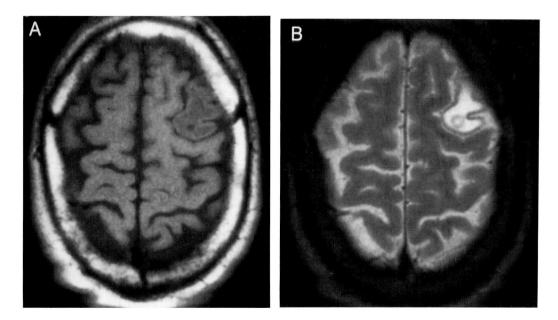

FIG. 5. Metastatic carcinoma, renal cell. **A:** TR 600, TE 25 msec. **B:** TR 2,000, TE 60 msec. Both sequences show vasogenic edema in the white matter exhibiting low signal intensity on the short TR and very high signal intensity on the long TR. Note the cystic nature of the metastatic nodule.

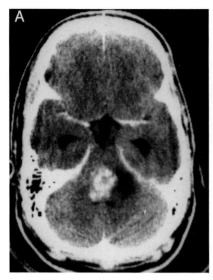

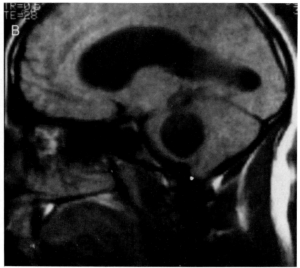

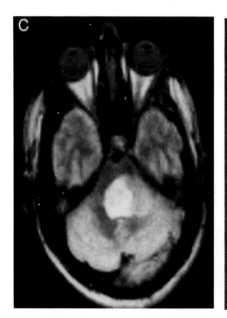

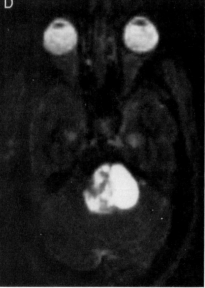

FIG. 6. Cystic brainstem glioma. **A:** CT scan with contrast. **B:** TR 500, TE 28 msec. **C:** TR 2,000, TE 40 msec. **D:** TR 2,000, TE 120 msec. The CT scan shows a solid component of the tumor, as evidenced by enhancement, with the cystic component more lateral on the left side. The short TR sequence shows the left-sided cystic component as having low signal intensity, due to the markedly prolonged T1 relaxation value (**B**). The early echo of the long TR sequence shows the cyst as having relatively low signal intensity when compared to the more edematous solid component, again due to the relatively long T1 value of the cystic lesion (**C**). The late echo shows relatively higher signal from the solid, edematous tumor when compared to the rest of the brain, but the cystic component has an even higher signal due to the markedly prolonged T2 relaxation value within the fluid when compared to the edematous lesion.

a focus for biopsy, to allow delineation of margins when total excision is planned, and to provide landmarks for planning radiation therapy. Because infiltrating astrocytomas and vasogenic edema may appear identical on either CT or MRI, both modalities may fall short of these goals. Edema is much less likely to spread across the corpus callosum to involve a contralateral hemisphere than aggressive glioma, a helpful differentiating feature (Fig. 3). Contrast enhancement may approximate tumor margins, but tumors need not be confined to such enhancing foci. Multifocal enhancement need not imply metastatic disease: True multicentric gliomas

occur 2.5% of the time (11), and even single, contiguous tumors may show several separate foci of enhancement (Fig. 4).

In our experience, MRI will often show different signal characteristics of the tumor nidus when compared to surrounding edema. On T2-weighted images, the edema appears more intense than the epicenter of the tumor. This may reflect the relatively greater water-filled extracellular space of the white matter when compared to the compact extracellular space in the highly cellular tumor (Fig. 5). Alternatively, if the tumor is necrotic or cystic, its signal is of very low intensity on T1-weighted images,

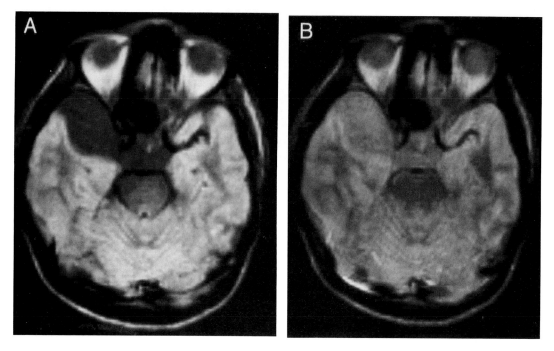

FIG. 7. Arachnoid cyst. **A:** TR 2,000, TE 28 msec. **B:** TR 2,000, TE 56 msec. Note that the signal intensity of the right-sided, middle fossa cyst matches that of the intraocular vitreous, the perimesencephalic space, and the cerebral aqueduct on both echos. This indicates the benign nature of the fluid collection.

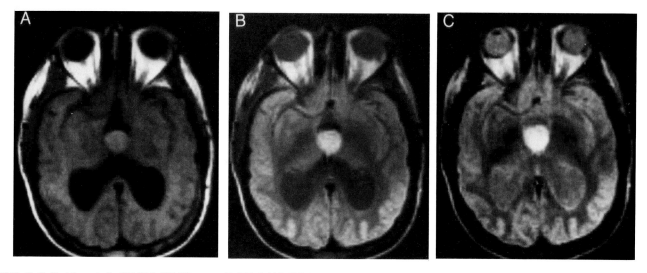

FIG. 8. Colloid cyst. **A:** TR 500, TE 28 msec. **B:** TR 2,000, TE 28 msec. **C:** TR 2,000, TE 56 msec. Note that the short TR sequence (**A**) reveals a somewhat hyperintense, round lesion. Capping of the lesion by the third ventricle indicates an intraventricular location for this tumor. The long TR sequence shows high signal intensity of the lesion on both echos.

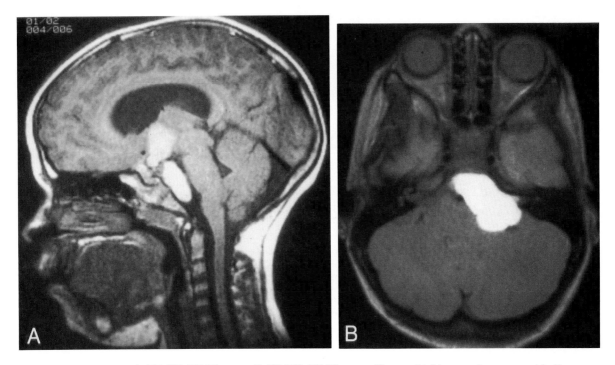

FIG. 9. Craniopharyngioma. **A:** TR 600, TE 25 msec. **B:** TR 200, TE 80 msec. The sagittal image shows a cyst in the suprasellar region effacing the third ventricle and a second loculation posterior to the dorsum. The axial image with the long TR shows persistent high signal in the cyst.

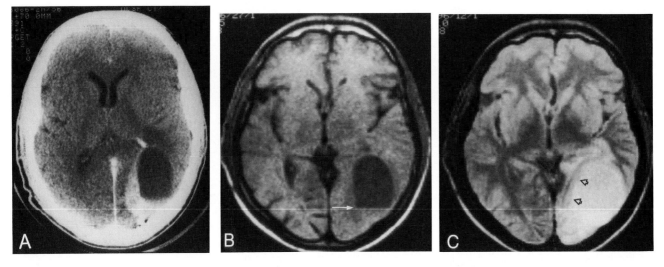

FIG. 10. Cystic glioma. **A:** CT scan with contrast. **B:** TR 500, TE 28 msec. **C:** TR 2,000, TE 28 msec. The cystic nature of the lesion is evident on CT, with a thickened, enhancing wall in the medial and posterior aspect, indicating the neoplastic nature of the cyst. MRI clearly depicts the fluid level within the cyst on the short TR sequence (**B;** *arrow*) as well as the irregular inner wall of the cystic cavity (**C;** *arrows*). Note that the very long T1 relaxation value of the cyst, as evidenced by low intensity on the short TR sequence, is not quite as long as that of CSF. This is proven on the long TR sequence, where the cyst fluid has a higher signal.

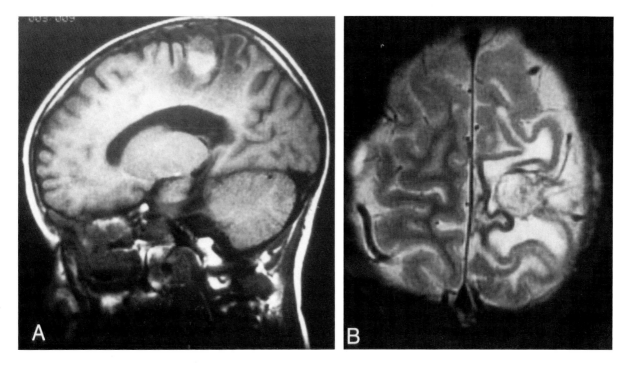

FIG. 11. Ependymoma with previous hemorrhage. **A:** TR 600, TE 25 msec. **B:** TR 2,000, TE 80 msec. The sagittal view suggests subacute hemorrhage in the high parietal convexity by virtue of some increased signal intensity on this short TR sequence in that location. The long TR sequence indicates a larger area of parenchymal abnormality corresponding to the location of the tumor. Note the relatively greater signal loss in the adjacent gyral surfaces attributable to hemosiderin deposition and preferential T2 shortening on that basis.

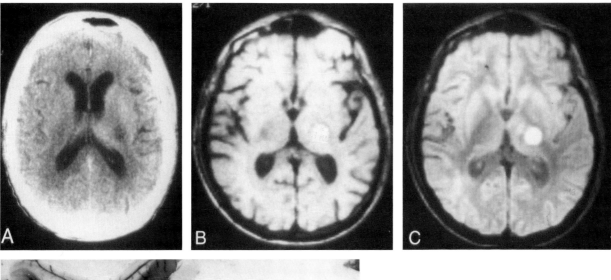

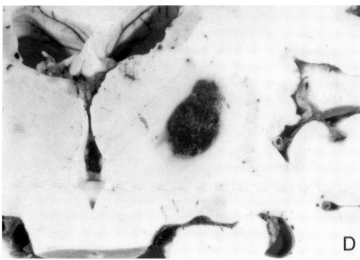

FIG. 12. Middle-aged musician with progressive dysfunction in right arm. **A:** CT without contrast. **B:** TR 500, TE 28 msec. **C:** TR 2,000, TE 28 msec. **D:** Pathologic specimen. The combination of low density on CT and high intensity on the short TR sequence (**A,B**) suggested an old focal hemorrhage. The lack of any surrounding edema on the long TR sequence also suggested a spontaneous bleed; however, the progressive history was worrisome for an underlying neoplasm. The patient died of cardiac causes shortly after the studies. The pathologic specimen verified the hemorrhage, but the histology revealed an underlying glioblastoma multiforme.

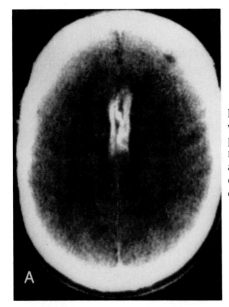

FIG. 13. Young man with progressive seizures, recently uncontrollable. **A:** CT without contrast. **B,C:** TR 2,000, TE 28, 56 msec, respectively. The CT scan shows prominent midline calcification without surrounding edema. No contrast enhancement was seen on the subsequent study. MRI depicts a much greater area of abnormal signal intensity throughout both paramedian hemispheric regions; however, the calcification is impossible to identify. Biopsy verified an anaplastic astrocytoma.

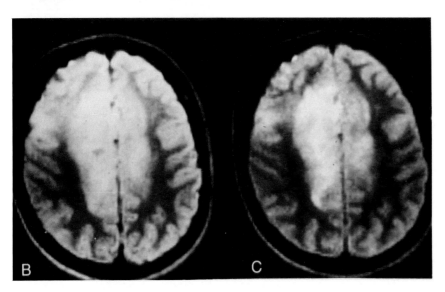

whereas the edema is better seen on routine T2-weighted images (Fig. 6). In such instances, a very late echo will show greater relative signal from the cystic component than the surrounding edematous brain.

Cyst Formation

A wide variety of neoplastic entities may produce cystic lesions within the brain. Benign developmental conditions, such as arachnoid or ependymal duplications, may cause cysts. Their hallmarks are uniformly thin walls, and the fluid within shows the characteristics of CSF—both features depicted by MRI (Fig. 7). Colloid cyst and craniopharyngioma, albeit benign, are clinically more ominous because of location and growth characteristics. The cyst contents of both lesions show wide variability that is reflected in the MR signal quality. Both lesions may show strong signal on T1-weighted images (Figs. 8 and 9).

Malignant tumors may show a wide variety of cystic morphology. Primary cysts may occur with tumors, or they may form secondarily due to central hemorrhage with subsequent liquifaction, central necrosis, entrapment of adjacent CSF space, or cavitation due to therapy. In general, malignant cysts demonstrate irregular walls, a fluid signal that differs markedly from CSF (having a shorter T1 relaxation value), and fluid levels

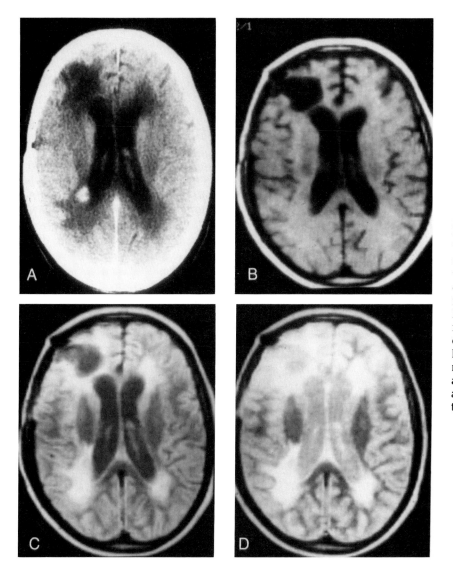

FIG. 14. Subependymal tumor spread, masked by underlying radiation leukoencephalopathy. Patient 2 years after resection of right frontal astrocytoma, progressive dementia. **A:** Contrast-enhanced CT. **B:** TR 500, TE 28 msec. **C:** TR 2,000, TE 28 msec. **D:** TR 2,000, TE 56 msec. The CT cannot completely exclude residual tumor at the site of resection; however, enhancement of a subependymal nodule indicating tumor spread is obvious. The MRI sequences show the site of tumor resection as a CSF-filled space. There is diffuse increase in signal intensity on the long TR images throughout the white matter indicating radiation reaction. This abnormal signal masks any focal alteration that would have been produced by the subependymal nodule seen on CT.

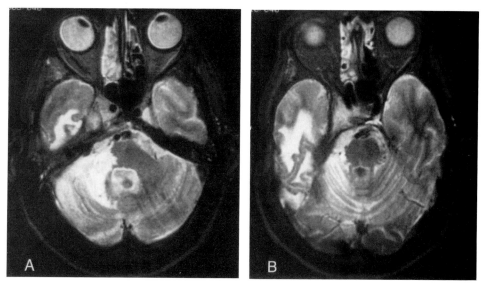

FIG. 15. Right paracavernous meningioma, status postradiation. **A,B:** TR 2,000, TE 80 msec. Adjacent sections. Note the abnormally high signal of the temporal lobe and right portion of the cerebellar middle peduncle. The meningioma is seen within the right cavernous sinus, as is medial deviation of the right globe caused by sixth nerve compression. The higher section shows the temporal lobe edema to better advantage. Also noted is increased soft tissue within the right ethmoid sinuses. The white matter change, confined to the right side of the brain at the same axial level as the meningioma, conformed to the radiation port used to treat this lesion.

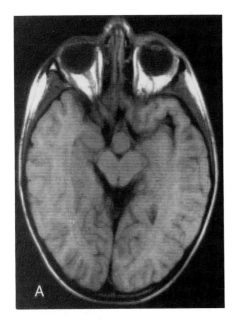

FIG. 16. Six-year-old girl with precocious puberty; hamartoma. **A:** TR 500, TE 30 msec. **B:** TR 2,000, TE 30 msec. **C:** TR 2,000, TE 60 msec. A well-circumscribed, isointense lesion is seen in the suprasellar cistern on the axial cuts. The long TR sequences show that the lesion at the tuber cinereum (**B;** *arrowheads*) remains isointense with brain on the two echos.

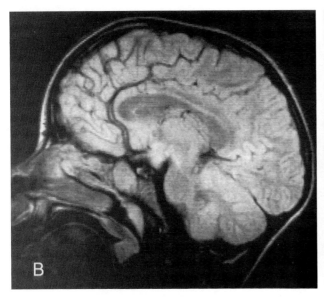

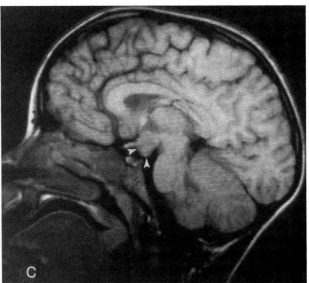

(Fig. 10). The fluid characterization capabilities of MRI are one of the particular advantages of MRI over CT when evaluating cystic neoplasms (12).

In CT and MRI, the sine qua non of cystic structures is the fluid/fluid level that changes orientation with gravity. This is caused by layering of the more heavy debris in the dependent portion of the fluid-filled cavity. The lesser proton density and shorter T2 in the layered component decrease its signal on T2-weighted images. On T1-weighted images, the very long T1 of the supernatant fluid portion shows it to be dark in comparison to the lower layer (but not quite as dark as CSF). Given multiple echos in a T2-weighted sequence, a proteinaceous cyst will eventually show less signal than pure CSF, the latter having the longest T2 relaxation of any biologic substance (see Chapter 1). However, given a very high proteinaceous component evenly distributed in a cyst or a very circumscribed solid tumor with a very high water content, the distinction between cystic and solid edematous tissue may sometimes be difficult. The judicious selection of instrument parameters (TR, TE) and slice thickness can help enhance signal differences between normal and proteinaceous brain fluid, can highlight septations (if any), and can show differential flow or pulsation phenomena in cysts compared to normal CSF spaces.

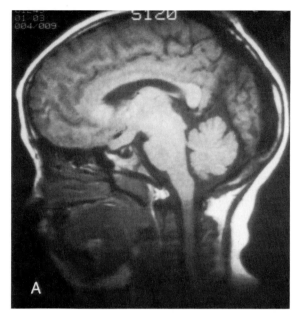

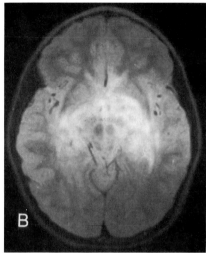

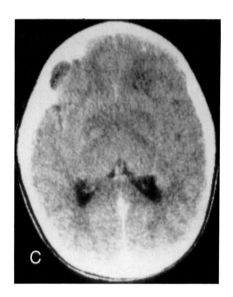

FIG. 17. Infiltrating optic glioma. **A:** TR 600, TE 25 msec. **B:** TR 2,000, TE 80 msec. **C:** CT scan with contrast. Thickening of the optic nerve leading to the chiasm is well demonstrated on the short TR sequence (**A**). The axial T2-weighted image reveals infiltration of the tumor along the optic radiations (**B**) to much better advantage than seen with CT (**C**).

Tumoral Hemorrhage

Bleeding into a tumor bed may occur primarily due to the disruption of the rich vascularity in such metastatic foci as those of hypernephroma, melanoma, choriocarcinoma, thyroid carcinoma, and others. Approximately 3% of all astrocytomas may present with symptoms of sudden bleeding (10), symptoms indistinguishable from other types of stroke. Infarction in the tumor bed as it outgrows its blood supply may also produce bleeding. In fact, silent hemorrhage within tumors may often go un

noticed, even on CT scans, because blood loses its high X-ray attenuation properties rather quickly (2–3 weeks). MRI on the other hand, exhibits the characteristic features of subacute or old hemorrhage for much longer periods of time. Usually, the hemorrhagic component is only a portion of the overall lesion. Even when the hemorrhage is large, the abnormal surroundings may indicate bleeding into pathologic tissue. Occasionally, the residue of hemorrhage from a tumor may be seen in the form of hemosiderin on the cortical surface near a tumor. This produces a striking shortening of T2, manifested as signal loss (Fig. 11). Rarely, however,

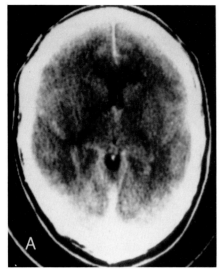

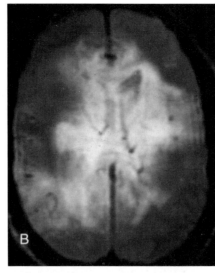

FIG. 18. Anaplastic astrocytoma. **A:** CT scan with contrast. **B:** TR 2,000, TE 80. Extensive tumor infiltration is seen in both hemispheres on the MRI study, as evidenced by the abnormal high signal intensity throughout the white matter and corpus callosum. Note the minimal amount of mass effect evidenced on both the MRI and CT despite the large area involved by tumor.

FIG. 19. Necrotic anaplastic astrocytoma. Elderly patient with progressive hemiparesis. **A:** TR 600, TE 25 msec. **B:** TR 2,000, TE 80 msec. Note the low intensity focus in the parietal region on the short TR image, consistent with marked prolongation of the T1 relaxation value of the necrotic core. The long TR image shows this area posteriorly within the relatively higher intensity zone of surrounding edema. Given the size of this lesion, note again the relatively mild mass effect.

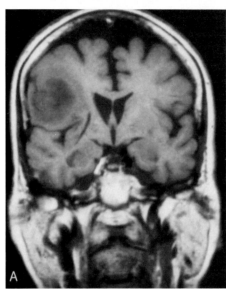

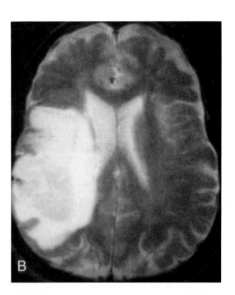

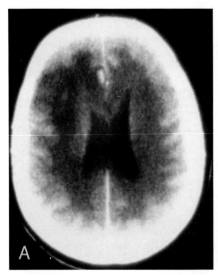

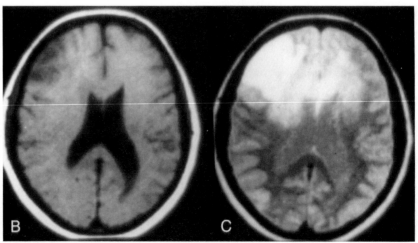

FIG. 20. Forty-five-year-old schoolteacher with recent memory loss and increasing difficulty with concentration. **A:** Contrast-enhanced CT. **B:** TR 500, TE 28 msec. **C:** TR 2,000, TE 56 msec. CT shows vague enhancement and surrounding low density in the right frontal region. The short TR image reveals focal low intensity in the periphery of the right frontoparietal cortex. The long TR image shows a much greater area of abnormality extending across the midline through the corpus callosum. Biopsy was directed at the region of low intensity on the T1-weighted image to yield the diagnosis of anaplastic astrocytoma.

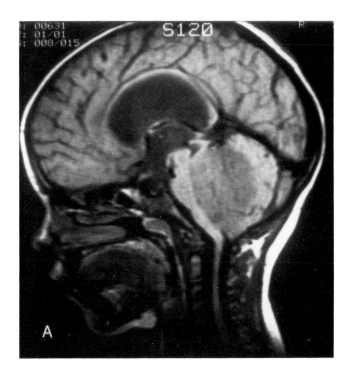

FIG. 21. Child with signs of hydrocephalus and cerebellar ataxia; juvenile pilocytic astrocytoma. **A:** TR 600, TE 25 msec. **B:** TR 2,000, TE 35 msec. **C:** TR 2,000, TE 80. A well-circumscribed, low-intensity lesion is seen in the cerebellar midline, compressing the fourth ventricle and brainstem from the dorsal aspect. Note the distortion of the quadrigeminal plate and aqueduct, resulting in hydrocephalus. The long TR sequences show the lesion as isointense with gray matter on the first echo, but of much greater intensity on the late echo (**C**). Note, incidentally, the engorged optic nerve sheaths filled with CSF, due to the hydrocephalus.

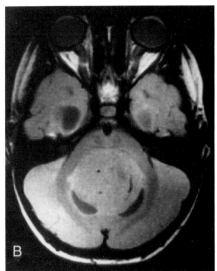

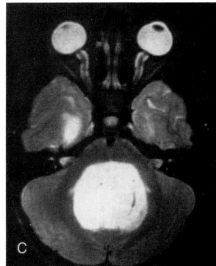

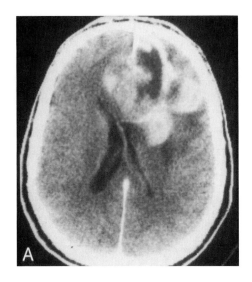

FIG. 22. Glioblastoma multiforme. **A:** CT scan with contrast. **B:** TR 1,000, TE 28, T1 420 msec. **C:** TR 2,000, TE 56 msec. The aggressive nature of the tumor is well depicted by CT, with enhancement in the left periventricular region, as well as both frontal lobes. The MRI study verifies the markedly prolonged T1 relaxation value, especially in the left frontal necrotic portion of the tumor. The T2-weighted image shows high intensity from the tumor and surrounding edema.

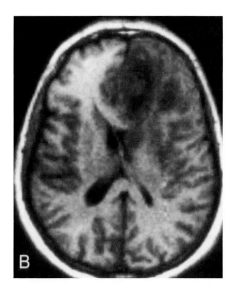

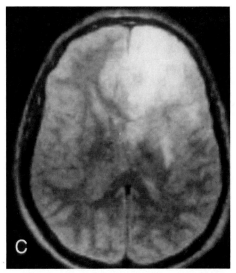

an even small hemorrhage may obliterate a tumor focus and simulate, for example, a hypertensive hemorrhage (Fig. 12).

Calcification

Punctate calcification leaves a signal void on MRI. Of course, partial volume effects dictate that a voxel that contains both a fleck of calcium and soft tissue will yield a signal, and the calcium may be missed unless these sections are used. Therefore, CT is more sensitive in characterizing certain lesions when punctate calcification is a quintessential feature of the histology. However, the counterpoint is that some lesions that seem

entirely calcified actually have a soft tissue matrix, which may be better detected with MRI (Fig. 13). Finally, certain ossified structures (e.g., crista galli) or lesions yield signal due to the presence of bone marrow and its fatty contents within the ossified matrix.

Lipomatous and Other Constituents

Fatty tumors of the CNS resemble other bodily fat in that their glyceride and cholesterol content is similar. Therefore, teratomas and lipomas will show a bright signal on T1-weighted sequences; however, the signal will fade from the first to the second echo of a T2-weighted sequence. Admixtures of lipomatous elements

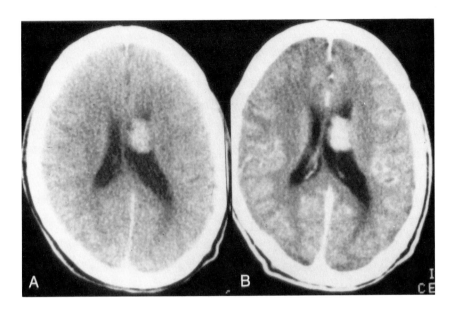

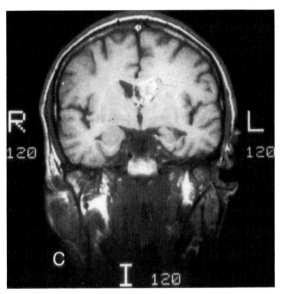

FIG. 23. Intraventricular ependymoma. **A,B:** CT without and with contrast. **C:** TR 600, TE 25 msec. **D,E:** TR 2,000, TE 40, 80 msec, respectively. The CT scan shows an inherently dense lesion within the left ventricle, which enhances. The inherent density is due to hemorrhage within the tumor, as shown by the coronal MRI image with the short TR (**C**). Note that the intraventricular tumor might be missed if only a late-echo, long TR sequence were obtained (**E**), without the benefit of an earlier echo.

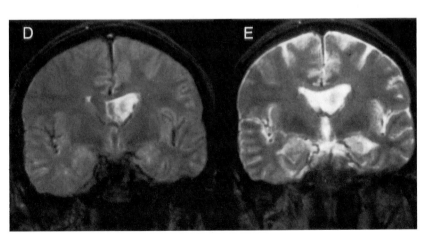

may rarely be found in such lesions as meningiomas and neurinomas that have undergone focal degeneration, sometimes resulting in punctate deposits of fat. Certain cystic lesions such as craniopharyngiomas may also accumulate cholesterol and triglycerides. Variable concentrations of these lipids, or the state of their hydration, as well as the presence of other substances, such as protein, paramagnetic species, and mucin, can effect diverse, and what are thought of as atypical, signal patterns on MRI. The direct explanations for the specific signal effects of these substances are not yet available.

Radiation Changes

In the evaluation of brain tumors with MRI, follow-up studies play a major role. One of the most difficult differential diagnostic questions on CT, that of tumor versus radiation necrosis, is not solved with proton MRI. Both lesions are dominated by the signal intensity from excess water (Fig. 14). Whole-brain radiation may cause the deep white matter to exhibit very strong signal intensity on MRI, thus, subependymal spread of tumor might be masked. The superior sensitivity of MRI means that foci of radiation damage are better detected than with CT, a helpful feature when symptoms from sites unrelated to the original tumor appear (Fig. 15).

Having considered some basic pathologic concepts in imaging of tumors with MRI, let us now consider some of the common tumor types that we are likely to encounter in clinical practice.

INTRAAXIAL LESIONS

Gliomas

These tumors arise from native glial elements of the brain. They vary from hamartomas and benign astrocytomas to anaplastic astrocytomas and glioblastoma multiforme. In general, the more benign the lesion, the more its signal intensity resembles brain. Thus, the tumor cinereum hamartoma, which produces precocious puberty in the first years of life (with much higher female predominance), is best appreciated by altered morphology of the suprasellar space, rather than by signal intensity changes (Fig. 16). This may be true of optic nerve or chiasm gliomas seen in children with neurofibromatosis; however, more aggressive astrocytomas contain blood vessels devoid of BBB and will yield higher signal on long TR sequences due to the increased water content of the extracellular space (vasogenic edema). Such aggressive gliomas grow slowly and infiltrate the brain along white matter tracts (Fig. 17).

In general, relatively little mass effect may be seen given the size of anaplastic astrocytomas (Fig. 18), com-

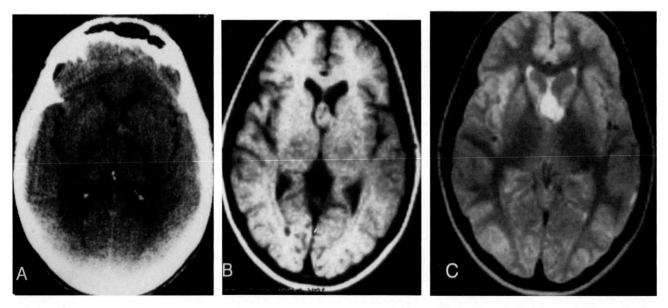

FIG. 24. Subependymal astrocytoma. **A:** CT scan without contrast. **B:** TR 500, TE 28 msec. **C:** TR 2,000, TE 56 msec. The relatively isointense signal on the short TR sequence distinguishes this subependymal astrocytoma from a colloid cyst (see Fig. 8). The characteristics of the lesion on the CT scan and on the long TR sequence are similar to that of a colloid cyst.

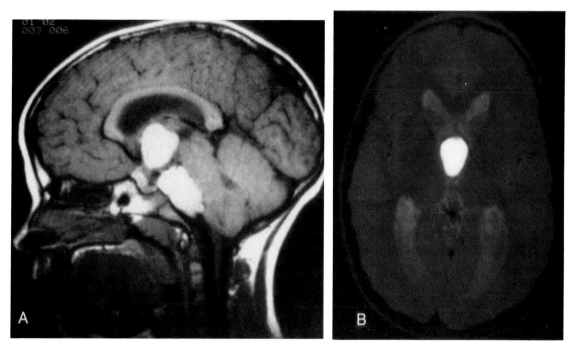

FIG. 25. Craniopharyngioma. **A:** TR 400, TE 24 msec. **B:** TR 2,000, TE 80 msec. The very high signal intensity of the supra- and retrosellar lesion on the short TR sequence indicates a very short T1 in the cyst fluid of this craniopharyngioma. This high intensity persists even on the late echo of the long TR sequence.

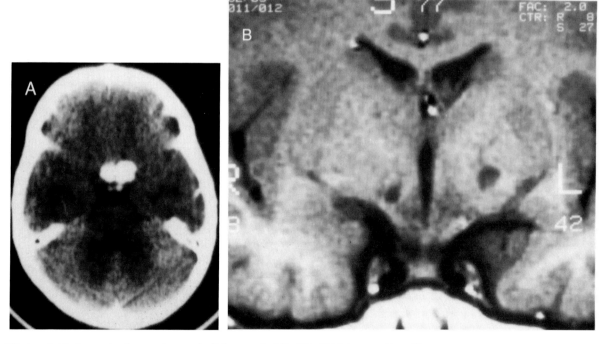

FIG. 26. A calcified craniopharyngioma. **A:** CT scan. **B:** TR 600, TE 25 msec. The CT scan shows a focal calcification in the suprasellar cistern. The MRI shows subtle narrowing of the inferior third ventricle and defacement of the normal structures in the suprasellar region; namely, the separation of the suprasellar cistern, optic chiasm, and hypothalamus is indistinguishable. Note the focal low signal intensities in the supralateral aspect of the hypothalamic region representing focal calcification. The diagnosis of a hypothalamic craniopharyngioma would be very difficult without the accompanying CT scan in this case.

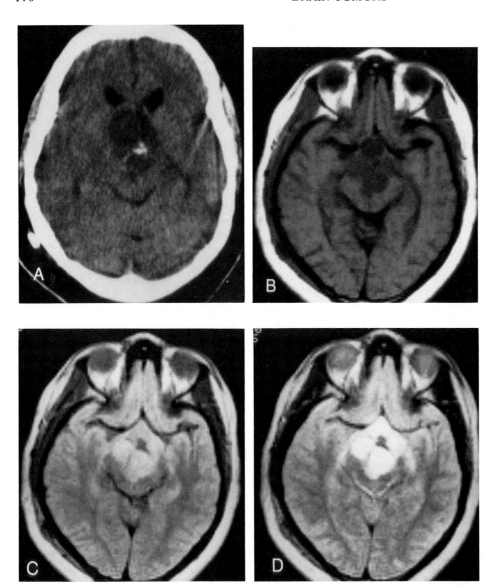

FIG. 27. Cystic craniopharyngioma. **A:** CT scan without contrast. **B:** TR 500, TE 28 msec. **C,D:** TR 2,000, TE 28, 56 msec, respectively. This CT scan shows a cystic lesion with focal calcification within, replacing the suprasellar and interpeduncular cisterns, with mild hydrocephalus. The short TR sequence illustrates the multiple loculations of the cystic lesion and the relationships of the anterior circle of Willis. Note that the long T1 of this cystic craniopharyngioma is opposite to that of Fig. 25. The long TR sequences help to prove that the fluid within the cyst is not like that of CSF, due to the very high signal intensity when compared to the temporal horns or orbital vitreous.

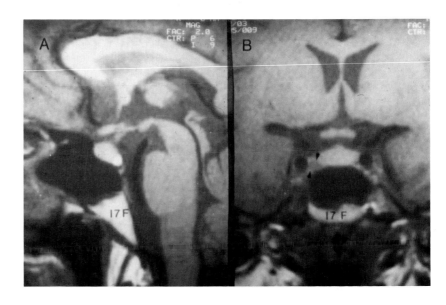

FIG. 28. Prolactinoma. Young woman with amenorrhea; galactorrhea. **A:** Sagittal 3-mm section, TR 600, TE 24 msec. **B:** Coronal section, same parameters as **A.** Note the upward convexity of the pituitary gland seen on both the sagittal and coronal images, with a focal, round lesion of low signal intensity seen in the right side of the gland on the coronal image (*arrowheads*). The stalk is deviated to the left. A 3-mm microadenoma was found at surgery.

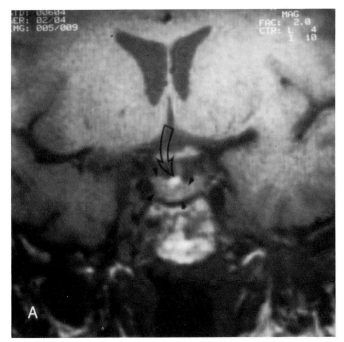

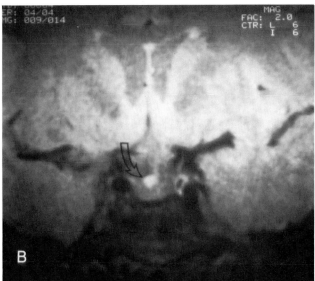

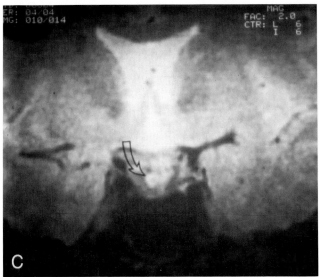

FIG. 29. Rathke's cleft cyst, and microadenoma. Patient with Cushing's disease. **A:** TR 600, TE 24 msec, 3-mm section. **B,C:** TR 2,000, TE 40, TE 80 msec, respectively. A focal, punctate lesion with high signal intensity is seen atop an enlarged right pituitary lobe (*arrows*). The high intensity is maintained from the short TR through the long TR sequences. This proved to be a Rathke's remnant cyst at surgery, where a microadenoma (*arrowheads*) was also found. Distinction from a hemorrhagic focus with these sequences was impossible.

FIG. 30. Pituitary macroadenoma. Young man with headaches; no hormonal abnormality. **A:** TR 500, TE 30 msec. **B:** Same as **A,** following administration of GD-DTPA. A large pituitary lesion is seen extending from the pituitary fossa up to the level of the third ventricle. Note the homogeneous enhancement of this lesion on the postcontrast sequence. The vascular relationships are well shown.

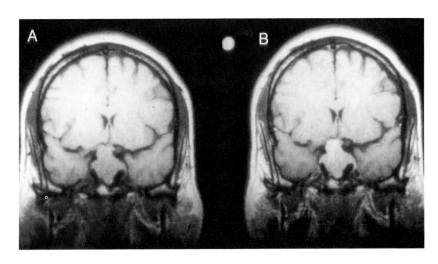

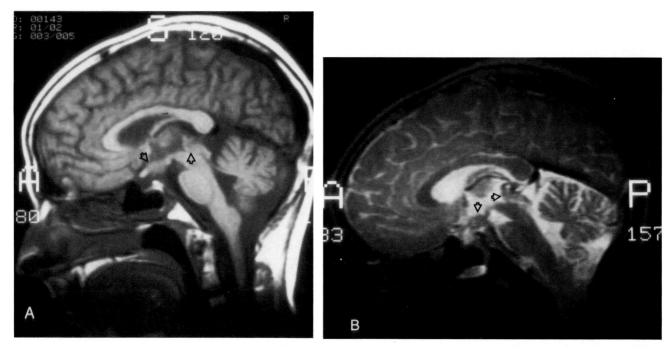

FIG. 31. Germinoma. Young man with diabetes insipidus. **A:** TR 600, TE 24 msec. **B:** TR 2,000, TE 80 msec. Distortion of the suprasellar cistern by a small, well-circumscribed isointense lesion is seen on the short TR sequence. A similar lesion is noted in the superior aspect of the quadrigeminal plate (*arrows*). The sequence with long TR and late echo again shows these two foci to be isointense and well outlined by the now highly intense CSF (*arrows*).

pared to similarly sized metastatic disease or regions of infection. However, if the associated vasogenic edema is extensive, the mass effect of primary brain tumors will be obvious.

Because the alteration of tissue contents within the tumor and the nontumoral region is similar, the separation of tumor margins from edema may be problematic. As discussed above, both tend to have elevated water content and may appear to be of lower or equal intensity relative to brain on T1-weighted images and higher than normal brain on T2-weighted images. It must be remembered that CT shares this limitation, especially in primary brain tumors. Iodinated contrast enhancement occurs only when such tumors produce an abnormal BBB. Even then, the enhancing component on CT need not correspond to tumor margins, since it only represents the region of greatest BBB disruption, and tumor may extend well beyond enhancing borders on CT. In general, the ability of MRI to distinguish the tumor's location from surrounding edema approximates that of CT. This ability is based on the capability of MRI to detect differences in tissue water content between the two abnormal regions. Truly cystic or centrally necrotic gliomas (or other types of tumor) will show marked pro-

longation of T1 and hence obvious hypointensity on T1-weighted, and even T2-weighted images, compared to the edematous surrounding brain (Fig. 19).

In our experience, also, when focal enhancement is gross on CT, MRI will show that region as a focus of greater water leakage, i.e., lower in intensity on T1-weighted images than the more peripheral border of vasogenic edema, even in the absence of frank cyst formation or necrosis; T2-weighted images invariably show a larger region of abnormality than the T1-weighted image alone. The central tumor may be hypointense, isointense, or hyperintense on these long TR sequences, but the surrounding edema is invariably hyperintense compared to brain, depending on the degree of T1 and T2 prolongation (Fig. 20), the TR and TE parameters, and the field strength of the imager used.

Given the above discussion regarding abnormal vascularity and central necrosis associated with greater degrees of malignancy in astrocytomas, we might expect a correlation between degree of malignancy and prolongation of T1 and T2 relaxation values in these tumors. This correlation is only partly valid. Certain histologic subtypes of relatively benign astrocytomas such as the juvenile pilocytic astrocytomas may also have very pro-

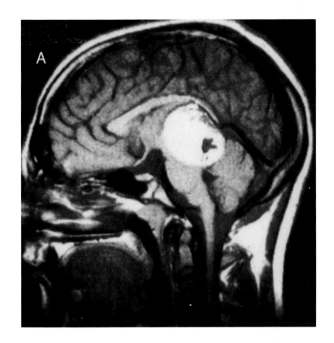

FIG. 32. Teratoma. **A:** TR 600, TE 24 msec. **B,C:** TR 2,000, TE 40, TE 80 msec, respectively. The high signal intensity of this circumscribed peripineal lesion on the short TR sequence is suggestive of fat, an impression verified by the loss of signal intensity over the two echos of the long TR sequence. Note that the posterior focus of low signal, representing a cystic focus, exhibits a chemical shift artifact (*arrows*).

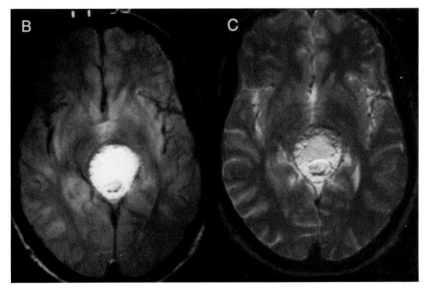

longed T1 and T2 values due to their tendency to exhibit microcystic degeneration. These lesions tend to have an almost cystic appearance on MRI and are relatively well circumscribed, with little surrounding edema (Fig. 21). Ganglioneuromas and gangliogliomas are rare benign lesions of the brain found in the early decades that may also appear ominous at first because of their cystic nature. However, the lack of significant edema and mass effect and their well-circumscribed appearance all suggest their relatively benign histology despite the long T1 and T2 relaxation values.

The most malignant and, unfortunately, the most common primary brain tumor is the glioblastoma multiforme. This tumor is most common in the fifth and sixth decades of life, has a predilection for the temporal and frontal lobes, and may spread across the corpus callosum, resulting in a "butterfly" appearance. In 5% of cases, this tumor is seen multifocally (11). The term *multiforme* reflects a varied appearance of this tumor both at necropsy and on MRI. The periphery generally shows a viable, granular tumor, whereas the core may show creamy necrotic material, hemorrhagic foci, and

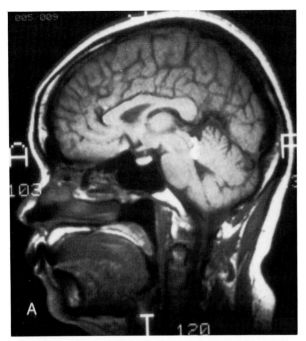

FIG. 33. Quadrigeminal plate lipoma. **A:** TR 600, TE 24 msec. **B,C:** TR 2,000, TE 40, TE 80 msec, respectively. The fatty nature of this incidental lesion is exhibited by these sequences, the signal intensity of fat fading over the two echos on the long TR sequence.

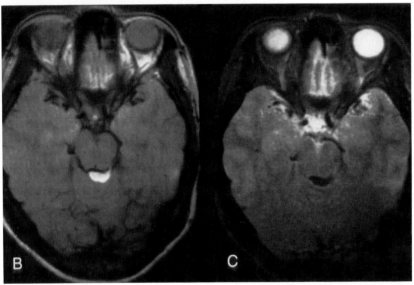

FIG. 34. Epidermoid. **A:** TR 600, TE 24 msec. **B:** TR 2,000, TE 80 msec. The tumor in the prepontine space is hard to seprate from CSF on the short TR sequence. The left fifth nerve is displaced. The long TR sequence suggests CSF-filled interstices in the tumor.

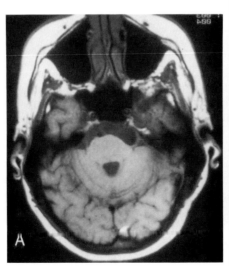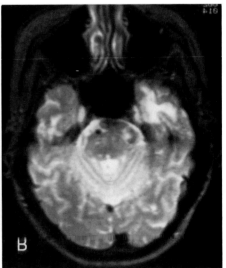

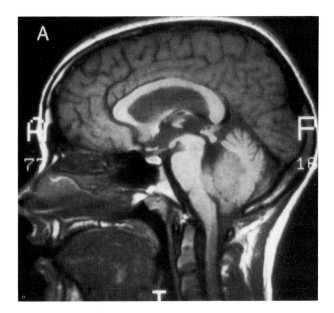

FIG. 35. Medulloblastoma. **A:** TR 600, TE 28 msec. **B,C:** TR 2,000, TE 40, TE 80 msec, respectively. A midline lesion of low signal intensity is seen in the dorsal aspect of the fourth ventricle, involving the obex and vermis. Note its separation from the brainstem and the associated hydrocephalus. The long T1 and T2 characteristics suggest malignancy. The location is very specific for medulloblastoma.

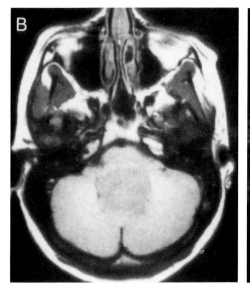

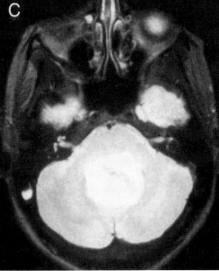

cyst(s) filled with xanthochromic fluid. Desite a circumscribed appearance on gross inspection, microscopic examination reveals the insidious invasive nature of this lesion, which lacks a capsule and extends deep into the white matter, well beyond its gross margins.

As with CT, MRI demonstrates the often cystic, necrotic nature of this lesion, the thick, irregular margins, as well as the variable degree of surrounding vasogenic edema (Fig. 22). If the tumor spreads deeply to reach the ventricular surface or superficially toward the gyri, seeding via the CSF is common (13).

Ependymomas constitute approximately 6% of all intracranial gliomas. These are relatively benign tumors of childhood and adolescence, arising from ependymal cells or the fibrillary neurologlia on which the ependyma rests; the latter subtype is termed *subependymoma*. The most common location of origin is the fourth ventricle, although any ependymal surface may give rise to the lesion. On MRI, the characteristic intraventricular location is well depicted (Fig. 23). Their well-circumscribed appearance and lack of invasiveness suggests the diagnosis. Occasionally, malignant degeneration produces aggressive behavior, and spread through the CSF pathway may occur.

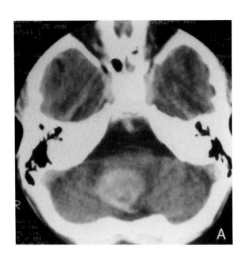
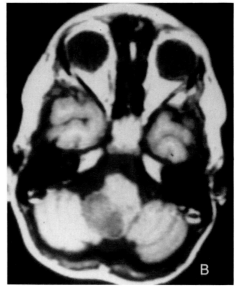

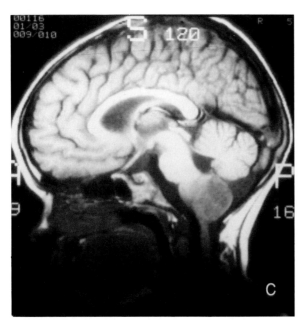

FIG. 36. Brainstem astrocytoma of childhood. **A:** CT scan with contrast. **B:** TR 600, TE 24 msec, sagittal. **C:** Same parameters, axial. The CT scan suggests a midline cerebellar tumor consistent with a medulloblastoma. The MRI indicates a brainstem origin for this somewhat exophytic mass with very long T1 characteristics. This proved to be a cystic astrocytoma.

A relatively uncommon tumor, the oligodendroglioma, needs mentioning in that its distinguishing feature, calcification, may be missed on MRI. More than 90% of these lesions contain calcium, which may be coarse or nodular (14). Although these tumors may present with seizures in their early, relatively benign stages, differentiation into more malignant histology is common. Therefore, the presence of calcium in a primary brain tumor does not preclude a malignant histology.

Midline Tumors

A variety of specific tumor types can be found in the midline of the supratentorial compartment. Colloid cysts represent only 2% of glial tumors (10), but their characteristic location at the foramina of monro in the third ventricle and the typical symptoms of positional headache make their diagnosis relatively easy. MRI shows these lesions as having hyperintense signal, not only on T2-weighted images, but also on T1-weighted images. The latter feature distinguishes them from an

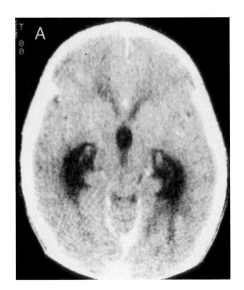

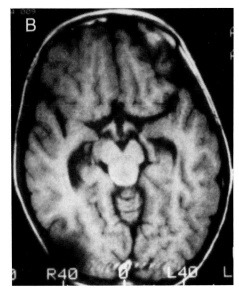

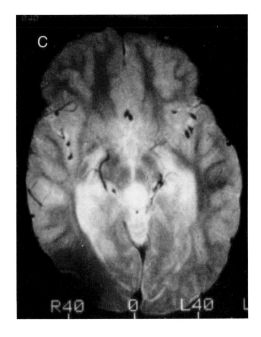

FIG. 37. Brainstem astrocytoma. Patient with neurofibromatosis; recent onset of ataxia and Parinaud's syndrome. **A:** Contrast-enhanced CT scan. **B:** TR 600, TE 24 msec. **C:** TR 2,000, TE 80 msec. The MRI images show a focal, well-circumscribed round lesion in the dorsal pons, effacing the aqueduct. Hydrocephalus is seen on both studies. The CT diagnosis was aqueductal stenosis, whereas the MRI identified the lesion for a biopsy.

occasional subependymal astrocytoma in this location (Figs. 8 and 24). The "colloid" in these cysts is really a mucinous fluid of variable viscosity secreted by the ependymal-like cuboidal cells that form their wall. Craniopharyngiomas may also exhibit striking signal intensity on T1-weighted images (Fig. 25). They present in childhood, with a second peak in late adulthood. The infundibular location of these lesions distinguishes them from colloid cysts, as does their frequent retrodorsal extension. As with CT, MRI may show a variety of signal patterns in these lesions. Craniopharyngiomas may

contain solid or cystic components or both. Calcification is a common feature seen in 80% of these lesions in children and in 40% in adults (15), but it might be difficult to pick up on MRI (Fig. 26). The cyst may be hyperintense on T1-weighted MRI or may show more typical long T1 values, i.e., low intensity, on such sequences (Fig. 27). Although histologically benign, surgical excision of this tumor may be difficult because of the tendency to adhere to adjacent vital structures.

Pituitary adenomas have only recently begun to be evaluated by MRI. Thin sections are necessary for the

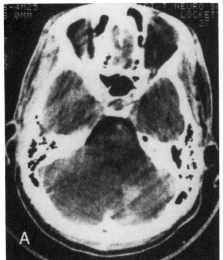
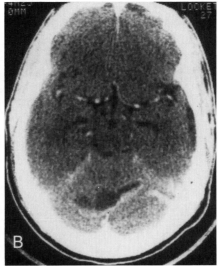

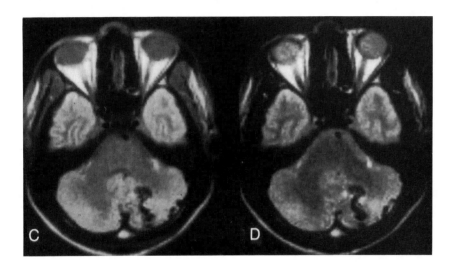

FIG. 38. Twenty-five-year-old man with an acute headache 2 months prior to admission; recent onset of cerebellar ataxia and occipital headache. **A,B:** Enhanced CT scan at two levels. **C:** TR 500, TE 28 msec. **D:** TR 2,000, TE 28 msec. **E,F:** TR 2,000, TE 28, TE 56 msec, respectively. **G:** Arteriogram. The CT scan suggested a posterior fossa enhancing mass, with edema superiorly. The MRI study at the higher level indicates that a hemorrhagic focus is responsible for the low density seen on CT. This is indicated by the high signal intensity (on both the short TR and long TR sequences) in the lesion. The vascular nature of this lesion is well depicted on MRI at the level of the enhancing CT focus. The angiogram verifies the presence of a hemangioblastoma. It had presumably bled 2 months earlier, when the patient developed an acute headache.

optimal delineation of the microadenoma. Preliminary experience suggests that only short TR sequences are needed for their demonstration. An upwardly convex gland harboring a low-intensity focal lesion, with contralateral deviation of the stalk (all best seen on coronal images), is the typical MRI appearance of the prolactinoma (Fig. 28). Not infrequently, a very small high-intensity lesion may be seen in the gland. At surgery, this may represent a hemorrhagic microadenoma; however, Rathke's pouch cysts may also have this appearance (Fig. 29). Macroadenomas are easily appreciated with the direct multiplanar capability of MRI. As with CT, these lesions show prominent enhancement with intravenous agents (Fig. 30). The role of such paramagnetic agents in evaluating microadenomas has only begun to be investigated as of this writing.

Pineal region tumors encompass a variety of pathologic entities. Aqueductal obstruction is the most common early complication that brings patients who harbor these lesions to medical attention because of the accompanying hydrocephalus. Parinaud's syndrome, a vertical gaze palsy, is present to some extent in most patients at the time of diagnosis. Certain astrocytomas, ependymomas, and metastases may occur in this location; however, the true pineal lesion generally falls into two major categories: tumors of germ cell origin and tumors of pineal cell origin (16,17). The latter are generally nonspecific, circumscribed lesions seen relatively rarely. The former, of germ cell origin, are of two major subtypes: the germinomas and the teratomas. Germinomas tend to be well defined, isointense with brain (Fig. 31), are seen more often in males, and may have a second focus

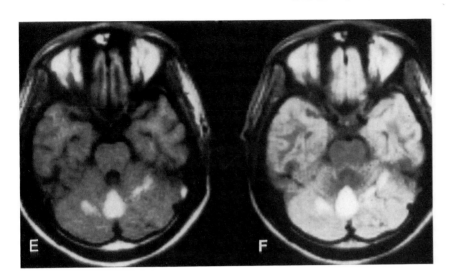

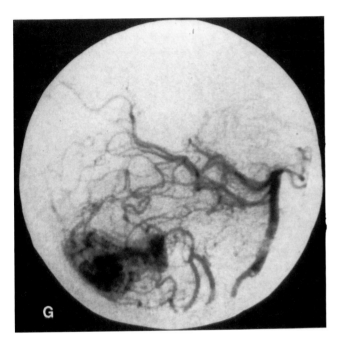

FIG. 38. (continued)

in the suprasellar region. Early pineal calcification is often seen in their presence. Teratomas, by their nature, almost always exhibit calcific, lipomatous, or cystic foci, making their MRI diagnosis relatively easy (Fig. 32).

Congenital Tumors

Lipomas are not an unusual incidental finding on MRI. They generally occur in the midline of the brain and exhibit the characteristic high signal on T1-weighted images, with fading on T2-weighted images (Fig. 33). Epidermoids, on the other hand, may show very long T1

and T2 relaxation features, making their distinction from the CSF spaces that they inhabit difficult (Fig. 34). Their favorite locations include the cerebellopontine angle, parasellar region, perimesencephalic spaces, and the intraventricular spaces.

Posterior Fossa Tumors

Medulloblastoma is a tumor that predominates in childhood. Classically, it is located in the midline behind the fourth ventricle, often compressing it. A minority may be found laterally in the hemispheres. These lateral

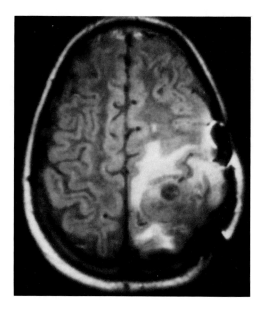

FIG. 39. Metastatic neuroblastoma, status postbiopsy (TR 2,000, TE 40 msec). Note that the tumor mass is of relatively equal intensity when compared to the white matter. The surrounding edema is easily identified, as is the interface between the two. The focus of very low signal intensity within the tumor represented calcification on the CT.

tumors are more often seen in the adult. The tumor is of neuroepithelial origin, very cellular, and moderately well demarcated from the cerebellar tissues. Cystic foci and calcification are rare, and central necrosis is seen only in the very large lesions. These features render a homogenous, well-circumscribed appearance on MRI, with long T1 and T2 relaxation characteristics (Fig. 35). Recurrence can be seen along any CSF surface, often remote from the original site. The characteristic location of this tumor helps to distinguish it from brainstem and cerebellar astrocytomas, which may also be seen in childhood (Fig. 36) and which have similar signal characteristics. The brainstem astrocytoma may be relatively occult on CT, causing only hydrocephalus. Owing to the known association of such lesions with neurofibromatosis, any patient with this entity and signs of hydrocephalus should have an MRI examination (Fig. 37). Hemangioblastomas are more unusual tumors, associated with Von Hippel–Lindau disease, and exhibit abnormal vascularity, cyst formation, and hemorrhage as common features on MRI (Fig. 38). Multiplicity is another hallmark of these lesions. Their presence in the posterior fossa should prompt screening of the spinal cord as well.

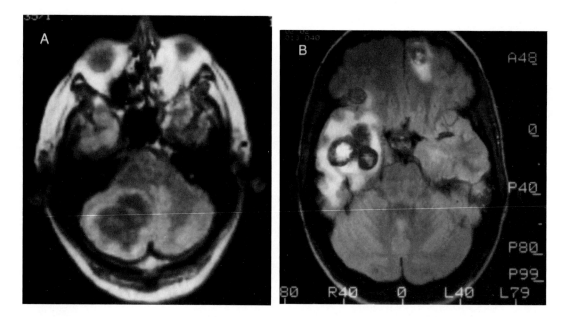

FIG. 40. Two examples of metastases with low signal on T2-weighted sequences. **A:** TR 2,000, TE 28 msec; metastatic mucinous adenocarcinoma. **B:** TR 2,000, TE 80 msec; metastatic melanoma. Note the low signal intensity of these lesions on the long TR sequences, consistent with a paramagnetic effect. The melanoma metastases exhibit central high intensity suggestive of recent hemorrhage (verified on the short TR sequence); however, no evidence of hemorrhage was found in the mucinous adenocarcinoma lesion following excision.

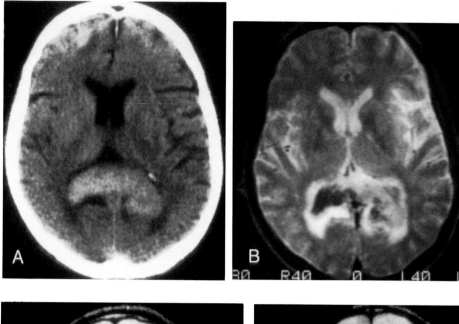

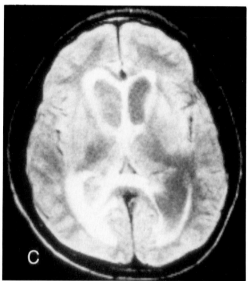
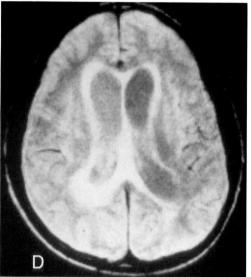

FIG. 41. Lymphoma. **A:** CT scan with contrast. **B:** TR 2,000, TE 80 msec. **C,D:** TR 2,000, TE 40 msec; two sections in another patient. Note the periventricular nature of these lymphomatous lesions. In the first patient (**A,B**), a low signal intensity along the right atrium is seen, suggesting a paramagnetic effect. Patient 2 exhibits more typical features of subependymal spread of tumor, with asymmetric involvement of the ventricular surfaces.

Metastases

Metastatic disease may mimic primary brain neoplasm when a single lesion is seen, but multiple lesions offer a strong clue due to the etiology. Also, the amount of vasogenic edema and mass effect tends to be greater with these lesions than with primary tumors of similar size. Finally, the demarcation between tumor and the surrounding edema is often easier in metastases than in primary tumors (Fig. 39). Unusual signal characteristics have been noted in mucinous adenocarcinoma and in melanoma metastases. These tumor types may exhibit a rather low signal intensity on heavily T2-weighted images, presumably due to paramagnetic effects (Fig.

40). Such abnormal signal decrease has also been noted in some focal lymphomatous lesions of the brain. The latter disease tends to have a periventricular location. It may spread along the subependymal surface (Fig. 41). Other primary and metastatic malignancies may also spread in this fashion.

EXTRAAXIAL LESIONS

Meningioma

This lesion represents the most common extraaxial neoplasm in adults, accounting for 15% of all brain

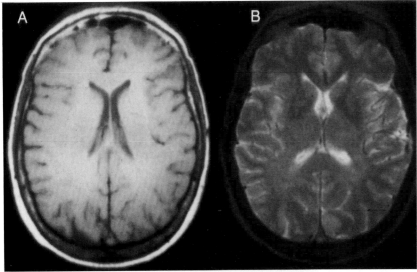

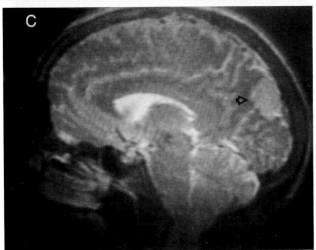

FIG. 42. Meningioma. Patient studied for retinal ischemia. **A:** TR 600, TE 24 msec. **B:** TR 2,000, TE 80 msec. **C:** TR 2,000, TE 120 msec; sagittal. The relatively isointense lesion in the left occipital pole is seen best on the longest echo image (**C;** *arrow*).

tumors. The pediatric age group may be affected, especially in the context of neurofibromatosis; however, the typical age of presentation is between 40 and 60 years, with women affected twice as often as men. The cerebral convexities (both laterally and along the falx) represent the most common location of the tumor. The dura along the sphenoid wings, body, and clinoids provides the other most common origin. The tentorial notch, posterior fossa, and foramen magnum play host to less than 10% of these tumors.

Morphologically, the meningioma is well encapsulated and indents the surface of the brain, producing symptoms by pressure rather than by invasion. The underlying brain atrophies with the slow expansion of the tumor; thus, little mass effect may be seen. The lesion tends to be isointense to brain on both T1- and T2-weighted sequences; therefore, anatomic distortion is the key to the MRI diagnosis. A thin rim of low intensity may separate the tumor from adjacent brain. Mottled nonuniform signal or focal signal void, representing calcification, may be seen, as may be thickening of the calvarial signal void, reflecting hyperostosis (8). Slight hyperintensity of the tumor on T2-weighted techniques can be emphasized by late-echo acquisitions (Fig. 42). Vasogenic edema may be seen, making the lesion easier to identify (Fig. 43). Paramagnetic contrast agents clearly help in depicting these lesions on MRI (Fig. 44).

Neurinomas

This term is ambiguous and has been used to describe the most common histologic types: the solitary schwan-

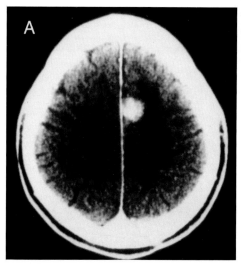

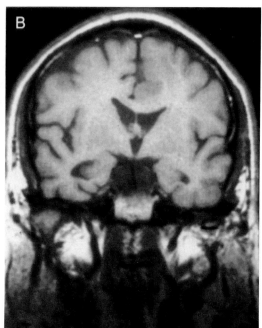

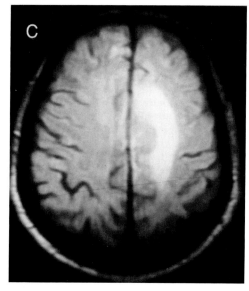

FIG. 43. Meningioma with edema. **A:** CT scan with contrast. **B:** TR 600, TE 24 msec. **C:** TR 2,000, TE 40 msec. The CT defines the enhancing, parafalcine lesion well and shows adjacent low density. The MRI study suggests a mass with subtle low intensity, compressing the roof of the left lateral ventricle. The sequence with the long TR depicts the vasogenic edema.

FIG. 44. Meningioma, paramagnetic contrast enhancement. Same patient as Fig. 42. **A:** CT with contrast. **B:** TR 500, TE 30 msec with GD-DTPA. Both iodinated and paramagnetic contrast agents enhance meningiomas in a similar fashion.

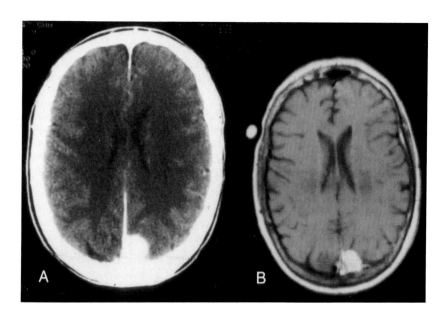

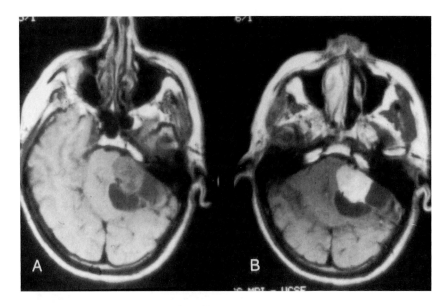

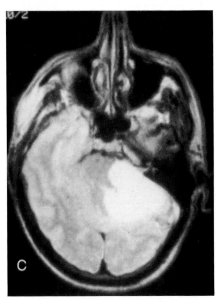

FIG. 45. Elderly man with left-sided hearing loss, nausea, and vomiting. A: TR 500, TE 30 msec. B: Same parameters as A, with GD-DTPA. C: TR 2,000, TE 60 msec. A lesion with relatively low signal intensity on short TR sequence is seen to enhance with gadolinium. Note the surrounding CSF loculations. The sequence with a long TR shows high signal intensity from the lesion and the loculations (prior to GD-DTPA).

noma and the neurofibroma of Von Recklinghausen's disease. The neurofibroma is distinguished grossly from the former by its more diffuse character, in continuity with a nerve already thickened by neoplasia, and by its soft (rather than elastic) nature. In fact, both types of lesions may be seen in Von Recklinghausen's disease. The MRI appearance of these lesions resembles meningiomas in their extraaxial, well-circumscribed morphology; however, neurinomas are much more likely to exhibit high signal on T2-weighted sequences than do meningiomas. Also, often there is an associated loculation of the adjacent CSF space next to the neurinoma. Prominent enhancement of these lesions with paramagnetic contrast agents has been noted (Fig. 45), as has the classic bone remodeling effect when the tumor is located adjacent to the auditory or other canal transmitting the

nerve of origin. Neurinomas of the vestibuloacoustic bundle are most common, but other cranial nerves may occasionally be involved (Fig. 46).

SUMMARY

This brief overview of tumor imaging with MRI reveals once again some of the early misconceptions with regard to this modality. MRI is *not* specific in differentiating neoplasms from other lesions. Knowledge of presenting signs and symtoms, biologic behavior, and incidence of tumors must be coupled with the MRI appearance for the optimal diagnostic use of this modality. Even then, differentiation of tumor from nonneoplasmatic etiology may be impossible.

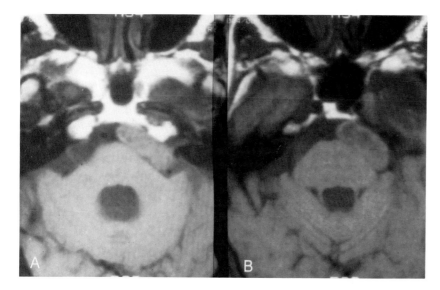

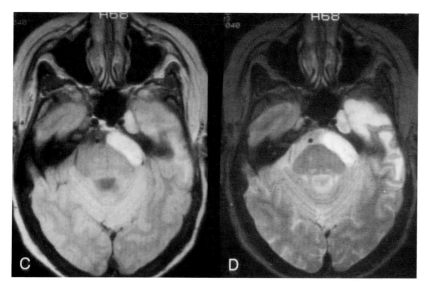

FIG. 46. Fifth nerve neurinoma. **A,B:** TR 600, TE 24 msec; two adjacent 3-mm sections. **C,D:** TR 2,000, TE 40, TE 80 msec, respectively. A discrete, cystic lesion is seen in the left prepontine cistern, entering Meckel's cave, and emerging in the cavernous sinus. The focal low-intensity round cysts are well depicted on the upper section of the short TR sequence. The long TR sequence verifies the abnormality in both locations.

REFERENCES

1. Bydder GM, Steiner RE, Young IR, et al. Clinical MR imaging of the brain: 140 cases. *AJR* 1982;139:215–36.
2. Weinstein MA, Modic MT, Pavlicek W, Keyser CK. Nuclear magnetic resonance for the examination of brain tumors. *Semin Roentol* 1984;19:139–47.
3. Brant-Zawadzki M, Badami JP, Mills CM, et al. Primary intracranial tumor imaging: a comparison of magnetic resonance and CT. *Radiology* 1984;150:436–40.
4. Brant-Zawadzki M, David PL, Crooks LE, et al. NMR demonstration of cerebral abnormalities: comparison with CT. *AJNR* 1983;4:117–24.
5. Randell CP, Collins AG, Young IR, et al. Nuclear magnetic resonance imaging of posterior fossa tumors. *AJR* 1983;141:489–96.
6. Daniels DL, Herfkens R, Loehler PR, et al. Magnetic resonance imaging of the internal auditory canal. *Radiology* 1984;151:105–8.
7. Bradley WG, Waluch W, Yadley RA, Wycoff RR. Comparison of CT and MR in 400 patients with suspected disease of the brain and cervical spinal cord. *Radiology* 1984;152:695–702.
8. Brant-Zawadzki M, Norman D, Newton TH, et al. Magnetic resonance of the brain: the optimal screening technique. *Radiology* 1984;152:71–7.
9. Brant-Zawadzki M, Berry I, Osaki L. Role of Gd-DTPA in MRI of the brain. I. Intraaxial lesions. *AJNR* 1986 (*in press*).
10. Russell DS, Rubinstein LJ. Deformations of other structural changes produced by intracranial tumors. In: *Pathology of tumors and the nervous system,* 4th ed. Baltimore: William and Wilkins. 361–70.
11. Kieffer SA, Salibi NA, Kim RC, et al. Multifocal glioblastoma: diagnostic implications. *Radiology* 1982;143:709–10.
12. Kjos BO, Brant-Zawadzki M, Kucharczyk W, Kelly WM, Norman D, Newton T. Cystic intracranial lesions: magnetic resonance imaging. *Radiology* 1985;155:363–9.
13. McGeachie RE, Gold LHA, Latchaw RE. Periventricular spread of tumor demonstrated by computed tomography. *Radiology* 1977;125:407–10.
14. Vanofakos D, Marcu H, Hacker H. Oligodendrogliomas. CT patterns with emphasis on features indicating malignancy. *JCAT* 1979;3:783–8.
15. Fitz CR, Wortzman G, Harwood-Nash C, et al. Computed tomography in craniopharyngiomas. *Radiology* 1978;127:687–91.
16. Jooma R, Kendall BE. Diagnosis and management of pineal tumors. *J Neurosurg* 1983;58:654–65.
17. Futrell NW, Osborn AG, Cheson BD. Pineal region tumors: computed tomographic–pathologic spectrum. *AJR* 1981;137:951–6.
18. Zimmerman RD, Fleming CC, Saint-Louis LA, et al. MRI in intracranial meningiomas. *AJNR* 1985;6:149–57.

CHAPTER 12

The Pituitary Gland and Sella Turcica

Walter Kucharczyk

The investigation of pituitary pathology has undergone significant changes during the past two decades. In the mid-1970s, computed tomography (CT) replaced pluridirectional tomography, pneumoencephalography, and angiography. CT permitted direct visualization of the sella turcica and its soft tissue contents in a noninvasive manner (1–4). Magnetic resonance imaging (MRI) now offers significant advantages over CT without intravenous contrast or radiation exposure. There is substantially greater soft tissue contrast as well as excellent definition of adjacent vascular structures. The direct multiplanar capability of MRI permits the patient to be positioned supine, thereby improving patient comfort. Unlike CT, dense bone at the skull base and dental hardware do not cause streak artifacts. These advantages have resulted in the rapid, widespread acceptance of MRI for the investigation of many intracranial and spinal disorders. Early magnetic resonance (MR) systems were only capable of relatively course spatial resolution, typically 7- to 10-mm-thick sections and a 128^2 matrix. Such resolution was simply inadequate for the evaluation of small lesions or intricate anatomy. With the current generation of MR systems, much improved spatial definition is possible. Modern units can provide contiguous 3- to 4-mm-thick sections and pixel sizes less than 1 mm^2 with routine multislice two-dimensional Fourier transform imaging (2DFT). Three-dimensional Fourier transform (3DFT) techniques allow even thinner slices (1.5 mm or less) but are less commonly used, primrily because they are more time consuming. Thus, the spatial resolution of MRI is now competitive with CT. In view of the many other advantages described, MRI is superceding CT as the modality of choice for evaluating the sella turcica (5–9).

MAGNETIC RESONANCE IMAGING TECHNIQUE

The pituitary gland and sella turcica are small structures with a complex relationship to the surrounding anatomy. Optimal MR evaluation requires careful patient positioning and excellent scanning technique. Multiple high-contrast contiguous thin sections with fine spatial resolution need to be obtained in a clinically "acceptable" imaging time. Often, multiple planes are required. Unfortunately, compromises need to be made if an acceptable imaging time is to be maintained. A brief description of the possible variables provides an overview of the trade-offs involved.

A circumferential head coil should be used. The patient's head should be positioned symmetrically at 0° to the canthomeatal line. Surface coils provide no advantage because of the central position of the sella turcica. A sagittal localizing image with a short repetition time (TR), short echo time (TE), and a single excitation is acquired to evaluate head position for subsequent diagnostic sequences.

Contiguous multislice 3-mm-thick sections, a 20-cm field of view (FOV), and a 256 × 256 matrix are used. Voxel dimensions of 3 × 0.8 × 0.8 mm are achieved.

Images are acquired in the sagittal and coronal planes. Coronal images are the diagnostically most useful because they allow optimal assessment of gland symmetry. There is also no partial volume artifact from the flow void of adjacent carotid arteries, which may occur in sagittal images. Sagittal images demonstrate the tuberculum and the dorsum sellae to best advantage, as well as the relationships of the pituitary stalk and the optic chiasm.

The operator-chosen variables TR and TE are the principal determinants of image contrast; that is, whether T1, T2, or spin-density images are created. For most intracranial imaging, T2-weighted images (T2-WI) have generally been accepted as the optimal screening method, with T1-weighted images (T1-WI) reserved for anatomic detail and further characterization of specific abnormalities (10). In imaging the sella the reverse is true.

T1-WI are the best for displaying morphology of the gland, the infundibulum, and optic chiasm, particularly their interfaces with the CSF in the suprasellar cistern.

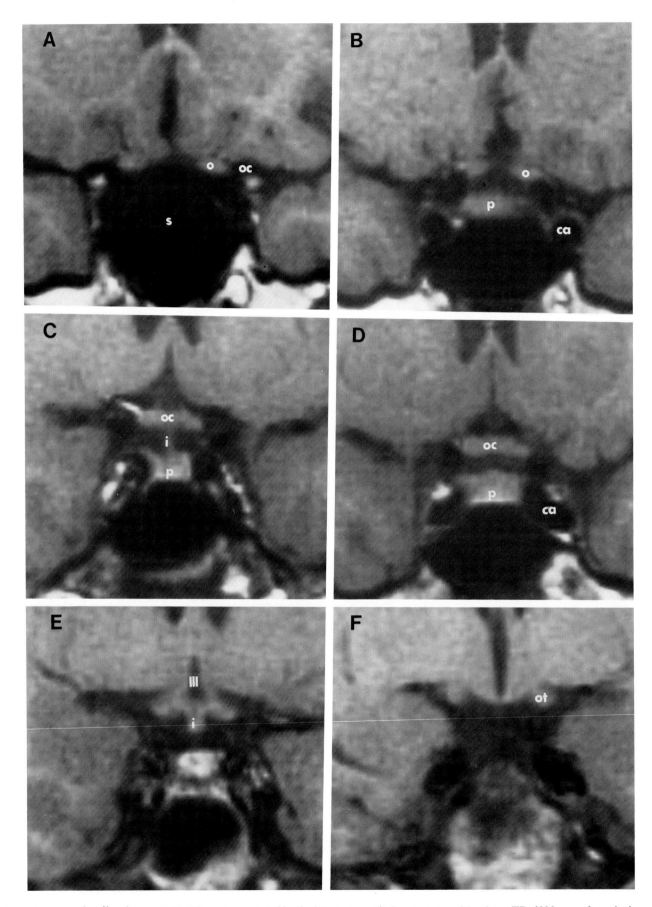

FIG. 1. Normal sella. Coronal (**A–F**) and sagittal (**G–J**) (*facing page*) 3-mm cuts with short-TR (600 msec) technique demonstrate the normal structures of interest: (o) optic nerve; (c) clinoid; (s) sphenoid; (ps) planum sphenoidale; (p) pituitary gland; (oc) optic chiasm; (i) infundibulum; (ca) carotid artery; (ot) optic tract; (m) mammillary body; (III) third ventricle. Where paired, only the left-sided structure is labeled. On the sagittal images, the *arrow* points to a low-intensity structure representing partial volume effect with the adjacent carotid artery. This should not be mistaken for a microadenoma.

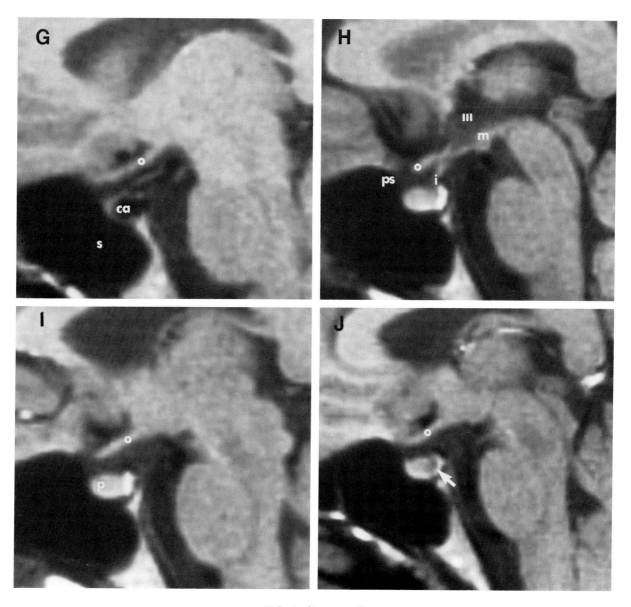

FIG. 1. *(Continued)*

With T1-weighting, the low signal intensity of the CSF sharply contrasts the interfaces of these solid structures (Fig. 1). On T2-WI, the signal intensity of CSF is substantially greater than adjacent structures. This in itself would not be problematic because the contrast would merely be reversed; however, the matter is complicated by the fact of pulsatile cisternal CSF motion. The spatial misregistration (ghosting) that this causes, and the reduced signal available on delayed echoes, considerably degrades edge definition, especially on thin sections (Figs. 2–4). Most important is that intraglandular pathology appears to be more readily recognized on T1-WI. In our own series we have not seen an adenoma on the T2-WI that could not be seen on the T1-WI. Thus, it has become our practice to obtain only T1-WI

to screen the gland. T2-WI are reserved to a supplementary role for further characterization of detected lesions or, if indicated, to examine the remainder of the brain.

Interslice gaps should be minimized or eliminated. For T1-WI a 0% to 20% gap is recommended. There is a penalty of reduced signal-to-noise ratio and reduced contrast when this is done owing to slice cross excitation, but its effect on T1-WI is small. If thin-slice T2-WI are used, at least a 20%, and preferably 50%, gap should be used (the effect of cross excitation is more significant). Since the pituitary gland is so small, in addition to thin slices, small voxels and small FOVs serve to increase spatial detail. All of these operator selectable variables serve to reduce signal. Therefore, to maintain high-quality images, the number of excitations must be

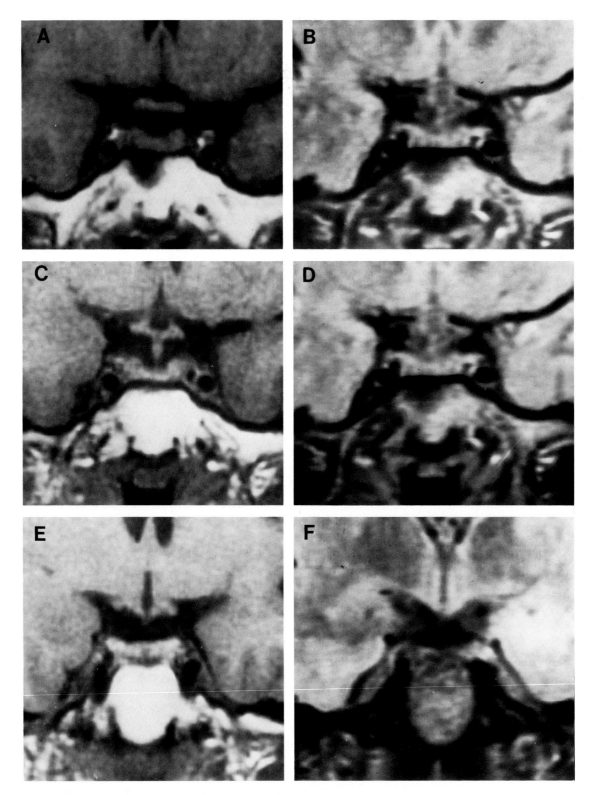

FIG. 2. T1-weighted (TR = 600 msec; TE = 20 msec) and T2-weighted (TR = 2,000 msec; TE = 20 msec) coronal images of the normal sellar and suprasellar cistern. Note loss of definition of the suprasellar structures, including the stalk and optic chiasm. T2-weighted image does present some improved definition of suprasellar vessels.

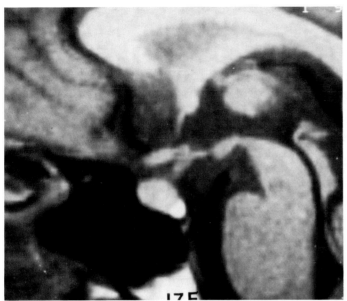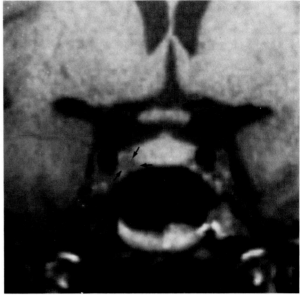

FIG. 3. A 17-year-old woman with Cushing's disease. Coronal image (TR = 600 msec; TE = 25 msec) reveals focal low-intensity lesion in the far right portion of gland measuring 3 mm in diameter (*arrows*). At surgery, a 3-mm microadenoma was removed. "Plump" appearance of gland in both sagittal and coronal images is a normal finding in pubertal and pregnant women.

increased. Four to six excitations usually result in excellent images. This by necessity increases imaging time.

Recommended imaging parameters are summarized in Table 1. A complete basic examination of the pituitary requires 20 to 30 min.

NORMAL ANATOMY

The sella turcica is a central saddle-shaped depression in the body of the sphenoid bone. It contains the pitu-

TABLE 1. *MRI technique*

Parameter	T1 sagittal	T1 coronal	T2 coronal[a]
TR (msec)	600	600	2,000
TE (msec)	20	20	70
Matrix	256	256	128 or 256
No. of excitations	4–6	4–6	2
Thickness (mm)	3	3	3
Slice spacing (mm)	0	0	1.5
No. of slices	9	9	20[b]
Distance covered (mm)	27	27	90
Field of view (cm)	20	20	20
Imaging time (min)	10–15	10–15	8–16

[a] The 70-msec (or later) echo can be acquired as part of a multiecho series.

[b] Up to 20 slices may be acquired, but only the center 3–5 slices incorporate the sella.

itary gland and the inferior end of the pituitary infundibulum. It is bordered superiorly by the diaphragma sella, laterally by the cavernous sinuses, and anteriorly, inferiorly, and posteriorly by sphenoid bone. Above the diaphragma, the CSF of the suprasellar cistern contains the superior portion of the infundibulum, the optic nerves and chiasm, the supraclinoid carotid arteries and the circle of Willis. The contents of the cavernous sinuses include the carotids and cranial nerves III, IV, V_1, V_2, and VI. The sellar floor is continuous with the tuberculum sellae anteriorly and the dorsum sellae posteriorly. The air-containing sphenoid sinus is directly below and anterior to the sella (11). All these structures can be visualized in every patient evaluated.

The anterior pituitary gland (adenohypophysis) is of homogeneous, intermediate intensity on both T1- and T2-weighted sequences. It is of similar intensity to cerebral white matter, which can be used as a reference (Fig. 1).

It is not entirely clear whether the posterior pituitary gland can be seen as a distinct entity. Most, but not all, T1-weighted examinations reveal a high-intensity, crescent-shaped structure oriented along the posterior-inferior margin of the gland (Fig. 1, midline sections). One group believes this to be fat in the sella turcica but outside the gland ("the sella fat pad") (12). Our own dissections [nine (U.C.S.F.)] have failed to substantiate the presence of intrasellar fat in this location; however, we have found intracellular fat within the neurohypophysis

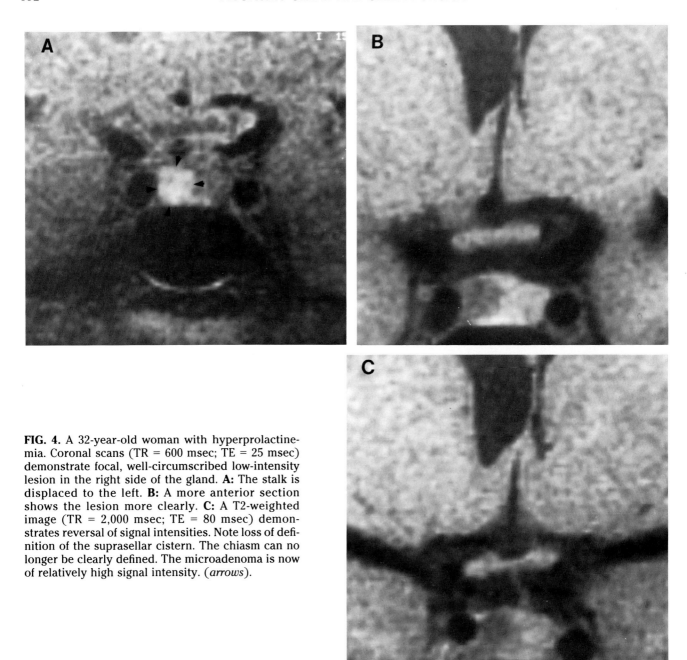

FIG. 4. A 32-year-old woman with hyperprolactine-mia. Coronal scans (TR = 600 msec; TE = 25 msec) demonstrate focal, well-circumscribed low-intensity lesion in the right side of the gland. **A:** The stalk is displaced to the left. **B:** A more anterior section shows the lesion more clearly. **C:** A T2-weighted image (TR = 2,000 msec; TE = 80 msec) demon-strates reversal of signal intensities. Note loss of defi-nition of the suprasellar cistern. The chiasm can no longer be clearly defined. The microadenoma is now of relatively high signal intensity. (*arrows*).

(J. deGroot and J. Kucharczyk, *personal communica-tion*). It thus appears that this high signal is fat, but in the posterior pituitary gland itself. As expected for signal emanating from fat, it is associated with chemical shift artifact (in the frequency-encoding direction) and has a relatively short T2. Its relative intensity is substantially reduced on T2-WI.

The gland occupies the inferior sella turcica. Normal gland height is variable and ranges from 3 to 8 mm. The gland shape is elliptoid on both sagittal and coronal images except for the superior surface, which is usually flat or concave upward. In young adult women or in pregnant women, the gland may exceed these dimen-sions, attaining 9 or even 10 mm in height and may bulge superiorly; however, symmetry with respect to the midline is maintained. Asymmetric upward bulges should always be suspect.

The pituitary infundibulum can be identified in both sagittal and coronal planes in all normal individuals. It is a midline structure, 1 to 1.5 mm thick, and of the same intensity as the adenohypophysis. It originates from the median eminence of the hypothalamus and traverses the

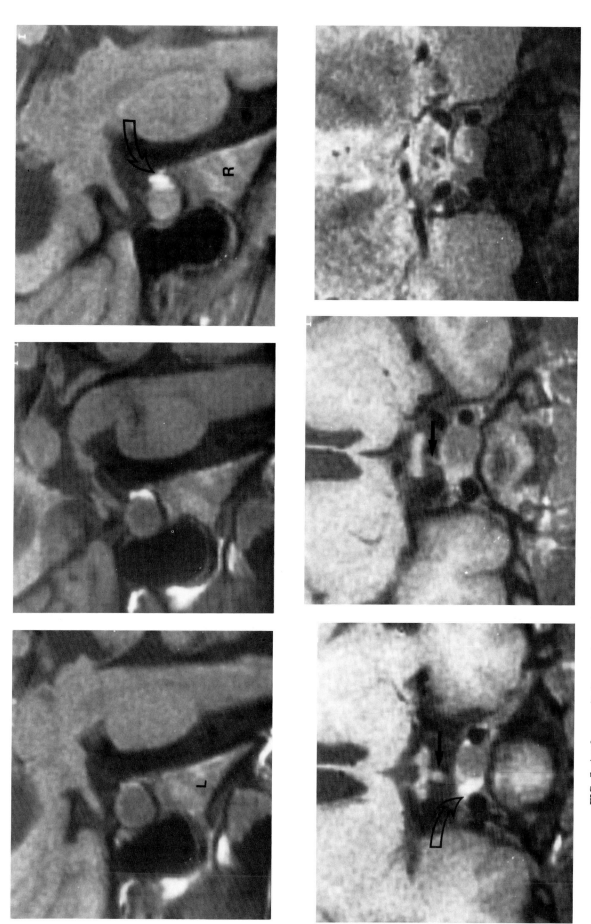

FIG. 5. An 8-mm pituitary microadenoma demonstrated in saggital (*top*) and coronal (*bottom*) images from a patient with hyperprolactinemia. (Imaging parameters were TR = 600 msec; TE = 20 msec, except for *bottom right:* TR = 2,000 msec; TE = 35 msec.) The adenoma is situated in the left side of the gland, displacing the normal pituitary and the stalk to the right (*black arrow*). *Curved arrow* points to high signal intensity of the posterior pituitary, also displaced to the right. Note that on the T2-weighted coronal image (*bottom right*), the adenoma shows increased signal intensity. The T2-WI provides no additional useful diagnostic information.

suprasellar cistern, sloping anteriorly as it descends. The stalk passes posterior to the optic chiasm and inserts on the dorsal surface of the pituitary gland. Inability to identify the stalk, thickening of the stalk, or significant deviations from a midline position should be regarded as abnormal.

The diaphragma sellae is a dural infolding that forms the roof of the sella. It is a fibrous structure positioned a variable distance above the sellar floor. It is not visualized with MRI.

The bony walls of the sella turcica cannot be directly visualized owing to the absence of resonating protons in cortical bone. The signal void of cortical bone results in an inability to distinguish the sella floor from the air-containing sphenoid sinus unless there is thickening of the mucosa in the sinus. Posteriorly, the dorsum sellae is visible as a narrow high-intensity line due to fat within a small marrow space.

The optic nerves are readily identified as they emerge from the optic foramina. Posteriorly they are more medial in position and are closely applied to the inferior surface of the frontal lobes. In the suprasellar cistern, the chiasm forms anterior to the stalk. From the chiasm the optic tracts extend posterolaterally to their connections

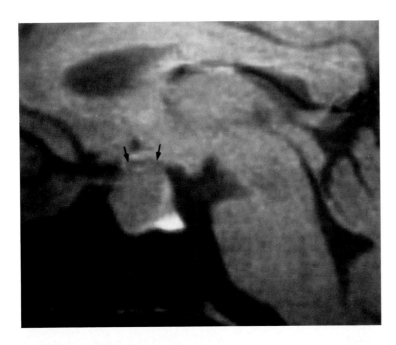

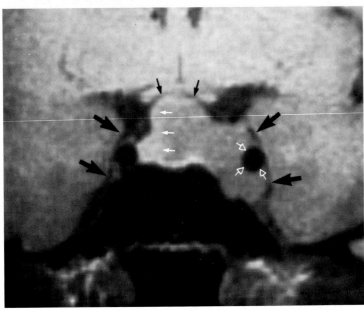

FIG. 6. Macroadenoma with suprasellar and left parasellar extension. Note the higher intensity of the normal gland displaced to the right (*solid white arrow*). The mass fills the left cavernous sinus and encircles the left internal carotid (*open white arrows*). Suprasellar extension compresses the chiasm (*small black arrows*). *Large arrows* point to the lateral dural wall of the cavernous sinus.

in the lateral geniculate bodies. The signal intensity of these structures throughout their course is very similar to cerebral white matter.

The cavernous sinuses form the lateral borders of the sella. The only structure that can be consistently visualized within the sinus is (by virtue of the signal void) the carotid artery. The remainder of the sinus has a speckled appearance of slightly greater signal intensity than the pituitary. The thin medial wall and the contained cranial nerves cannot be visualized as distinct structures. The thicker lateral wall appears as a vertically oriented low-intensity line. The signal void defining the carotid arteries can be followed from the cavernous sinus to the suprasellar cistern. The most distal portions of the carotid as well as the proximal portions of the anterior and middle cerebral arteries are easily identified.

DISEASES OF THE PITUITARY GLAND

Pituitary Adenoma

Pituitary adenomas are common histologically benign tumors that arise from the adenohypophysis. They represent approximately 15% of intracranial neoplasms (12). Symptoms are caused by virtue of hormonal activity or by compression of adjacent structures. Many are asymptomatic and are only discovered incidentally at autopsy (13,14).

Adenomas can be classified by size and endocrine function. Tumors less than 10 mm are considered microadenomas; those larger than 10 mm, macroadenomas. Classification on the basis of function separates nonsecreting from secreting types, based on the absence or presence of hormone production. The secreting (or "functioning") variety may be further subdivided by type of hormone overproduction: prolactin, growth hormone (GH), adrenocorticotropic hormone (ACTH), and a variety of other, much rarer types. The ability to detect minute quantities of plasma and tissue hormones by radioimmunoassay and immunocytologic procedures has greatly facilitated this classification system (12).

The clinical signs and symptoms of adenomas depend on the functional status of the tumor, its size, and its extrasellar extent. Functioning adenomas present with symptoms of hormone overproduction. The tumor may be only a few millimeters in diameter. Nonfunctioning adenomas do not present until their compressive effects compromise the function of the remaining normal gland, interfere with the transport function of the infundibulum and its surrounding portal venous network, or compress or invade parasellar or suprasellar structures. Thus, nonfunctioning tumors often attain a substantial size before clinical presentation.

The MRI appearance of adenomas reflects these basic differences in modes of presentation. The functioning tumors are usually microadenomas confined to the sella

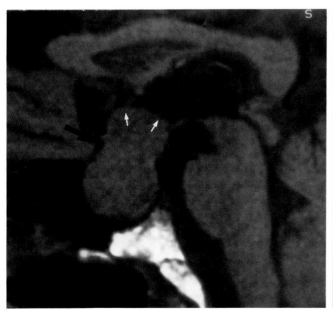
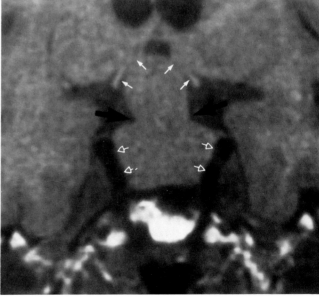

FIG. 7. A 50-year-old man presenting with visual loss. MRI (TR = 600 msec; TE = 25 msec) demonstrates large isointense intrasellar mass. The tumor fills the suprasellar cistern and effaces the anterior recesses of the third ventricle and elevates and compresses the optic chiasm (*solid white arrows*). Note narrowing of the tumor at the level of the diaphragma (*black arrows*). The intracavernous carotid arteries are displaced laterally (*open white arrows*).

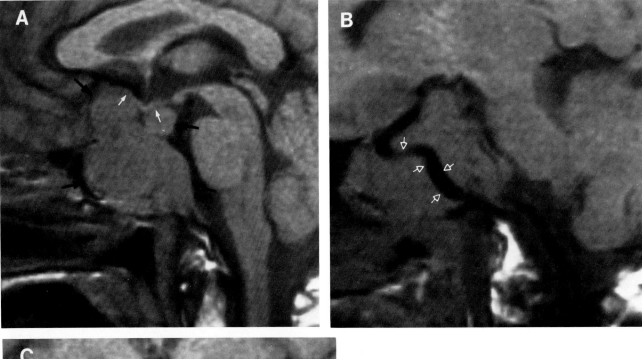

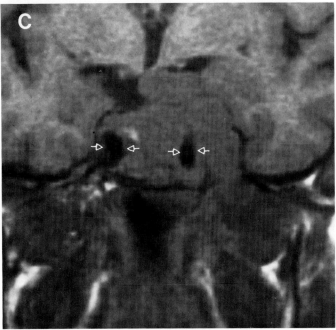

FIG. 8. Large intra- and suprasellar mass. The tumor displaces and attenuates the chiasm (*solid white arrows*). Note on the sagittal section that the adenoma spills posteriorly into the prepontine cistern. On the parasagittal section (**B**), the intercavernous portion of the carotid artery can be seen to be encased by the tumor. The lumen of the vessel is not compromised (*open white arrows*). On the coronal section, both carotid arteries are enveloped rather than displaced by tumor. There is minimal lateral displacement of the vessels.

turcica. Most are laterally situated. They are visible in many cases simply as a focal area of hypointensity in the otherwise uniformly intense pituitary gland (Figs. 3 and 4). Occasionally, no focal hypointensity can be identified. Asymmetric expansion of one of the gland surfaces (upward and downward bulge) or contralateral displacement of the stalk may also be seen (Fig. 5). ACTH-secreting tumors, which cause Cushing's disease, may be very small. Experience with very small microadenomas is too limited to state what the sensitivity of MRI will be

for such small lesions. Early results are encouraging, demonstrating good correlation between imaging and operatively confirmed findings (6).

Although hormonally active tumors may attain considerable size prior to clinical presentation, more commonly "macroadenomas" are nonfunctioning. Macroadenomas compress adjacent pituitary tissue, resulting in impairment of pituitary tropic hormone production, or compress the optic chiasm, cavernous sinuses, or carotid arteries, with the subsequent symptoms such involvement causes. As with smaller tumors, the diagnosis is often established in advance of imaging. In this context MRI is an excellent means of confirming the clinical diagnosis, of accurately delineating tumor extent, and defining the involvement of parasellar structures.

Macroadenomas have MRI characteristics very similar to their smaller counterparts: a mass arising from the pituitary gland that is hypointense on T1-WI. Adenomatous tissue can at times be separated from normal pituitary tissue on the basis of this lower intensity (Fig. 6). In other cases, the adenoma may be so large that normal pituitary tissue cannot be identified (6).

One of the most important roles of MRI in the diagnosis of macroadenomas is the delineation of extrasellar extent. The multiplanar capability of MRI and its excellent visualization of vital parasellar structures facilitates thorough preoperative evaluation (Fig. 7).

Superior extension is particularly well delineated. The intermediate-intensity tumor margin is distinctly identifed within the near-black pool of CSF on T1-WI. In some cases, the position and the size of the diaphragmatic opening can be inferred by the waist formed around the tumor. More important, the separation between the adenoma and the optic chiasm is much more clearly visualized than is possible with CT (Fig. 7). With larger tumors, the optic nerves and chiasm can be seen draped over the tumor. With very large tumors, the floor of the third ventricle can be invaginated, and obstructive hydrocephalus may result.

Lateral extension results in cavernous sinus involvement. The medial wall of the sinus is quite thin and cannot usually be distinguished from adjacent tissue. It is usually impossible to judge whether tumor is invading this wall or simply displacing it. With pronounced lateral extension, tumor can then be seen extending in continuity from the sella, encircling the carotid artery, and bowing the lateral cavernous sinus wall outward (Figs. 6–8). Even with this appearance, the tumor may simply be pushing these structures laterally rather than invading them. The lateral wall is anatomically thicker than the medial wall and is seen as a vertically oriented, low-intensity band. Breach of the lateral wall, although rare, may therefore be more dependably evaluated.

Although cavernous sinus involvement is not infrequent, constriction or occlusion of the intracavernous carotid artery is. The laterally extended adenoma typically is seen around the vessel, but almost invariably the vessel retains its normal luminal diameter (Fig. 8). The high contrast provided by the signal void of rapidly flowing blood within the carotid is a quality unique to MRI in evaluating this region. The need for angiography to define the relationship of the carotids to the sella and to the adenoma is eliminated.

In the evaluation of inferior extension, CT demonstrates expansion of the bony sella or pressure erosion of the floor. Although MRI fails to demonstrate the osseous changes, it directly demonstrates tumor extension into the sphenoid sinus. It is difficult, however, to deter-

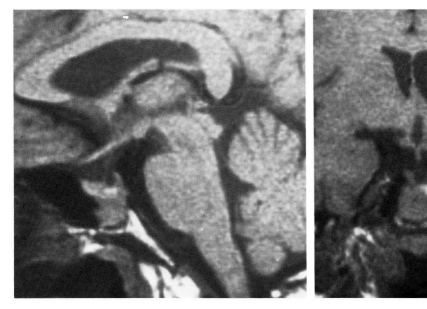

FIG. 9. Pituitary adenoma with infrasellar extension only. On the sagittal image, the inferior contours of the gland seem to be preserved except posteriorly, where tumor has eroded through the sella floor into the sphenoid sinus. Coronal images (*right*) tend to be less useful in identifying infrasellar extension because the presence or absence of the sella floor cannot be easily determined, since bone and air have similar signal intensities.

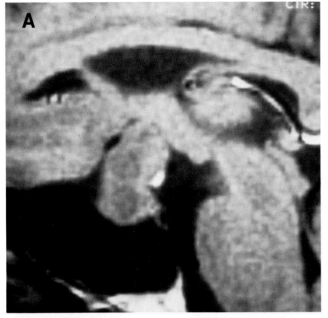

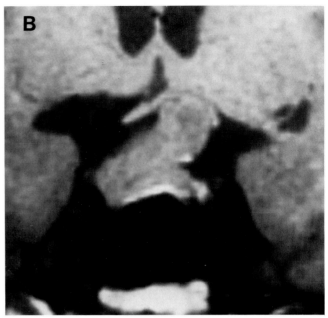

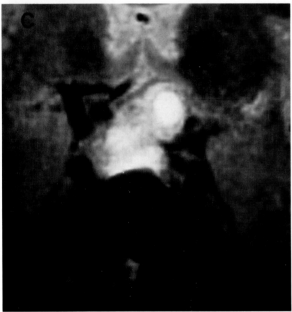

FIG. 10. Intrasellar pituitary macroadenoma with lobulated suprasellar extension. **A,B:** Within the tumor are well-circumscribed areas of cystic degeneration that appear as regions of relatively low signal intensity on T1-WI (TR = 600 msec; TE = 25 msec). **C:** On the T2-weighted coronal images (TR = 2,000 msec; TE = 70 msec), there is marked increase in signal in the cystic components of the tumor.

mine whether such a tumor may have eroded into the sphenoid sinus, as opposed to remodeling the floor of the sinus (Fig. 9).

Intratumoral changes, such as cystic degeneration or hemorrhage, are encountered more frequently in larger tumors. In cystic degeneration, sharply defined regions of low signal intensity on T1-WI and marked hyperintensity on T2-WI are seen (Fig. 10). The presence of a fluid-fluid level is a much more specific sign (Fig. 11). Intensity values of some noncystic adenomas may mimic cysts. Caution must therefore be exercised in the diagnosis of a cyst on the basis of intensity alone.

Hemorrhage into an adenoma is a rare, but well-recognized, complication. Intratumoral hemorrhage can

have a catastrophic clinical presentation with severe headache, sudden visual loss, and acute pituitary insufficiency. The MRI appearance is pathognomonic. On both T1-WI and T2-WI, hyperintense material (blood) is seen within an intermediate-intensity tumor. The sella turcica may be expanded from the preexisting tumor. If visual loss is present, the optic nerves/chiasm are seen to be compressed by the tumor (Fig. 12).

Post-Therapeutic Evaluation

Primary therapy of symptomatic pituitary adenomas is either surgical or medical. Radiotherapy is usually

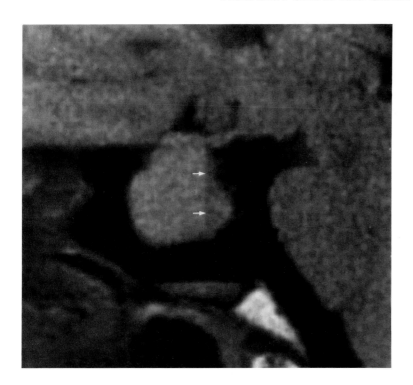

FIG. 11. Pituitary macroadenoma. Fluid-fluid level (*arrows*) indicates that this lesion is at least partially cystic. At surgery, a large cystic pituitary adenoma was removed.

reserved for treatment of large inoperable tumors or as an adjunct to primary surgical resection. Clinical or biochemical evidence of recurrence usually results in repeat evaluations of the gland and sella turcica.

The postoperative assessment of the sella turcica can be difficult because normal landmarks and symmetry may be lost. In most cases, a baseline postoperative scan is not available. The surgical approach to the majority of pituitary tumors is transphenoidal, the intracranial route being reserved for tumors with marked supra- or parasellar extension. Typically, after transphenoidal resection of a pituitary adenoma, the normally pneumatized sphenoid sinus contains either fluid, muscle, or fat graft, and there is a defect in the sellar floor. With the exception of the bone defect, MRI reflects these operative changes. If the patient is scanned within a few months of surgery, the fat graft can be identified as high-intensity material on T1-WI in the sphenoid sinus (Fig. 13). A year or more after surgery, the fat usually loses this appearance and approximates muscle in intensity. It is not certain exactly when this transition takes place, since very few patients are scanned serially.

The appearance of the sella itself very much depends on the size of the tumor previously resected, whether the tumor bed was packed with soft tissue, and of course on the presence or absence of recurrent tumor. Because of these factors, neither the shape and symmetry of the intrasellar soft tissue nor the position of the infundibulum can be used as diagnostic guidelines. Clearly, if there is soft tissue outside the anatomic confines of the sella, recurrent or residual tumor is present. The difficulty lies in assessing intrasellar recurrence. At the present time, there is no reliable method of doing so without the aid of a baseline postoperative MRI. If a baseline study is available, any increase in mass effect within the sella turcica is ascribed to tumor. Intraoperative soft-tissue packing is expected to retract with interval follow-up, and hence mass effect should be reduced. MR intensity characteristics do not allow soft-tissue grafts to be reliably separated from recurrent tumors because both are usually of intermediate intensity, and either may be somewhat heterogeneous.

Medical therapy is usually reserved for prolactinomas and occasionally GH-secreting tumors. The dopamine analog, bromocriptine, is the drug most commonly used. Its mechanism of action is controversial, but it probably is not tumoricidal. It appears to decrease adenoma size by causing a reduction in cellular volume, both nuclear and cytoplasmic (15). Biochemically, it acts as a prolactin-inhibiting factor. Serial studies with CT have shown that most prolactinomas diminish in size with regular continued administration of the drug. These changes have been observed as early as 1 week after initiation of drug therapy (16). Reports of MRI changes with bromocriptine use are few and scattered (8,17). There is every reason to suspect that parallel observations to that of CT will occur with regard to tumor bulk. It is open to speculation whether MRI intensity characteristics will change. Some interesting theories have been advanced (17). Personal experience is limited to three patients who had MRI both before and after treatment. Two of three showed regression in tumor size

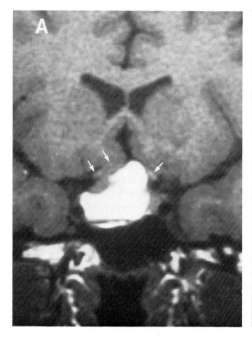
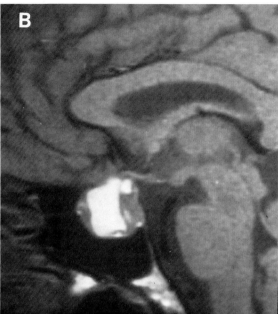

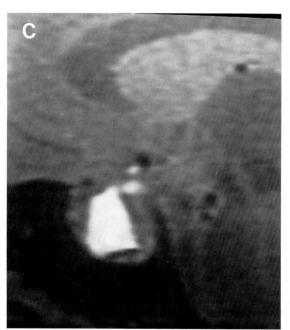

FIG. 12. Hemorrhagic pituitary macroadenoma. Subacute and chronic hemorrhagic material (methemaglobin) is of relatively high signal intensity on both T1-WI (TR = 600 msec; TE = 25 msec) (**A** and **B**) and T2-WI (TR = 1,500 msec; TE = 80 msec) (**C**). Note chiasmatic compression (*arrows*).

at 3- to 4-month follow-up. None demonstrated any change in internal characteristics.

Benign Intrasellar Cysts and Epithelial Rests

Cystic lesions of the sellar and suprasellar region constitute a diverse group of pathologic entities. These include solid tumors that degenerate and become secondarily cystic and others that are primarily cystic in origin. This latter group is the subject of this section.

Benign intrasellar cysts usually originate from one of two sources: from arachnoid membrane or from epithelial rests along the migratory path of Rathke's cleft. Arachnoid cysts are extra-axial lesions seen in a variety of intracranial locations. The most common locations are the anterior portion of the middle cranial fossa, the posterior fossa in and around the foramen magnum, and in the suprasellar cistern. Suprasellar cysts arise from the arachnoid membrane lying on or near the diaphragma sellae. These may have an intrasellar com-

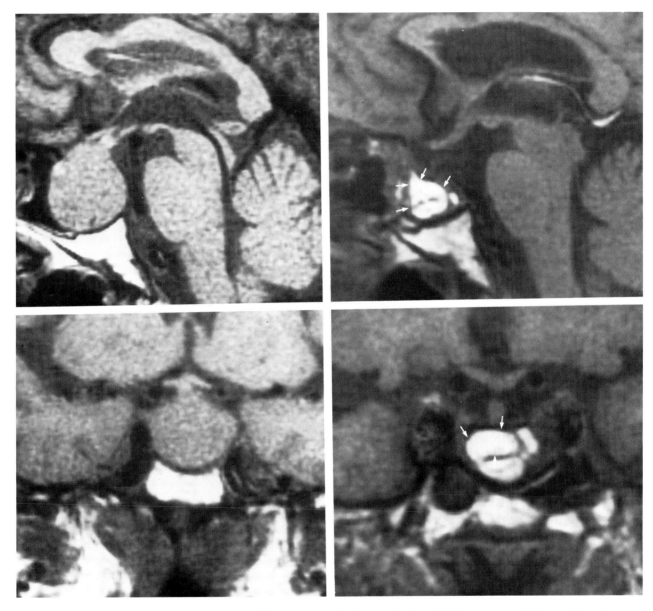

FIG. 13. Macroadenoma (TR = 600 msec; TE = 25 msec) pre- (*left*) and post- (*right*) transsphenoidal resection. The tumor was completely removed. Following resection, the sphenoid and floor of the sella are packed with muscle and fat. *Arrows* point to fat packing. The elliptically shaped area of high intensity below the packing on the coronal image is marrow within the clivus.

ponent if they grow or prolapse through a sufficiently large defect in the diaphragma. Rarely, they may be entirely intrasellar. Pituitary dysfunction may develop because of compression of the stalk or the pituitary gland; however, the bulk of the cyst is almost always in the suprasellar cistern. The cyst contains cerebrospinal fluid (CSF). The MRI appearance is characteristic. A homogeneous well-circumscribed lesion is seen centered in the cistern. Its internal intensity is identical to that of ventricular CSF on both T1-WI and T2-WI (Fig. 14). The wall of the cyst is often too thin to be visualized.

Because there may be little image contrast between the cyst and cisternal CSF, the best signs are often compression and/or displacement of adjacent structures, the floor of the third ventricle, the chiasm, the infundibulum, or the pituitary gland. It is particularly important to visualize the stalk traversing the cistern to the pituitary gland in order to distinguish a space-occupying arachnoid cyst from the normal variant, "empty sella." Whereas cysts displace or obliterate the stalk, in an empty sella, the stalk maintains its normal course to insert in the midline of a typically flattened pituitary

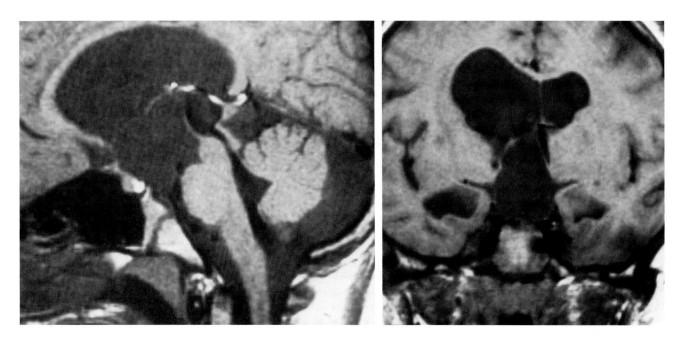

FIG. 14. Benign suprasellar subarachnoid cyst (TR = 600 msec; TE = 25 msec) obstructing the foramen of Monro, causing secondary hydrocephalus. The cyst is of CSF signal intensity. Note normal intrasellar pituitary gland below the cyst.

gland located posteroinferiorly in a slightly enlarged sella turcica (Figs. 15–17).

In contradistinction to arachnoid cysts, epithelial cysts found in or near the sella turcica are thought to be derivatives of Rathke's cleft. Other names that have

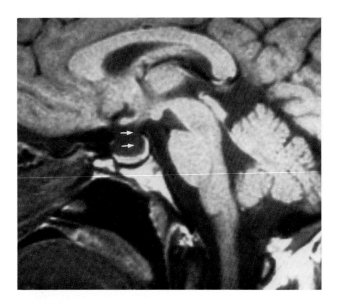

FIG. 15. Empty sella (TR = 600 msec; TE = 25 msec). The pituitary gland is flattened against the inferior and posterior margins of the sella turcica. The stalk maintains its normal course (*arrows*),

been used for this same lesion are pars intermedia cysts, intrasellar colloid cysts, and Rathke's pouch cysts. These lesions may differ in their location with respect to the gland or in their contents, but the histology of their walls is identical. The term "Rathke's cleft cyst" can be used to describe all such cysts.

Embryologically, invagination of Rathke's pouch cephalad results in the formation of the anterior and intermediate pituitary lobes. Very small vesicles and/or epithelial rests, remnants of the cleft, commonly persist into adulthood in or between these lobes. These rests are the cellular precursors for future cysts.

The wall of Rathke's cleft cyst is a single cell layer that is composed of cuboidal, columnar, or squamous epithelium. Goblet cells are present in variable numbers and account for secretory activity. Their contents may be serous or mucoid. Cysts may enlarge because of such secretion but most remain small (3 mm or less).

Symptomatic Rathke's cleft cysts are rare. Prior to the use of high-resolution CT for the investigation of pituitary disorders, most were only discovered at autopsy. On CT, they have been observed as small, low-density lesions in or near the pars intermedia (1). MRI also has demonstrated a large number of these cysts. Based on MR signal intensity, two distinct types appear to exist. One type has an intensity pattern indistinguishable from arachnoid cysts (intensity equal to CSF on both T1-WI and T2-WI). It differs in location from an arachnoid cyst in that it is predominantly within the pituitary gland,

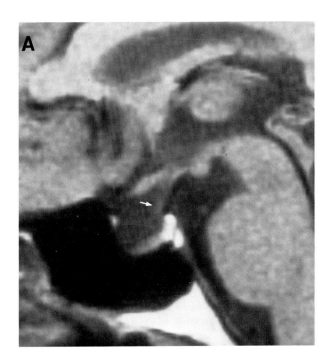

FIG. 16. Empty sella (TR = 600 msec; TE = 25 msec). Sagittal section demonstrates the stalk extending into the floor of the sella where the gland is flattened against the floor and the dorsum. On a relatively posterior coronal section (**B**), the entire length of the stalk can be identified. Superior to the stalk is the optic chiasm. In the midline superiorly is the chiasmatic recess of the third ventricle. Inferiorly, there is asymmetric expansion of the floor of the sella. On the left there is a 3-mm-diameter focal area of low signal intensity, which at surgery proved to be a prolactin-secreting adenoma (*black arrows*). The high signal intensity to the right is due to partial volume averaging with the high-signal-intensity marrow within the clivus and dorsum. On the more anterior coronal section (**C**), the sella fossa is almost completely empty. The gland is flattened against the floor and lateral walls.

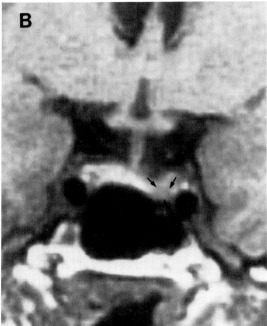

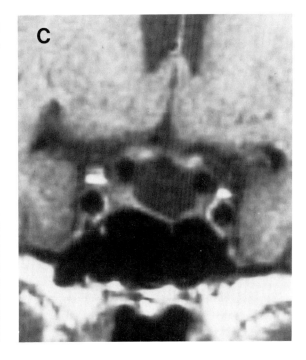

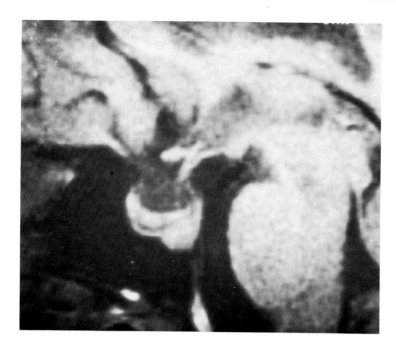

FIG. 17. Partially enlarged empty sella with pituitary adenoma extending posteriorly and inferiorly. In this case, the adenoma can be clearly separated from the normal gland.

not the cistern (Figs. 18 and 19). The other type is high intensity on both sequences (Fig. 20). Both types are homogeneous and well circumscribed. Because these small cysts are incidental findings, surgical confirmation is available in only a few symptomatic cases. In these it has been found that the CSF-like type of cyst has clear, serous fluid contents; the other type, mucoid contents. It may seem a discrepancy that a single common appearance is not observed, but it must be remembered that although the histology of the walls is similar (or identical) with both types, with MRI it is not the wall that is seen but the contents, and hence, the difference in appearance for histologically similar lesions is due to the differing cyst contents.

A unique finding with MRI is that several patients have been found to have a small (2–3 mm) high-intensity focus on the dorsal surface of the gland with a strong predilection for the anterior aspect of the inferior portion of the stalk, just at its insertion to the gland (Fig. 21). The etiology of this focal finding has not been surgically substantiated, but correlation with the results of previous autopsy series suggests that these high-intensity areas are probably small squamous remnants or cysts of Rathke's cleft (18,19). As such they should be recognized and treated as incidental findings. They certainly are distinctly different from adenomas. The only potentially confusing differential diagnosis is with a small craniopharyngioma.

The incidence of pituitary cysts in the normal population is uncertain. At autopsy they are very common,

although most of these are tiny. It is therefore expected that many of these will be seen as focal lesions within the pituitary with the increasing clinical use of MRI. It is for this very reason that MRI must be used in close conjunction with clinical and biochemical evaluation and not as a screening test.

Other Intrasellar Lesions

Adenomas and nonneoplastic cysts are by far the most common lesions within the sella turcica. A variety of uncommon disorders also occur, many of which are only briefly discussed here. These may be broadly considered as neoplastic, inflammatory, or vascular lesions.

Intrasellar neoplasms (apart from adenomas) are rare except as extensions from a primarily extrasellar process. Pituitary carcinoma and metastases to the region have been described, but there are no such reports describing MRI findings. One would expect to see a destructive mass, but to comment on the MR intensity would be speculative. Purely intrasellar craniopharyngiomas are the most common intrasellar tumor after pituitary adenoma. These often have highly suggestive MR features: a high-intensity cyst on T1-WI, a signal void denoting calcification, and a soft-tissue component. Meningiomas have also been known to be entirely confined to the sella. There is no reason to suspect that their MR characteristics will differ from meningiomas elsewhere.

The only vascular disorders of importance in this area

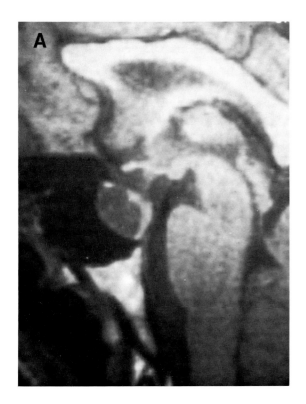

FIG. 18. Intrasellar Rathke's cleft cyst. T1-weighted (TR = 600 msec; TE = 25 msec) sagittal image (**A**). There is a cystic low-intensity lesion displacing the normal pituitary gland cephalad and posteriorly. On the coronal image (**B**) the gland is seen to be draped over the cystic structure. On a T2-weighted (TR = 2,000 msec; TE = 35 msec) coronal image (**C**), the cyst intensity is identical to that of CSF. Surgically proven Rathke's cleft cyst, "low-signal-intensity type."

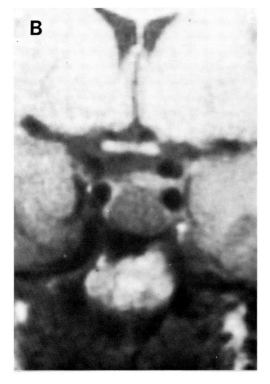

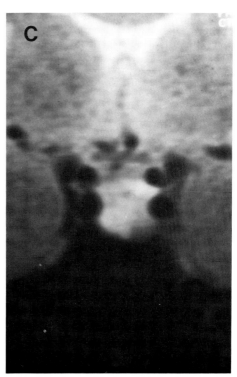

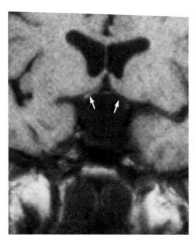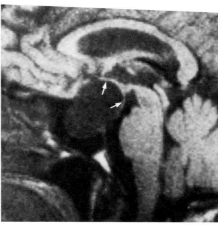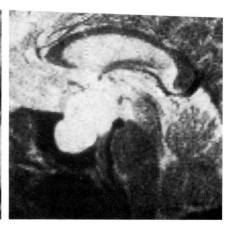

FIG. 19. Large Rathke's cleft cyst, which is of low signal intensity on the T1-WI (TR = 600 msec; TE = 25 msec) and exhibits signal intensity similar to CSF on the T2-weighted image (TR = 2,000 msec; TE = 35 msec). Note the gland draped over the apex of this large cystic lesion (*arrows*).

are intrasellar aneurysms and aberrant carotid arteries. Transphenoidal surgery on either can be catastrophic. Both are easily recognized by visualization of a vascular flow void within the sella. Conversely, the course of the carotid arteries can be delineated without need for angiographic study.

Inflammatory lesions may be idiopathic (adenohypophysitis) or infectious (abscess); both are rare. Pituitary abscess may occur after surgery. It presents as an intrasellar mass. Lymphocytic adenohypophysitis is thought to be an autoimmune disorder of the pituitary gland, usually seen in postpartum women. In the one case we have examined, the gland was diffusely and symmetrically enlarged without any significant change in signal intensity (Fig. 22).

Parasellar Lesions

Many other tumors, infiltrative processes, and vascular abnormalities have a predilection for the parasellar and suprasellar region. Craniopharyngioma, meningioma, optic chiasm glioma, and aneurysms of the circle of Willis are but a few examples of the more common ones. (A much more extensive list is available in most radiology texts.) The MRI features of these specific disease entities are discussed in other chapters in this volume. From the standpoint of the pituitary gland, these lesions do not usually invade it directly, but any may cause pituitary dysfunction by compression of the stalk or gland. The MRI will clearly show the pathology to be extrasellar.

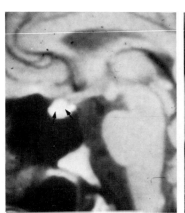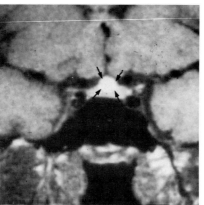

FIG. 20. High-signal-intensity intrasellar Rathke's cleft cyst (*arrows*) (TR = 600 msec; TE = 25 msec).

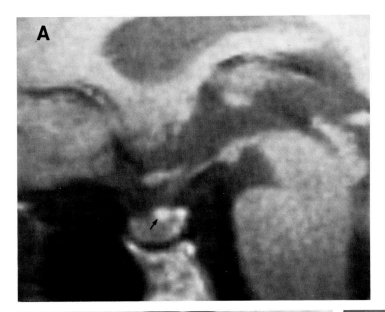

FIG. 21. A 2-mm-diameter bright spot at the base of the stalk seen on both T1-WI (TR = 600 msec; TE = 25 msec) and T2-WI (TR = 2,000 msec; TE = 25 msec). This is believed to represent a remnant of Rathke's cleft cyst.

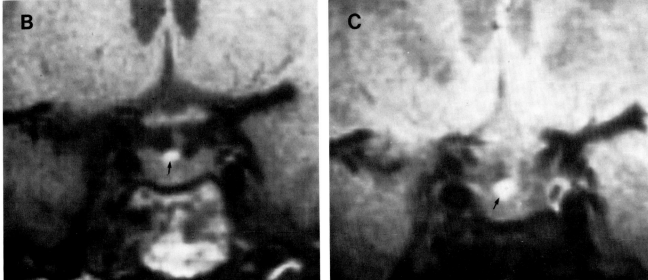

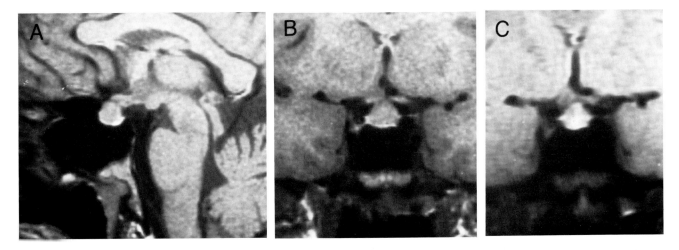

FIG. 22. Surgically proven adenohypophysitis. Note symmetrical gland enlargement on T1-WI (TR = 600 msec; TE = 25 msec) and increased signal of the gland on T2-WI (TR = 1,500 msec; TE = 40 msec).

REFERENCES

1. Chambers EF, Turski PA, LaMasters D, Newton TH. Regions of low density in the contrast-enhanced pituitary gland: normal and pathologic processes. *Radiology* 1982;144:109–13.
2. Davis PC, Hoffman JC, Tindall GT, Braun IF. CT-surgical correlation in pituitary adenomas: evaluation in 113 patients. *AJNR* 1985;6:711–6.
3. Roppolo HMN, Latchaw RE, Mayer JD, Curtin D. Normal pituitary gland: microscopic anatomy-CT correlation. *AJNR* 1983;4:927–35.
4. Syversten A, Haughton VM, Williams AL, Cusick JF. The computed tomographic appearance of the normal pituitary gland and pituitary microadenomas. *Radiology* 1979;133:385–91.
5. Bilaniuk LT, Zimmerman RA, Wehrli FW et al. Magnetic resonance imaging of pituitary lesions using 1.0 to 1.4 T field strength. *Radiology* 1984;153:415–8.
6. Kucharczyk W, Davis DO, Kelly WM et al. Thin-section, high resolution imaging of pituitary adenomas at 1.5 tesla. *Radiology 1987 (in press).*
7. Lee BCP, Deck MDF. Sellar and juxtasellar lesion detection with MR. *Radiology* 1985;157:143–7.
8. Pojunas KW, Daniels DL, Williams AL, Haughton VM. MR imaging of prolactin-secreting microadenomas. *AJNR* 1986;7:209–13.
9. Wiener SN, Rzesotarski MS, Droege RT, et al. Measurement of pituitary gland height with MR imaging. *AJNR* 1985;6:717–22.
10. Brant-Zawadzki M, Norman D, Newton TH, et al. Magnetic resonance imaging of the brain: the optimal screening technique *Radiology* 1984;152:71–7.
11. Rhoton AJ. Microsurgical anatomy of the sella region. In: Wilkins RH, Rengachary SS, eds. *Neurosurgery.* New York: McGraw-Hill, 1985:811–21.
12. Kovacs K, Horvath E, Asa SL. Classification and pathology of pituitary tumors. In: Wilkins RH and Rengachary SS, eds. *Neurosurgery.* New York: McGraw-Hill, 1985:834–42.
13. Burrow GN, Wortzman G, Rewcastle WB, et al. Microadenomas of the pituitary and abnormal sellar tomograms in an unselected autopsy series. *N Engl J Med* 1981;304:156–8.
14. Parent AD, Bebin J, Smith RR. Incidental pituitary adenomas. *J Neurosurg* 1981;228–31.
15. Rengachary SS, Tomita T, Jeffries BF, et al. Structural changes in human pituitary tumor after bromocryptine therapy. *Neurosurgery* 1982;10:251–2.
16. Thorner MO, Martin WH, Rogol AD, et al. Rapid regression of pituitary prolactinomas during bromocryptine therapy. *J Clin Endocrinol Metab* 1980;51:438–45.
17. Weissbuch SS. Opinion. Explanation and implications of MR signal changes within pituitary adenomas after bromocryptine therapy. *AJNR* 1986;7:214–6.
18. Carmichael HT. Squamous epithelial rests in the hypophysis cerebri. *Arch Neurol Psychiatr* 1931;26:966–75.
19. Svein HJ. Surgical experiences with craniopharyngiomas. *J Neurosurg* 1965;23:148–55.
20. Mark L, Pech P, Daniels DL, et al. The pituitary fossa: a correlative anatomic and MR study. *Radiology* 1984;153:453–7.
21. Oot R, New PFJ, Buonanno FS, et al. MR imaging of pituitary adenomas using a prototype resistive magnet: preliminary assessment. *AJNR* 1984;5:131–7.

CHAPTER 13

Vascular Disease: Hemorrhage

David Norman

An understanding of the role of magnetic resonance (MR) in detection and characterization of vascular lesions is evolving. Improvements in spatial detail suggest great promise in delineation of structural vascular lesions (1), and insights into the appearance of evolving intraparenchymal hematoma have broadened the applications (2,3).

PRINCIPLES

Flowing Blood

Flow effects are described in greater detail in Chapters 4 and 5. In the commonly used spin-echo sequences, rapidly flowing blood usually causes a high-velocity signal loss. On T2-weighted images in which CSF is of relatively high signal intensity, there is sharp contrast between cisternal CSF and the signal void of blood flowing rapidly through the vessel lumen. Slowly flowing blood (venous) usually appears as relative signal void as well. On entry slices, however, slowly flowing blood will have a relatively high signal. The entry slices in the case of veins are the most cephalad sections in tissue volumes imaged above the heart and the most caudal sections in tissue volumes imaged below the heart. Slowly flowing blood may also appear as high signal in situations in which there is even-echo rephasing or pseudogating (4) (see Chapter 4). Imaging techniques are currently being developed in which flowing blood yields very high relative signal intensity (1). These techniques permit short scan times without compromise of spatial detail and are therefore useful in imaging vessels.

Hemorrhagic Lesions

The MR appearance of intraparenchymal hematoma has been elegantly elucidated by Gomori et al. (3) (Fig. 1). Acute hematomas (1–7 days old) are isointense, or slightly hypointense, to gray matter on T1-weighted images (TR < 600 msec). On T2-weighted images (TR > 1500 msec), the signal intensity of the central portion of the clot is very low. This corresponds to the dense portion of the hematoma identified on computed tomography (CT) scans. In hematomas layer, the dependent portion is of low signal intensity on MR and high attenuation on CT. Parenchymal edema adjacent to the hematoma is detectable at 24 to 48 hr and is iso- or hypointense on T1-weighted images and hyperintense on T2-weighted images. This peripheral hyperintensity resolves over a period of several weeks.

Few studies have been performed on hyperacute hematomas (<24 hr). Early investigations suggest that these early hematomas are actually of high signal intensity on T2-weighted images (5).

Subacute Hematoma

The more peripheral portion of the hematoma develops a high signal intensity on short-TR images at approximately 7 (±2) days. This region of high signal intensity is medial to the peripheral edematous reaction described above. The hyperintensity persists and extends centripetally during a 2- to 3-week period. The same series of events occurs on the T2-weighted images but lags slightly behind the T1-weighted images. Hyperintensity of hematomas may persist for more than 1 year.

At approximately 1 week, a ring or capsule develops about the hematoma. This ring is iso- or hypointense on T1-weighted images and markedly hypointense on T2-weighted images, contrasting sharply with the now high signal intensity of the peripheral portion of the hematoma and the high signal intensity of the edema beyond the hematoma. This low signal intensity ring persists indefinitely. It corresponds to the enhancing ring seen on CT in subacute and chronic hematomas, which represents a collagenous capsule (6) that is hemosiderin laden.

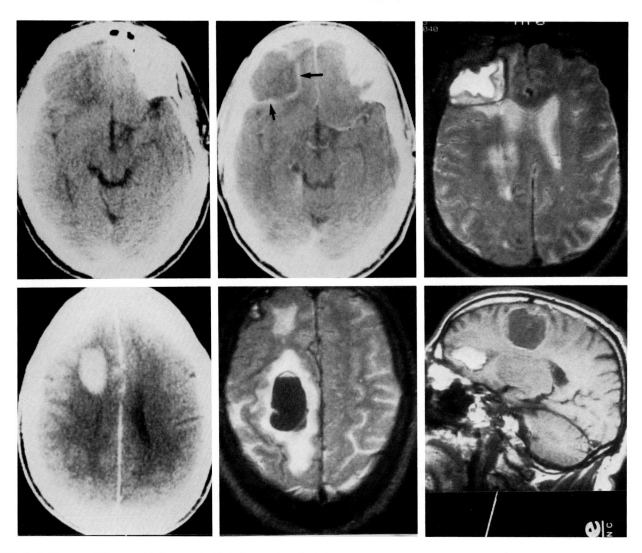

FIG. 1. A 62-year-old man with hemorrhagic infarcts. One is 3 days old; the second is 14 days old. The acute lesion (**bottom row**) in the right parietal region appears as an area of high density on CT. The subacute lesion (**top row**) in the subfrontal region appears as an area of low density with an enhancing ring following contrast injection (*arrows*). On the T1-weighted sagittal MR image (TR = 600 msec; TE = 20 msec) (**bottom right**), both lesions can be identified. The acute lesion appears as an area of relatively low signal intensity that reflects a preferential T2 shortening associated with deoxyhemoglobin. The subacute lesion appears as high signal intensity with a surrounding rim of low signal intensity. The high signal intensity is due to methemoglobin, the low signal intensity to hemosiderin. On the T2-weighted axial images (TR = 2,000 msec; TE = 20 msec), the high parietal acute bleed (**bottom row, center**) appears as an area of low signal intensity, reflecting the presence of a large quantity of deoxyhemoglobin. There is a fluid-fluid level with a small area of high signal intensity, representing methemoglobin in the apical portion of the lesion. The thin rim of low signal intensity in the apical portion of the lesion represents an early hemosiderin capsule. High intensity beyond the hematoma represents parenchymal edema. The subacute low frontal lesion (**top row, right**) exhibits high signal intensity representing methemoglobin. The hemosiderin capsule is of low signal intensity, reflecting a preferential T2 shortening due to hemosiderin. The capsule is much thicker than that seen in the acute lesion. (Courtesy, Betsy A. Holland, M.D., Marin General Hospital)

PATHOPHYSIOLOGY

When blood extravasates into the brain substance, clotting begins within 2 to 3 hr. Centrally, the red blood cells (RBCs) are hemoconcentrated. Their cell walls are intact; the intracellular oxyhemoglobin is converted to deoxyhemoglobin. Breakdown of the clot and clot re-

sorption occur initially at the periphery. The RBC wall breaks down; a chocolate-brown semiliquid material evolves, composed primarily of methemoglobin. A rim forms in the most peripheral portion of the clot. Macrophages in the capsular rim region engulf RBCs with resultant deposition of hemosiderin in the capsule. The peripheral portion eventually evolves to a hemosiderin-laden slit, which is orange in color. The hypointensity centrally and peripherally is most pronounced on T2-weighted images and reflects preferential T2 proton relaxation. In the central portion of the hematoma, intracellular Fe^{2+} deoxyhemoglobin with four unpaired electrons has pramagnetic qualities that are responsible for the preferential T2 proton relaxation on T2-weighted images (3). This effect is proportional to the square of the magnetic field strength and is therefore more readily detected and characterized on higher field strength units. The low signal intensity in the peripheral rim seen primarily on T2-weighted images is also due to a preferential T2 proton relaxation that is caused by the hemosiderin deposited by the macrophages within the hematoma rim. The greater the quantity of blood phagocytized and deposited, the thicker the rim (3).

The hyperintensity seen in the subacute hematoma converges from the periphery toward the central portion of the hematoma. It is caused by, and correlates with, the appearance of methemoglobin in the aging hematoma. Intra- or extracellular methemoglobin causes a shortening of T1 relaxation by a mechanism similar to that of paramagnetic contrast agents (3). Prolongation of T2 is associated with the presence of extracellular methemoglobin. (Intracellular methemoglobin will cause a preferential T2 proton relaxation.) As intraparenchymal hematoma evolves, the hyperintensity on the T1-weighted images precedes that seen on the T2-weighted images. This suggests that RBC lysis lags behind methemoglobin production (3). The appearance of the high signal intensity associated with methemoglobin does not appear to be significantly influenced by field strength.

The peripheral hyperintensity surrounding the hema-

TABLE 1. *Changes occurring over time in the evolution of components of intraparenchymal hemorrhage from acute to subacute to chronic stages*

	T1-weighted image	T2-weighted image
Center	Isointense ↗	Low ↗
Periphery	Isointense ↗	Isointense ↗
Rim	Isointense	Isointense ↘
Adjacent white matter	Isointense	High ↘

Arrows indicate change over time.

toma on T2-weighted images is distributed in white matter and represents vasogenic edema. The above events are illustrated diagramatically in Fig. 2 and Table 1.

Subarachnoid Hemorrhage

Acute subarachnoid hemorrhage is not as readily detected with MR. In the small number of patients who have undergone MR imaging following acute subarachnoid hemorrhage, there does not seem to be any alteration in signal on T1- and T2-weighted images. Absence of significant signal alteration may reflect absence of sufficient lowering of oxygen tension to result in deoxyhemoglobin formation (7). In the subacute phase, the extravasated blood becomes bright both on T1- and T2-weighted images. This presumably reflects methemoglobin formation (2,8).

SPECIFIC DISEASE PROCESSES

Spontaneous Intraparenchymal Hemorrhage

Hypertension is the most common cause of spontaneous intracerebral hemorrhage. The MR appearance of intraparenchymal hematoma is described above. In practice, patients who suffer significant hemorrhage are usually not good candidates for MR exams because they exhibit varying degrees of obtundation and are therefore unable to cooperate adequately. CT is a practical and effective means of detecting, characterizing, and quantifying significant quantities of acute intraparenchymal hemorrhage. As described above, MR is more sensitive than CT in defining subacute and chronic intraparenchymal hemorrhage. The residua of very old hematomas are characterized by a hemosiderin laden cicatrix (Fig. 3).

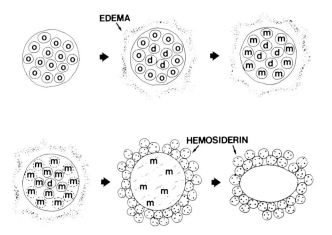

FIG. 2. Various stages of evolution of intraparenchymal hematoma on MR: (o) oxyhemoglobin; (d) deoxyhemoglobin; (m) methemoglobin; (*circles*) intact RBCs; (*dashed circles*) lysed RBCs; (*dotted circles*) macrophages laden with hemosiderin granules. (From ref. 3.)

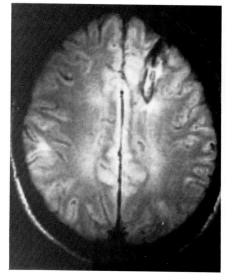
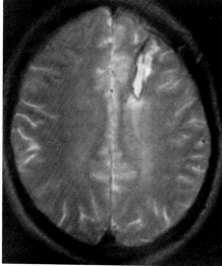

FIG. 3. A 56-year-old woman who had a left frontal hemorrhage 3 years previously. Elliptical lesion in the left frontal lobe represents the residua of the hematoma cavity (TR = 2,000 msec; TE = 40/80 msec). The low-signal-intensity rim is due to hemosiderin deposition in the walls of the remaining cicatrix.

Spontaneous Subarachnoid Hemorrhage: Aneurysms

Aneurysms are the most common cause of spontaneous subarachnoid hemorrhage. In the acute phase, CT is the most sensitive technique. Patient handling is less problematic than in MR imaging. Approximately 20% of aneurysmal hemorrhages have associated intraparenchymal hemorrhage (9). MR is useful in patients who are suspect for a subarachnoid hemorrhage at an earlier time and in whom the CT scan is negative, either because the quantity of blood is small or because the subarachnoid blood has evolved to a point where it is isodense with surrounding tissue. In these cases, MR becomes quite useful because of the high signal intensity exhibited by subacute and chronic subarachnoid blood on both T1- and T2-weighted images. Evidence of very old subarachnoid hemorrhage (spontaneous, traumatic, or iatrogenic) may be evidenced on MR in the form of superficial siderosis. Hemosiderin deposits on the brain surface appear as linear areas of marked T2 shortening (10) (Figs. 4 and 5).

Magnetic resonance may be of additional use in the cooperative patient in detecting the actual aneurysm (Fig. 6). High spatial detail permits detection of flow

FIG. 4. Superficial siderosis; T2-weighted images (TR = 2,200 msec; TE = 70 msec) obtained in a 1.5-tesla (T) unit. The patient is 2 years post-surgical resection of a posterior fossa ependymoma. The low-signal-intensity (*black*) rimming of the belly of the pons, margins of the cerebellum, and walls of the fourth ventricle reflect deposition of hemosiderin.

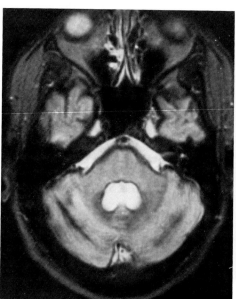
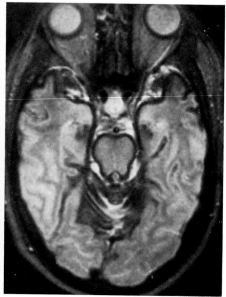

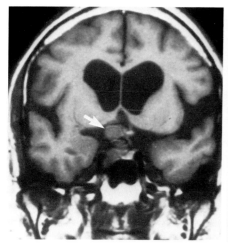
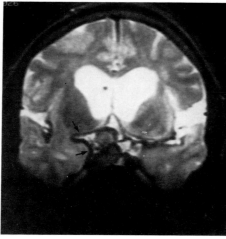

FIG. 5. A 40-year-old woman status post previous resection of a tuberculum meningioma. T1-weighted MR examination (TR = 600 msec; TE = 20 msec) demonstrates recurrent tumor (*white arrow*). The T2-weighted image (TR = 2,000 msec; TE = 35 msec) shows a thick rind of low signal intensity outlining the right temporal lobe and sylvian cistern (*arrows*). These are not vascular structures; rather, they represent hemosiderin deposition. (Courtesy, San Francisco Magnetic Resonance Center.)

void within the aneurysm. Increased signal intensity associated with thrombus (methemoglobin) within all or a portion of the aneurysm may also be seen. In giant aneurysms, complex signal intensities result from an admixture of flowing blood at varying velocities and degrees of turbulence, thrombus in various stages of organization and age, and calcium and hemosiderin deposits (Figs. 7 and 8). Location, morphology, and mixed signal intensities in a concentric lamellar arrangement often create an image that is usually specific.

Vascular Malformations

Arteriovenous malformations (AVMs) can cause subarachnoid hemorrhage or intraparenchymal hemor-

rhage or both. Approximately 50% of AVMs present with intracerebral hematoma. MR detects the intraparenchymal hemorrhage and is equivalent, and perhaps superior to, CT in demonstrating the racemose entanglement of arteries and veins (Figs. 9 and 10). CT requires intravenous contrast. Arteries and veins can occasionally be distinguished on MR by the second-echo rephasing phenomena seen in slowly flowing venous blood.

Venous malformations may best be regarded as anomalous venous drainage. When they occur in the

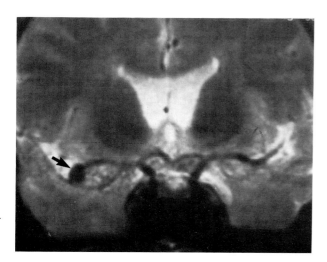

FIG. 6. Incidental 6-mm right middle cerebral artery aneurysm (*arrow*) identified on T2-weighted (TR = 2,000 msec; TE = 70 msec; coronal MR examination). The supraclinoid carotid arteries, the anterior communicating arteries, and the horizontal portions of the middle cerebral arteries are clearly defined as well.

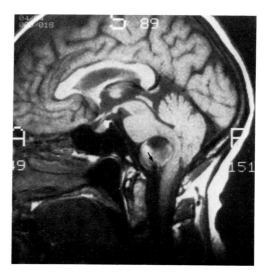

FIG. 7. A 65-year-old woman with progressive cranial nerve palsies. Axial CT demonstrated a well-circumscribed enhancing pontine mass. T1-weighted (TR = 600 msec; TE = 25 msec) sagittal MR examination clearly defines a $2\frac{1}{2}$ cm in diameter aneurysm compressing and distorting the brainstem. Note jet effect at the neck of the aneurysm (*arrow*). Mixed signal within the lumen of the aneurysm reflects turbulent flow. (Courtesy, San Francisco Magnetic Resonance Center and Leon Kasoff, M.D., Peninsula Hospital.)

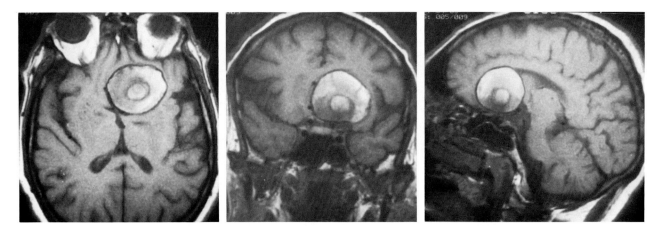

FIG. 8. Axial, coronal, and sagittal T1-weighted (TR = 600 msec; TE = 25 msec) images demonstrate a left supraclinoid giant internal carotid artery aneurysm in a 55-year-old man. Mixed signal intensities within the lumen of the aneurysm represent turbulent flow and methemoglobin deposition in the periphery of the thrombus. Low-signal-intensity rim reflects hemosiderin deposition in the wall of the aneurysm.

supratentorial compartment, they are rarely a cause of patient symptoms and/or hemorrhage. In the posterior fossa, they can occasionally be associated with spontaneous intracerebral hemorrhage. Venous malformations in the posterior fossa should not be excised. These veins represent the primary route of venous drainage of the tissue in which they are located. On MR, the morphology of venous malformations is similar to that which has been described on CT scans (Figs. 11 and 12). There is a linear area of signal void that may have a stellate collec-

tion of vessels at the more medial or deeper aspects. Occasionally, because of slow flow, there may be even-echo rephasing.

Cryptic Vascular Malformations

Cryptic vascular malformations (CVMs) represent vascular malformations that, at angiography, show no vascular abnormalities and may or may not exhibit an

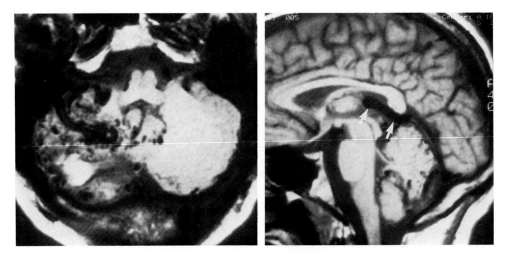

FIG. 9. A 23-year-old woman with a large cerebellar AVM with clinical symptoms suggesting recent hemorrhage. Axial T1-weighted (TR = 600 msec; TE = 25 msec) image shows multiple serpiginous areas of mixed signal intensity, primarily flow void, reflecting a multitude of vascular channels with laminar and turbulent flow. A region of high signal intensity in the inferior lateral aspect of the cerebellum on the right represents a small subacute intraparenchymal hematoma that was not appreciated on CT scan. Sagittal image demonstrates markedly enlarged straight sinus (*arrows*) as well as enlarged vascular channels within the inferior and posterior aspect of the cerebellum in the midline.

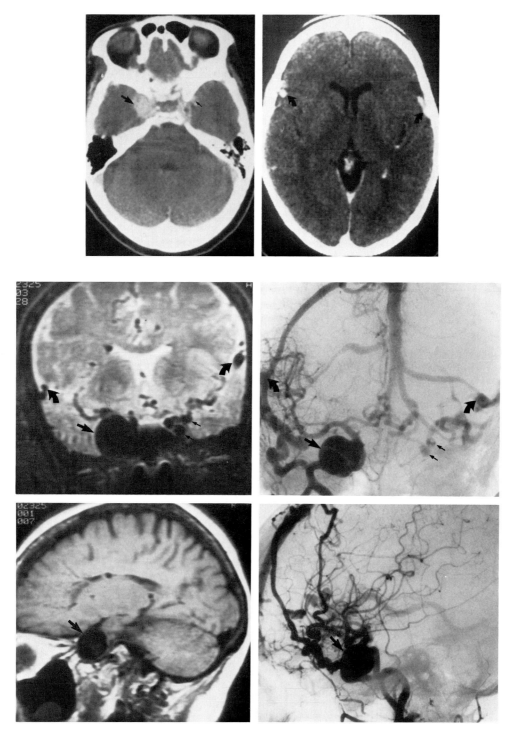

FIG. 10. Complex case of right giant internal carotid aneurysm and bilateral dural vascular malformations. Post-contrast-axial CT shows a paracavernous enhancing lesion (*large straight arrow* on the right) and a region of tubular-type enhancement on the anterior inferomedial aspect of the left temporal lobe (*small arrow*). At a higher level, bilateral tubular-shape areas of enhancement adjacent to the surface of the brain (*curved arrows*) are identified. The abnormalities are much better characterized on the coronal and sagittal MR scans. The giant aneurysm appears as an area of signal void (*large straight arrow*). The dural veins at the floor of the middle fossa on the left appear as smaller rounded areas of signal void (*small arrows*) and the convexity veins again as bilateral areas of signal void (*curved arrows*). These same findings are identified in a similar fashion on the anteroposterior and lateral angiograms. (Courtesy, F. Chaney Li, M.D., Kaiser Permanente Hospital, Redwood City, California.)

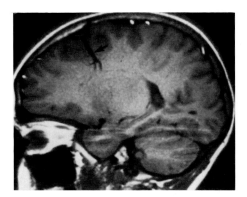

FIG. 11. Sagittal T1-weighted (TR = 600 msec; TE = 20 msec) image demonstrating a venous angioma. The single large draining vein (*arrow*) appears as an area of signal void. Smaller radiating vessels drain into the larger vessel.

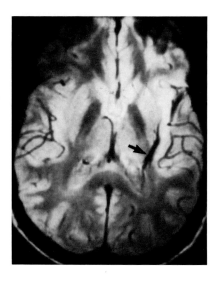

FIG. 12. Deep left temporoparietal venous angioma (TR = 2,000 msec; TE = 70 msec). (Courtesy, San Francisco Magnetic Resonance Center.)

associated mass effect. On CT, they exhibit some degree of calcification, variable enhancement, and mass effect. Cryptic vascular malformations may be AVMs, venous malformations, telangiectasias, and/or cavernous angiomas. These four types may be distinguished only with a histologic specimen.

The appearance of CVMs on CT is nonspecific and often indistinguishable from slowly growing tumors. On MR, CVMs appear as mixed signal intensity on both T1- and T2-weighted images (11,12). There are always some tissue elements that have both short T1 and prolonged T2 (Figs. 13–16). Unique to the lesions are areas of signal void that represent calcium or hemosiderin or both. These lesions uniformly, however, appear to be surrounded by a rim of very low signal intensity most pronounced on T2-weighted images, representing hemosiderin. The MR appearance of CVMs appears to be relatively specific (11). MR has proven to be more sensitive than CT in the detection of CVMs, and MR is now the examination of choice in both detecting and characterizing CVMs.

Venous Sinus Thrombosis

Venous sinus thrombosis may occur spontaneously, usually in association with dehydration, or may be a

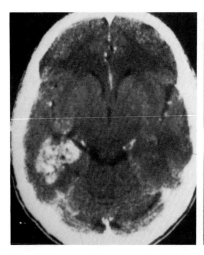
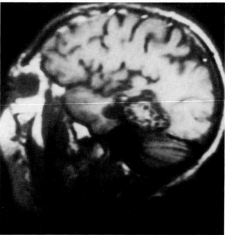
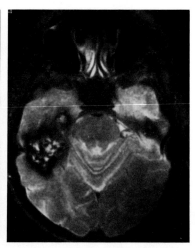

FIG. 13. A CVM. Axial CT demonstrates partially calcified enhancing lesion above the petrous apex on the left. T1-weighted sagittal MR (TR = 600 msec; TE = 20 msec) shows a lesion of mixed signal intensity with thick surrounding low-intensity hemosiderin rim. On the T2 weighted axial image (TR = 2,000 msec; TE = 70 msec), the preferential T2 shortening of hemosiderin is again demonstrated. Findings are characteristic for CVM.

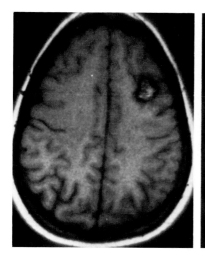
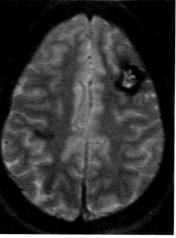

FIG. 14. Incidentally discovered high-convexity left frontal CVM. T1-weighted image on the left (TR = 600 msec; TE = 20 msec) demonstrates a high-signal-intensity central portion, reflecting subacute and old clot, and a surrounding rim of low signal intensity reflecting hemosiderin. T2-weighted image on the right (TR = 2,000 msec; TE = 70 msec) exhibits similar findings.

FIG. 15. A CVM: 48-year-old woman with frontal headache. CT scan demonstrated a nonenhancing calcified lesion. Coronal and axial MR images (TR = 2,000 msec; TE = 70 msec) demonstrate lesion with a central portion of mixed signal intensity and a thick hemosiderin-laden rim of low signal intensity. Note the absence of any surrounding edema. Findings are typical for a CVM.

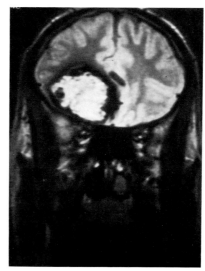
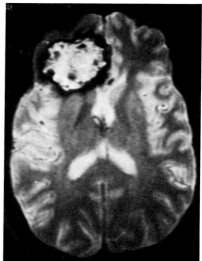

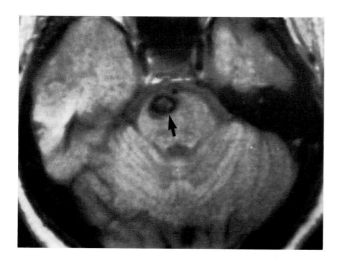

FIG. 16. Cryptic pontine vascular malformation (*arrow*).

sequel to local or generalized sepsis of the central nervous system. The sinus most frequently involved is the superior sagittal sinus, occasionally in combination with the transverse or sigmoid sinuses. Patients with spontaneous thrombosis may be conveniently divided into infantile and adult groups. In the infantile group, thrombosis may occur during a systemic illness when dehydration or malnutrition are present. In the adult group, most cases are seen during the puerperium or in association with head injury or, rarely, with ulcerative colitis. MR is uniquely sensitive in detecting and characterizing venous sinus thrombosis (Figs. 17 and 18). In the acute phase, the involved sinus will appear isointense on T1-weighted images and hypointense on T2-weighted images. This is explained on the same basis as described earlier for intraparenchymal clot. In the subacute phase,

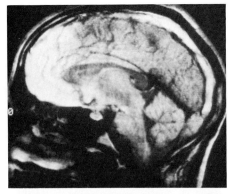

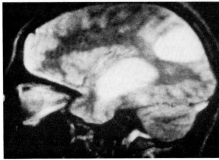

FIG. 17. Patient with sagittal sinus thrombosis and secondary venous infarction. Midsagittal image (TR = 2,000 msec; TE = 25 msec) shows high signal intensity along the posterior two-thirds of the superior sagittal sinus extending to the torcula, indicating subacute thrombus within the sinus. Parasagittal image demonstrates two large areas of increased signal intensity, representing secondary venous infarction.

signal intensity of the sinus becomes very bright both on T1- and T2-weighted images (13,14).

Arterial Dissection

Subintimal hemorrhagic dissection may be post-traumatic or spontaneous in nature. Cystic medial necrosis may be present. Occasionally there is an association with fibromuscular dysplasia. The presentation is that of an acute or subacute neurologic deficit. The only useful imaging technique prior to MR has been angiography, on which either an intimal flap and/or vessel narrowing, often irregular in contour, can be identified. On MR, we can now identify both the luminal narrowing and the associated subintimal hemorrhage, which appear as high signal intensity on T1- and T2-weighted images (Figs. 19 and 20). The high signal intensity represents the development of methemoglobin in the evolving hematoma.

Trauma

Hemorrhagic lesions post-trauma range from large to petechial in size. The large hemorrhagic lesions may be detected by CT or MR or both. Small petechial hemorrhages not detected by CT are readily demonstrated by MR (Fig. 21). Small shear injuries at the junction of gray and white matter are also more readily detected. Practical problems of patient handling must be overcome be-

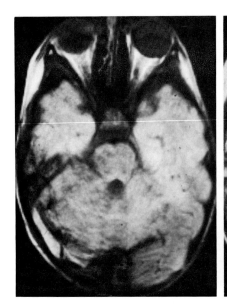
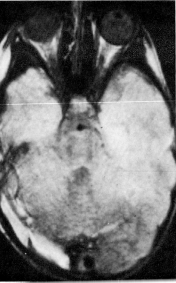

FIG. 18. Transverse sinus thrombosis secondary to mastoiditis ("otitic meningitis"). Axial scan (TR = 2,000 msec; TE = 25 msec) demonstrates a high-signal-intensity subacute thrombus in the right transverse sinus. Note the signal void in the midline, representing normal blood flow through the region of the torcula. Intermediate signal intensity in the right mastoid air cells represents inflammatory tissue. Normally, the mastoids appear as areas of signal void owing to the presence of bone and air.

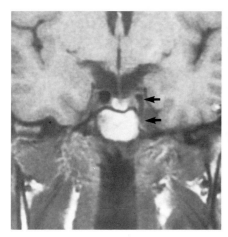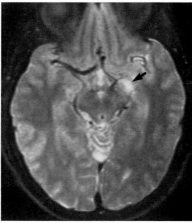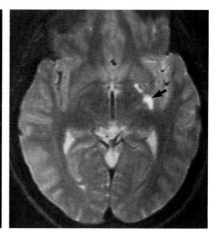

FIG. 19. A 35-year-old man with acute onset of right hemiparesis. MR (TR = 600 msec; TE = 20 msec) demonstrates marked narrowing of the caliber of the supraclinoid left internal carotid artery (*arrows*). On the T2-weighted (TR = 2,200 msec; TE = 70 msec) axial images, the horizontal portion of the middle cerebral artery is not visualized. Areas of high signal intensity in the left basal ganglia reflect focal infarction secondary to dissection of the origins of the lenticulostriate arteries.

fore widespread application of MR to the acutely traumatized patient is possible.

Subacute subdural hematomas, which may be isodense on CT, are hyperintense on both T1- and T2-

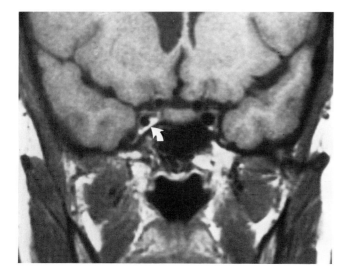

FIG. 20. T1-weighted (parasagittal, TR = 600 msec) coronal scan of 36-year-old woman with acute onset of left hemiparesis. Sections of the paracavernous portions of the internal carotid artery demonstrate subacute subintimal hematoma in the inferolateral aspect of the right internal carotid artery (*arrow*).

weighted MR images (Fig. 22). MR is therefore the more sensitive examination in patients suspect for a subacute post-traumatic extraaxial collection (15,16).

SUMMARY

Magnetic resonance detects and depicts acute intraparenchymal hemorrhagic lesions as areas of relative isointensity on T1-weighted images and low signal intensity on T2-weighted images. These findings are more pronounced at higher field strengths. Subacute intraparenchymal hemorrhage appears as high signal intensity on both T1- and T2-weighted images. MR is insensitive in the detection of acute subarachnoid hemorrhage. In the subacute stage of subarachnoid or subdural hemorrhage, MR is more sensitive than CT. The collections are bright on both T1- and T2-weighted images.

For practical purposes, MR is the best modality for evaluating cooperative patients who may have suffered acute or subacute intraparenchymal hemorrhage. For those with subarachnoid hemorrhage, CT is currently the most appropriate examination for detecting acute hemorrhage and MR the most appropriate for detecting subacute hemorrhage. In patients in whom a CVM is suspect, MR is the most sensitive and specific modality available.

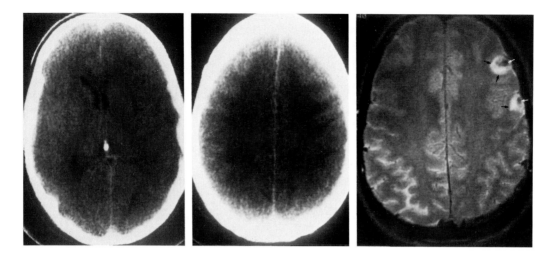

FIG. 21. A 39-year-old man status post motor vehicle accident. Noncontrast CT scan demonstrates a mild mass effect, with no evidence of hemorrhagic lesions. MR examination (TR = 2,000 msec; TE = 70 msec) demonstrates hemorrhagic cortical lesions with low signal representing deoxyhemoglobin (*white arrows*) and high signal representing methemoglobin or edema or both (*black arrows*). No capsule has formed. (Courtesy, Betsy A. Holland, M.D., Marin General Hospital.)

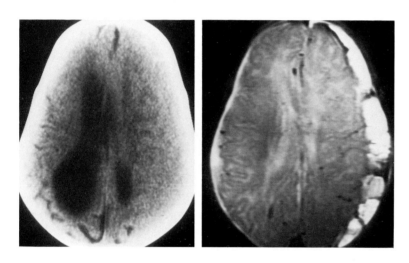

FIG. 22. Bilateral subdural hematomas, which are isodense on CT. The collection on the right was not appreciated on the CT scan. The collections are more readily detected on MR because of the high signal intensity associated with methemoglobin formation.

REFERENCES

1. Wedeen VJ, Meuli RA, Edelman RR, Geller SC, Frank LR, Brady TJ, Rosen BR. Projective imaging of pulsatile flow with magnetic resonance. *Science* 1985;230:946–8.
2. Bradley WG Jr, Schmidt PG. Effect of methemoglobin formation on the MR appearance of subarachnoid hemorrhage. *Radiology* 1985;156:99–103.
3. Gomori JM, Grossman RI, Goldberg HI, Zimmerman RA, Bilaniuk LT. Intracranial hematoma: imaging by high-field MR. *Radiology* 1985;157:87–92.
4. von Schulthess GK, Higgins CB. Blood flow imaging with MR: spin-phase phenomena. *Radiology* 1985;157:687–95.
5. Zimmerman RD, Snow RB, Heier LA, Lin C, Deck MDF. MRI of acute intracranial hemorrhage. *AJNR* 1987 (*in press*).
6. Enzmann DR, Butt RH, Lyons BE, Buxton JL, Wilson DA. Natural history of experimental intracerebral hematoma: sonograph, computed tomography and neuropathology. *AJNR* 1981;2:517–26.
7. Kemp SS, Grossman RI, Ip CY, Fishman JE, Joseph DM, Asakura T. The importance of oxygenation in the appearance of acute subarachnoid hemorrhage on high field magnetic resonance imaging. *Acta Radiol.* 1986 (*in press*).
8. DeLaPaz RL, New PFJ, Buonanno FS, et al. NMR imaging of intracranial hemorrhage. *J Comput Assist Tomogr* 1984;8:599–607.
9. Heros RL, Zervas NT. Subarachnoid hemorrhage. *Ann Rev Med* 1983;34:367–75.
10. Gomori JM, Grossman RI, Bilaniuk LT, Zimmerman RA, Goldberg HI. High-field MR imaging of superficial siderosis of the central nervous system. *J Comput Assist Tomogr* 1985;9:972–3.
11. Gomori JM, Grossman RI, Goldberg HI, Hackney DB, Zimmerman RA, Bilaniuk LT. Occult cerebral vascular malformations: high-field MR imaging. *Radiology* 1986;158:707–13.
12. Lemme-Plaghos L, Kucharczyk W, Brant-Zawadzki M, Uske A, Edwards M, Norman D, Newton TH. MRI of angiographically occult vascular malformations. *AJR* 1986;146:1223–8.
13. McMurdo SK Jr, Brant-Zawadzki M, Bradley WG Jr, Chang GY, Berg BO. Dural sinus thrombosis: study using intermediate field strength MR imaging. *Radiology* 1986;161:83–6.
14. Macchi PJ, Grossman RI, Gomori JM, Goldberg HI, Zimmerman RA, Bilaniuk LT. High field MR imaging of cerebral venous thrombosis. *J Comput Assist Tomogr* 1986;10:10–3.
15. Moon KL Jr, Brant-Zawadzki M, Pitts LH, Mills CM. Nuclear magnetic resonance imaging of CT-isodense subdural hematomas. *AJNR* 1984;5:319–22.
16. Zimmerman RA, Bilaniuk LT, Hackney DB, Goldberg HI, Grossman RI. Head injury: early results of comparing CT and high field MR. *AJNR* 1986;7:757–64.

CHAPTER 14

Vascular Disease: Ischemia

Michael Brant-Zawadzki and Walter Kucharczyk

Magnetic resonance imaging (MRI) offers unique advantages for the evaluation of cerebral ischemia in the clinical (and experimental) setting. Ischemia, even in its earliest stages, is associated with the changes in brain water content. Because of the inherent sensitivity of MRI to alterations in tissue free-water content, it can detect ischemic insult to the brain earlier than any other diagnostic method available; indeed, these changes can be seen within 1 hr of their onset (1–6). Looking to the future, imaging of other nuclei, particularly sodium, is also potentially promising in that ischemia effects an early, marked increase in tissue sodium concentration (7). Also, future developments in magnetic resonance (MR) spectroscopy may allow the combination of anatomic imaging and analysis of fundamental cellular processes (8), as discussed elsewhere in this volume. Because MRI and MR spectroscopy can be done by the same instrument, this technology may eventually offer an unprecedented ability to detect and monitor the progression of acute ischemia, as well as evaluate the effect of various therapeutic interventions. Finally, the fact that MR allows the study of vasculature both in an atomic and quantitative fashion (9–18) means that a single modality may eventually be used to study not only the anatomic and biochemical alterations produced by ischemia in the brain, but also the derangements of blood supply that cause the ischemia in many cases.

Understanding the appearance and distribution of brain ischemia as evaluated by MRI and the clinical context in which this modality might be used is facilitated by a review of the pathophysiology of ischemia and infarction in the brain.

PATHOGENESIS OF CEREBRAL ISCHEMIA AND INFARCTION

The brain, despite its small volume relative to the rest of the body, demands 20% of the cardiac output and 25% of the blood's glucose supply for its metabolic needs. When a reduction of blood flow occurs diffusely or to a focal region of the brain, cellular dysfunction begins within minutes. If the reduction of blood flow is of sufficient degree and duration, even the restoration of flow will not prevent the ensuing irreversible cellular damage and cell death.

Generalized reduction of cerebral perfusion is most often caused by dysfunction in the rhythm or force of the cardiac pump, leading to decreased output or diffuse occlusive disease of the carotid and vertebrobasilar systems, including their small intracranial branches. Such a generalized reduction of perfusion means that the compensatory collateral pathways available when focal ischemia is present are themselves deprived of flow and are ineffectual.

Most often, cerebral ischemia is a regional event, occurring in the territory of one of the major intracerebral vessels. The cause is probably a combination of factors, including preexisting myocardial inefficiency, underlying compromise of the lumen of the parent vessel, change in the oxygen content of the blood, viscosity, or coagulability, all of which may lead to in situ thrombosis. Another common event is embolization from a cardio- or extracraniovascular source.

Once cerebral perfusion drops below the critical threshold, a cascade of biochemical alterations is set in motion (19–23). Initially, the loss of oxygen interrupts oxidative phosphorylation, the most efficient way the cell has to produce adenosine triphosphate (ATP) from glucose, and anaerobic glycolysis supervenes. This latter metabolic pathway produces much less ATP per molecule of glucose and yields excess amounts of lactic acid, a metabolite potentially harmful to normal cellular integrity. Also, the depletion of ATP disrupts the function of the cell's sodium–potassium pump, which normally maintains the cellular electrolyte homeostasis. As a result, ions are released from intracellular binding sites, extracellular sodium leaks into the cell, and potassium is lost to the extracellular space. Water fluxes parallel sodium in these first hours of ischemia; the osmotic gradient created by the intracellular increase in sodium and lactate leads to accumulation of water within the cell (cytotoxic edema). Phospholipid catabolism occurs early during ischemia, leading to free fatty acid production, which further increases tissue osmolarity, aggravating the shift of water from the vascular to the extracellular and then intracellular space. All this occurs within the first 30 min of ischemia, with the overall increase of water content 3% to 5% during this time frame (19–20). Further progression produces irreversible damage to mitochondrial and cytoplasmic membranes of the brain cells and begins to grossly damage the endothelial cells as well. By 6 hr, the blood–brain barrier begins to break down, with progressive leakage of water and protein from the intravascular compartment. This latter phase of edema is termed *vasogenic edema,* and it continues to increase during the first few days, provided that collateral perfusion or reperfusion of the affected vascular bed is available. Obviously, the lack of any blood flow precludes progression of vasogenic edema, although compartmental shifts (extra- to intracellular) may continue to occur.

In the typical case, however, progressive vasogenic edema produces a mass effect that may further compromise the vasculature in or on the periphery of the ischemic region. The infarct can thus propagate centripetally despite reestablishment of blood flow; also, if ischemically damaged endothelium is again faced with the perfusion pressure of a healthy vascular bed, a greater risk of

hemorrhage is present. In view of these two factors, therapeutic intervention in the face of acute infarction is generally aimed more at decreasing the edema rather than surgical improvement of perfusion, although the latter approach might be viable in the first 6 to 8 hr after the onset of ischemia (24).

Once infarction is present, the morphologic characteristics of the lesion result from the edema and mass effect, both of which are present in acutely ischemic as well as infarcted tissue, albeit to a much lesser degree in the former. It therefore may be impossible to distinguish reversible ischemia from frank infarction based on MRI alone. By the second and certainly third week, the mass effect and edema subside, and the atrophic process with cell drop-out and variable gliosis begins. Cystic foci of variable size may develop as the end stage of the process.

One controversial aspect of ischemic infarcts is their tendency to hemorrhage, and this has therapeutic implications as well as pertinence to imaging.

The pathologic literature has cited a much higher incidence of secondary hemorrhage in infarction than has the CT literature. This is probably due to the retrospective, nonserial nature of many of the CT studies. More recently, a prospective serial CT study of patients with acute hemorrhage has documented a 43% incidence of secondary hemorrhage within the first 4 weeks of infarction (mostly in the second week), with worsening of clinical symptoms in only 10% of those who bled. Those with large, embolic infarcts were more likely to develop

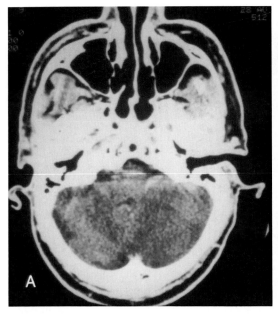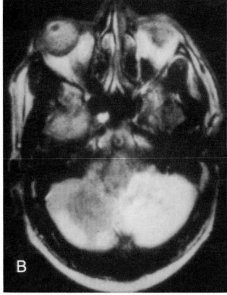

FIG. 1. Acute onset of ataxia 16 hr prior to diagnostic imaging. **A:** Noncontrast CT. **B:** TR 2,000, TE 60 msec. The CT scan shows a vague region of low density in the left cerebellar hemisphere. The MR study reveals a definite area of high signal intensity throughout the left cerebellar hemisphere, as well as peripheral abnormality of a similar nature in the right cerebellar hemisphere.

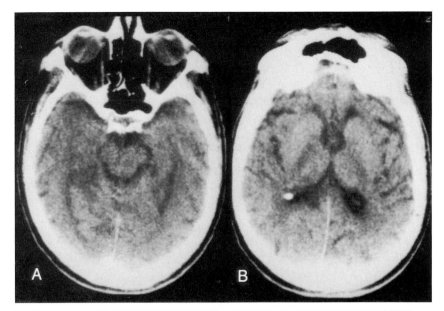

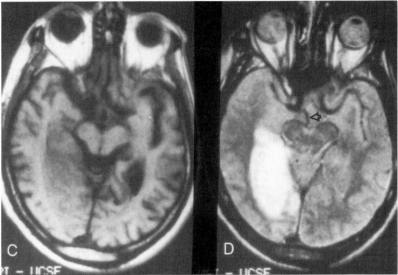

FIG. 2. Elderly man with acute onset of left homonomous hemianopsia and weakness, 12 hr prior to imaging. **A,B:** Noncontrast-enhanced CT, two adjacent sections. **C:** TR 500, TE 30 msec. **D:** TR 2,000, TE 60 msec. The CT scan shows only a vague area of low density in the hippocampus of the right hemisphere. The MR study shows a well-circumscribed area of high signal intensity on the long TR–long TE image. Note the lack of significant decrease in intensity on the short TR image. Incidentally, good visualization of the internal carotid–middle cerebral artery complex is seen bilaterally, with a prominent right posterior communicating artery (*arrow*); therefore, in this patient, embolization of the posterior cerebral territory could have arisen from an internal carotid source.

true hematomas in the first week, whereas more patchy, irregular, and even cortical petechial hemorrhages were seen in nonembolic infarcts, usually 2 or more weeks after onset, and were clinically inconsequential (25).

Finally, in this discussion of pathophysiology, it should be pointed out that many small infarcts are clinically silent, and chronic multifocal ischemia may be responsible for observed senescent changes in cerebral tissue (26). In the normal adult, the perfusion of the cerebral cortical mantle is threefold that of the deep hemispheric white matter. The deep regions depend on the relatively sparse long, thin perforating vessels. Overall, cerebral blood flow decreases with aging (27–29). Autoregulatory vasodilitation can compensate for decreased perfusion to a certain extent; however, flow re-

duction due to a combination of various factors, such as extracranial cerebrovascular occlusive disease, intracranial microangiopathy due to hypertension or other cause, diminished cardiac output, and transient hypotensive periods of a physiologic nature, may become first manifest in the relatively hypoperfused white matter. Such small, deep hemispheric infarcts may be of no clinical significance unless a sufficient aggregate of these occurs.

MAGNETIC RESONANCE IMAGING

Proton MRI is directly based on the presence and distribution of hydrogen nuclei in tissue. In the brain, the resonating nuclei that yield MR signals are essen-

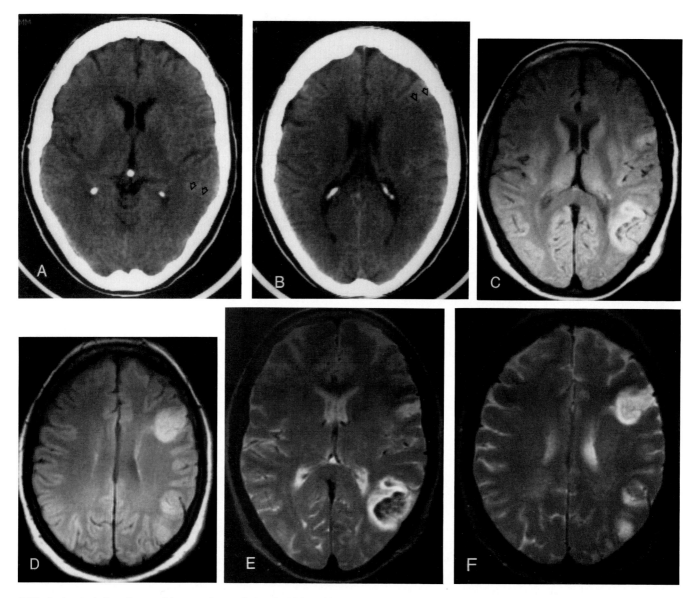

FIG. 3. Acute infarction and hemorrhage. Aphasia 12 hr prior to CT. History of atrial fibrillation. **A,B:** Noncontrast CT; two sections. **C–F:** TR 2,000; **C,D:** TE 20 msec; **E,F:** TE 80 msec. The CT scan shows subtle hypodensity in the region of Wernicke's area and the anterior operculum, with sulcal effacement (*arrows*). The MR study was obtained 2 days later (patient was on heparin). Note that two areas of infarction are shown. Also, there is obvious signal decay within the posterior infarct, best seen on the late-echo images (**E,F**). This is due to the preferential T2 shortening caused by deoxyhemoglobin, indicating recent hemorrhage.

tially those of water. Therefore, the major advantage of MRI in ischemia is its ability to detect better the early and subtle changes in the concentration of tissue water produced by the ischemic insult. Such subtle changes are insufficient to alter significantly X-ray attenuation, but will alter the MR signal intensity pattern to produce an obvious change in the image (Fig. 1). Numerous clinical studies have documented the superiority of MRI in detecting cerebral infarcts when compared to CT (30–36).

Indeed, experimental models have suggested that ischemia might be detected within 1 hr of onset by MRI (6).

Experimental evidence suggests that the prolongation of the T1 and T2 relaxation values is greatest in the early stages of ischemia, when water free of proteins is accumulating, prior to the disruption of the blood–brain barrier. This initially small (3–5%) increase in the tissue water content causes relatively increased signal intensity on the long TR sequences and relatively decreased signal

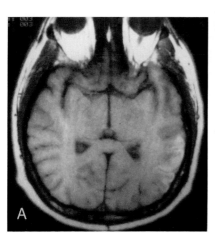
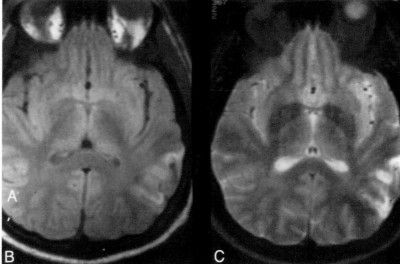

FIG. 4. Subacute infarct with secondary petechial hemorrhage. **A:** TR 600, TE 20 msec. **B:** TR 2,000, TE 35 msec. **C:** TR 2,000, TE 70 msec. The short TR image shows a gyriform pattern of high signal intensity in the posterior temporal cortical mantle. The long TR images show a larger region of high signal intensity in, and subjacent to, the cortex. The high signal on the short TR image is due to subacute hemorrhage and the resultant methemoglobin formation. The altered signal on the long TR sequences is also contributed to by the associated edema.

intensity on those obtained with a short TR. The images obtained with long TR and long TE settings have proven the most sensitive. Those obtained with a short TR, which tends to lessen the intensity of infarcts, have the finite TE time and proton density working to raise the intensity of infarcts (see Chapter 1). These conflicting effects may cancel intensity differences between normal and infarcted tissue (Fig. 2). After the vasogenic phase allows leakage of plasma proteins into the infarcted region, the T1 and T2 values begin to return to normal. Accumulation of sodium, which parallels that of water in this early phase of ischemia, is of investigational interest. The imaging of sodium is hampered by the fact that the signal is 4,000 times weaker than proton-based signal (7).

One of the clinical issues critical to MRI of infarction is the ability to separate acute ischemic infarction from hemorrhagic stroke due to hypertensive bleed, that from rupture of arteriovenous malformations, bleeds into small tumors, etc. Both infarction and early hemorrhage may show a high signal on midfield images obtained with a long TR, with low to isointense signal when a short TR is used. Recent experience has suggested, however, that acute hemorrhage exhibits a preferential shortening of T2 relaxation values, producing a relative signal void in the hemorrhagic focus. This preferential

decay of signal is thought to be due to the magnetic susceptibility of deoxyhemoglobin inside of inhomogeneously distributed red cells, an effect that accelerates signal decay in direct proportion to the strength of the magnetic field (37). This signal void of acute hematomas is especially obvious on long TR–long TE images (Fig. 3) and has been noted at intermediate fields but should be seen more reliably on high field imagers. This signal feature, when present, would easily distinguish acute hematoma from infarct. Subacute hematoma is accurately identified with MRI. The paramagnetic effect of methemoglobin on T1 shortening effects a high signal on images obtained with a short TR setting; thus, a subacute hemorrhage is easily identified within an infarct (Fig. 4).

As discussed above, up to 43% of ischemic infarcts may be complicated by a secondary hemorrhage sometime in their course. Certain forms of ischemia, however, are more likely to present with an acute hemorrhagic event. Inflammatory vasculitis is especially likely to produce such primary hemorrhagic infarcts, as is vasculopathy with *moyamoya* collateral development (Fig. 5). The finding of multiple, punctate bland infarcts in the region of the gray–white junction or in the deep hemispheric watershed zone, with a hemorrhagic focus (typically in the basal ganglia), should prompt the con-

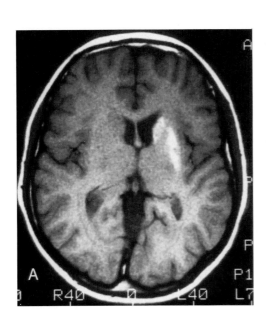
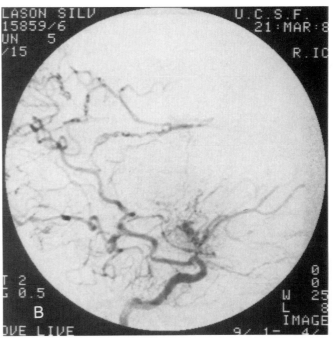

FIG. 5. Hemorrhagic infarction due to underlying vasculopathy. **A:** TR 600, TE 20 msec. **B:** Left carotid arteriogram. The MR study shows a high signal abnormality in the head of the caudate and in the lenticular nucleus. This is consistent with hemorrhagic infarction of these structures. The patient was a poorly controlled juvenile diabetic. The subsequent arteriogram shows occlusion of the internal carotid artery in its supraclinoid portion, with development of collateral vascularity both through the perforator route and the convexity branches of the posterior cerebral artery.

sideration of vasculitis as the underlying etiology. Conversely, hemorrhage in the subarachnoid space may produce vascular spasm and ischemia in a watershed territory (Fig. 6). Clearly, the sensitivity of MRI to the specific alterations produced by blood products makes it likely that it will help fuel the clinical controversy with regard to anticoagulation in the face of hemorrhagic components of infarction (38).

Chronic infarcts are generally seen as well-circumscribed regional areas of altered signal intensity. The adjacent brain will show signs of atrophy (enlarged ventricular and/or sulcal CSF spaces). True micro- or macroscopic cyst formation may occur, with the fluid essentially identical to CSF in signal characteristics (Fig. 7). Old hemorrhage in a previous infarct is seen as a feathery or irregular focus of signal loss on long TR–long TE images, due to the magnetic susceptibility effects of hemosiderin. Distinction from dystrophic calcification is only possible on morphologic criteria, when the calcium is seen as a large clump.

As briefly mentioned above, the aging brain is especially subject to the risk of ischemia, especially in the deep hemispheric region. Indeed, studies have shown that up to 30% of patients over the age of 65 studied by MRI exhibit multifocal regions of high signal on long TR–long TE images (26–39). This is thought to be due to small, clinically silent infarcts or perhaps to diffuse ischemic change (Fig. 8). Autopsy studies have shown that small infarcts are commonly seen in the deep hemispheres of otherwise normal brains taken from elderly subjects (40). Of course, hypertensive disease and other types of microangiopathy (e.g., systemic lupus erythematosus, radiation vasculopathy) will predispose the brain to such changes, even in the younger age groups (Fig. 9). Although white-matter disease such as multiple sclerosis may enter the differential diagnosis in such cases, the involvement of the basal ganglia makes ischemia a much more likely etiology (Fig. 10). Prior to MRI, antemortem diagnosis of many such small, subclinical infarcts was not appreciated.

The diagnosis of small infarcts in the posterior fossa is also facilitated by MRI; CT has been especially unrewarding in this region. The small size of these infarcts, the relative lack of edema, and the presence of bone streak artifacts all pose major hurdles to their CT diagnosis. As with other lesions in the posterior fossa, MRI is

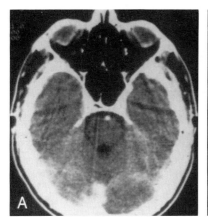

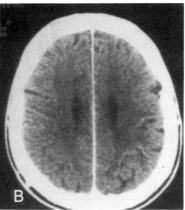

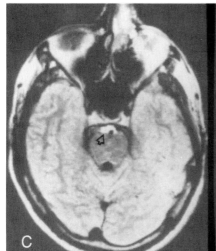

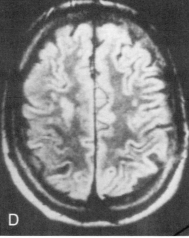

FIG. 6. Acute left hemiparesis several days after a severe headache was noted. At that time, lumbar puncture documented subarachnoid bleeding. **A,B:** A CT scan with contrast. **C,D:** TR 2,000, TE 30 msec. **E:** TR 500, TE 30 msec. **F:** Vertebral arteriogram; Towne projection. Despite the negative CT scan, the MR study (done within 2 hr of the CT scan) documents several foci of high signal intensity in the centrum semiovale, more prominent on the right. Also seen is a collection of high signal intensity around the patent basilar artery in the prepontine cistern (**C,E;** *arrows*). The short TR image (**E**) verifies that this collection represents a subacute clot. The arteriogram documents spasm of the basilar artery in this location. The high signal foci in the watershed perforating distribution presumably were caused by hypoperfusion secondary to the spasm.

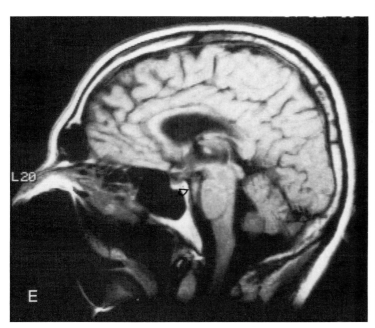

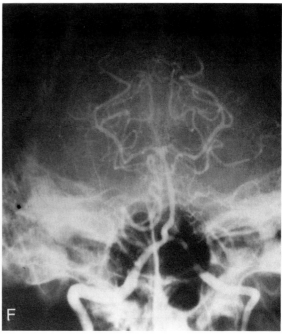

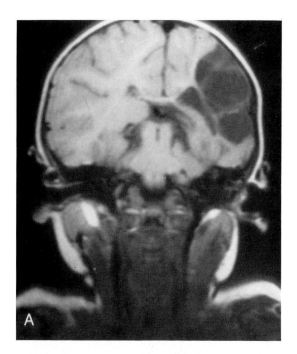

FIG. 7. Chronic infarct; left middle cerebral artery distribution. **A:** TR 600, TE 20 msec, coronal. **B:** TR 2,000, TE 35 msec. **C:** TR 2,000, TE 70 msec. The MR study documents a multiloculated abnormality in the region of the left middle cerebral artery. The signal intensity within the abnormal region is similar to that of CSF. Also, there is an apparent enlargement of the ipsilateral ventricular system indicating atrophy. An acute onset of right hemiparesis several months prior to the study was known to have occurred.

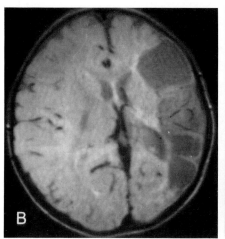

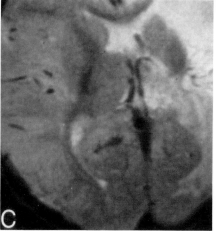

FIG. 8. A 79-year old woman; no significant medical history. **A:** TR 2,000, TE 28 msec. **B:** TR 2,000, TE 56 msec. Multiple foci of high signal intensity are seen throughout the white matter of both hemispheres, separate from and subjacent to the ventricular ependyma. No history of cardiovascular risk factors was present in this patient. Such foci most likely represent subclinical ischemic damage (see text).

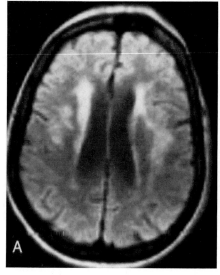

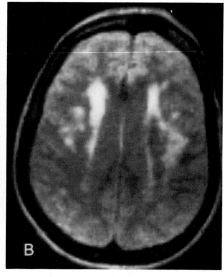

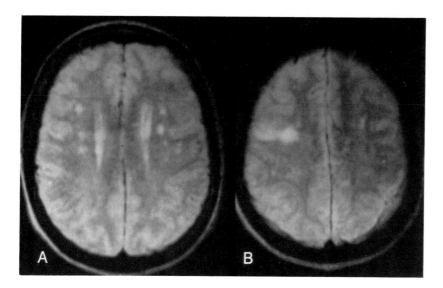

FIG. 9. Thirty-three-year-old woman with lupus erythematosus. **A,B:** TR 2,000, TE 28 msec; two adjacent sections. Multiple punctate foci of high signal intensity are seen in the deep hemispheric white matter consistent with ischemia, presumably due to the small-vessel abnormalities known to occur in certain patients with lupus.

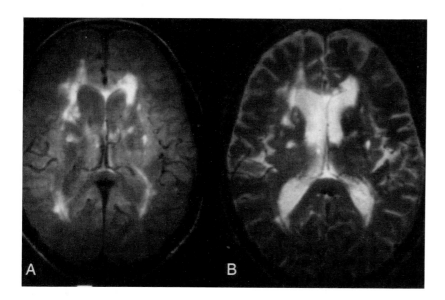

FIG. 10. Elderly woman with hypertension; previous episodes of infarction. **A:** TR 2,000, TE 40 msec. **B:** TR 2,000, TE 80 msec. Multiple foci of high signal intensity are seen throughout the periventricular white matter, as well as in the caudate nuclei, lenticular nuclei, and internal capsule. Such findings are consistent with infarction on the basis of hypertensive vasculopathy involving the small perforating branches to these regions.

the procedure of choice in the depiction of such infarcts (Fig. 11). The spinal cord may be another structure in which ischemia will be detected relatively easily by MRI.

LIMITATIONS OF MRI IN ISCHEMIA

It should be evident by this point that a topic not yet addressed by current experience is the potential ability of MRI to separate reversible ischemia from permanent infarction. This point is generally raised in the context of diagnostic evaluation of transient ischemic attacks. These are by definition clinical episodes of focal neurologic dysfunction with resolve within 24 hr. It should be stressed that clinical reversibility does not equate with pathologic reversibility. Because silent infarcts occur,

infarcts associated with only transient symptoms also occur. Thus, parenchymal changes may be observed on MRI in regions corresponding to where transient clinical dysfunction may have originated (Fig. 12).

The functional territory of the brain affected may be large initially during an acute episode, accounting for the manifest deficit, but with clinical resolution, the majority of this territory functionally recovers. Whether or not truly reversible ischemia (in the pathologic sense) can be detected with MRI alone is difficult to prove and has yet to be reported. Reversible MRI changes have been described in presumed ischemia secondary to lupus vasculitis (41,42).

Clearly, the ability of MRI to date the ischemic insult is limited. Increased water content is readily seen with MRI but accompanies all stages of ischemia, from the

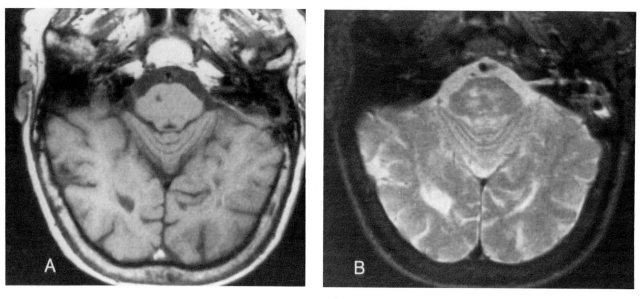

FIG. 11. Brainstem infarction. Acute-onset right facial palsy 1 month previous, with slow clinical improvement since: CT scan was normal. **A:** TR 600, TE 24 msec. **B:** TR 2,000, TE 80 msec. Multiple foci of high signal document ischemia of the brainstem on the long TR image. Only the largest lesion is seen on the short TR image.

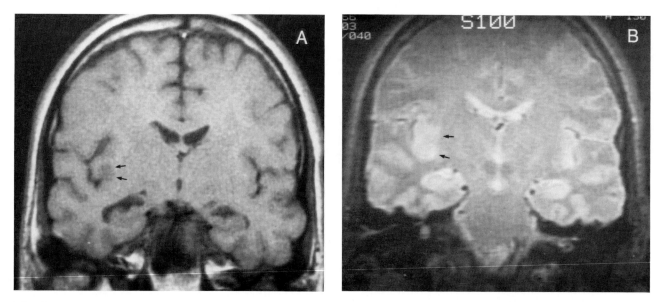

FIG. 12. Elderly man with sudden left-arm weakness 1 week earlier, which resolved during 24 hr. **A:** TR 600, TE 20 msec. **B:** TR 2,000, TE 80 msec. A focal lesion of high signal intensity is seen in the right middle cerebral artery distribution on the long TR image, corresponding to the smaller focus of low intensity on the short TR image (*arrows*). Despite the transient nature of the clinical findings, the permanence of the MRI lesion suggests true infarction.

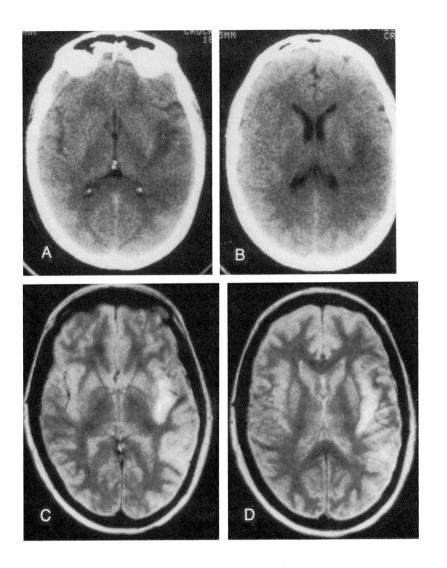

FIG. 13. Elderly woman with several week's history of confusion, loss of verbal fluency, and mild right hemiparesis. **A,B:** CT scan without contrast. **C,D:** TR 2,000, TE 60 msec. The corresponding sections at two levels show a well-circumscribed area of low density in the left upper opercular region on the precontrast CT scan. After contrast, the low density was no longer appreciated. The MR study shows high signal abnormality in the opercular region and less well-defined high signal in the posterior temporal lobe. The vague nature of the symptoms, the unusual appearance of the lesion, and the concern of the clinician prompted biopsy, which revealed subacute infarction and not tumor (as initially suspected on the clinical criteria). This case points out the nonspecific nature of MRI and CT.

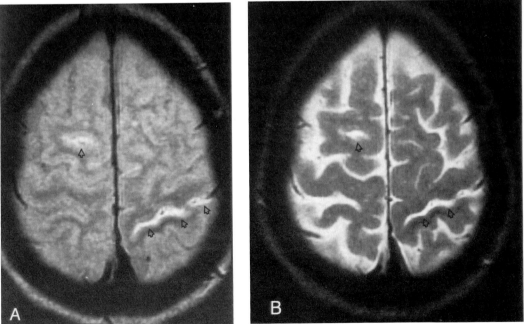

FIG. 14. Cortical infarction. **A:** TR 2,000, TE 35 msec. **B:** TR 2,000, TE 80 msec. Note the difficulty in separating the cortical infarction on the long TR–long TE study, where the infarcts simulate a large CSF-filled sulcus. The long TR–short TE image depicts the infarcted gyri as distinctly separate from the CSF space (*arrowheads*).

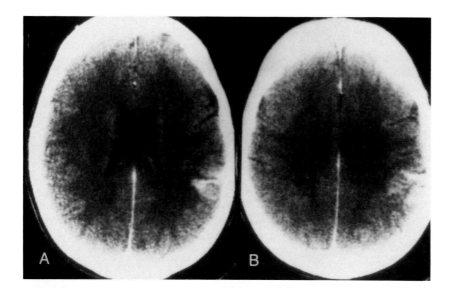

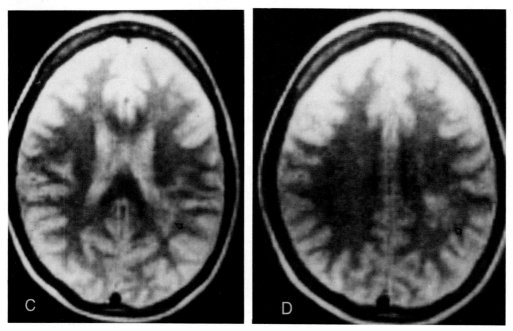

FIG. 15. Subacute infarction, "luxury" perfusion on CT. **A,B:** CT scan with contrast; two adjacent sections. **C,D:** TR 2,000, TE 60 msec corresponding sections. The gyral enhancement seen on CT in the left parietal cortex has no counterpart on the MRI image. However, the CT scan misses the ischemic lesion in the underlying white matter shown on MRI (*arrows*).

early, potentially reversible stage to the late stage of encephalomalacia. Indeed, most processes in the brain produce edema, and given an atypical appearance of the lesion or an unusual distribution and the lack of appropriate clinical history, distinction of infarction from another process may be impossible (Fig. 13). Another limitation of MRI is the ability to detect cerebral infarcts confined in the cortical mantle (43). The normal gray matter already has a relatively high water content. The increment by which ischemia raises the water content of the gray matter is relatively small; thus, the choice of instrument parameters for detecting ischemic versus normal gray matter is more critical. Too little T2 weighting keeps the ischemic tissue similar in signal to the gray matter; too much T2 weighting makes it similar to the adjacent sulci filled with CSF (Fig. 14). On CT, detection is aided by the gyral enhancement with contrast agents of the cortical lesion. This may be due to leakage of the agent across the blood–brain barrier or to excess agent in the vascular space due to "luxury" perfusion or arteriovenous shunting around the ischemic zone. The leaky capillary bed allows excess water in the extracellular space to alter the MRI signal, but luxury perfusion as such has no MRI counterpart (Fig. 15).

Contrast agents for MRI are under clinical investigation; however, the present generation does not seem to enhance the arterial or capillary space (see Chapter 6). Therefore, luxury perfusion may not be shown even with contrast-enhanced MRI; however, enhancement of gray-matter infarction after blood–brain barrier break-down occurs should be analogous to that seen with CT.

SUMMARY

The brief overview of the pathophysiologic and MRI aspects of cerebral ischemia offered above suggests that the major strength of MRI is the sensitivity of this modality to the presence of edema produced by ischemia. Also, as discussed elsewhere in this volume, the ability to evaluate major vessels going to the brain affords us information with regard to not only the end-organ itself, but its nutrient supply routes as well (Fig. 6) (16). This superior sensitivity should help in investigations aimed at evaluating various forms of therapy or even prophylaxis of ischemia. In the clinical setting, patients who present with acute "stroke" may not be the best candidates for MRI, since they may require life-support equipment difficult to place into a high magnetic field environment. Also, further experience with separating acute hematoma from ischemic infarction on MR images at various field strengths is necessary to be sure that optimal patient management can be based on the MRI results. Nevertheless, the availability of MRI should expand our understanding of both acute and chronic cerebral ischemia to a much greater extent.

REFERENCES

1. Brant-Zawadzki M, Norman D, Newton TH, et al. Magnetic resonance of the brain: The optimal screening technique. *Radiology* 1884;152:71–7.
2. Bradley WG, Waluch V, Yadley RA, Wycoff RR. Comparison of CT and MR in 400 patients with suspected disease of the brain and cervical spinal cord. *Radiology* 1979;512:695–702.
3. Bydder GM, Steiner RE, Young IR, et al. Clinical MR imaging of the brain. 140 cases. *AJNR* 1982;3:475–80.
4. Naruse S, Horikawa Y, Tanaka C, Hirakawa K, Nishikawa H, Yoshizaki K. Proton nuclear magnetic resonance studies on brain edema. *J Neurosurg* 1982;56:747–52.
5. Brant-Zawadzki M, Bartkowski HM, Ortendahl DA, et al. NMR in experimental and clinical cerebral edema. *Noninvasive Med Imag* 1984;1:43–7.
6. Brant-Zawadzki M, Pereira B, Weinstein P, Moore S, Kucharczyk W, Berry I, McNamara M, Derugin N. MRI of acute experimental ischemia in rats. *AJNR* 1986;7:7–11.
7. Hilal SK, Maudsley AA, Simon HE, Perman WH, Bonn J, Mawad ME, Silver AJ, Ganti SR, Sane P, Chien IC. *In vivo* NMR imaging of tissue sodium in the intact cat before and after acute cerebral stroke. *AJNR* 1983;4:245–9.
8. Bottomley PA, Hart HR, Edelstein WA, et al. Anatomy and metabolism of the normal human brain studied by MR at 1.5 tesla. *Radiology* 1984;150:441–6.
9. Wedeen VJ, Rosen BR, Chesler D, Brady TJ. MR velocity imaging by phase display. *JCAT* 1985;9(3):530–6.
10. Bryant DJ, Payne JA, Firmin DN, Langmore DB. Measurement of flow with NMR imaging using a gradient pulse and phase difference technique. *JCAT* 1984;8(4):588–93.
11. Wehrli FW, McFall JR, Shutts D, et al. Approaches to in plane and out-of-plane flow. *Non-invasive Med Imag* 1984;1:127–36.
12. Wherli FW, Shinakawa A, McFall JR, et al. MRI of venous and arterial flow by a selective saturation-recovery spin–echo method. *JCAT* 1985;9:537–45.
13. Bradley WG, Waluch V. Blood flow: magnetic resonance imaging. *Radiology* 1985;154:443–50.
14. Bradley WG, Waluch V. NMR even echo rephasing in slow laminar flow. *JCAT* 1984;8:594–8.
15. VonSchultheiss GK, Higgins CB. Blood flow imaging with MR: Spin-phase phenomena. *Radiology* 1985;157:687–95.
16. Edelman RR, Weeden VJ, Davis KR, et al. MR angiography of carotid arteries. Presented at American Society of Neuroradiology Annual Meeting, San Diego, January, 1986.
17. Goldberg HL, Spagnoli MV, Berkowitz H, et al. MRI characteristics of carotid artery atherosclerotic disease. Presented at American Society of Neuroradiology Annual Meeting, San Diego, January 1986.
18. Hinshaw DB, Holshouser B, Hasso AN, et al. High resolution MRI of carotid bifurcations using surface coils. Presented at American Society of Neuroradiology Annual Meeting, San Diego, January, 1986.
19. Gotoh O, Asano T, Koide T, Takakura K. Ischemic brain edema following occlusion of the middle cerebral artery in the rat. I: The time courses of the brain water, sodium and potassium contents and blood–brain barrier permeability to I-125-albumin. *Stroke* 1985;16(1):101–9.
20. Hossmann KA, Shuier FJ. Experimental brain infarcts in cats. I. Pathophysiological observations. *Stroke* 1980;11(6):583–92.
21. Schuier FJ, Hossmann KA: Experimental brain infarcts in cats. II. Ischemic brain edema. *Stroke* 1980;11(6):593–601.
22. Marcy VR, Walsh FA. Correlation between cerebral blood flow and ATP content following tourniquet-induced ischemia in cat brain. *J Cereb Blood Flow Metab* 1984;4:362–7.
23. Welsh FA. Review regional evaluation of ischemic metabolic alterations. *J Cereb Blood Flow Metab* 1984;4:309–16.
24. Weinstein PR, Anderson GG, Teller DA. Neurological deficit and cerebral infarction after temporary middle cerebral artery occlusion in unanesthetized cats. *Stroke* 1986;17(2):318–24.
25. Hornig CR, Dorndof W, Agnoli AL. Hemorrhagic cerebral infarction—A prospective study. *Stroke* 1986;17(2):179–85.
26. Bradley WG, Waluch V, Brant-Zawadzki M, Yadley RA, Wycoff RR. Patchy, periventricular white matter lesions in the elderly: A common observation during NMR imaging. *Noninvas Med Imag* 1984;1:35–41.
27. Melamad E, Lavy S, Bentin S, Cooper YR, Rinot Y. Reduction in regional cerebral blood flow during normal aging in man. *Stroke* 1980;11(1):31–6.
28. Shaw TG, Mortel KF, Meyer JS, Rogers RL, Hardenberg J, Cataia MM. Cerebral blood flow changes in benign aging and cerebrovascular disease. *Neurology* 1984;34:855–62.
29. Naritomi H, Meyer JS, Sakai F, Yamaguchi F, Shaw T. Effects of advancing age on regional cerebral blood flow. *Arch Neurol* 1979;36:410–6.
30. Bryan RN, Willcott MR, Scheiders NJ, Ford JJ, Derman HS. Nuclear magnetic resonance evaluation of stroke. A preliminary report. *Radiology* 1983;149:189–92.
31. Sipponen JT. Uses of techniques. Visualization of brain infarction with nuclear magnetic resonance imaging. *Neuroradiology* 1984;26:387–91.
32. Kistler JP, Buonanno FS, DeWitt LD, David KR, Brady TJ, Fisher CM. Vertebral-basilar posterior cerebral territory stroke—Delineation by proton nuclear magnetic resonance imaging. *Stroke* 1984;15(3):417–26.
33. Pykett IL, Buonanno FS, Brady TJ, Kistler JP. True three-dimensional nuclear magnetic resonance neuroimaging in ischemic stroke: correlation of NMR, x-ray CT and pathology. *Stroke* 1983;14(2):173–7.
34. Sipponen JT, Kaste M, Ketonen L, Sepponen RE, Katevuo K, Sivula A. Serial nuclear magnetic resonance (NMR) imaging in patients with cerebral infarction. *JCAT* 1983;7(4):585–9.
35. Brant-Zawadzki M, Solomon M, Newton TH, Weinstein P, Schmidley J, Norman D. Basic principles of magnetic resonance imaging in cerebral ischemia and initial clinical experience. *Neuroradiology* 1985;27(6):517–20.

36. Swanson RA, Schmidley JW. Amnestic syndrome and vertical gaze palsy: early detection of bilateral thalamic infarction by CT and NMR. *Stroke* 1985;16(5):823–7.

37. Gomori JM, Grossman RI, Goldberg HI, Zimmerman RA, Bilaniuk LT. Intracranial hematomas: imaging by high-field MR. *Radiology* 1985;157:87–93.

38. Hart RFG, Lockwood KI, Hakim AM, Koller R, Davneport JG, Coull BM, Brey R, Furlan AJ, O'Neill BJ, Pettigrew LC, Nath A, Yatsu FM, Sherman DG, Easton JD, Miller VT. Immediate anticoagulation of embolic stroke: brain hemorrhage and management options. *Stroke* 1984;15(5):779–89.

39. Brant-Zawadzki M, Fein G, Van Dyke C, Kiernan R, Davenport L, DeGroot J. Magnetic resonance imaging of the aging brain: patchy white matter lesions and dementia. *AJNR* 1985;675–682.

40. Peress NS, Kane WC, Aronson SM. Central nervous system findings in a tenth decade autopsy population. In: Ford DE, ed., *Neurobiological aspects of maturation and aging.* New York: Elsevier, 1973:253–65. (Progress in brain research; vol. 40.)

41. Aisen AM, Gabrielsen TO, McCune WJ. MR imaging of systemic lupus erythematosus involving the brain. *AJNR* 1985;6:197–201.

42. Vermess M, Bernstein RM, Bydder GM, Steiner RE, Young IR, Hughes GRV. Nuclear magnetic resonance (NMR) imaging of the brain in systemic lupus erythematosus. *JCAT* 7(3):461–7.

43. Weinstein MA, LaValley A, Rosenbloom SA, Duchesneau, PM. Limitations of MRI for the detection of gray matter lesions. Presented at American Society of Neuroradiology Annual Meeting, San Diego, January, 1986.

44. Macchi PJ, Grossman RI, Gamori JM, et al. High field MRI of cerebral venous thrombosis. *JCAT* 1986;10(1):10–5.

CHAPTER 15

Intracranial Infection

Robert A. Zimmerman, Larissa T. Bilaniuk, and Gordon Sze

The advent of computed tomography (CT) revolutionized the diagnostic evaluation of the patient in whom intracranial infection was suspected (1). CT provided information about the presence or absence of a mass, its location, its effect on the ventricular system and subarachnoid pathways, and with the use of intravenous radiographic contrast agents, the state of the blood–brain barrier (BBB). The CT information supplanted that obtained from more invasive imaging studies (ventriculography, pneumoencephalography, and arteriography). In little more than a decade following the introduction of CT, magnetic resonance imaging (MRI) has become a clinical tool. The question is now, Will MRI alter the role of CT in the evaluation of intracranial infections and if so, for what reasons?

The experience with MRI in the evaluation of intracranial infections has thus far been restricted because of an insufficient number of scanners and their limited availability for inpatients. Moreover, this new technique is still under development, and any data accumulated are preliminary. Thus, the literature on the application of MRI to intracranial infections has so far been sparse (2,3). The aim of this chapter is to put into perspective our initial experience with MRI in intracranial infections.

Assuming that both imaging modalities, MRI and CT, are equally available in a hospital-based setting, which of the two would be the study of choice? An attempt to answer this question shall be made as specific disease entities are discussed. The answer might differ even within the same disease category, depending on the patient's condition (4). The stable patient who is cooperative and who does not have any contraindications to MRI (such as a cardiac pacemaker) can be examined provided that he or she is not claustrophobic. In the patient who is not cooperative, because of illness or age (infancy or senility), or who is in extremis or is rapidly deteriorating, or who requires major monitoring and support, the following must be kept in mind. Computed tomography is rapid. A single section takes on the order of 5 sec, and so long as motion does not occur during that time, that section is interpretable. With MRI, scan times are on the order of minutes, and motion during a portion of that scan time results in a degraded or uninterpretable image. However, it must also be noted that in 5 sec, the CT provides only one section, whereas in 2 to 10 min, the MRI provides from several to many (even 40) images. It is possible to perform MRI on a patient under general anesthesia, and it is possible to monitor patients within the MRI environment. Intubation devices, respirators, intravenous pumps, and other devices can be dealt with so as not to distort the magnetic field and not to be pulled into the magnet. However, it is significantly more difficult to take care of the ill patient within the MRI scanner room than it is at the CT scanner.

Given the inherent difficulties in performing MRI on very ill patients—a common situation with intracranial infectious diseases—What then are the differences between the information derived from MRI and CT? CT studies are done primarily in the axial plane. Coronal images can be accomplished by hyperextending the head in either the prone or supine position. Direct coronal sections done in this manner require the cooperation of the patient. In patients with intracranial infection, coronal sections are usually not easily achieved. Coronal and sagittal sections can be reconstructed from multiple thin axial sections, but they typically suffer from image degradation. Magnetic resonance imaging requires no alteration of the patient's position. Direct axial, coronal, and sagittal sections are obtained without uncomfortable positioning of the patient. With MRI, there is no image degradation from plane to plane.

With CT, radiographic contrast agents can be administered intravenously so that disturbances in the BBB are demonstrated, and the neovascularity within the connective tissue of the abscess capsule is enhanced. The iodinated contrast agent enters the substance of the inflammatory lesion through the disruption in the BBB and produces increased density on CT scans due to higher X-ray attenuation of the contrast agent. With MRI, paramagnetic contrast agents that cross the BBB are in clinical trials. Such an agent is gadolinium DTPA (Fig. 1) (5); however, it has not yet been approved for clinical use by the Food and Drug Administration (FDA). Thus, with MRI there is no available BBB agent

for routine use. In situations in which CT contrast enhancement is crucial (such as in demonstrating involvement of the basilar meninges in tuberculous meningitis), MRI is not yet competitive. Conversely, contrast enhancement is needed for CT in order to identify an abscess capsule and to separate it from the surrounding edema. With MRI, thus far, we have been successful in showing the mature abscess capsule as a structure of different signal intensity, distinct from the abscess contents and the surrounding edema. It has not always been

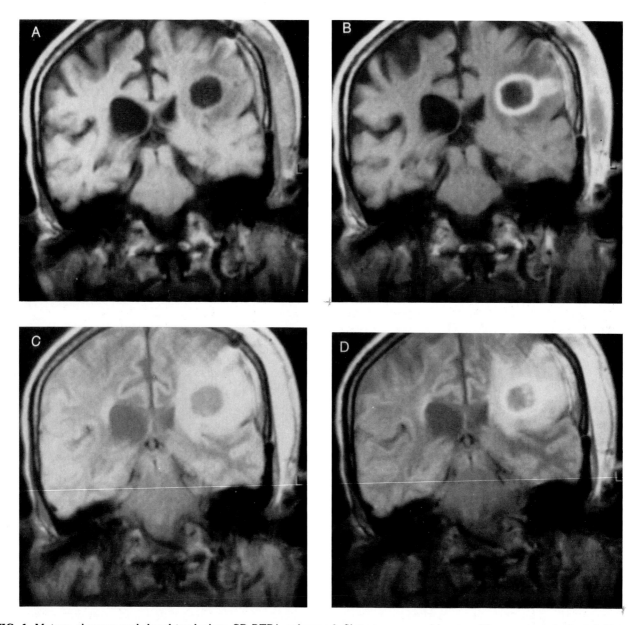

FIG. 1. Mature abscess and daughter lesion; GD-DTPA enhanced. Sixty-two-year-old man with severe periodontal disease who developed slurred speech and right-sided weakness. **A:** TR 600, TE 24 msec; pre-GD-DTPA. **B:** TR 600, TE 24 msec; post-GD-DTPA. **C:** TR 2,000, TE 40 msec; pre-GD-DTPA. **D:** TR 2,000, TE 40 msec; post-GD-DTPA. The central necrotic core of the main abscess cavity, the rim (representing a capsule), and the surrounding edema are well shown by the pre-GD-DTPA images (**A,C**); however, the incipient daughter abscess is depicted as separate from the edema only after the contrast agent is administered (**B,D**). The biopsy tract may have contributed to the location of the daughter lesion.

possible with CT to predict how completely the abscess capsule is formed, because reactive brain change around a forming capsule can show ring enhancement. It is hoped that MRI will help to characterize better the maturity of the capsule and thus indicate the optimum time for drainage and excision.

Depicting calcification is an advantage of CT. Calcification significantly attenuates the X-ray beam and shows up on the scan as an area of increased density. As far as MRI is concerned, calcified tissue contains few mobile protons so that no signal is produced (6). In order for these calcifications to be seen on MRI, the calcifications have to occupy the full thickness of the slice and not be interspersed in tissue composed of mobile protons (7). When partial voluming of the calcification and adjacent tissue occurs, or when the calcification is small, a signal is returned, often obscuring the signal void that would be expected from the calcification. Calcification is important in the diagnosis of the dead larval stage of cerebral cysticercosis and in other chronic infections and the end stages of congenital infections (8). Studies of cysticercosis with MRI have shown that MRI is relatively insensitive in identifying these calcifications (3).

A hallmark of inflammatory reaction within the brain is often the presence of an increase in water content at the affected site. CT shows gross areas of vasogenic edema as a zone of decreased density. MRI shows not only gross vasogenic edema well, but smaller and less obvious (by CT) areas of inflammatory change. The high signal intensity on T2-weighted images identifies these areas, and the multiplanar sections graphically localize them.

CT is highly sensitive in demonstrating the increased density of acute hematomas. As hemoglobin breaks down, the density decreases, and the hematoma becomes first isodense and then hypodense (9). High-field [1.5 tesla (T)] MRI is sensitive in detecting acute, subacute, and chronic hematomas (10). MRI is able to show small intraparenchymal hematomas long after they cease to be obvious on CT. Demonstration of areas of hemorrhage helps to characterize more fully infectious diseases that are heterogeneously spread, such as mycotic vasculopathy with rupture; cerebritis; bacterial abscesses; disseminated infections, such as tuberculomas; and necrotizing encephalitis, such as herpes simplex.

As can be seen from the foregoing discussion, both CT and MRI have their advantages and disadvantages. Is one better than the other? It depends on the circumstances and the information sought. It is clear that MRI is more sensitive to lesions that are marked by increased water content and that CT is more sensitive to lesions that are denoted by calcification. CT with contrast injection is better able to characterize active disturbances in the BBB than is MRI until gadolinium DPTA is FDA approved. Is one technique more specific than the other?

The answer again depends on the information that is needed in order to make the diagnosis. If we need to know that calcifications are present, as in cysticercosis, then CT should be used. If we need to detect abnormality in the medial temporal lobes and isle of Reil in the insular region, as in herpes simplex encephalitis, then MRI is more sensitive. With both CT and MRI, the clinical information including age, sex, symptoms, physical findings, and initial clinical course is vital to the intelligent interpretation of the findings and to the correct use of the imaging information in the care of the patient. Either technique interpreted out of the context of the clinical situation is less useful.

SPECIFIC DISEASES

Bacterial Infections

CEREBRITIS

Cerebritis is the earliest form of purulent brain infection. Pathologically, the involved area is often ill-defined, edematous, with petechial hemorrhages, and vascular congestion. CT shows cerebritis most often as a poorly delineated, low-density area that has mass effect and slight heterogeneous enhancement (11). The CT manifestations are nonspecific, but in the appropriate clinical context they indicate a need for further diagnostic evaluation and treatment. Magnetic resonance is superior to CT in showing areas of edematous cerebritis as high-signal-intensity abnormalities on T2-weighted images (Figs. 2 and 3). If the petechial hemorrhages are of sufficient magnitude, these will also be seen on T1- and T2-weighted images as abnormal signal intensity depending on the chemical state of the blood (10). Mass effect is well demonstrated with MRI as displacement of ventricles and compression of sulci and fissures (Figs. 1 and 2). The presence of multiple areas of involvement by cerebritis will be better demonstrated with MRI than by CT. Cerebritis is a condition that may respond to medical management with appropriate antibiotics. Resolution of the process can occur over a period of weeks to months. MRI may prove superior in following the resolution of mass effect and of signal abnormality as the treatment proves effective.

BRAIN ABSCESS

If cerebritis is not successfully treated, liquefaction occurs. The host responds by forming fibroblasts that migrate into the area surrounding the cerebritis in an attempt to wall it off. The fibroblasts are derived from endothelial cells in the blood vessels (12). The wall that they help to build is the capsule of the abscess. The wall consists of an inner lining of granulation tissue, a middle

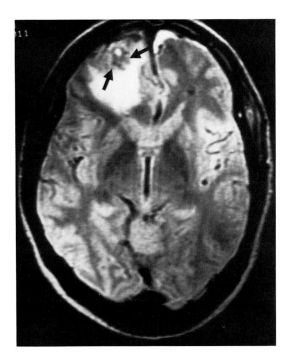

FIG. 2. Cerebritis, subdural empyema. Middle-aged woman with headaches, fever, and personality changes. Axial T2-weighted image (TR = 2,500 msec, TE = 40 msec) of 5-mm-thick section shows hyperintense edematous zone in the white matter of the right frontal lobe surrounding a sub-cortical area of more mixed signal intensity (*arrows*). The frontal horn of the right lateral ventricle is posteriorly displaced, and the medial aspect of the right frontal lobe is herniated beneath the anterior falx. A small extracerebral high-intensity pyogenic fluid collection is present over the left frontal lobe. On antibiotic therapy, the areas of mixed intensity signal and surrounding edema subsequently developed into a well-formed abscess. The collection over the left frontal lobe at surgery proved to be a small subdural empyema.

layer of collagen, and an outer layer of reactive glial tissue. It is the middle collagen layer that is formed by the migrating fibroblasts. The abscess capsule tends to be the weakest on its inner aspect facing the white matter in the direction of the ventricles. This is because the fibroblasts arise from more superficial vessels in the cortical gray matter, and the distance they have to migrate is greatest at the inner aspect of the abscess. As a result of this weakness, daughter abscesses tend to occur along the weaker inner wall toward the white-matter side. There is danger of rupture of the abscess into the ventricle, leading to acute pyogenic ventriculitis and death.

The organisms responsible for brain abscesses have evolved since the preantibiotic era. Currently, abscesses secondary to traumatic or iatrogenic causes tend to be due to staphylococci, and those hematogenously disseminated are more often due to mixed aerobic and anaerobic organisms (13). Staphylococci, pneumococci, and streptococci remain important because they are re-

sponsible for CNS infections in children. Of the hematogenously disseminated abscesses, more than half are solitary and are usually located in the vascular distribution of the anterior and middle cerebral arteries. The frontal lobes are the most common site of involvement, with the temporal lobes next in frequency. Abscesses are most typically found at the corticomedullary junctures of the brain, the site at which hematogeneously spread infection is physically stopped because of a decrease in vascular luminal size. In the late stages of cerebritis, contrast-enhanced CT will show a thin ring. With more collagen deposited in the wall, a more distinct ring enhancement is identified. Evolution of the abscess in various stages of capsule formation has been detailed by Enzmann (14). A thin-walled, ring-enhancing lesion on CT, surrounded by edema, has been taken to be reasonably characteristic of a brain abscess (Fig. 4A). Unfortunately, a multitude of other disease processes, including malignant and metastatic brain tumors, infarctions, and resolving hematomas, can show similar findings on CT. The degree of enhancement seen with CT in brain abscesses is decreased by the use of steroids and to some extent by antibiotic therapy. The false-negative rate for CT in identifying abscesses greater than 1 cm in diameter is small. There has been an effort to avoid surgery in cases where lesions are deep, multiple, or when the patient is a poor surgical candidate (15). The CT information, when taken with the clinical situation, has led to early conservative management of these patients by means of antibiotics.

With MRI, the abscess capsules have been identified as one of two types: hemorrhagic or nonhemorrhagic. The hemorrhagic abscess capsules will have a signal intensity that depends on the state of hemoglobin (Fig. 5). MRI has been very sensitive in showing vasogenic edema surrounding the abscess capsule and the central pyogenic material. The pyogenic contents are of high signal intensity in the early abscess stage on the T2-weighted image (Fig. 5D), but the intensity may decrease as the abscess becomes sterile (Fig. 1). On the T1-weighted image, the higher signal intensity of the edema and contents allows their separation from the less intense nonhemorrhagic abscess capsule. Mass effect, number of abscesses, and the presence or absence of daughter abscesses are well shown by MRI. Multiplanar scanning gives precise anatomic localization. Ventriculitis can occur when the abscess ruptures into the ventricular space or can be iatrogenically produced. The CSF will alter its signal based on the degree of purulence introduced (Fig. 6). In most cases, such a development heralds a grave prognosis.

TUBERCULOSIS

By the year 1900, tuberculomas were the most common cause of an intracranial mass, more common than

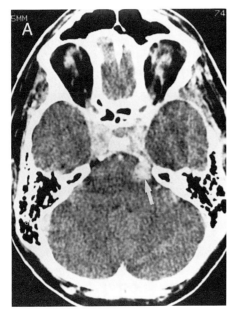

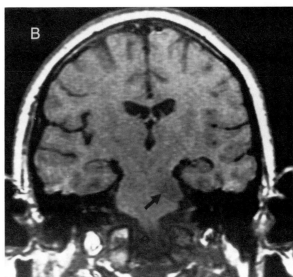

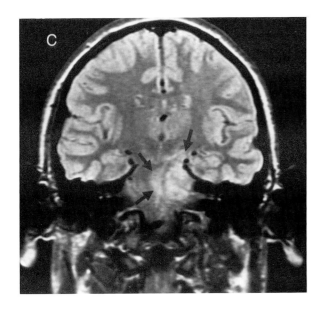

FIG. 3. Cerebritis. Young adult on antibiotic treatment for actinomycosis of the sphenoid sinus, cavernous sinuses, and suprasellar area. The patient developed fifth nerve pain on the left. **A:** Contrast CT shows an enhanced mass (*arrow*) in the pons along the course of the fifth cranial nerve from the cavernous sinus. **B:** Coronal T1-weighted image (TR = 600 msec, TE = 25 msec) of 5-mm-thick section shows a zone of hypointensity (*arrow*) in the lateral aspect of the left pons. **C:** Coronal T2-weighted image (TR = 2,500 msec, TE = 30 msec) shows an abnormal area of hyperintense signal (*arrow*) involving a greater portion of the pons than is suggested by either the T1-weighted image or the CT scan.

brain neoplasms (13). In the affluent parts of the world today, tuberculomas and tuberculous meningitis are uncommon. Tuberculomas remain a relatively common problem in the less well-developed areas, including India, Mexico, Egypt, and other economically deprived countries.

In general, there has been an inclination to tuberculous meningitis in infants and young children, but it can be found at any age. In the young, the onset is often insidious, as it may be in the older patient. Weight loss, apathy, fever, and nonspecific symptoms may be present for weeks to months. Seizures and focal neurological deficits occur as a result of coexisting tuberculomas or infarctions secondary to vasculitis.

Intracranial tuberculomas result from hematogenous spread of *Mycobacterium tuberculosis,* a small Gram-

positive rod. Primary focus is characteristically in the lungs. The pulmonary focus may be quite small and not easily identified on routine chest radiographs. The tuberculoma is a form of granuloma and as such grows to form initially a small, round, discrete mass. Growth of the mass produces neurological deficits depending on location and size. Pathologically, tuberculomas are characterized by a central zone of caseous material surrounded by reactive epithelioid cells, Langerhan's giant cells, and lymphocytic cells (13). Rupture of the tuberculoma into the CSF can produce tuberculous meningitis.

On CT, the tuberculoma may be solitary or multiple and present with or without evidence of concomitant tuberculous meningitis. The most typical appearance of the tuberculomas on CT is that of a discrete, plaque-like,

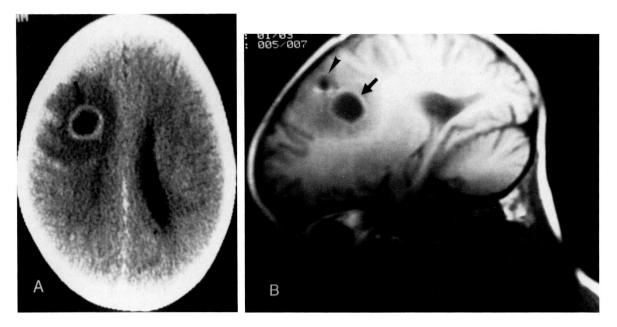

FIG. 4. Brain abscess. Child with headaches, fever, seizures, and left hemiparesis. **A:** Contrast-enhanced CT shows a discrete, thin-walled contrast-enhancing ring lesion (*arrow*) in the white matter of the right frontal hemisphere; it is surrounded by edema, and there is compression of the body of the right lateral ventricle. **B:** T1-weighted image (TR = 800 msec, TE = 20 msec) of 5-mm-thick section shows an isointense, thin-walled ring lesion in the frontal white matter surrounded by an area of relative hypointensity, with a more hypointense central portion. Note a second abscess (*arrowhead*) more superiorly.

contrast-enhancing lesion (Fig. 7), often at the cortico-medullary juncture (16,17). However, the lesion may attain considerable size and may also present as a ring-enhancing lesion. When it presents without tuberculous meningitis, the CT differential diagnosis includes that of metastatic disease or other solitary or multiple contrast-enhancing masses.

A gross pathologic characteristic of tuberculous leptomeningitis is a diffuse gray opacity of the leptomeninges owing to thick, gelatinous infiltrates around the base of the brain (13). Multinucleated giant cells, lymphocytes, and plasma cells are scattered throughout this material. Tuberculous bacilli are seen in large numbers. Blood vessels running through the involved CSF spaces may be affected by the inflammatory exudate with resulting thrombosis and brain infarction. Interference with reabsorption of CSF produces a communicating hydrocephalus.

Tuberculous meningitis is seen on CT as marked contrast enhancement of thickened basilar meninges, enlargement of CSF spaces, hydrocephalus (communicating or obstructive), and coexisting tuberculomas (Fig. 7) (18,19). The presence of thick contrast-enhancing basilar cisterns and small, discrete, nodular intraparenchymal lesions should suggest the combination of tuberculoma and tuberculous meningitis. MRI has been disappointing in the demonstration of inflammatory changes in the meninges and subarachnoid space. Without the use of a BBB contrast agent, it has not been

possible to demonstrate findings analogous to those demonstrated with enhanced CT. Distention of the subarachnoid space is well shown by MRI in the axial and coronal planes (Fig. 7E). Tuberculomas have appeared as areas of high signal intensity on T2-weighted images (Fig. 7D). In several instances, the site of the tuberculoma, reflecting its hematogenous dissemination, has shown focal hemorrhage as seen in an embolic infarct. This presented as a high signal area on T1-weighted images with even higher signal on the T2-weighted image (methoglobin) (Figs. 7C and D). The combination of nodular lesions of abnormal signal intensity in association with communicating hydrocephalus in the appropriate clinical setting suggests the diagnosis of tuberculoma with tuberculous meningitis.

BACTERIAL MENINGITIS

Leptomeningitis is an inflammatory process that involves the meningeal coverings of the brain and spinal cord. Specifically, it involves the pial covering of the brain and the arachnoid lining of the dura. Depending on the duration of the infection and its treatment, the process may be labeled acute, subacute, or chronic; depending on the nature of the infectious agent, it may be labeled suppurative or nonsuppurative. Acute suppurative leptomeningitis is seen with hemophilus influenza and staphylococcal pneumonia among others. Hemophilus influenza is seen in children from months to several

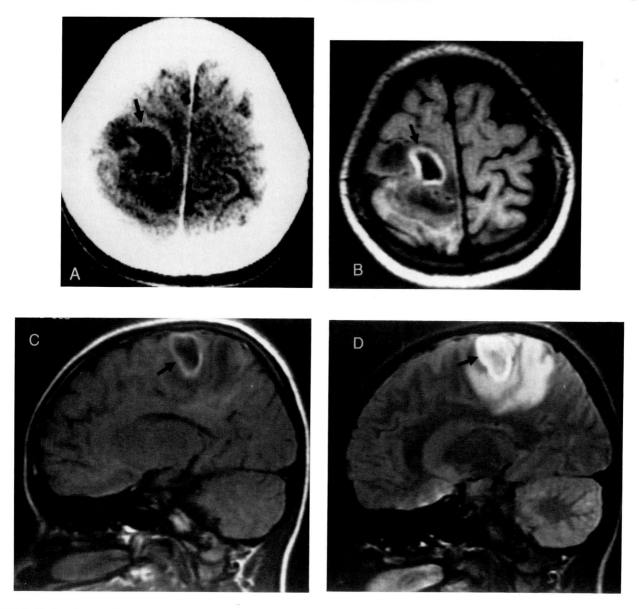

FIG. 5. Brain abscess. Teenage girl who developed seizures several days after esophageal dilatation. **A:** Contrast CT shows a thin-walled, enhancing cystic lesion (*arrow*) in the right parietal subcortical region. **B:** T1-weighted image (TR = 600 msec, TE = 25 sec) of 5-mm-thick axial section shows a thin-walled hyperintense rim abscess, with surrounding hypointensity. Note (in comparison to the opposite side) effacement of sulci on the right. **C:** Sagittal T1-weighted image (TR = 600 msec, TE = 25 msec) of 5-mm-thick section shows the hyperintense, thin-walled abscess (*arrow*). **D:** Sagittal T2-weighted image (TR = 2,500 msec, TE = 30 msec) of 5-mm-thick section shows a hyperintense abscess wall (*arrow*), with high-signal contents (pus) and high-signal surrounding edema.

years of age. In the newborn period, infection is more often due to Gram-negative rods, such as *Escherichia coli* and *citrobacter*. These organisms are accompanied by an outpouring of polymorphonuclear neutrophils (PMN). The pia and arachnoidal membranes become congested and hyperemic and the subarachnoid space distended by the exudate (13). Blood vessels passing through the inflammatory exudate may become involved in an obliterative process, leading to thrombosis. As a result, infarction of the subpial tissues may occur.

Cerebral edema with mass effect and herniation can develop acutely, whereas subacutely, hydrocephalus may result from blockage of the CSF pathways by the inflammatory exudate. In the more chronic process, fibrin acts to produce dense scar tissue.

The CT manifestations of meningitis vary from the sublime to the overwhelming. In its earliest manifestations, meningitis appears as distention of the subarachnoid space. Contrast enhancement of the meninges may be demonstrated on CT, a finding that does not harbor

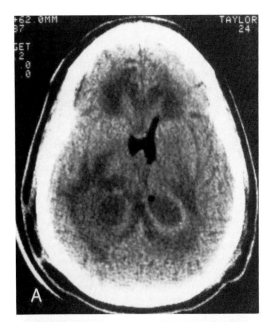

FIG. 6. Ventriculitis. Twenty-two-year-old woman with a history of benign aqueductal stenosis, shunted 20 years ago. Since then, the patient has suffered repeated bouts of *Staphylococcus epidermidis* and *Staphylococcus aureus* ventriculitis and meningitis. The current scans were precipitated because of mental status changes. Pathology: *S. aureus* ventriculitis. **A:** Noncontrast CT scan shows enlarged ventricles with visible rims, surrounded by edema. Due to purulent infectious exudate, the CSF has increased density. A recent shunt revision is most likely responsible for the air within the ventricles. **B,C:** On the long TR images (TR = 2,000, TE = 30, 60 msec), diffuse high intensity secondary to edematous changes surrounds the ventricles. High intensity is also present within the ventricles, again secondary to purulent exudate. The ependyma, in this case, appears as an isointense ring (**C**).

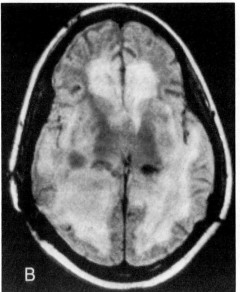

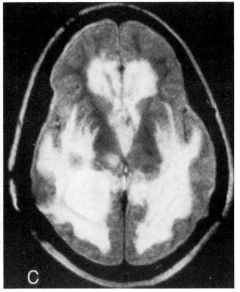

ill for the patient, provided that treatment is prompt and effective (20). Hydrocephalus may be seen at any time during the course and may be communicating or obstructive. Involvement of arteries and veins in the subarachnoid space leads to infarction. The pia is a resistant barrier to the spread of infection from the CSF space; however, following infarction of the cortex and disruption of the pial barrier, infection can extend into the involved tissues (Fig. 8).

Necrosis of the arachnoid leads to subdural collections (see below). If the infectious disease process has been controlled, then the collection is likely to be sterile; however, when the infectious process has not been controlled, a subdural empyema may be formed. Contrast-enhanced CT is effective in demonstrating the subdural membrane. Pyogenic subdural collections appear to be slightly higher in density than CSF. In the neonate, as in the adult, ventriculitis accompanying meningitis produces a thickening of the ependyma, with marked contrast enhancement and a periventricular decrease in density of the white matter.

The application of MRI to bacterial meningitis has been limited, primarily because of the neurological status of the patient with meningitis. MRI shows the distention of the subarachnoid space (Fig. 8) and the enlargement of the ventricles. Narrowing or occlusion of the aqueduct of Sylvius is clearly shown with thin sagittal sections (Fig. 9). Periventricular accumulation of CSF around the obstructed ventricle can be seen but may not be easily differentiated from the changes asso-

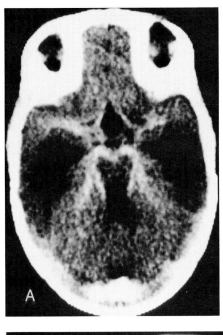

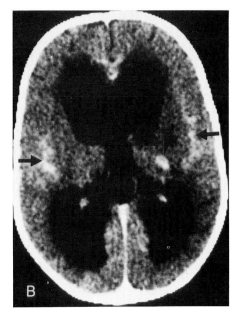

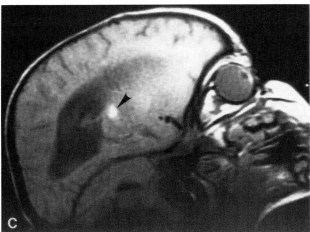

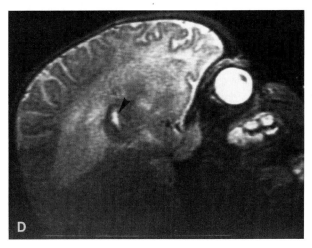

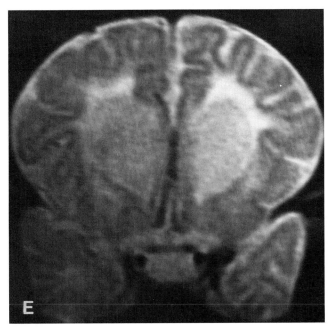

FIG. 7. Tuberculous meningitis and tuberculomas. Infant with failure to thrive, fever, and recent obtundation. **A:** Contrast CT shows both marked enhancement of the basilar meninges and hydrocephalus. **B:** Higher section of contrast CT shows marked enhancement of the meninges of the Sylvian fissures (*arrows*), hydrocephalus, and an enhancing tuberculoma (*arrowhead*) in the left thalamus. **C:** Sagittal T1-weighted image (TR = 600 msec, TE = 25 msec) of 5-mm-thick section shows a hyperintense, hemorrhagic focus at the site of the tuberculoma in the thalamus (*arrowhead*). Ventricular enlargement is present consistent with hydrocephalus. **D:** Sagittal T2-weighted image (TR = 2,000 msec, TE = 75 msec) shows distention of the subarachnoid space and hyperintensity at the site of the tuberculoma (*arrowhead*). **E:** Coronal T2-weighted image (TR = 2,000 msec, TE = 75 msec) of 5-mm-thick section shows distention of the subarachnoid space and ventricular system. Note high signal intensity at the upper margins of the lateral ventricles due to reabsorption of CSF from the obstructed ventricles.

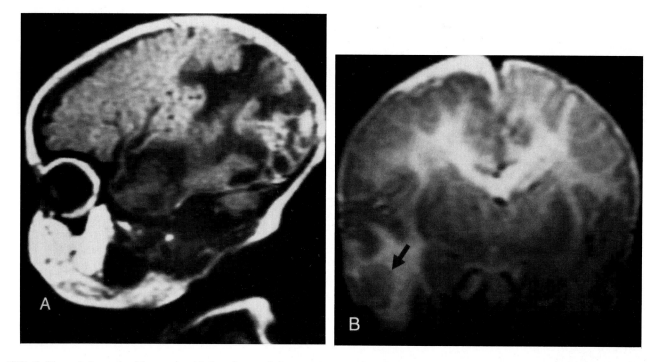

FIG. 8. Neonatal meningitis cerebral infarction and abscess formation. Neonate with failure to thrive and seizures. **A:** Sagittal T1-weighted image (TR = 600 msec, TE = 25 msec) of 5-mm-thick section shows marked hypointensity of brain edema in the right temporal parietal and occipital lobes. Focal hyperintense cortex in the right posterior temporal occipital region represents hemorrhagic infarction. Edematous change in the anterior temporal lobe outlines a slightly hypointense intra-temporal area of early abscess formation. **B:** Coronal T2-weighted image (TR = 2,000 msec, TE = 70 msec) of 5-mm-thick section shows distended subarachnoid space, superiorly, more on the right than on the left due to meningitic exudates and bilateral edematous white matter in the semicentral centrum ovale, with edema in the right temporal lobe outlining a left hypointense early abscess (*arrow*).

ciated with ependymitis. Cortical and subcortical infarction as a result of occlusion of vessels can also be identified. The hemorrhagic nature of such cortical infarctions is well shown (Fig. 8). Loculation of the subdural space by pyogenic infection following necrosis of the arachnoid can also be shown with MRI.

Subdural and Epidural Empyemas

The arachnoid and dura are adherent but a potential space, the subdural space, exists between them. Dura is the periosteum of the inner table of the skull. As such, the dura is an effective barrier to the spread of infection other than penetration by venous channels. Infections of the intracranial epidural or subdural space may arise by direct contiguity, such as osteomyelitis of the calvarium or sinus wall (21,22). Necrosis of the arachnoid due to meningitis can lead to subdural space infection. In addition, spread of infection along the venous channels passing through the potential epidural and subdural spaces can lead to infection (23). Septic phlebitis may occur as a result of increased pressure within infected paranasal sinuses or mastoid air cells, helping to transmit infection

retrograde along venous channels that are not protected by valves.

Experience has shown that the majority of subdural and epidural empyemas arise as a complication of paranasal sinusitis, and most occur during the adolescent years. Headache, fever, focal seizures, and a change in mental status raise concern in the patient with a history of sinusitis, otitis, mastoiditis, or other paranasal sinus inflammatory disease process. The principal diagnostic method of evaluation in the patient suspected of sinusitis with cerebral complications has been CT. Empyemas of the extracerebral space are evidenced on CT as extra-axial collections that are slightly greater in density than CSF and are separated from the falx or the inner table of the skull by a contrast-enhancing membrane (Fig. 10A) (22,23). Not infrequently, edema in the underlying brain signifies venous thrombosis or accompanying cerebritis. Extracerebral collections are well shown by MRI in the coronal and axial planes, along with their associated mass effect and edematous changes in the cerebral parenchyma (Figs. 10B and C). The T2-weighted image shows the collections as having increased signal but usually not as high as that of the edematous brain. MRI also shows the margin of reactive

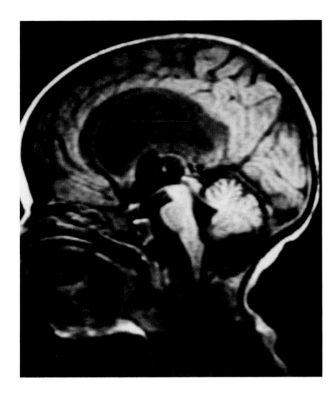

FIG. 9. Postmeningitic hydrocephalus. Infant successfully treated with antibiotics for Haemophilus Influenza meningitis who developed an increasing head size. Sagittal T1-weighted image (TR = 600 msec, TE = 25 msec) of 5-mm-thick section shows marked enlargement of the lateral and third ventricles and stretching of the anterior cerebral artery over the corpus callosum. There is a lack of distention of the cerebral aqueduct, which appears filled in by slightly increased signal-intensity material.

brain that can occur adjacent to such collections. Magnetic resonance imaging is highly sensitive in identifying inflammatory changes within the paranasal sinuses as areas of high signal intensity on T2-weighted images (Fig. 11).

VIRAL INFECTIONS

Viral infections produce a wide spectrum of changes in the brain tissue from nonapparent to necrosis, hemorrhage, edema, and vascular congestion (24). All of these four components may be found in various proportions. At the microscopic level, the inflammatory response to viruses varies from inapparent to more conventional inflammatory responses. In the more typical response, PMN leukocytes are found surrounding vessels. Subsequently, the nature of the cell reaction changes to mononuclear and lymphoid cells. Superimposed on this is the development of vascular congestion and of small conglomerates of inflammatory cells in a nodular fashion. These changes may be overshadowed by a more destructive necrotizing or thrombotic process, resulting

in edema and tissue loss. The histologic picture depends on both the infective agent and the host response. The representative viral infection in this section is herpes simplex. Cytomegalovirus (CMV) is referred to in the discussion on AIDS.

Herpes Simplex Virus

Herpes simplex type 2 (HSV-2) occurs mostly as a genital infection and may be transmitted to the newborn at the time of birth. HSV-2 is less prevalent than *Herpes simplex* type 1 (HSV-1). HSV-1 is a ubiquitous virus that produces cold sores around the oral cavity. HSV-1 is the more common agent in the production of encephalitis in the child and adult and appears to be a reactivation of a latent infection. Herpes encephalitis may present with a flu-like prodroma and a recurrence of cutaneous herpetic eruption. The neurological manifestations often involve personality and behavior changes as well as other manifestations. Prognosis becomes grave in those patients who progress to coma.

The classic gross pathological changes associated with HSV-1 are those of a hemorrhagic, necrotizing involvement of one or both frontal and/or temporal lobes (24). Computed tomography often shows poorly defined areas of hypodensity in the anterior and medial aspects of the temporal lobe. This low density extends medially into the isle of Reil. Such changes are usually not seen before the fifth day on a CT scan (25,26). Involvement of the opposite frontal and temporal lobes can be seen. Contrast enhancement due to disruption of the BBB occurs but usually not until somewhat after the appearance of low-density zones (27). Thus, contrast enhancement is unusual before the second week. Hemorrhage, a finding often seen microscopically, is not usually seen with CT. CT has been hampered in the diagnosis of the early stages of herpes simplex involvement of the temporal and frontal lobes by partial volume and beam-hardening artifacts.

MRI appears quite sensitive and capable of early detection of the disease by demonstrating high signal abnormalities in the inferior frontal and temporal lobes with T2-weighted images (Fig. 12A). Involvement of the medial temporal lobes with extension into the isle of Reil, but with sparing of the putamen, is well shown both in the axial and coronal planes (Fig. 12B). Our initial experience suggests that MRI has the potential of becoming the diagnostic method of choice in the patient suspected of herpes simplex encephalitis and in whom motion can be controlled. It is possible that the pattern of involvement may contain characteristic if not pathognomonic information.

In passing, it might be useful to point out that herpes Zoster in the distribution of the fifth cranial nerve is

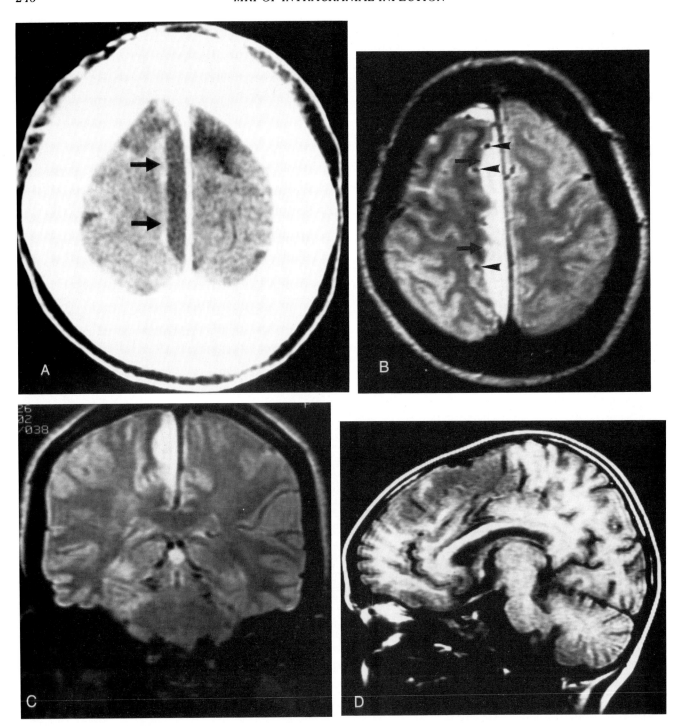

FIG. 10. Subdural empyema. Woman in her late 40s. History of sinusitis, now with obtundation. **A:** Contrast-enhanced CT shows a parafalcine extracerebral collection on the right with a contrast-enhancing membrane (*arrows*). **B:** T2-weighted image (TR = 2,500 msec, TE = 35 msec) shows a hyperintense collection paralleling the right side of the falx (*arrow*), displacing cortical blood vessels (*arrowheads*) laterally along with the cortex. **C:** Coronal T2-weighted image (TR = 2,000 msec, TE = 35 msec) shows the same hyperintense extra-axial collection paralleling the right side of the falx, displacing the hemisphere laterally. **D:** T1-weighted image (TR = 600 msec, TE = 25 msec) shows a hypointense process in the interhemispheric fissure. Although there is some suggestion of mass effect in the form of effacement of gyri, the sagittal T1-weighted image is not satisfactory for outlining the collection or its mass effect.

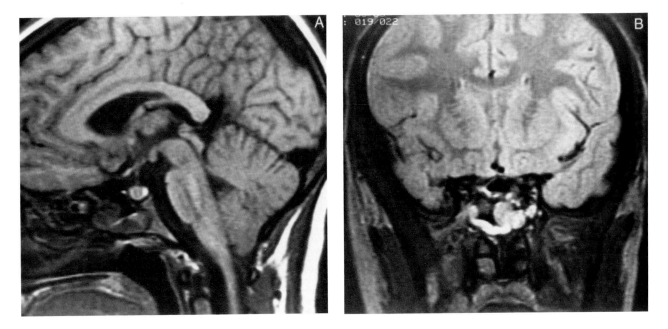

FIG. 11. Sphenoid sinusitis. Teenage girl with upper respiratory infection, fever, and headaches. **A:** Sagittal T1-weighted image (TR = 600 msec, TE = 20 msec) of 5-mm-thick section shows slightly hypointense mucosal thickening within the sphenoid sinus. **B:** Coronal T2-weighted image (TR = 2,500 msec, TE = 35 msec) shows hyperintense mucosal sinus thickening.

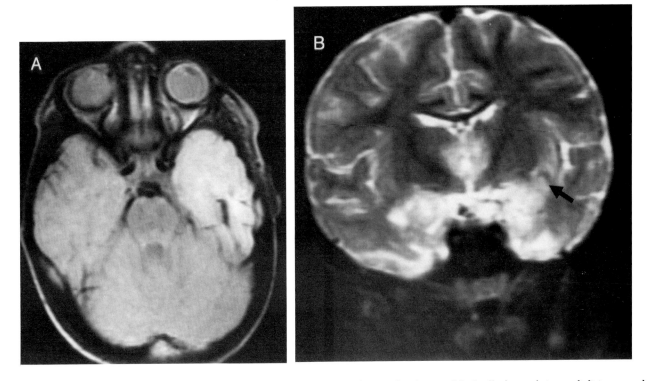

FIG. 12. Herpes Simplex encephalitis. **A:** Young child with obtundation and seizures. Markedly hyperintense left temporal lobe on the T2-weighted image (TR = 2000 msec, TE = 35 msec). **B:** Coronal T2-weighted image (TR = 2,500 msec, TE = 80 msec) of 5-mm-thick section shows involvement of the medial temporal lobes in the region of the unci and hippocampal gyri by abnormal tissue of high signal intensity. Note involvement of the isle of Reil at its base on the left (*arrow*) and involvement of both thalami.

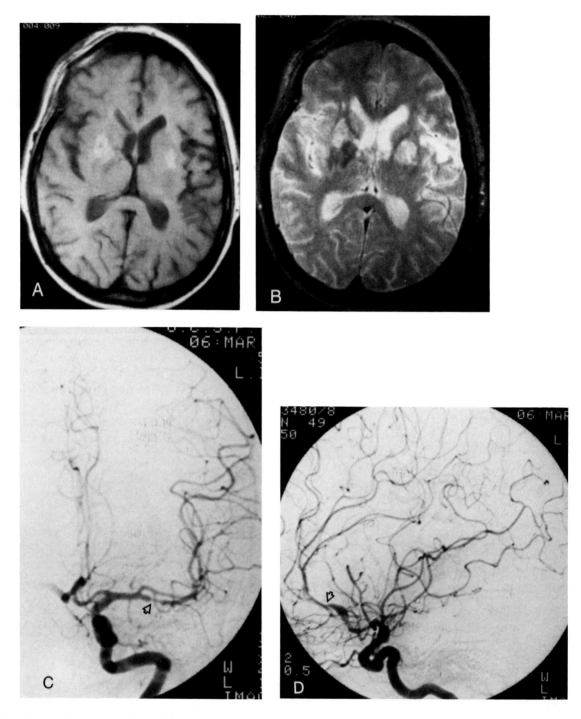

FIG. 13. Herpes Zoster vasculitis. Sixty-two-year-old woman; four-month history of Herpes Zoster ophthalmicus; recent hemiparesis. **A:** Axial T1-weighted image (TR = 600 msec, TE = 24 msec) shows bilateral foci of high signal in the region of the basal ganglia, suggesting hemorrhage. **B:** The T2-weighted image (TR = 2,000 msec, TE = 80 msec) verifies the bilateral hemorrhagic infarcts. **C,D:** Anteroposterior and lateral digital subtraction arteriogram documents the multiple stenoses (*arrowheads*) representing the vasculitic process.

occasionally associated with acute neurological signs. These, however, are the results of an associated vasculitis (presumably immune-mediated) and not a herpes encephalitis (Fig. 13).

PARASITIC DISEASES

Parasitic diseases of the central nervous system are rare in the United States but frequent in less developed nations of the world, especially those in which sanitation is poor and the climate conducive to the propagation of the life cycle of the parasite. In the United States, these diseases are seen in immigrants from countries in which the diseases are endemic and in patients who have been tourists in such countries. Toxoplasmosis, toxocariasis canis, and cysticercosis are only a few of the many parasitic diseases. Of these, the most likely to be encountered in the United States is cysticercosis, endemic in Mexico. Immigrants in the United States of Mexican extraction may have already contracted the disease, whereas tourists traveling on vacation through Mexico are possible victims. In this chapter, cysticercosis and toxocariasis canis are used as examples.

Toxocariasis Canis

The adult worm lives in the intestine of dogs, and its eggs are excreted in the stool (28). The ovum develops into an infective larva, which may be ingested by other dogs. Prenatal transmission to the fetus can occur, producing a congenital infection. Toxocariasis more often infects puppies than adult dogs. The ova excreted by the puppy can contaminate the hand of a child or items that

the child puts into his or her mouth, allowing ingestion of the ova. Larva emerge within the intestine, penetrate the bowel wall, invade the portal vein, and infect the liver and lungs. Larva within human tissue produces granulomas. In addition to the liver and lungs, the eye and the brain can be involved. Brain involvement is rather uncommon, and when it occurs may result in convulsions, lethargy, and signs of meningeal inflammation. In neural tissue, toxocariasis produces granulomas that possess phagocytes, lymphocytes, plasma cells, and reactive astrocytes (29).

Computed tomography shows the granulomas as calcifications surrounded by decreased density in the white matter. Necrotic cavities may occur at sites of involvement. MRI T2-weighted images show high signal intensity of the white matter at sites of inflammatory involvement. The calcifications at the site of granuloma formation are sometimes seen as a focal signal void (Fig. 14). Neither the CT picture nor the MRI picture can be considered to be specific for this disease. Given the environment of a child, the poor sanitation, the presence of a puppy or dog, and the clinical suspicion, the imaging findings are then consistent with the disease process. An intradermal skin test for toxocariasis has been developed, but cross-reactions occur with other metazoans. Liver biopsies have been successful in some cases in demonstrating inflammatory granulomas due to the migration of the parasites.

Cysticercosis

Cysticercosis is caused by the larval form of the pork tapeworm, *Taenia solium.* The definitive host, man

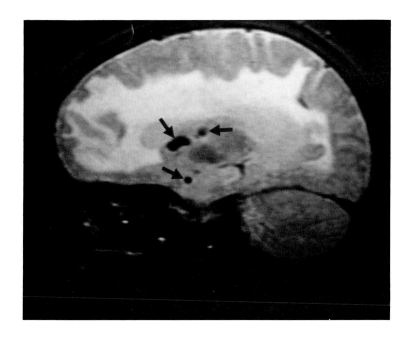

FIG. 14. *Toxocara Cani.* Teenage boy with seizures and retardation. Sagittal T2-weighted image (TR = 2,000 msec, TE = 70 msec) 5-mm-thick section shows marked hyperintense signal change in the white matter surrounding the lateral ventricle, which is of lesser signal intensity, and at least three discrete areas of marked hypointensity (*arrows*) in the basal ganglia due to calcifications.

harbors tapeworm in the intestine. Eggs are eliminated in the feces and are ingested by the intermediate host, the pig. Man becomes infected following the ingestion of pork that has been insufficiently cooked. The consumed organism develops a scolex that attaches to the jejunal mucosa, develops into the adult worm, completing the life cycle. Larvae or oncospheres, reingested by the host through contamination of the fingers or food products, penetrate the intestine and permit invasion of other tis-sues outside the gastrointestinal tract. This produces mature cysticerci, which appear as oval, translucent cysts, containing a single scolex with four suckers. Muscle, brain, eyes, liver, lung, and subcutaneous tissues are the primary sites of involvement (13). Cysticerci in skel-etal muscles may be tender or painful, with the cysts eventually calcifying. Brain is the second most common organ, after the skeletal muscle, to be involved. In gen-eral, the clinical manifestations occur after the parasite

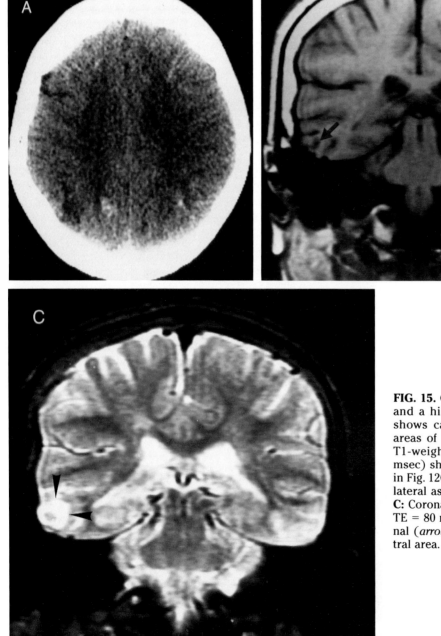

FIG. 15. Cysticercosis. Teenage girl with seizures and a history of travel to Mexico. **A:** Plain CT shows calcification in the cortical–subcortical areas of both cerebral hemispheres. **B:** Coronal T1-weighted image (TR = 600 msec, TE = 20 msec) shows, in retrospect after review of image in Fig. 12C, an area of hypointensity in the inferior lateral aspect of the right temporal lobe (*arrow*). **C:** Coronal T2-weighted image (TR = 2,500 msec, TE = 80 msec) shows a zone of hyperintense sig-nal (*arrowheads*) surrounding a less intense cen-tral area.

dies, and as a result may occur many years after the onset of infection.

Cysticerci are found primarily in the cerebral gray matter, within the subarachnoid space adherent to the meninges, and within the ventricular system. Intraparenchymal cysticerci produce an inflammatory response with fibroconnective tissue, granulation tissue, and chronic inflammatory cells consisting of monocytes, plasma cells, lymphocytes, and eosinophils (13). The cysticercus itself is a bladder larva, from 0.5 to 2 cm in size. The cyst fluid is transparent in live cysts, and jelly-like following the death of the organism. The scolex and its connection, the spiral canal (which contains calcareous corpuscles) form a small mural nodule, several millimeters in size, on one wall of the cyst. Following death of the organism, a more marked inflammatory response occurs, leading to calcification of the organism. These calcifications can be identified radiographically

(30). Many of the apparent intracortical cysticerci actually are located in the depth of the sulcus from which they may burrow into the cortex. In addition to these 1-cm or slightly larger cysts found within the ventricle or subarachnoid space, there are also larger racimose cysts of several centimeters in size found within the subarachnoid space. These lack a viable scolex. As a result of involvement of the CSF spaces, obstructive or communicating hydrocephalus may be produced. Arteritis has also been reported as a result of vascular adventitial involvement by the cysticercus.

At present, the most reliable study for the diagnosis of cysticercosis of the brain is the CT scan. CT shows the acute intraparenchymal phase of cysticercosis as a low-density zone of higher absorption than CSF (31). Following contrast injection, these zones may enhance homogenously or in a ring-like pattern (31). Following death of the organism, a calcified lesion remains (Fig.

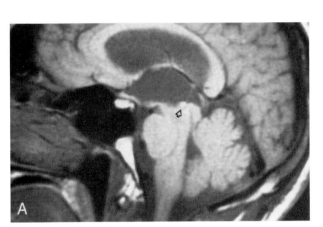

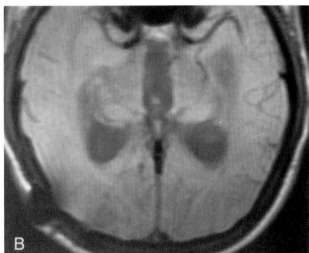

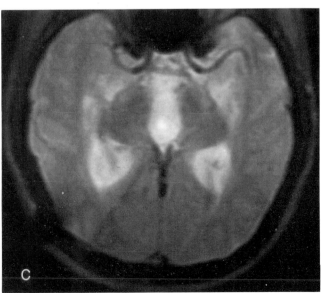

FIG. 16. Intraventricular cysticercosis. Thirty-eight-year-old man with signs of increased intracranial pressure; proven third ventricular cysticercosis. A: Sagittal (TR = 600 msec, TE = 24 msec) image shows a small nodule (arrow) at the entrance to the aqueduct (most likely representing scolex) and a thin strand attached to it superiorly, representing cyst wall. B,C: Axial (TR = 2,000 msec, TE = 40, and 80 msec) images verify hydrocephalus; CSF and cyst fluid are indistinguishable.

15A) (8). The intraventricular and subarachnoid cyst contents are of the same density as CSF. Their membranes are thin, and do not usually show enhancement, although they may. The obstruction that they produce at the foramen of Monro, cerebral aqueduct or outlets of the fourth ventricle, or within the basilar cisterns is usually obvious. The instillation of Metrizamide by ventriculography, or when hydrocephalus is absent by cisternography for the basal cisterns, can outline these cysts. Demonstration of calcifications in the cortical or subcortical regions in the appropriate clinical setting indicates the likelihood of infection. Confirmation can be obtained by immunologic studies on the CSF and serum and by the presence of elevated CSF protein, eosinophilia, and low glucose levels. Radiographs of the extremities for calcified larvae are also useful (32). A new form of chemotherapy, Praziquentel, is currently under investigation (32).

Marvella et al. (3) reported the MRI findings of cysticercosis. Cysts and live cystercerci within the brain have reasonably characteristic configurations on MRI. The picture consists of a low-intensity cystic lesion with signal intensity properties paralleling CSF and within it a much smaller mural high-intensity nodule that represents the scolex. Following death of the organism and its subsequent calcification, CT is superior in demonstrating the calcified focus. MRI may show the calcification as a signal void and may also show reactive changes on T2-weighted images in the surrounding brain as a high signal intensity zone that helps to outline the dead organism (Fig. 15). MRI may be effective in some instances in showing the intraventricular and subarachnoid cysts, more so than CT without Metrizamide (Fig. 16). It can also show evidence of ependymal attachment of the cyst, which makes surgical excision difficult (Fig. 17).

FUNGAL INFECTIONS

Fungal infections of the brain are distributed either geographically or ubiquitously. Aspergillosis, brucellosis, cryptococcosis, and candidiasis are examples of conditions caused by ubiquitous fungi that become manifest in the susceptible patient. Susceptibility accompanies diseases or therapies that suppress the body's immunity. Chemotherapy, steroid therapy, and ac-

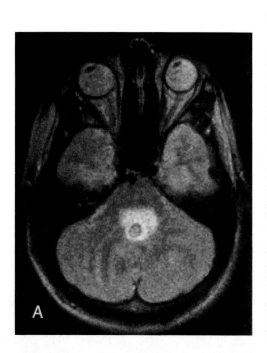 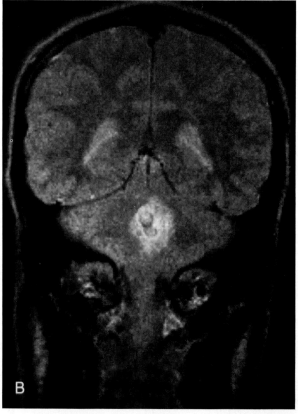

FIG. 17. Intraventricular cysticercosis. Thirty-five-year-old man with headache and papilledema. Axial (**A**) and coronal (**B**) T2-weighted images (TR = 2,000 msec, TE = 80 msec) show a multilocular cyst with a hypointense rim located in the fourth ventricle. High signal intensity around the fourth ventricle suggests ependymitis and edema due to cyst attachment in the wall.

quired immunodeficiency syndrome (AIDS) are among some of the more prevalent situations that allow the ubiquitous mycoses to become manifest. Geographically distributed fungi are represented by coccidioidomycoses and blastomycoses, among others. Coccidioidomycosis is an endemic disease of the southwestern United States, as well as parts of Central and South America. It may be seen in people from the eastern part of the United States or others who have traveled to endemic areas and returned.

The type of pathologic findings resulting from fungal infections depends on the nature of the fungal structure and its mode of introduction into the tissue. It also depends on the susceptibility of the host to respond to the innoculum. Organisms that because of their small size (micra) gain access to the microcirculation penetrate the fine vessels that feed the meninges, leading to acute and chronic leptomeningitis (13). Such responses are seen in cryptococcosis and candidiasis, among others. Organisms that form larger structures, such as hyphal fungi, are capable of obstructing arteries and produce septic infarcts—aspergillosis, for example. Organisms with pseudohyphae, structures that are larger than yeasts and smaller than true hyphae, occlude smaller blood vessels, producing tissue breadown and subsequent microabscess formation. This is seen in a variety of fungal disorders, including cerebral candidiasis.

Aspergillus, an ubiquitous fungus, presents in the patient with normal immunity most often as a cause of sinus mucosal inflammation. In the immunocompromised patient, *Aspergillus* may extend directly through the walls of the paranasal sinuses to involve contiguous structures, such as the cavernous sinus (including the intracavernous internal carotid artery and the cavernous

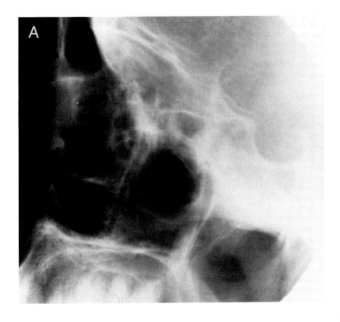

FIG. 18. Aspergillosis of the sphenoid sinus with intracranial extension involving the anterior cerebral arteries with infarction. Middle-aged woman with leukemia, abrupt loss of vision, and obtundation. **A:** Lateral sinus radiograph shows increased density in the region of the sphenoid sinus. **B:** Coronal CT section shows opacification of the right sphenoid sinus and mucosal thickening within the left. Note that there is bony destruction of the floor and roof of the left sphenoid sinus (*arrowheads*). **C:** Sagittal T2-weighted image (TR = 2,000 msec, TE = 80 msec) of 5-mm-thick section shows hyperintense signal changes within the sphenoid sinus and within the contiguous inferior aspect of the frontal lobe. Ethmoid sinuses are also involved.

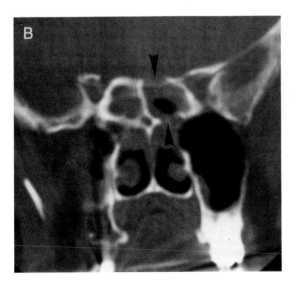

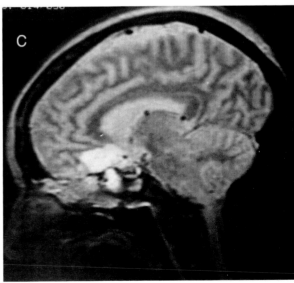

venous plexus) and the subarachnoid space (including CSF-enveloped blood vessels, such as the anterior and middle cerebral arteries and the distal internal carotid artery). With invasion of blood vessels, secondary thrombosis and infarction can occur. Hematogenously disseminated aspergilli can lodge in vessels, produce infarction, and grow through the vessel walls to produce a fungal brain abscess. Extension of the *Aspergillus* to the subarachnoid space produces meningitis and meningoencephalitis. The hematogenously spread *Aspergillus* often produces hemorrhagic infarction owing to its vasculopathic nature.

The immunocompromised patient's inability to respond to the infection permits rapid spread, with CT showing a pattern of involvement that is often very non-specific. The aspergillosis abscess often lacks the ring enhancement seen in abscesses in patients with normal defense mechanisms. MRI shows well both hemorrhagic and nonhemorrhagic infarction. The presence of sinus inflammation, a process well shown by MRI (Figs. 11 and 18) in conjunction with contiguous cerebral involvement (Fig. 18) suggests *Aspergillus* in the appropriate clinical setting. It is important to remember that aspergilli may involve the cerebral tissues by spread from pulmonary foci, in which case cerebral parenchymal involvement may be present without evidence of sinus disease (33,34).

Acquired Immunodeficiency Syndrome

Aquired immunodeficiency syndrome (AIDS) appears to be due to HTLV-III virus, which produces a dysfunction of cell-mediated immune system characterized by inversion of the normal T-helper/T-suppressor cell ratios. Humoral immunity appears to be intact.

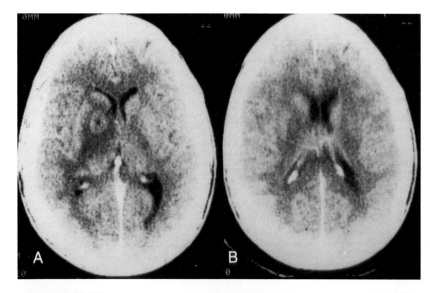

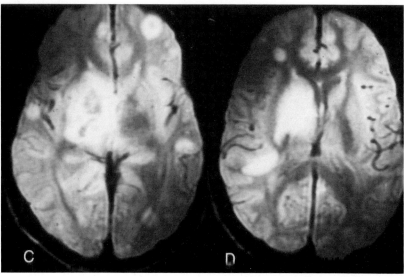

FIG. 19. Acquired Immune Deficiency syndrome; toxoplasmosis. Young adult man with recent onset of confusion and known AIDS. **A,B:** Contrast-enhanced CT at two adjacent levels shows a ring-enhancing lesion in the right basal ganglia. **C,D:** Axial MR (TR = 2,000 msec, TE = 40 msec) images at corresponding levels show much more extensive disease.

Population at risk includes homosexual men; bisexual men; intravenous drug abusers; patients requiring multiple transfusions, such as hemophiliacs and other rare multiple-transfusion patients; and, in the past, Haitians. The most common infectious disease processes are not of the CNS but of other organs (13), such as the lungs, with pneumocystic carinii pneumonia in 55%. Approximately 26% develop Kaposi's sarcoma, and another 15% of patients have other opportunistic infections, including viral or fungal, with many involving the CNS. Depending on the series reported, 10% or more of patients with AIDS have involvement of the CNS (35).

The neurological manifestations of these various infectious agents in the AIDS patient are highly variable. They depend on the location, number, and rate of progression of the disease process. Infectious agents producing multiple parenchymal lesions include *Toxoplasma gondii, Cryptococcus neoformans, Candida albicans,* and cytomegalovirus (CMV) (36,37). The etiology of meningitis–meningoencephalitis is often cryptococcosis.

Toxoplasmosis is an obligate intracellular protozoan that in the immunologically intact patient produces subclinical and benign infections that are self-limited,

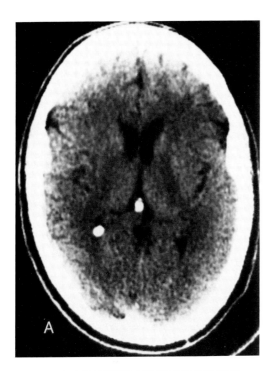

FIG. 20. Acquired Immunodeficiency syndrome with subacute encephalitis. Young adult man with recent onset of dementia. **A:** Axial CT shows minimal prominence to CSF spaces. **B:** Axial T2-weighted image of 7-mm-thick section shows marked hyperintense signal change throughout the white matter in both cerebral hemispheres. **C:** Coronal T2-weighted image of 7-mm-thick section shows both cerebral and cerebellar white-matter hyperintense signal changes.

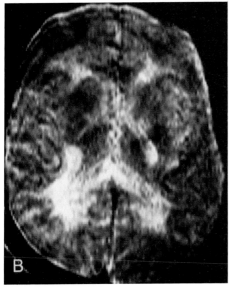

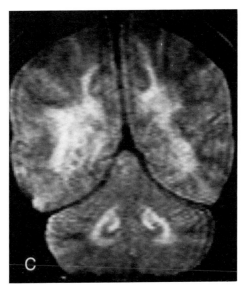

often in the form of adenopathy and fever. In the AIDS patient, *Toxoplasma gondii* tends to produce brain abscesses (37). CMV virus is a member of the herpesvirus family, and is found in a large percentage of adults. With reactivation in the immunologically intact patient, it produces a subclinical, mild infection resembling mononucleosis. In the AIDS patient it produces microabscesses.

Patients with AIDS and suspected neurological disease are currently evaluated with CT. Focal parenchymal brain lesions appear on CT in the form of ring or nodular enhancing lesions (Fig. 19). *Toxoplasma gondii* appears to be the most frequent cause of ring or nodular enhancing lesions at the corticomedullary junctures or within the basal ganglia (37). These are usually associated with mass effect and edema. They frequently have multiple central areas of lucency within an individual lesion, and when the lesions are multiple, they often vary in size (38). Although not specific of infection in an immunosuppressed patient, magnetic resonance is much more sensitive than CT, showing variation in size of the multiple lesions as opposed to the more uniform size and central necrosis seen in metastatic disease.

Cryptococcal meningitis presents most often as ventricular and basilar cisternal enlargement, appearing as either hydrocephalus or atrophy (36). This may be accompanied by periventricular white-matter hypodensity. These patients tend to manifest an encephalopathic picture of dementia, a situation not usually reversible.

Subacute encephalitis is now recognized as an important, distinct form of encephalopathy presenting with dementia in patients with AIDS. The consistent findings within this group are cerebral atrophy of a moderate to marked degree, sparing of cortical gray matter but involving the white matter, basal ganglia, cerebellum, and brainstem. Perivascular and parenchymal collections of macrophages and multinucleated giant cells, diffuse astrocytosis, and perivascular lymphocytic infiltrates are found in the white matter. A proportion of these patients will show CMV inclusions, but recent evidence of finding the nucleic acid of HTLV-III suggests that direct infection of the brain tissue by the AIDS virus may be the etiologic source of subacute encephalitis. Computed tomographic findings are those of enlargement of the CSF spaces and of central white-matter high signal abnormality on T2-weighted image, with some involvement of the deep basal ganglionic and cerebellar tissue (Fig. 20). In the AIDS patient with contrast-enhancing parenchymal lesions, consideration must be given not only to infectious etiologies but to neoplastic ones. There is a relatively high incidence of primary brain lymphoma and of metastatic Kaposi's sarcoma. In our experience, the lesions of lymphoma tend to be a more solid contrast-enhancing mass. It is important to note

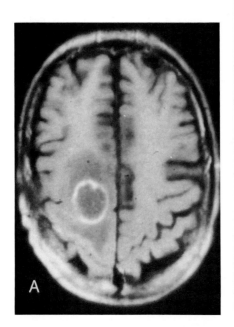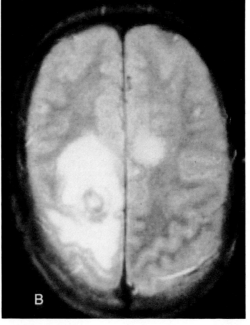

FIG. 21. Acquired Immunodeficiency syndrome: lymphoma and toxoplasmosis. **A:** Enhanced (Gd-DTPA) magnetic resonance T1-weighted image (TR = 500 msec, TE = 30 msec) shows a ring lesion with surrounding low intensity in the right centrum semiovale. **B:** Nonenhanced T2-weighted image (TR = 2,000 msec, TE = 60 msec) shows the lesion, surrounded by edema, and two other abnormal foci contralaterally. Despite the similarity of the enhancing lesion to an abscess, it proved to be lymphoma at biopsy. The left-sided lesion proved to be due to toxoplasmosis. Note the superior sensitivity of the T2-weighted image.

that both neoplastic and infectious lesions may coexist in the same patient and may not be easily differentiated by contrast-enhanced CT or by MRI (Fig. 21). MRI appears to be much more sensitive than CT in the detection of parenchymal brain lesions. T2-weighted images show high signal intensity at the sites of involvement by tumor or infection. Although MRI has been highly successful in identifying involvement of the brain tissue, it has not contributed to specificity.

REFERENCES

1. Zimmerman RA, Patel S, Bilaniuk LT. Demonstration of purulent bacterial intracranial infections by computed tomography. *AJR* 1976;127:155–65.
2. Davidson HD, Steiner RE. Magnetic resonance imaging in infections of the central nervous system. *AJNR* 1985;6:499–504.
3. Suss RA, Maravilla KR, Thompson J. MR imaging of intracranial cysticercosis: comparison with CT and anatomopathologic features. *AJNR* 1986;7:235–42.
4. Zimmerman RA, Bilaniuk LT. Applications of magnetic resonance imaging in diseases of the pediatric central nervous system. *Magnetic Resonance Imaging* 1986;4:11–24.
5. Runge VM, Schoerner W, Niendor HP, et al. Initial clinical evaluation of gadolinium DTPA for contrast-enhanced magnetic resonance imaging. *Magnetic Resonance Imaging* 1985;3:27–35.
6. Holand BA, Kucharczyk W, Brant-Zawadzki M, et al. MR imaging of calcified intracranial lesions. *Radiology* 1985;157:353–6.
7. Zimmerman RA, Bilaniuk LT, Schut L, Packer RJ, Sutton L, Bruce D. Medical imaging of pediatric brain tumors. In: *Proceedings of the symposium on pediatric neuro-oncology, Kobe, Japan (in press).*
8. Byrd SE, Locke GE, Biggers S, Percy AK. The computed tomographic appearance of cerebral cysticercosis in adults and children. *Radiology* 1982;144:819–23.
9. Dolinskas CA, Bilaniuk LT, Zimmerman RA, et al. Computed tomography of intracerebral hematomas: I. transmission CT observations on hematoma resolution. *Radiology* 1977;129:681–8.
10. Gomori JM, Grossman RI, Goldberg HI, Zimmerman RA, Bilaniuk LT. Intracranial hematomas: imaging by high-field MR. *Neuroradiol* 1985;157:87–93.
11. Zimmerman RA, Bilaniuk LT, Shipkin PM, et al. Evolution of cerebral abscess: correlation of clinical features with computed tomography: a case report. *Neurology* 1977;27:14–9.
12. Enzmann DR, Britt RH, Yeager AS. Experimental brain abscess evolution: computed tomographic and neuropathologic correlation. *Radiology* 1979;133:113–22.
13. Parker JC, Dyer ML. Neurologic infections due to bacteria, fungi, and parasites. In: Davis RL, Robertson DM, eds. *Textbook of neuropathology.* Baltimore: Williams & Wilkins, 1985:632–703.
14. Enzmann DR, Britt RH, Placone R. Staging of human brain abscess by computed tomography. *Radiology* 1983;146:703–8.
15. Rosenblum ML, Hoff JT, Norman D, Edwards MS, Berg BO. Nonoperative treatment of brain abscesses in selected high-risk patients. *J Neurosurg* 1980;52:217–25.
16. Whelan MA, Stern J. Intracranial tuberculoma. *Radiology* 1981;138:75–81.
17. Peatfield RC, Shawdon HH. Five cases of intracranial tuberculoma followed by serial computerized tomography. *J Neurol Neurosurg Psychiatry* 1979;42:373–9.
18. Rovira M, Romeno F, Torrent O, et al. Study of tuberculosis meningitis by CT. *Neuroradiol* 1980;19:137–41.
19. Scott Casselman E, Hasso AN, Ashwal S, Schneider S. Computed tomography of tuberculous meningitis in infants and children. *J Comput Assist Tomogr* 1980;4:211–6.
20. Bilaniuk LT, Zimmerman RA, Brown L, Yoo HJ, Goldberg HI. Computed tomography in meningitis. *Neuroradiol* 1978;16:13–4.
21. Smith HP, Hendrick EB. Subdural empyema and epidural abscess in children. *J Neurosurg* 1983;58:392–7.
22. Carter BL, Bankoff MS, Fisk JD. Computed tomographic detection of sinusitis responsible for intracranial & extracranial infections. *Radiology* 1983;147:739–42.
23. Zimmerman RA, Bilaniuk LT. CT of orbital infection and its cerebral complications. *AJR* 1980;134:45–50.
24. Leestmo JE. Viral infections of the nervous system. In: Davis RL, Robertson DM, eds. *Textbook of neuropathology.* Baltimore: Williams & Wilkins, 1985:704–87.
25. Davis JM, Davis KR, Kleinman GM, et al. Computed tomography of Herpes Simplex encephalitis with clinicopathological correlation. *Radiology* 1978;129:419–27.
26. Enzmann DR, Ranson B, Norman D, et al. Computed tomography of *Herpes simplex* encephalitis. *Radiology* 1978;129:419–25.
27. Zimmerman RD, Russel EJ, Leeds NE, Kaufman D. CT in the early diagnosis of Herpes Simplex encephalitis. *AJN* 1980;134:61–6.
28. Sprent JF. Observations on the development of Toxocara Canis (Werner, 1782) in the dog. *Parasitology* 1958;48:184–209.
29. Mikhael NZ, et al. Toxocara Canis infestation with encephalitis. *Can J Neurol Sci* 1974;1:114–20.
30. Bradsford JF. Cysticercus cellulosae—its radiographic detection in the musculature and the central nervous system. *Br J Radiol* 1941;14:79–93.
31. Rodriguez-Carvajal J, Salgado P, Gutierrez-Alvarado R, Escobar-Izquierdo A, Aruffo C, Palacios E. The acute encephalitic phase of neurocysticercosis: computed tomographic manifestations. *AJNR* 1983;4:51–5.
32. Sotelo J, Escobedo F, Rodriguez-Carvajal J, Torres B, Rubio-Donnadieu F. Therapy of parenchymal brain cysticercosis with proziquantel. *N Engl J Med* 1984;310:1001–7.
33. Grossman RI, Davis KR, Taveras JM, Flint Beal M, Phillip O'Carroll C. Computed tomography of intracranial Aspergillosis. *J Comput Assist Tomogr* 1981;5:646–50.
34. Enzmann DR, Brant-Zawadzki M, Britt RH. CT of central nervous system infection in immunocompromised patients. *AJNR* 1980;1:239–43.
35. Jaffe HW, Bregman DJ, Selik RM. Acquired Immune Deficiency Syndrome in the United States; the first 1000 cases. *J Infect Dis* 1983;148:339–45.
36. Post MJD, Hensley GT, Moskowitz LB, Fischl M. Cytomegalic inclusion virus encephalitis in patients with AIDS: CT, clinical and pathologic correlation. *AJNR* 1986;7:275–80.
37. Toxoplasma encephalitis in Haitian adults with Aquired Immuno Deficiency Syndrome: a clinical-pathologic CT correlation. *AJNR* 1983;4:155–62.
38. Kelly WM, Brant-Zawadzki M. Acquired Immuno Deficiency Syndrome: neuroradiologic findings. *Radiology* 1983;149:485–91.

CHAPTER 16

Diseases of White Matter

Betsy A. Holland

The diagnosis of white matter abnormalities was revolutionized by the advent of computed tomography (CT), which provided a noninvasive method of detection and assessment of progression of a variety of white matter processes. However, the inadequacies of CT were recognized early, including its relative insensitivity to small foci of abnormal myelin in the brain when correlated with autopsy findings and its inability to image directly white matter diseases of the spinal cord (1). Magnetic resonance imaging (MRI), on the other hand, sensitive to the slight difference in tissue composition of normal gray and white matter and to subtle increase in water content associated with myelin disorders, is uniquely suited for the examination of white matter pathology. Its clinical applications include the evaluation of the normal process of myelination in childhood and the various white matter diseases, including disorders of demyelination and dysmyelination.

DETERMINANTS OF NORMAL GRAY-WHITE CONTRAST

Radiographic contrast between gray and white matter, whether by CT or MRI, depends on minor differences in their respective chemical composition. Since the protein and electrolyte content of gray and white matter are essentially identical, the major differentiating factors arise from water and lipid content. Gray matter is richer in water; white matter, in lipid (Table 1).

Tissue contrast in CT depends on differences in photoelectric absorption or X-ray attenuation. The X-ray attenuation of a tissue is directly related to the atomic number of its constituents. Simplistically put, lipids are rich in carbon, an element with a relatively low atomic number ($N = 6$). Water is rich in oxygen, an element with an intermediate atomic number ($N = 8$). Consequently, lipids attenuate X-rays less effectively than water. Since white matter is richer in lipids and gray matter, in water, white matter attenuates X-rays less

effectively and has a lower CT density number than gray matter (2).

Tissue contrast in magnetic resonance (MR) depends on differences in mobile hydrogen density. Although lipids are a rich source of hydrogen protons, the hydrogen protons in brain lipid are immobile. In fact, high-resolution spectra obtained from studies of proton spin relaxation and proton density in animals have demonstrated that the hydrogen protons in myelin, tightly bound in fatty acid chains, do not contribute directly to white matter signal or gray-white discrimination (3–5). However, lipid concentration may indirectly affect contrast by changing the relaxation times of adjacent water protons. Conversely, water is rich in mobile hydrogen. In comparison to gray matter, white matter is relatively poor in water (a substance rich in mobile hydrogen protons) and relatively rich in myelin lipids (a substance lacking mobile hydrogen). White matter, therefore, has T1 and T2 relaxation times that are shorter than gray matter.

BRAIN MATURATION

Development of the human brain is incomplete at birth (6,7). Myelination of the central nervous system (CNS) proceeds rapidly in the perinatal period, occurring first in the peripheral nervous system, then the spinal cord, and last in the brain. The brain is not fully myelinated until late in the second decade. The gradual

TABLE 1. *Chemical composition of gray and white matter*

Component	Gray matter (total %)	White matter (total %)	Myelin (total %)
Water	82	72	40
Lipid	6	16	30
Protein	11	11	29
Electrolytes	1	1	1

myelination of the brain results in sequential major changes in its chemical composition, especially during the first year of life. Since myelin is rich in protein (30%) and poor in water (40%) compared with gray and white matter (Table 1), myelination results in a decrease in brain water and an increase in brain protein and lipid content. Water content decreases rapidly initially, from 88% at birth to 82% at 6 months, and then at a much slower rate through age 8 to 10 years (Fig. 1). In the first 6 months of life, cholesterol levels double, with a more gradual steady rise through age 4 to 5 years (6) (Fig. 2).

By CT, the very high water and low protein content of the neonatal white matter results in an accentuation of gray-white differentiation. With advancing age, the gray-white matter density difference decreases due to an increase in white matter attenuation. This change in white matter attenuation is attributable to the gradual decrease in water and increase in protein content associated with myelination (9). Correlative studies performed in the baboon confirm that the increase in white matter attenuation on CT directly parallels the increase in myelin on histologic examination (10).

In the adult, gray-white differentiation on MR stems from the higher water content (higher spin density) of gray matter compared with white. In the absence of myelin, the proton spin density of gray and white matter is relatively equal. Consequently, in the unmyelinated neonate, no gray-white differentiation is seen on T2-weighted spin-echo sequences. Furthermore, the very high water content of the perinatal brain results in a marked prolongation of both T1 and T2 relaxation values, approaching those of cerebrospinal fluid. During the first year of life, a rapid decline in the relaxation times is seen, followed by a more gradual decrease dur-

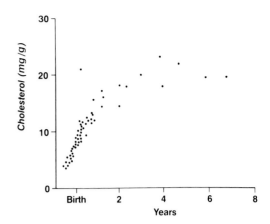

FIG. 2. Concentration of cholesterol per unit weight in whole brain according to age. (Adapted from ref. 8.)

ing the next few years (11) (Fig. 3). This decline in relaxation values parallels the decrease in water content observed in autopsy studies (6) (Fig. 1).

In the unmyelinated neonate, the lack of gray-white differentiation on T2-weighted spin-echo sequences renders the brain almost featureless (Fig. 4A). Subcortical white matter can first be differentiated from gray at 3 to 6 months; then white matter is transiently of higher signal intensity than gray matter on T2-weighted images (Fig. 4B). This is a reversal of the relative signal intensities seen in the adult and reflects the higher water content of the unmyelinated white matter compared with gray in the infant. The internal capsule can first be identified as a low rather than high signal intensity structure at 6 months of age. These changes occur first in the posterior limb and then the anterior limb. The corpus callosum is well defined by 9 months (Fig. 4C). At 9 months to 1 year of age, the periventricular white matter is less intense than gray, but centrally confined (Fig. 4C). During the ensuing years, the myelinated white matter tracts gradually extend more peripherally toward the cortex, with progressively finer branching, and decrease in signal intensity (Fig. 4D and E). Although the brain assumes a fairly adult appearance by 3 years of age, due to minor refinements, full brain maturation is not attained until early adolescence (Fig. 4F). The time course and sequence of changes demonstrated by magnetic resonance are similar to those observed in the pediatric brain at autopsy.

Awareness of the normal age-related appearance of the brain is a prerequisite to the evaluation of children with suspected abnormal or delayed myelination. A significant delay in the age-related degree of myelination may be detected in association with diffuse cerebral insults, such as perinatal asphyxia and infection (12-14). In addition, in a minority of children presenting with idiopathic delayed motor or speech development or

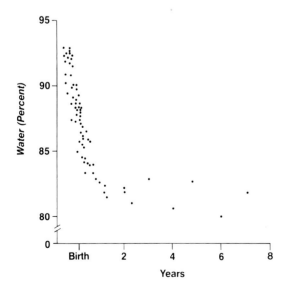

FIG. 1. Percentage of water in whole brain according to age. (Adapted from ref. 8.)

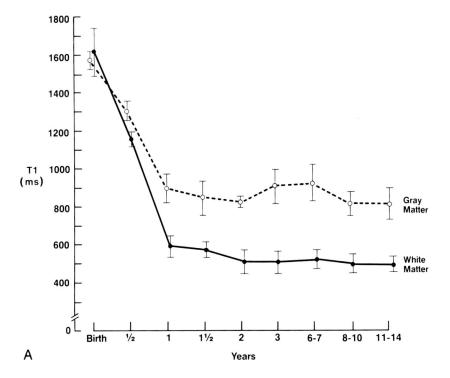

A

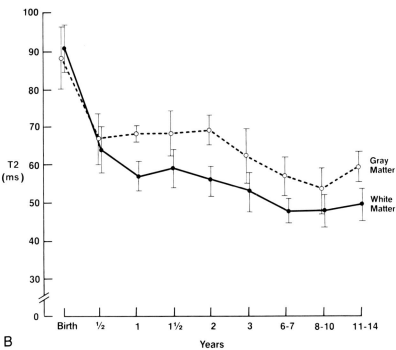

B

FIG. 3. T1 (**A**) and T2 (**B**) relaxation values of gray and white matter by age. (From ref. 11.)

learning disabilities, MR demonstrates significantly delayed myelination for age (15) (Fig. 5). The apparent delay in myelination correlates only roughly with the degree of clinical developmental delay. The prognostic significance of this finding and the ensuing brain maturation in these children remains to be elucidated by longitudinal studies.

MYELINOCLASTIC DISEASES

The myelinoclastic or demyelinating diseases are those in which myelin is formed normally but is later destroyed. Such diseases may be primary, of unknown etiology (such as multiple sclerosis) or secondary, associated with a variety of infectious, toxic, or vascular

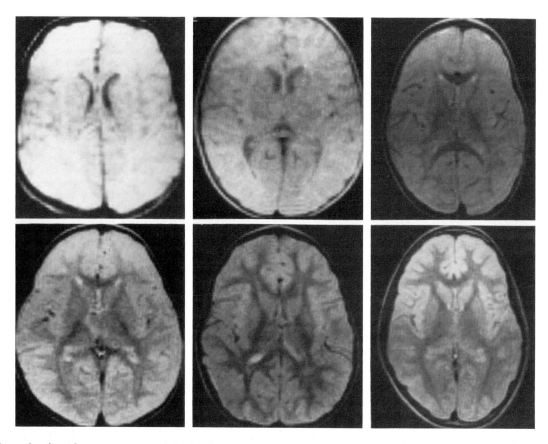

FIG. 4. Normal spin-echo appearance of the brain at the ventricular level with increasing age (TR = 2,000 msec; TE = 56 msec): (**A**) 2 weeks; (**B**) 6 months; (**C**) 1 year; (**D**) 2 years; (**E**) 3 years; and (**F**) 14 years. (From ref. 11.)

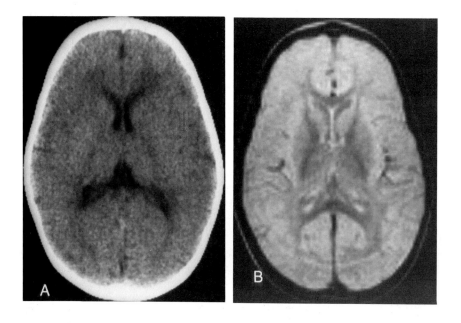

FIG. 5. Three-year-old boy with developmental delay. **A:** CT scan is normal. **B:** MR scan (TR = 2,000 msec) shows myelination of only internal capsule and periventricular white matter. This degree of myelination is similar to that of a 1-year-old (Fig. 4C), rather than a 3-year-old (Fig. 4E).

TABLE 2. *Myelinoclastic diseases*

Primary: multiple sclerosis
Secondary
   Infectious
      Progressive multifocal leukoencephalopathy (PML)
      Subacute sclerosing panencephalitis (SSPE)
      Acute disseminated encephalomelitis (ADE)
   Toxic-Anoxic
      Radiation
      Central pontine myelinolysis (CPM)
      Marchiafava-Bignami
      Subcortical arteriosclerotic encephalopathy (SAE)
      Anoxia

insults (Table 2). Distinctive pathologic features include destruction of the myelin sheaths of nerve fibers, relative sparing of axis cylinders, and perivascular inflammatory infiltration.

Multiple Sclerosis

Multiple sclerosis (MS) is the most common of the demyelinating disorders. Clinical features include acute episodes of focal CNS deficits, remissions of variable extent, and subsequent exacerbations. Paresis, paresthesias, impaired vision, and diplopia are among the classic symptoms. Two-thirds of cases occur in females, with a peak incidence in the third and fourth decades. The prevalence of MS has a geographic distribution, with the highest frequency in northern Europe and the United States, followed by southern Canada and Australia.

Pathologic findings include multiple focal lesions of demyelination, varying in size from 1 mm to several centimeters, predominantly perivenular in location. Acute lesions demonstrate variable degrees of myelin loss, with sparing of axis cylinder, phagocytic microglia, and perivascular infiltration with lymphocytes and mononuclear cells. Chronic lesions are relatively acellular, with fibroglial tissue and rarely persistent white cell infiltration. Three-fourths of MS plaques are in white matter; a minority in cortical and deep gray matter. Although the lesions may be widely distributed, in approximately 50%, the plaques are adjacent to the lateral ventricles, particularly near the angles.

Diagnosis is based on the characteristic clinical presentation, with a chronic relapsing course of symptoms localized to at least two anatomic regions of the CNS (16); however, it is not surprising that diagnosis based on clinical criteria alone is often hampered by an atypical course, particularly in the early stages. Paraclinical tests, such as visual evoked responses and brainstem auditory evoked responses, are moderately sensitive, particularly to lesions of the spinal cord, brainstem, and optic nerves (17). Analysis of cerebrospinal fluid for oligoclonal bands, myelin basic protein, and immunoglobulin G, are of similar diagnostic utility. Computed tomography demonstrates characteristic lesions in up to 25% to 50% of patients with definite and 0% to 20% of patients with probable MS. Double-dose delayed CT scans demonstrate significantly more lesions than a routine contrast-enhanced scan; however, CT is relatively insensitive when directly compared to autopsy findings (1).

Magnetic resonance is widely recognized as the most sensitive method for the diagnosis of MS (18–22), positive in 76% to 100% of patients with definitive MS (18,20,21). In patients with probable MS, however, MR is not significantly more sensitive than CT. In the acute phase, characteristic plaques will be demonstrated in 60% to 93%; in the chronic phase or in remission, in 75% to 82% (18,21). The most important factor in determining MR sensitivity is sequence selection. Of T1- and T2-weighted spin-echo, partial saturation, and inversion recovery sequences, a moderately T2-weighted sequence (TR = 2,000 msec; TE = 70 msec) is most sensitive for demonstrating the full extent and the largest number of lesions. The signal-to-noise ratio and the contrast between normal and abnormal white matter are high. On more heavily T2-weighted sequences, periventricular plaques may be indistinguishable from the high signal intensity of adjacent cerebrospinal fluid. On T1-weighted spin-echo sequences (TR = 500 msec; TE = 30 msec) or partial saturation sequences, contrast between normal and abnormal white matter is reduced or lost (Fig. 6). Inversion recovery sequences are difficult to interpret, particularly in the supraventricular region, and at the gray-white junction, where lesions are sometimes indistinguishable from partial volume averaging of cortical sulci (20,23). However, such sequences may be more sensitive for the detection of lesions in the internal capsule and brainstem. In fact, no one imaging sequence is consistently superior, presumably due to variability in the relaxation times of MS plaques. T1 and T2 values probably depend on the degree of demyelination, gliosis, and edema.

The characteristic MR findings on spin-echo sequences are high signal intensity foci, a few millimeters to a few centimeters in diameter. In the vast majority, at least two lesions can be identified, not uncommonly with a unilateral predominance (Fig. 6). The lesions are most commonly located in the cerebral hemispheres, usually contiguous with the lateral ventricles (Fig. 7). Additionally, plaques may be identified in the subcortical white matter, the internal capsule, and the white matter of the temporal lobes (Fig. 8). In slightly less than half of patients, concomitant lesions will be demonstrated in the posterior fossa, usually in the pons or cerebellar white matter (Fig. 8). Occasionally, a single lesion in an atypical location may be the only abnormality, rendering a specific diagnosis by MR impossible

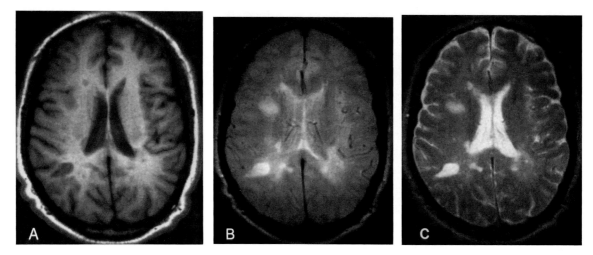

FIG. 6. Multiple sclerosis in a 46-year-old woman. **A:** On a T1-weighted sequence, the periventricular plaques of demyelination appear as foci of variably diminished signal intensity compared with normal white matter (TR = 600 msec; TE = 20 msec). **B:** On a mildly T2-weighted sequence, the plaques appear as foci of increased signal intensity (TR = 2,000 msec; TE = 40 msec). **C:** On a moderately T2-weighted sequence, the plaques are more discrete and of even greater signal intensity compared with adjacent normal white matter (TR = 2,000 msec; TE = 80 msec). Therefore, even punctate lesions are easily identifiable. Note that as is typical for MS, involvement is bilateral but asymmetric, with, in this case, a predominance of lesions on the right.

(Fig. 9). In advanced disease, MR may show diffuse cerebral atrophy in addition to focal white matter abnormalities (Fig. 10).

The MR findings in MS correlate only roughly with clinical disease, with respect to both lesion localization and disease activity. In the supratentorial compartment, the majority of patients with clinical symptoms localized to the cerebral hemispheres will have a corresponding lesion on MR scans; however, almost half of patients with periventricular abnormalities on MR will have no correlative symptoms. In the posterior fossa, fewer than half the patients with clinical symptoms localized to the brainstem or cerebellum will have a corresponding lesion on MR; however, most patients with posterior fossa MR findings will suffer corresponding symptoms (18,21).

It does not appear that acute and chronic MS plaques can be distinguished by MR without the benefit of para-

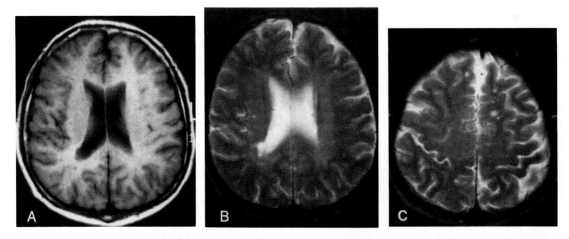

FIG. 7. Multiple sclerosis in a 39-year-old man with acute neurologic symptoms. **A:** The focus of demyelination adjacent to the occipital horn of the right lateral ventricle is difficult to distinguish from the ventricle, since on a T1-weighted sequence (TR = 400 msec; TE = 20 msec), both have prolonged relaxation times. **B:** On a moderately T2-weighted sequence (TR = 2,000 msec; TE = 80 msec), the plaque adjacent to the right lateral ventricle is demonstrated as a discrete lesion. **C:** Typical punctate lesions of demyelination are shown in the centrum semiovale bilaterally.

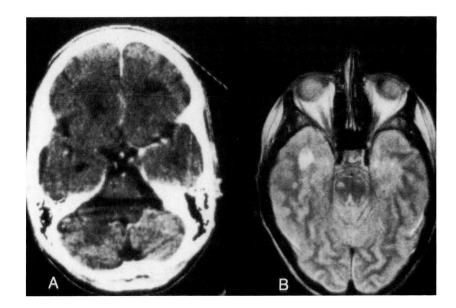

FIG. 8. Multiple sclerosis in a 35-year-old woman. **A:** Contrast-enhanced CT demonstrates no abnormalities in the posterior fossa or white matter of the temporal lobe. **B:** Discrete lesions of abnormal signal intensity are shown in the pons and the right temporal tip white matter, presumably corresponding to areas of demyelination (TR = 2,000 msec, TE = 28 msec).

magnetic contrast agents. The appearance and relaxation values are similar in all stages of the disease (Figs. 7, 9, and 11). Rarely, the appearance of a chronic MS plaque will have a distinctive central low signal intensity, perhaps secondary to fibroglial changes (Fig. 12). Anecdotal data indicate that intravenous gadolinium

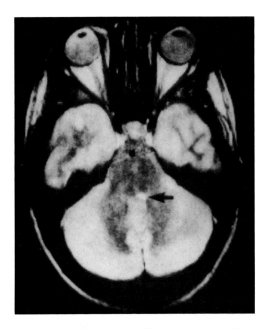

FIG. 9. Multiple sclerosis in a 26-year-old female medical student, presenting with acute dysconjugate gaze. A small focus of increased signal intensity in the posterior pons (*arrow*) is the only abnormality demonstrated. The site of the lesion, in the medial longitudinal fasciculus, a relay pathway between the extraocular muscles and the vestibular nuclei, accounts for her symptoms.

DTPA results in enhancement of acute but not chronic plaques. The mechanism of the enhancement is a blood-brain barrier permeability similar to that seen with iodinated contrast on CT. If patients are followed with successive MR scans, both apparent progression and regression of disease may be demonstrated (24).

The spinal cord is a common site for MS plaques at autopsy. Characterized pathologically by an elongated configuration, such lesions usually occur in the dorsal and lateral segments, without respect for gray-white matter boundaries. Using T2-weighted sequences, such plaques may be detected in 18% to 50% of MS patients (17,20,25). In slightly less than half of patients, two or three separate lesions may be detected. Their signal intensity characteristics are similar to cerebral plaques (Fig. 13). Cord atrophy has also been described. Only rarely are the findings confined to the spinal cord without brain involvement. No reliable correlation has been demonstrated between MR and clinical findings in cord disease.

INFECTIOUS DEMYELINATION

A variety of viral infections result in extensive white matter demyelination due to the effects of the virus itself and viral-induced immune complexes. The former group is typified by progressive multifocal leukoencephalopathy (PML) and subacute sclerosing panencephalitis (SSPE), the latter by acute disseminated encephalomyelitis (ADE). The latency is variable. ADE may present 1 week after exposure to varicella or influenza. SSPE may present clinically as much as 6 years after exposure to the measles virus. The clinical course in most of these diseases typically progresses to coma

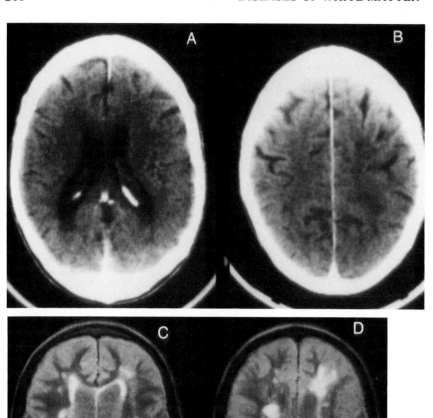

FIG. 10. Chronic changes of MS in a 41-year-old woman. **A:** Cerebral atrophy with enlargement of cortical sulci and lateral ventricles is shown by contrast-enhanced CT. No discrete white matter abnormalities are seen. **B:** At the level of the centrum semiovale, a single low-density lesion is shown on the left posteriorly. **C,D:** MR scans (TR = 2,000 msec; TE = 28 msec) demonstrate multiple foci of abnormal signal intensity throughout the periventricular and subcortical white matter, in addition to the atrophy shown by CT.

and, often, death. The pathologic findings are usually characterized by perivascular white cell infiltration and confluent perivenous areas of demyelination involving both gray and white matter. The corresponding CT and MR findings are nonspecific, including focal abnormalities in subcortical white matter and cortical and deep gray matter (26–28).

Progressive multifocal leukoencephalopathy is, of late, one of the more commonly occurring infectious demyelinating disorders. PML strikes the immunocompromised host, afflicting patients receiving immunosuppressive therapy, as well as patients with lymphoma, leukemia, and, recently, acquired immunodeficiency syndrome (AIDS). PML is caused by infection with the DNA papovavirus. Pathologic changes include focal areas of demyelination, with enlarged distorted oligodendroglia, the cells responsible for the formation of the myelin sheath (29). Minimal inflammatory changes

occur. The areas of demyelination vary from microscopic to massive. They tend to begin in the subcortical white matter. CT scans in PML demonstrate subcortical white matter lucency, often scalloped peripherally. The lesions are often asymmetric and in a parieto-occipital distribution. The MR findings are confluent areas of abnormal signal intensity affecting subcortical white matter in a similar distribution to that shown by CT (Fig. 14). In patients with AIDS, similar or more diffuse white matter changes may occur because of infection with cytomegalovirus, the AIDS virus, HTLV-III, or the papovavirus of PML (Fig. 15).

TOXIC-ANOXIC DEMYELINATION

Focal or widespread demyelination may occur secondary to a host of exogenous insults. Radiation, even

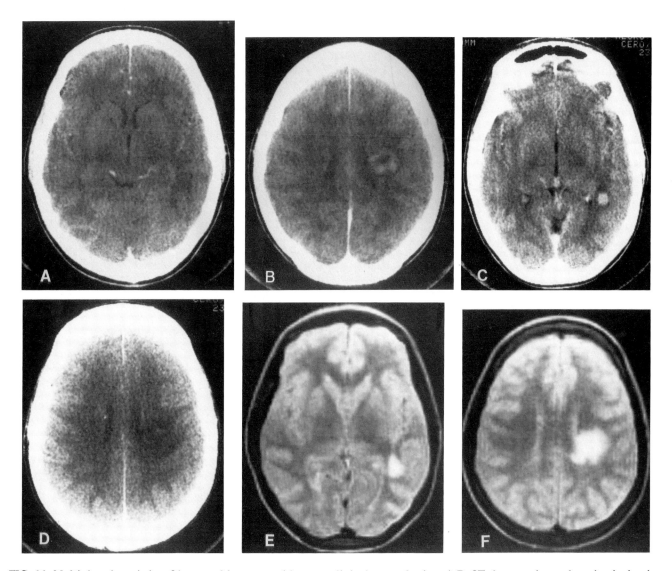

FIG. 11. Multiple sclerosis in a 31-year-old woman with acute clinical exacerbation. **A,B:** CT shows a ring-enhancing lesion in the left centrum semiovale. Such enhancement indicates an active focus of demyelination with blood-brain barrier breakdown. No other abnormalities are seen. **C,D:** Three months later, the lesion in the centrum semiovale is predominantly low in density with only minimal enhancement, implying almost complete restoration of the blood-brain barrier. However, interval development of an enhancing lesion in the deep white matter of the left temporal lobe is shown, a new area of active demyelination. **E,F:** By MR, performed at the same time as the second CT, both lesions are similar in appearance and signal intensity. The acute lesion cannot be distinguished from the more chronic plaque.

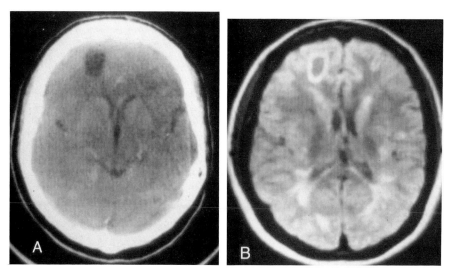

FIG. 12. Multiple sclerosis in a 27-year-old woman, transiently asymptomatic. **A:** A well-defined, low-density frontal lobe white matter lesion is shown by CT. Its low density and lack of enhancement are consistent with a chronic plaque. **B:** On a T2-weighted MR scan (TR = 2,000 msec; TE = 28 msec), the lesion is atypical, low in signal intensity centrally, with a rim of high signal intensity peripherally. This appearance, presumably due to fibroglial changes in a long-standing lesion, is not specific and may also be seen in areas of remote infarction.

FIG. 13. Multiple sclerosis of the spinal cord in a 56-year-old man with a 20-year history of intermittent lower extremity paresthesias and paresis. **A:** On a mildly T2-weighted sequence (TR = 2,000 msec; TE = 20 msec), focal cord atrophy is seen at the C2 and C7 levels. **B:** On a more heavily T2-weighted sequence (TR = 2,000 msec; TE = 70 msec), a corresponding focus of increased signal intensity is shown in the dorsal cord.

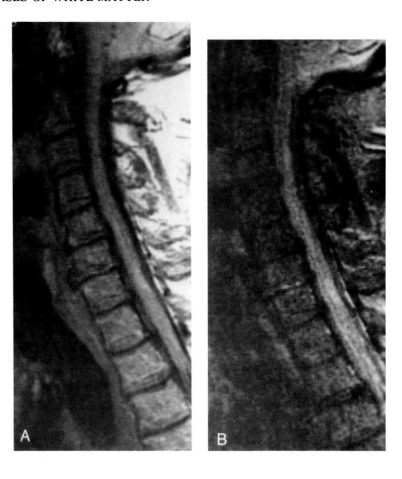

in the therapeutic range, may result in irreversible myelin destruction. Nutritional factors, electrolyte abnormalities, and alcohol may play a role in the development of central pontine myelinolysis (CPM) and Marchiafava-Bignami disease. Anoxia, whether global or focal, may result in severe myelin damage.

Therapeutic irradiation for brain tumors and skull lesions results in both transient and permanent CNS changes. The transient complications are of limited consequence. The delayed effects include not only focal radionecrosis, but also diffuse white matter abnormalities. Factors affecting the development of radiation injury are the total dose received, the time course of administration, and the number and size of the fractions of irradiation (30,31). In widespread white matter injury, the histologic changes are nonspecific. White matter demyelination and vacuolation, interstitial edema, and fibrillary gliosis have been described. The underlying

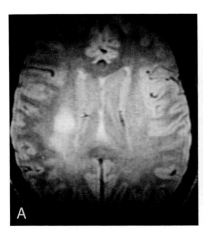
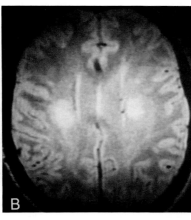

FIG. 14. Progressive multifocal leukoencephalopathy in a 38-year-old man with AIDS. **A,B:** MR shows bilateral lesions of increased signal intensity in the periventricular parietal white matter bilaterally, the classic but not invariable, distribution for PML.

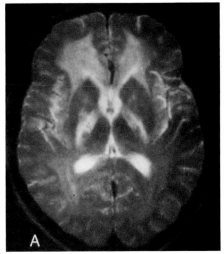 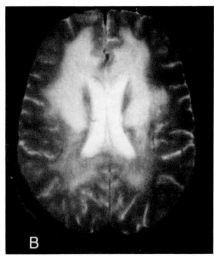

FIG. 15. Thirty-one-year-old man with AIDS. **A,B:** MR scans show a diffuse increase in signal intensity in the frontal and parietal white matter, as well as in the posterior limb of the internal capsule. The etiology of these changes was unclear and presumed to be secondary to either cytomegalovirus or the HTLV-III AIDS virus.

pathogenesis is assumed to be vascular, secondary to arteriolar hyalinization and wall thickening. Consequently, the most severe changes occur in the deep, poorly vascularized periventricular white matter (32).

In the presence of widespread radiation-induced white matter injury, CT scans may demonstrate decreased attenuation, either diffuse or focal. More commonly, cortical atrophy is seen, with dilatation of ventricular and subarachnoid spaces and no definite white matter abnormality (24,33,34). Three MRI patterns of white matter change have been described: (a) focal, corresponding to the radiation port (Fig. 16); (b) focal, adjacent to the lateral ventricles (Fig. 17A and B); and (c) diffuse (Fig. 17C and D) (35,36). In the diffuse pattern, high signal intensity on T2-weighted sequences has a scalloped margin laterally, abutting the cortical gray matter, due to arcuate or U-fiber damage. In all three patterns, the corpus callosum is usually spared. In the

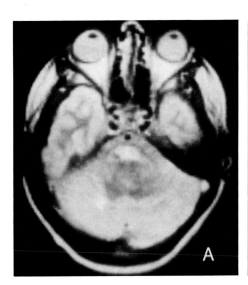 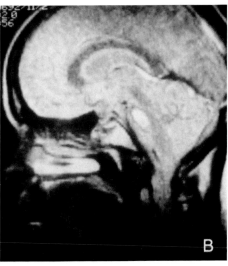

FIG. 16. Focal pontine radiation lesion in a 24-year-old man, 18 months after receiving a full course of radiotherapy for a craniopharyngioma. Axial (**A**) and sagittal (**B**) scans (TR = 2,000 msec; TE = 56 msec) show a single focus of increased signal intensity in the central pons.

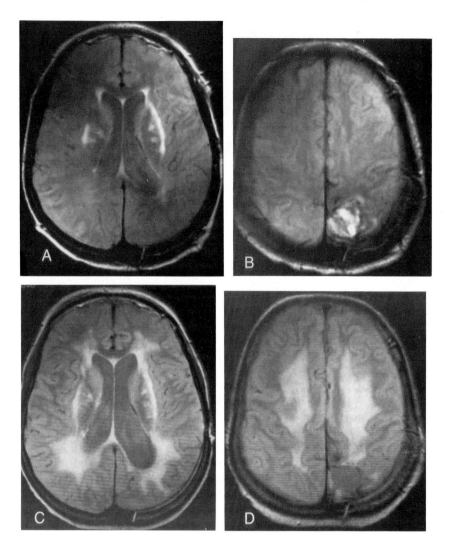

FIG. 17. Diffuse radiation change in a 63-year-old after resection of a left parietal astrocytoma. **A,B:** Initial MR scan (TR = 2,000 msec; TE = 40 msec) shortly after surgery and the beginning of radiotherapy demonstrates high signal intensity in the periventricular white matter and the external capsules. The increased signal intensity in the tumor bed is due to post-surgical changes. **C,D:** Fifteen months later, after a full course of radiotherapy, the interval development of diffuse white matter abnormalities extending along U fibers almost to the cortex is shown. Note that the parietal lesion is now of similar signal intensity characteristics as cerebrospinal fluid compatible with encephalomalacia without evidence of residual tumor.

FIG. 18. Subependymal tumor spread obscured by diffuse radiation lesions in a 32-year-old, 2 years after surgery and radiation therapy for a frontal anaplastic astrocytoma. **A:** CT scan shows a focus of contrast enhancement along the wall of the occipital horn of the right lateral ventricle due to subependymal tumor recurrence. Also seen is a frontal region of low density due to encephalomalacia in the tumor bed and low density throughout the periventricular white matter secondary to radiation damage. **B:** MR (TR = 2,000 msec; TE = 28 msec) shows only the frontal low-signal-intensity area of encephalomalacia and the widespread white matter abnormalities; however, the high signal intensity of the periventricular white matter obscures the underlying focus of subependymal tumor spread.

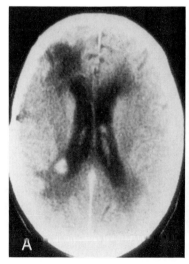
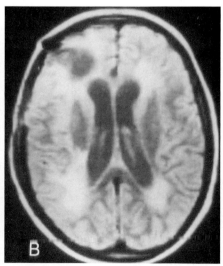

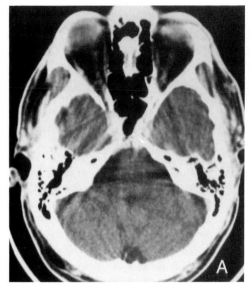
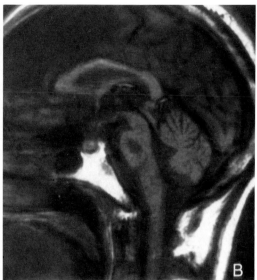
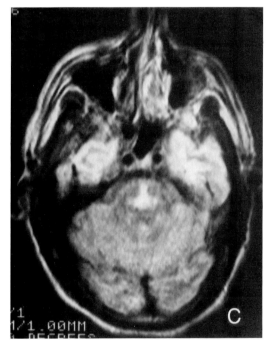

FIG. 19. Central pontine myelinolysis. **A:** The CT scan is normal. Examination of the pons is degraded by interpetrous artifacts. **B:** T1-weighted (TR = 600 msec; TE = 20 msec) sagittal MR scan demonstrates a discrete area of diminished signal intensity in the central pons. **C:** T2-weighted axial scan (TR = 2,000 msec; TE = 56 msec) demonstrates a large pontine lesion of increased signal intensity. Note that the pons is normal in size, and no associated hydrocephalus is seen, distinguishing this lesion from a brainstem neoplasm.

few patients studied with radiation-induced atrophy, underlying focal or diffuse white matter demyelination was demonstrated by MR, although not seen by CT (35). The prolonged T1 and T2 relaxation parameters of radiation lesions are no different from the white matter lesions of MS, infarcts, or periventricular edema (36). In fact, the high sensitivity and low specificity of MR in the detection of radiation effects is a potential shortcoming, since clinically important abnormalities, such as tumor recurrence or subependymal spread of tumor, may be masked by the widespread high signal intensity radiation effect (Fig. 18).

Central pontine myelinolysis is characterized by a focus of demyelination in the pons. The lesion, variable in extent, ranges from a few millimeters to 1 cm in diameter (37). Microscopically, the myelin sheaths of the central pontine nerve fibers are destroyed in a single symmetrical focus (38). Clinical manifestations may be profound. Mental status is depressed and is followed by the rapid onset of pseudobulbar palsy and flaccid quadriplegia, usually progressing to death within 1 month. More commonly, patients demonstrate no brainstem symptoms because of either the small size of the pontine lesion or coma related to metabolic abnormalities (38). CT demonstrates a focal area of pontine low density with variable enhancement and without brainstem en-

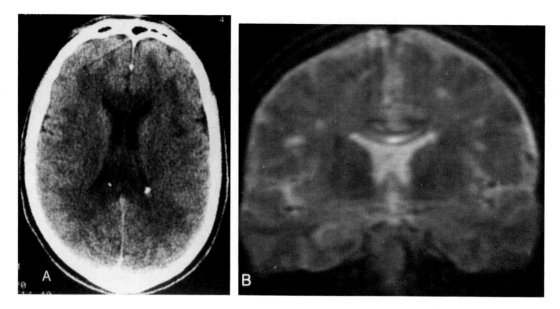

FIG. 20. Marchiafava-Bignami in a 42-year-old alcoholic. **A:** Contrast-enhanced CT shows slightly diminished density in the corpus callosum and periventricular white matter. **B:** Coronal MR scan (TR = 2,000 msec; TE = 80 msec) demonstrates a linear focus of increased signal intensity extending through the middle lamina of the corpus callosum, as well as small lesions in the subcortical white matter peripherally.

largement. In patients who survive, resolution of the pontine abnormality may be demonstrated over the course of weeks or years (39,40). MR shows a variable-size region of prolonged T1 and T2 in the central pons

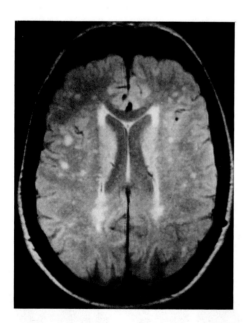

FIG. 21. Age-related white matter changes in a 78-year-old with no cognitive dysfunction. A few punctate lesions of increased signal intensity are seen, the largest in the right anterior limb of the internal capsule and the left occipital periventricular white matter (TR = 2,200 msec, TE = 55 msec). The findings are mild in degree for age.

(Fig. 19). Differential diagnosis includes brainstem infarction, MS, glioma, and encephalitis.

Marchiafava-Bignami disease is characterized by a single midline focus of demyelination in the corpus callosum. Microscopically, demyelination of the middle lamina of the corpus callosum occurs with relative sparing of the axis cylinders. Other lesions may occur in the white matter of the cerebral hemispheres as well as the cerebellar peduncles. Clinical features are variable, including seizures, progressive dementia, hemiparesis, and coma. Spontaneous remission is not unusual (41). In the acute phase, CT demonstrates decreased density throughout the corpus callosum (Fig. 20A). In the chronic phase, cortical and corpus callosum atrophy develop (42). Spin–echo MR scans show a linear focus of increased signal intensity on T2-weighted sequences through the middle layer of the corpus callosum (Fig. 20B). Other small foci of demyelination may be detected in the subcortical and periventricular white matter.

The effects of anoxia are usually more striking in gray than white matter because of its higher metabolic requirements; however, in 20% to 50% of elderly patients, focal areas of brain softening are demonstrated in the periventricular and subcortical white matter, as well as in the basal ganglia at autopsy (43,44). This white matter gliosis is attributed to atherosclerotic changes in deep perforating arteries, with intimal fibrosis, medial hypertrophy, and extensive hyalinization. The clinical sequelae of these lesions is unclear; however, these lesions tend to be more extensive in patients with dementia and subcortical arteriosclerotic encephalopathy (SAE) (45).

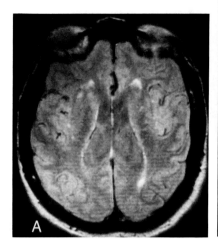
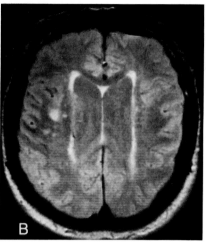

FIG. 22. Age-related white matter changes in a 67-year-old man. Multiple white matter lesions of increased signal intensity compared with normal brain are shown in the periventricular and subcortical white matter (TR = 2,200 msec; TE = 35 msec). Note the predominance of lesions along the optic radiations centrally and at the gray-white junction peripherally, as opposed to the more strictly periventricular location of the plaques of MS.

Although periventricular lucency has been described with CT in the elderly (46), MR is far more sensitive to the detection of the white matter changes of aging. In fact, central white matter foci of increased signal intensity on T2-weighted spin–echo sequences are seen in 20% to 30% of people over age 65 years (Fig. 21) (8). The deep white matter of the centrum semiovale and the optic radiations are the most commonly affected (Fig. 22) (47,48). Concomitant basal ganglia involvement is not unusual (Fig. 23). These white matter lesions of aging may be similar in appearance and distribution to those of MS. The differentiating features rest on clinical grounds, including the age at presentation and clinical course. The lesions associated with aging are less likely than those of MS to abut directly the ventricular wall and are more commonly peripheral in location, near the gray-white junction (Fig. 22). Preliminary results suggest an association among the severity of these white matter lesions, cerebrovascular risk factors, and cognitive loss (47).

THE DYSMYELINATING DISEASES

The dysmyelinating diseases are those in which normal myelin is not formed or, once formed, is not maintained, often due to a specific enzyme deficiency. The dysmyelinating disorders can further be subdivided into those affecting solely white matter, the leukodystrophies, and those affecting gray matter additionally or primarily (49). The peripheral nervous system is spared, with the exception of metachromatic leukodystrophy and Krabbe's disease (50).

The dysmyelinating diseases are a mixed group, sharing several features. Most are due to a single enzymatic defect, resulting in abnormal myelin catabolism and lipid storage. In metachromatic leukodystrophy, the most common of these rare diseases, aryl-sulfatase A deficiency, results in the accumulation of sulfatides. Krabbe's disease is caused by a lack of galactocerebroside β-galactosidase and is characterized by the accumulation of galactocerebroside breakdown products in

FIG. 23. Elderly man with profound dementia. **A,B:** MR scans (TR = 2,200 msec; TE = 80 msec) show many lesions of variable size in the corona radiata and subcortical white matter. Although some are confluent with the walls of the lateral ventricles, similar in distribution to the plaques of MS, the basal ganglia involvement is characteristic of small-vessel disease.

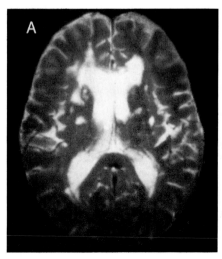
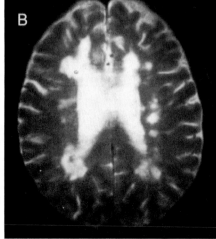

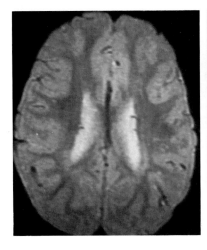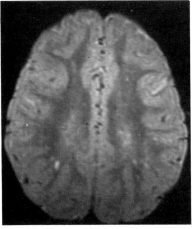

FIG. 24. Adrenoleukodystrophy (type I) in a 6-year-old boy. Axial MR scans (TR = 2,000 msec; TE = 35 msec) show abnormally increased signal intensity in the parieto-occipital white matter bilaterally.

macrophages. In adrenoleukodystrophy, the enzymatic abnormality is incompletely identified but appears to rest in an abnormality of long-chain fatty acid metabolism. Canavan's disease and the hyperammonemias, including maple syrup urine disease, are caused by an abnormality of amino acid metabolism, including deficiency of various urea cycle enzymes as well as errors of branch-chain amino acid catabolism. The most common are inherited as an autosomal recessive, including metachromatic leukodystrophy, Krabbe's disease, Canavan's disease, and Leigh's disease. Adrenoleukodystrophy is unique in that it is inherited as a sex-linked recessive.

Symptoms are usually nonfocal and ultimately devastating. Patients usually progress from weakness and intellectual decline to frank dementia, spasticity, and unresponsiveness. In most of the dysmyelinating syndromes, the clinical presentation is within the first 2 years of life; however, several of these disorders may present later in the first decade, including metachromatic leukodystrophy, adrenoleukodystrophy, and Leigh's disease. The pathologic findings may be nonspecific. In the leukodystrophies, extensive demyelination is demonstrated, particularly in the centrum semiovale, with severe loss of oligodendroglia. In those with predominant gray matter involvement, gliosis and necrosis may be identified in the basal ganglia, cortical gray matter, and brainstem. Several of these diseases can be distinguished by the presence of distinctive cell types: the globoid cell (macrophages containing myelin breakdown products) in Krabbe's disease; spongy degeneration (lipid-filled glial cells) in Canavan's disease and the hyperammonemias; lipid-filled PAS-staining inclusions in macrophages in adrenoleukodystrophy; and Rosenthal bodies (eosinophilic hyaline bodies in astrocytes) in Alexander's disease.

The CT findings are usually nonspecific, particularly in the later stages, demonstrating diffuse cerebral atro-

FIG. 25. Leigh's disease in an 11-year-old boy. MR scan (TR = 2,000 msec; TE = 56 msec) demonstrates multiple foci of increased signal intensity involving both gray and white matter. In addition to the lentiform nuclei abnormalities frequently documented by CT, lesions are shown in the brainstem and cortical gray matter.

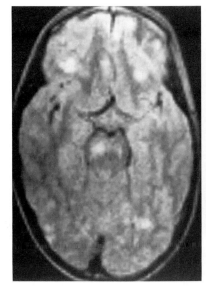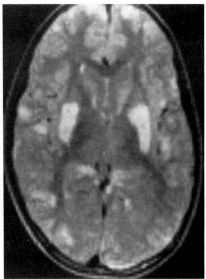

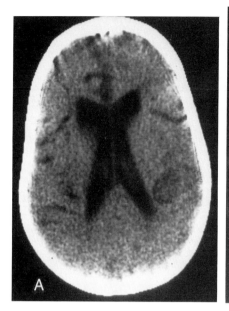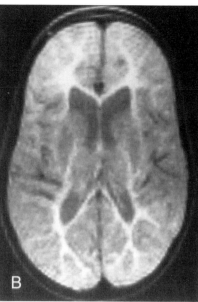

FIG. 26. Pelizaeus-Merzbacher in a 7-year-old boy. **A:** CT scan shows diffuse atrophy with enlarged lateral ventricles. **B:** The MR scan (TR = 2,000 msec; TE = 56 msec) demonstrates a diffuse increase in white matter signal intensity.

phy and widespread diminished white matter attenuation. In the early stages, however, distinguishing features may be identified in some cases. In Krabbe's disease, intrinsically increased density may be demonstrated in the thalami, caudate, and corona radiata. In adrenoleukodystrophy type I, decreased white matter attenuation occurs predominantly in a parieto-occipital distribution, with gradual caudorostral progression and contrast enhancement along its anterior margin. In type II adrenoleukodystrophy, marked contrast enhancement of various white matter tracts, such as the internal capsule, forceps major, and centrum semiovale, may be seen. In Alexander's disease, the white matter changes are often most severe in the centrum of the frontal and temporal lobes. In Leigh's disease, lesions of decreased density are seen in the lentiform nuclei and occasionally in the head of the caudate.

The MR findings in the dysmyelinating disorders have been described only anecdotally; however, in the early stages, the distribution of abnormalities is similar to that described in the autopsy and CT literature (Figs. 24 and 25). In the late stages, the most common MR findings are cortical atrophy and widespread white matter changes, with an increase in signal intensity on T2-weighted spin–echo sequences (Fig. 26). It is unlikely that MR will prove more specific than CT in the evaluation of the leukodystrophies, but its increased sensitivity should permit earlier diagnosis (23,51–53).

A PRACTICAL APPROACH TO WHITE MATTER DISEASE

Schemes 1 and 2 represent an approach (perhaps simplistic) to white matter diseases.

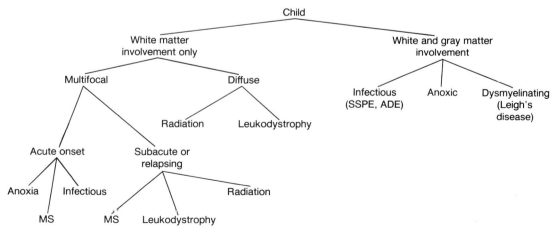

SCHEME 1

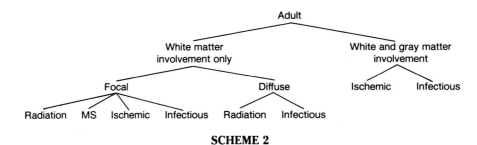

SCHEME 2

REFERENCES

1. Haughton WM, Ho KC, Williams AL, et al. CT detection of demyelinated plaques in multiple sclerosis. *AJR* 1979;132:213–15.
2. Brooks RA, DiChiro G, Keller MR. Explanation of cerebral white-gray contrast in computed tomography. *J Comput Assist Tomogr* 1980;4:489–91.
3. Bottomley PA, Hart HR Jr, Edelstein WA, et al. Anatomy and metabolism of the normal human brain studied by magnetic resonance at 1.5 tesla. *Radiology* 1984;150:441–6.
4. Kamman RL, Go KG, Muskiet FAJ, Stomp GP, Van Dijk P, Berendsen HJC. Proton spin relaxation studies of fatty tissue and cerebral white matter. *Magnetic Resonance Imaging* 1984;2:211–20.
5. Pykett IL, Rosen BR. Nuclear magnetic resonance: *in vivo* proton chemical shift imaging. *Radiology* 1983;149:197–201.
6. Dobbing J, Sands J. Quantitative growth and development of human brain. *Arch Dis Child* 1973;48:757–67.
7. Yakolev PI, Lecours AR. The myelogenetic cycles of regional maturation in the brain. In: Minkowski A, ed. *Regional development of the brain in early life.* Oxford: Blackwell, 1967:3–69.
8. Bradley WG, Waluch V, Brant-Zawadzki M, Yadley RA, Wycoff RR. Patchy, periventricular white matter lesions in the elderly: common observation during NMR imaging. *Noninvasive Med Imaging* 1984;1:35–41.
9. Penn RD, Trenko B, Baldwin L. Brain maturation followed by computed tomography. *J Comput Assist Tomogr* 1980;4:614–6.
10. Quencer RM. Maturation of the normal primate white matter: computed tomographic correlation. *AJNR* 1982;3:365–72.
11. Holland BA, Haas DK, Norman D, Brant-Zawadzki M, Newton TH. MRI of normal brain maturation. *AJNR* 1986;7:201–8.
12. Davidson HD, Steiner RD. Magnetic resonance imaging in infections of the central nervous system. *AJNR* 1985;6:499–504.
13. Johnson MA, Pennock JM, Bydder GM, et al. Clinical NMR imaging of the brain in children: normal and neurologic disease. *AJNR* 1983;4:1013–26.
14. Johnson MA, Pennock JM, Bydder GM, et al. *AJR* 1983;141:1005–18.
15. Holland BA, Haas DK, Norman D, Brant-Zawadzki M, Newton TH. MRI of brain maturation [Abstract] *Proceedings of the Annual Meeting of the Western Neuroradiological Society,* Monterey, California, 1985.
16. Poser CM, Paty DW, Scheinberg L, et al. New diagnostic criteria for multiple sclerosis: guidelines for research protocols. *Ann Neurol* 1983;13:227–31.
17. Bartel DR, Markand ON, Kolar OJ. The diagnosis and classification of multiple sclerosis: evoked responses and spinal fluid electrophoresis. *Neurology* 1983;33:611–7.
18. Jackson JA, Leake DR, Schneider S, Rolak LA, Kelley GR, Ford JJ, Appel SH, Bryan RN. Magnetic resonance imaging in multiple sclerosis: results in 32 cases. *AJNR* 1985;6:171–6.
19. Lukes SA, Crooks LE, Aminoff MJ, et al. Nuclear magnetic resonance imaging in multiple sclerosis. *Ann Neurol* 1983;13:592–601.
20. Runge VM, Price AC, Kirschner HS, Allen JH, Partain CL, James AE Jr. Magnetic resonance imaging of multiple sclerosis: a study of pulse-technique efficacy. *AJNR* 1984;5:691–702.
21. Sheldon JJ, Siddharthan R, Tobias J, Sheremata WA, Soila K, Viamonte M Jr. MR imaging of multiple sclerosis: comparison with clinical and CT examinations in 74 patients. *AJNR* 1985;6:683–90.
22. Young IR, Hall AS, Pallis CA, Bydder GM, Legg NJ, Steiner RE. Nuclear magnetic resonance imaging of the brain in multiple sclerosis. *Lancet* 1981;2:1063–6.
23. Young IR, Randell CP, Kaplan PW, James A, Bydder GM, Steiner RE. Nuclear magnetic resonance (NMR) imaging in white matter disease of the brain using spin-echo sequences. *J Comput Assist Tomogr* 1983;7:290–4.
24. Runge VM, Price AC, Kirschner HS, Allen JH, Partain CL, James AE Jr. The evaluation of multiple sclerosis by magnetic resonance imaging. *RadioGraphics* 1986;6(2):203–12.
25. Maravilla KR, Weinreb JC, Suss R, Nunnally RL. Magnetic resonance demonstration of multiple sclerosis plaques in the cervical cord. *AJNR* 1984;5:685–9.
26. Carroll BA, Lane B, Norman D, Enzmann D. Diagnosis of progressive multifocal leukoencephalopathy by computed tomography. *Radiology* 1977;122:137–41.
27. Duda EE, Huttenlocher PR, Patronas NJ. CT of subacute sclerosing panencephalitis. *AJNR* 1980;1:35–8.
28. Lukes SA, Norman D. Computed tomography in acute disseminated encephalomyelitis. *Ann Neurol* 1983;13:567–72.
29. Weiner LP, Herndon RM, Narayon O. Isolation of virus relation SV40 from patients with progressive multifocal leukoencephalopathy. *N Engl J Med* 1972;286:385–90.
30. Kramer S, Lee KF. Complications of radiation therapy: the central nervous system. *Semin Roentgenol* 1974;9:75–83.
31. Sheline GE, Wara WM, Smith V. Therapeutic irradiation and brain injury. *Int J Radiat Oncol Biol Phys* 1980;6:1215–28.
32. Courville CB, Myers RO. The process of demyelination in the central nervous system. II. Mechanism of demyelination and necrosis of the cerebral centrum incident to x-irradiation. *J Neuropathol Exp Neurol* 1958;17:158–81.
33. Kingsley DPE, Kendalle BE. CT of the adverse effect of therapeutic radiation of the central nervous system. *AJNR* 1981;2:453–60.
34. Wang AM, Skias DD, Rumbaugh CL, Schoene WC, Zamani A. Central nervous system changes after radiation therapy and/or chemotherapy: correlation of CT and autopsy findings. *AJNR* 1983;4:466–71.
35. Curnes JT, Laster EW, Ball MR, Moody DM, Witcofski RL. *AJNR* 1986;7:389–94.
36. Dooms GC, Hecht S, Brant-Zawadzki M, Berthiaume Y, Norman D, Newton TH. Brain radiation lesions: MR imaging. *Radiology* 1986;158:149–55.
37. Adams RD, Victor M. *Principles of neurology.* 2nd ed. New York: McGraw-Hill Book Co. 1981:720–3.
38. Wright DG, Laureno R, Victor M. Pontine and extrapontine myelinolysis. *Brain* 1979;102:361–85.
39. Anderson TL, Moore RA, Grinnell VS, Itabashi HH. Computerized tomography in central pontine myelinolysis. *Neurology* 1979;29:1527–30.
40. Rosenbloom S, Buchholz D, Kumar AJ, Kaplan RA, Mossess H III, Rosenbaum AE. Evolution of central pontine myelinolysis on CT. *AJNR* 1984;5:110–2.
41. Adams RD, Victor M. *Principles of neurology.* 2nd ed. New York: McGraw-Hill Book Co. 1981:722–3.
42. Rancurel G, Gardeur D, Thibierge M, et al. Computed tomography of Marchiafava-Bignami disease. *Proceedings of the Twelfth Annual Neuroradiologicum Symposium, Washington, D.C., Oct. 10–16, 1982.*

43. Tomlinson BE, Blessed G, Roth M. Observations on the brains of non-demented old people. *J Neurol Sci* 1968;7:331–56.

44. Wisniewski HM, Terry RD. Morphology of the aging brain, human and animal. *Prog Brain Res* 1973;40:167–86.

45. Caplan LR, Schoene WC. Clinical features of subcortical arteriosclerotic encephalopathy (Binswanger disease). *Neurology* 1978;28:1206–15.

46. Goto K, Ishii N, Fukasawa H. Diffuse white-matter disease in the geriatric population. *Radiology* 1981;141:687–95.

47. Brant-Zawadzki M, Fein G, Van Dyke C, Kiernan R, Davenport L, de Groot J. MR imaging of the aging brain: patchy white-matter lesions and dementia. *AJNR* 1985;6:675–82.

48. Zimmerman, RD, Fleming CA, Lee BCP, Saint-Louis LA, Deck MDF. Periventricular hyperintensity as seen by magnetic resonance: prevalence and significance. *AJNR* 1986;7:13–20.

49. Poser C. Dysmyelination revisited. *Arch Neurol* 1978;35:401–8.

50. Malone MJ. The cerebral lipidoses. *Pediatr Clin North Am* 1976;23:303–26.

51. Geyer CA, Sartor KJ, Prensky AJ, Abramson CA, Hodges FJ III, Gado MH. Leigh's disease (subacute necrotizing encephalopathy): CT and MRI findings in 5 cases. American Society of Neuroradiology, San Diego, California, 1986.

52. Rutledge JN, Hillal SK, Silver AJ, Bello JA. MRI of dystonic states. American Society of Neuroradiology, San Diego, California, 1986.

53. Holland BA, Haas DK, Norman D, Brant-Zawadzki M, Newton TH. MRI of normal and abnormal brain maturation. American Society of Neuroradiology, New Orleans, Louisiana, 1985.

54. Wilson GH, Byfield J, Hanafee WN. Atrophy following radiation therapy for central nervous system neoplasms. *Acta Radiol Ther Phys Biol* 1972;11:361–8.

CHAPTER 17

Strategies for Efficient Imaging of the Lumbar Spine

Bent O. Kjos and David Norman

The ability to perform high-quality magnetic resonance (MR) examinations of the lumbar spine in as short a time as possible is of major importance. Many patients with spine abnormalities are unable to remain immobile for extended periods of time because of discomfort. Prolonged examination times lead to increased motion artifact and a subsequent degradation of image quality. The high cost of MR imaging equipment also dictates that examinations be performed as rapidly as possible, without sacrificing quality. Understanding the factors influencing image quality, signal-to-noise ratio (SNR), and imaging time is the key to limiting examination time without significantly compromising quality. This chapter discusses the factors affecting SNR and how these factors can be manipulated to develop efficient imaging strategies for the spine. The general principles can be applied to imaging other structures as well.

CHARACTERISTICS OF THE LUMBAR SPINE

There are several unique characteristics of the lumbar spine related to MR imaging.

1. Object contrast is high. Tissue types that must be distinguished include neural tissue, disc, bony cortex, cerebrospinal fluid (CSF), and fat. These tissues have widely different relaxation times and to a lesser extent different spin densities, which permit the use of a variety of pulse sequences to distinguish among anatomic components of the lumbar spine. Selection of imaging parameters can therefore be focused on SNR and imaging time considerations. This contrasts with brain imaging in which T2- or T1-weighted sequences are specifically indicated for differing abnormalities.

2. Elements of the lumbar spine are the largest in the spinal axis. Requirements for spatial detail are therefore not as critical as in imaging of, for example, the cervical spine. Higher spatial detail may in fact be undesirable because contrast is diminished.

3. Unlike imaging of the cervical spine, CSF motion is not generally a problem in imaging of the lumbar spine. Although signal void from CSF motion may be seen in some cases, especially in cases with large discs or spinal stenosis, this is usually easily recognized as such and does not cause artifacts that diminish the diagnostic utility.

REQUIREMENTS FOR LUMBAR SPINE IMAGING

Sequences selected must have adequate contrast resolution and be able to separate the different components of the spine on the basis of intensity differences. Spatial resolution in the range 0.8 to 1.5 mm is appropriate for most lumbar spine cases. Slice thickness should be no greater than 5 mm for axial scans and 3 mm for sagittal scans. Sections should not be so thick that volume averaging obscures pathology and/or anatomy. Finally, the patient must be comfortable and not overly anxious. Analgesics and anxiolytics may be necessary even if examination times are kept short.

FACTORS AFFECTING SNR

Maximizing SNR in a limited scan time requires understanding of the factors affecting SNR. These factors can be divided into (a) independent tissue characteristics that influence the SNR but cannot be varied; (b) choice of receiver coil; and (c) machine settings that can be directly controlled to affect SNR (Table 1).

Independent Tissue Characteristics

T1 relaxation time, T2 relaxation time, hydrogen density, and motion of tissue all affect SNR in that they determine the total signal intensity for any given se-

Tissue characteristic	Machine setting
T1	Pixel volume
T2	FOV
Spin density	Matrix size
Motion	Slice thickness
	Timing parameters
	TR
	TE
	NEX
	Type of receiver coil

quence. SNR in a given tissue is greater in sequences that result in higher signal intensity for that tissue as opposed to sequences that result in lower signal intensity. In spin-echo imaging sequences, longer repetition times (TR) and short-echo sampling times (TE) will give more SNR and are therefore preferable if there is also adequate tissue contrast and the imaging time is not too long.

Surface Coils

Appropriately designed coils dramatically improve spine image quality and reduce imaging time by preferentially receiving signal from the limited tissue volume immediately adjacent to the coil. The maximum advantage in SNR can be obtained by using a surface coil that is no larger than required to cover the desired anatomy. A larger coil receives additional noise from tissue outside the region of interest. This contributes to the total signal and thereby diminishes SNR. If the same region is imaged using two different-size coils but otherwise identical imaging parameters, the images using the smaller coil will be superior. If, for example, the entire lumbar spine and conus region are studied, a 5 × 10-in. rectangular coil is usually needed, whereas if only the lower three or four lumbar vertebral bodies are imaged, then a smaller 5-in. round coil can be used. The smaller coil has superior SNR characteristics and therefore fewer excitations and shorter imaging times are necessary. The radiologist must therefore determine the extent of spinal anatomy to be examined to optimize use of the imager.

Number of Excitations

A simple but inefficient method of improving SNR is to increase the number of excitations (NEX). SNR increases with the square root of NEX. Doubling the NEX doubles the imaging time and increases the SNR by 41%. Tripling the NEX triples the imaging time and increases the SNR by 73%. The effect of varying the

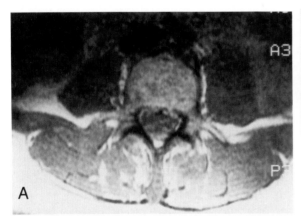
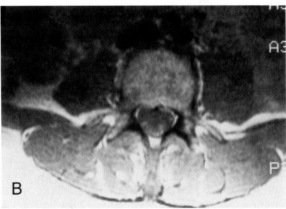
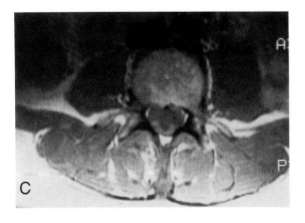

FIG. 1. Effect of varying NEX on SNR and image quality; 5-mm-thick axial 1,000/25 spin-echo scans were obtained on the same patient using 1 NEX (**A**), 2 NEX (**B**), and 4 NEX (**C**). Images were photographed using the same window and level settings. Note how images become less grainy with increasing NEX because of improving SNR. The most important improvement between the 1 NEX and 2 NEX images is the decrease in motion artifact from the aorta, which obscures visualization of the thecal sac on the single-NEX image. This motion-induced noise in the phase-encoding direction is random and is therefore improved by signal averaging. Interchanging the phase and frequency directions will change the orientation of this artifact to left right and may make a 1-NEX study more diagnostic.

NEX on actual image quality is shown in Fig. 1. An approach to efficient imaging is to optimize other parameters without increasing the NEX. Although increasing the NEX will improve image quality, it fails to improve efficiency.

Pixel Volume: Field of View, Matrix, and Slice Thickness

The key determinants of SNR over which the operator has great control are the factors controlling pixel size; namely, slice thickness, number of matrix elements, and field of view (FOV). SNR is directly proportional to the pixel volume. If the pixel volume is doubled and all other factors are unchanged, the SNR is also doubled. Imaging efficiency is optimized by adjusting pixel size so

that it is appropriate to the size of the structure being imaged. It should be neither too large nor too small. Achieving unnecessarily high spatial resolution (pixels too small) results in lower SNR and longer imaging times. Excessively large pixels result in high SNR but inadequate spatial resolution.

In lumbar spine imaging, the maximum acceptable slice thickness is 5 mm for axial images and 3 mm for sagittal images. Thinner sections will decrease SNR; more excitations will be required to compensate for this. In clinical situations where uncertainty is high or infants are involved, thinner sections may be appropriate.

Controlling the in-plane resolution or pixel area by varying the FOV and matrix size is the most important technique for improving scan efficiency. The in-plane resolution is simply calculated by dividing the FOV by the matrix size:

TABLE 2. *Relative SNR values calculated for various settings of matrix size, FOV, and NEX*[a]

Matrix (phase × frequency)	FOV (cm)	NEX	Pixel volume (mm^3)	SNR (normalized)	SNR/time (normalized)	Scan time (min) (TR = 1 sec)
Standard sequence (SNR and SNR/time = 1)						
128 × 256	16	2	0.78	1	1	4.27
Effect of varying matrix size						
128 × 128	16	2	1.56	2.00	2.00	4.27
128 × 192	16	2	1.04	1.33	1.33	4.27
128 × 256	16	2	0.78	1.00	1.00	4.27
192 × 192	16	2	0.69	1.09	0.73	6.40
192 × 256	16	2	0.52	0.82	0.54	6.40
256 × 256	16	2	0.39	0.71	0.35	8.53
Effect of varying NEX						
128 × 256	16	1	0.78	0.71	1.41	2.13
128 × 256	16	2	0.78	1.00	1.00	4.27
128 × 256	16	4	0.78	1.41	0.71	8.53
128 × 256	16	6	0.78	1.73	0.58	12.80
128 × 256	16	8	0.78	2.00	0.50	17.07
Effect of varying FOV						
256 × 256	12	2	0.22	0.40	0.20	8.53
256 × 256	16	2	0.39	0.71	0.35	8.53
256 × 256	20	2	0.61	1.10	0.55	8.53
256 × 256	24	2	0.88	1.59	0.80	8.53
256 × 256	32	2	1.56	2.83	1.41	8.53
Varying FOV with a 192 × 192 matrix						
192 × 192	16	2	0.69	1.09	0.73	6.40
192 × 192	20	2	1.09	1.70	1.13	6.40
192 × 192	24	2	1.56	2.45	1.63	6.40
Effect of proportional change in both FOV and matrix size						
128 × 128	12	2	0.88	1.13	1.13	4.27
128 × 256	12	2	0.44	0.56	0.56	4.27
256 × 256	24	2	0.88	1.59	0.80	8.53

[a] SNR/imaging time is a measure of scanning efficiency since it gives the amount of SNR achieved per unit of imaging time. SNR and SNR/time values are listed relative to the values for the standard sequence, shown in row 1, which are assigned the value 1.

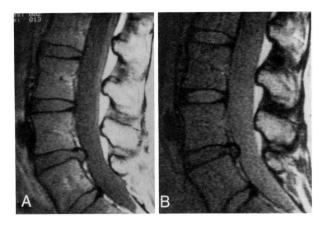

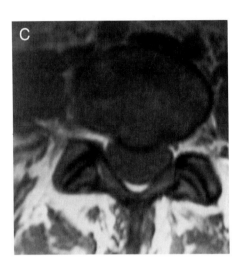

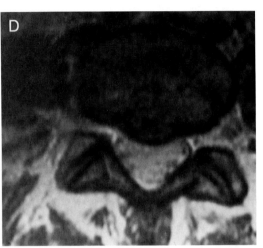

FIG. 2. Standard lumbar spine examination using the smaller 5-in. round surface coil. Positioning of the coil is first checked by a rapid "localizer" scan requiring less than 1 min (not shown). Accurate positioning is very important when using the smaller coil. Three-mm-thick sagittal scans are performed through the lower four intervertebral discs with 4 NEX, SE 1,000/20,50 (**A,B**), 128 × 256 matrix, and 16-cm FOV. Twenty-eight images (14 levels) are obtained in a scan time of 8 min, 35 sec. Five-mm-thick axial scans are performed from L2 to S1 with 2 NEX, SE 1,500/20,50 (**C,D**), 128 × 256 matrix, and 16-cm FOV. Forty images (20 levels) are obtained in a scan time of 6 min, 29 sec. Total examination time is approximately 25 min. Note the degeneration of the L4–L5 disc with diminished signal intensity within the disc and the midline posterior disc herniation. Spatial and contrast resolution are excellent despite a short examination time and lack of strong T2 weighting.

$$\text{Pixel diameter} = \text{FOV/matrix elements}$$

For example, a 24-cm FOV used in conjunction with a 256 × 256 matrix (phase-encoding axis × frequency axis) will yield an in-plane resolution of 240 mm/256 or 0.9 mm. In order to minimize scan time, the FOV should be made as small as possible while still covering the area of interest. A smaller FOV permits a proportionally smaller matrix to be used; this results in similar spatial resolution and SNR but decreased imaging time. In the example above, if a 12-cm FOV can be used instead of a 24-cm FOV, then a 128 × 128 matrix can be used instead of a 256 × 256 matrix; this will yield the same resolution and similar SNR in half the imaging time.

A list of various imaging sequences and their relative SNR values is shown in Table 2, which shows the effect on SNR of varying matrix size, FOV, and NEX. The signal-to-noise value of a sequence employing a 128 × 256 matrix and a 16-cm FOV is normalized to the value of 1.

SAGITTAL IMAGING

In sagittal imaging of the lumbar spine, the radiologist must decide if a large FOV should be used, to include the entire lumbar spine and conus region, or a small FOV, to include the lower three or four vertebral bodies. The larger FOV will double the examination time. The decision may be further influenced by the duration of examination time that the patient will tolerate.

A 24- to 32-cm FOV is usually required to include the conus region. Employing a 256 × 256 matrix with a 24-cm FOV yields a 0.9 × 0.9-mm² pixel that provides examinations of quality spatial and contrast detail. A 192 × 192 matrix with a 24-cm FOV would yield a 1.2 × 1.2-mm² pixel that would probably be optimal in SNR and spatial detail. This is currently not available in most instruments. In any case, a surface coil large enough to cover the entire lumbar spine is necessary.

If images of the lower lumbar spine are required, a 16-cm FOV will usually cover the intervertebral discs from L2 to S1. This smaller FOV allows use of a smaller

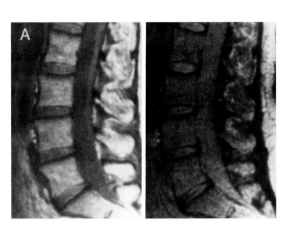

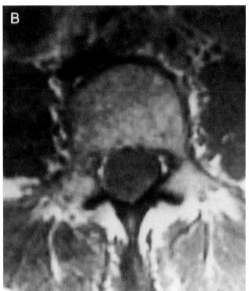

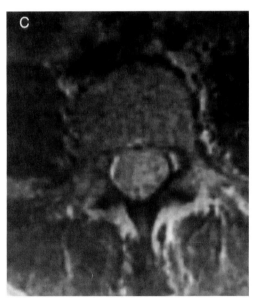

FIG. 3. Standard lumbar spine examination using the larger 5 × 10-in. rectangular surface coil. Positioning of the coil is first checked by a rapid localizer scan. Three-mm-thick sagittal scans are performed through the conus region and entire lumbar spine with 4 NEX, SE 1,000/20,50 (**A**), 256 × 256 matrix, and 32-cm FOV. Twenty-eight images (14 levels) are obtained in a scan time of 17 min, 7 sec. Five-mm-thick axial scans are performed from L2 to S1 with 2 NEX, SE 1,500/20,50 (**B,C**), 256 × 256 matrix, and 24-cm FOV. Forty images (20 levels) are obtained in a scan time of 12 min, 53 sec. Total examination time is approximately 40 min. Examination is essentially normal.

matrix size without compromise of spatial resolution. Utilizing the smaller 128 × 256 matrix halves imaging time compared to using a 256 × 256 matrix. Furthermore, this smaller FOV permits the use of a smaller surface coil that has comparatively superior SNR characteristics. It may therefore be possible to acquire a comparable quality scan using fewer NEX than would be possible with a larger coil. This can result in an additional factor of 2 reduction in total imaging time. Imaging only the lower three or four vertebral bodies in the lumbar spine will therefore decrease the imaging time by 50% to 75% because both a smaller coil and matrix can be used. The smaller coil can reduce imaging time by a factor of 2, and the smaller matrix will reduce imaging time by an additional factor of 2.

AXIAL IMAGING

In almost all patients a 16-cm FOV will completely cover the entire cross-sectional area of the spine and the dorsal soft tissues. Using a larger FOV than necessary increases scan time as well as the motion artifact from abdominal and pelvic structures. With a 16-cm FOV, acceptable spatial resolution can be achieved with the smaller 128 × 256 matrix. SNR resulting from a 16-cm FOV study with a 128 × 256 matrix can be improved without significantly increasing pixel size by either increasing the NEX or by increasing the FOV in conjunction with increasing the matrix size to 256 × 256. Both of these options increase imaging time. Doubling the NEX while retaining the 128 × 256 matrix will double

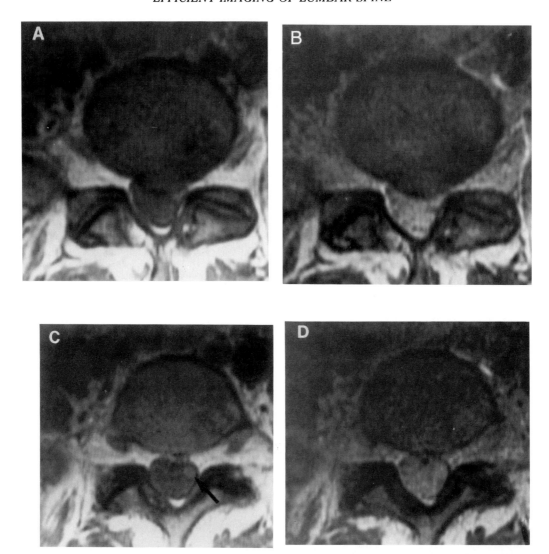

FIG. 4. Two cases of swollen nerves within the thecal sac secondary to distal disc disease. **A–D:** SE 1,500/20,50 axial images with 2 NEX, 16 FOV, 128 × 256 matrix requiring 6-min, 29-sec scan time. Left-sided L5-S1 disc herniation compresses the left S1 nerve root origin. This is seen on both SE 1,500/20 (**A**) and SE 1,500/50 (**B**) images. Note the higher CSF-disc contrast on the more T2-weighted SE 1,500/50 image. The swollen left S1 nerve (*arrow*) is seen within the thecal sac just superior to the herniated disc on the SE 1,500/20 image (**C**). The nerve was not identified on the second-echo (SE 1,500/50) image, which has poor CSF-nerve contrast (**D**). **E–H:** Five-mm-thick axial SE 1,300/20,50 scans with 4 NEX, 16 FOV, 128 × 256 matrix requiring 11-min, 10-sec scan time. Note the improved SNR on this 4-NEX exam. A left-sided L5-S1 herniated disc is again easily demonstrated on both SE 1,300/20 (**E**) and SE 1,300/50 (**F**) images. CSF-disc contrast is greater on the second-echo image (**G**). The swollen left S1 nerve (*arrow*) is seen within the thecal sac above the disc on the SE 1,300/20 image. The nerve was not identified on the 1,300/50 image (**H**).

the imaging time and raise the SNR by 41% (Table 2). Increasing the FOV to a 24-cm FOV and the matrix to 256 × 256 will also double the imaging time but will improve SNR by 59% (using the same coil). This latter sequence is more efficient and is especially useful for very large patients and for when the larger, less efficient surface coil is used.

Image quality with the 5-in. round coil, 16-cm FOV, 128 × 256 matrix, and 2 NEX is usually excellent. If the conus is to be included, the larger 5 × 10-in. coil is used, and additional signal is required to compensate for its

lower efficiency. Usually a 20- to 24-cm FOV, 256 × 256 image is obtained. Using the larger coil results in a doubling of examination time in both axial and sagittal planes (Fig. 2 and 3).

SNR IMPLICATION OF IMPROVING OR DECREASING RESOLUTION

Table 2 also demonstrates the large increase in scan time required to improve spatial resolution while maintaining the same SNR. If a 256 × 256 matrix is used

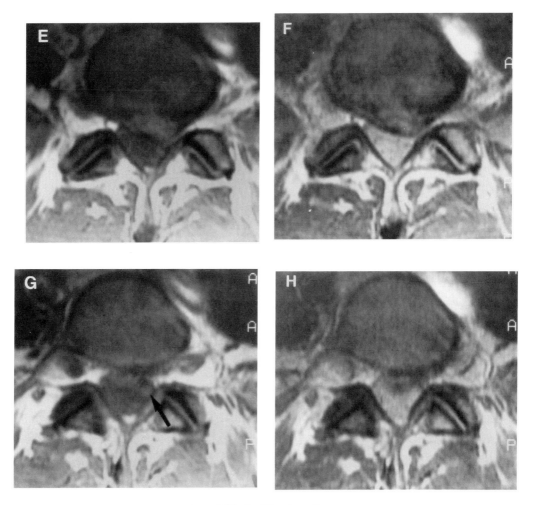

FIG. 4. *(Continued)*

instead of a 128 × 256 matrix while keeping the same FOV, the pixel volume is cut in half, the imaging time is doubled, and the SNR is decreased by 30% (Table 2). To overcome this drop in SNR the NEX must be doubled. Thus, to decrease the pixel area by a factor of 2 requires a fourfold increase in examination time. Switching from a 128 × 128 matrix to a 256 × 256 cuts the pixel area by a factor of 4 and necessitates a 16-fold increase in examination time to maintain the same SNR.

SNR may be increased by enlarging the pixel size and decreasing spatial resolution. Although not generally available on current imagers, a 128 × 128 matrix would be useful for this purpose. Using a 128 × 128 matrix instead of a 128 × 256 matrix would not change the imaging time but would increase SNR by 41%. Another method of improving SNR without increasing imaging time is to increase the FOV while keeping the matrix constant. Changing from a 16-cm to a 20-cm FOV will increase SNR by 56% but only decrease spatial resolution by 20%. These methods may be necessary in several clinical circumstances. In patients unable to lie immobile for more than 2 to 3 min, slightly decreasing spatial

resolution may make a rapid single-NEX study possible. Increasing the FOV is useful in obese patients in whom excess subcutaneous fat separates the spine from the surface coil, thereby worsening SNR. In these patients and in cases of diminished SNR for technical reasons (including poor machine calibration), using a slightly larger pixel size may enable performance of a diagnostic study that would otherwise not be possible.

TABLE 3. *Different spin-echo sequences with identical imaging times*

TR	NEX
2,000	1
1,000	2
500	4
400	5
200	10
100	20

[a] The sequences shown here have the same imaging time. If the matrix size is 256 × 256, then the imaging time will be ~8.5 min for each sequence.

The two protocols we routinely use for lumbar spine imaging are as follows.

Lumbar spine including conus

Large coil: 5 × 10 in. round.
    Axials: 20 to 24-cm FOV; 256 × 256 matrix; 2 NEX; 5 mm thick.
    Sagittals: 24 to 32-cm FOV; 256 × 256 matrix; 2 to 4 NEX; 3 mm thick.

Lower lumbar spine only

Small coil: 5 in. round.
    Axials: 16-cm FOV; 128 × 256 matrix; 2 NEX; 5 mm thick.
    Sagittals: 16-cm FOV; 128 × 256 matrix; 2 to 4 NEX; 3 mm thick.

Sequence Timing Parameters (TR, TE)

Adjusting TR and TE affects SNR by controlling the signal intensity of the tissues. Goals in optimizing these machine settings include maximizing signal, keeping the imaging time short, and maintaining tissue contrast. The equation for spin-echo imaging time is

Imaging time
    = TR × NEX × matrix size (in phase direction)

With a fixed imaging time and a predetermined matrix size,

$$TR \times NEX = constant$$

Therefore for a fixed imaging time, a short-TR sequence with many NEX, a long-TR sequence with few NEX, or something in between may be selected (Table 3). Increasing the NEX will increase SNR, but doubling the NEX will increase the SNR by only 41%. With continued increase in NEX, there is diminishing gain in SNR. Similarly, an increase in TR will increase SNR by allowing increased T1 relaxation; however, doubling TR does not double SNR, and continued increase in TR leads to diminishing gain in SNR.

In choosing the TR of an imaging sequence, it is important to consider the number of levels required to image the region of interest. In multiple-slice spin-echo (MSE) sequences, the number of possible levels is proportional to the TR. If a 600-msec TR sequence yields 10 levels, then a 1,200-msec TR sequence will yield 20 levels. If 20 levels are desired, performing either a single 1,200-msec TR sequence or two 600-msec TR sequences requires the same total imaging time, but the longer TR sequence will have a higher SNR. If overlapping slices or a more T1-weighted sequence are desired,

an interleaved, shorter TR series may be chosen, but these interleaved sequences will generally have lower SNR than a single, longer TR series.

In most adults, about fifteen 3-mm-thick sagittal scans performed at 3.6 mm intervals will span the lumbar spine. Depending on the machine specifications, this means that a TR of approximately 1,000 msec is needed to obtain enough levels. Approximately fifteen to twenty 5-mm-thick axial scans obtained at 6-mm intervals are required to image the lower three or four intervertebral discs. This requires a TR of 1,000 to 1,500 msec. With hardware and software modifications, most MR imagers will be able to perform 15 levels within 750 msec and 20 levels within approximately 1,000 msec.

For maximum SNR, the echo time (TE) should be as short as possible, because of high tissue contrast in the spine, an intermediate series with TR of approximately 1,000 msec and TE of 20 msec (1,000/20) will identify spine tumors and almost all disc herniations. The CSF usually has moderately low signal intensity, with solid nerve roots and tumors having higher signal intensity; the bony cortex and disc annulus have lower signal intensity than CSF. Performing scans with more T1 weighting, i.e., TR < 800 msec, may not be beneficial because it is difficult to distinguish the very low signal intensity of CSF from bony cortex, osteophytes, or annulus. In some cases, especially in studies with marginal SNR, it may be impossible to distinguish disc from CSF even on 1,000/20 spin-echo studies. For this reason, a more T2-weighted second-echo image, on which the CSF has much higher signal intensity than adjacent tissues, is required. Increasing TR and/or TE will increase T2 weighting; but increasing TE decreases the number of slices that can be obtained, and increasing TR increases imaging time. The amount of T2 contrast required must be determined. Usually, a 50-msec second echo will increase the relative signal intensity of CSF sufficiently to distinguish it from adjacent tissues. Later echoes in conjunction with longer TR will lead to greater CSF-disc or CSF-scar contrast but requires a longer imaging time. In most cases, a 2-NEX, 128 × 256 matrix, 1,000/20,50-msec study requiring 4.3 min will provide a diagnostic exam. A 2,000/20,70-msec study will improve SNR and T2 weighting; this doubles examination time to 8.5 min. Although the 2,000/70 image has greater CSF-disc contrast, there is less CSF-nerve contrast on the 2,000/20 image than on the 1,000/20 image. The choice of TR and TE depends on the SNR characteristics of the imager, the individual patient, and the radiologist (Fig. 4).

CONCLUSIONS

Understanding the factors affecting SNR is important in devising efficient imaging strategies of the lumbar spine. Adjustment of pixel size by minimizing FOV and matrix size is a very efficient way to keep scan times low while still maintaining spatial resolution and SNR. Using a surface coil just large enough to span the region of interest will enable one to minimize the NEX. Although larger TR and TE settings will yield highest CSF-disc contrast, this also requires longer imaging time. Adequate contrast may instead be achieved with intermediate TR and TE settings. Because patient size, clinical history, and signal-to-noise characteristics vary from patient to patient, standard imaging protocols should be modified for more efficient scanning of individual patients. This requires a working knowledge of the many factors affecting SNR.

With the rapid development of MR technologies, many new techniques are becoming available to lumbar spine imaging. Improved surface coils will allow scans to be performed with fewer NEX. Angled scans can be performed parallel to the individual endplates. Single-section scans can be acquired very rapidly using reduced flip-angle techniques with gradient-reversal echoes. This will be useful in patients unable to hold still, in further evaluating areas where the findings are not definite, and in obtaining initial images to check surface-coil position. In any case, the principles concerning SNR are the same, and an understanding of these principles will allow efficient application of these new technical improvements to lumbar spine imaging.

CHAPTER 18

The Spine

David Norman

High-resolution magnetic resonance imaging (MRI) of the spine promises to replace all other imaging modalities including plain films, computed tomography (CT), and myelography, in most disorders affecting the cord or canal. Stringent objective criteria of high-quality, high-resolution images have not been firmly established. Critical components revolve about optimization of signal to noise (S/N), good contrast, and good edge definition, the latter representing an important component of spatial detail. Signal-to-noise ratio is influenced by gradient coils, power supplies, preamps, fringe fields, eddy currents, software, etc.; and S/N also increases linearly with increasing field strength. A three- to five-fold increase in S/N can be achieved with surface receiving coils. Surface coils must be designed so that they are appropriate in size and impedance for the object being imaged and the size and weight of the patient. Depth resolution of surface coils is defined by the radius of the coil.

Other important components of image quality include data acquisition on a 256^2 matrix and data display on a 512^2 matrix. Image quality should be equivalent in all orthogonal and nonorthogonal planes. Artifacts from CSF and blood flow and respiratory motion should be minimized and/or compensated. Compensation may be accomplished with cardiac and/or respiratory gating, and/or a variant thereof.

THE MAGNETIC RESONANCE IMAGE: COMPARISON TO COMPUTED TOMOGRAPHY

The physical principles underlying the magnetic resonance (MR) image are considerably different from those of x-ray CT, and the image appearance is therefore also quite different. The contrast detail of MR surpasses that of CT severalfold, and the spatial detail is equivalent or superior, assuming a cooperative patient (Fig. 1A–D).

Osseous structures appear as areas of relative signal void, reflecting a paucity of mobile hydrogen protons. Cortical bone, which is dense (white) on CT, is low in intensity (black) on MR. Cancellous bone, due to marrow and fat within its interstices, is of relatively high signal intensity (white) on T1-weighted images and early echoes on T2-weighted images. In later decades, the blood-forming elements in marrow are frequently displaced by fat, resulting in a progressive increase in signal intensity within cancellous bone (1). This phenomenon is one of the few brighter events in the declining years. The contrast between cortical and cancellous bone results in excellent anatomic detail—albeit, a learning period is required to accommodate to this new gray-scale encoding used in the display of anatomic data.

Vertebral bodies, pedicles, facets, and laminae appear as structures of high-signal-intensity cancellous bone framed by a thin margin of low-signal-intensity cortical bone on T1-weighted images. On T2-weighted images, the signal in cancellous bone diminishes, and the distinction between cortical and cancellous bone is not as well defined (Fig. 2).

LUMBAR SPINE AND CANAL: IMAGING TECHNIQUES

Most of the images in this chapter were obtained with a GE Signa system operated at 1.5 tesla (T). All exams were performed with surface-receiving coils. Selection of imaging sequences must take into account the total time available for an exam. This should not exceed 1 hr because patients can rarely tolerate more. Issues of matrix size (spatial detail), S/N, and motion degradation must all be considered. For example, additional excitations performed to improve S/N may actually result in diminished image quality due to patient motion associated with prolonged examination time.

In patients with lumbar radicular symptoms, the fol-

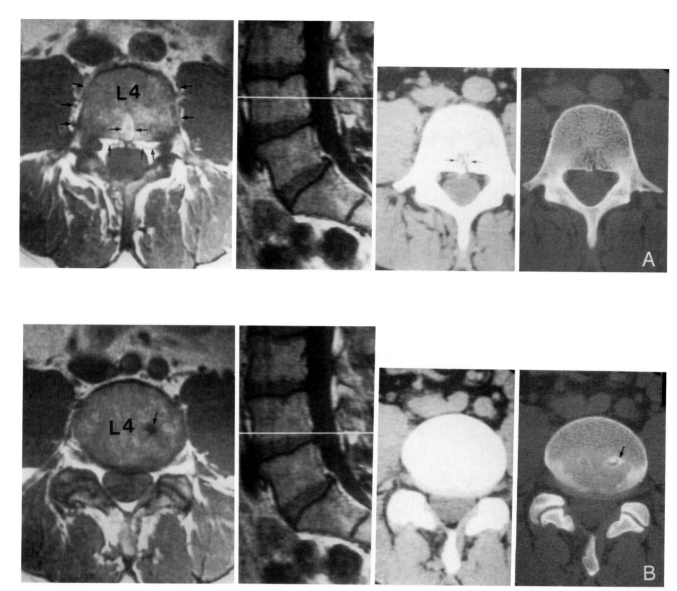

FIG. 1. Lumbar spine, normal anatomy: CT and MR scans on a 44-year-old asymptomatic man. The MR scans were acquired on a GE Signa System operating at 1.5 T. The MR scans are relatively T1-weighted (TR = 1,000 msec; TE = 20 msec) images. Section thickness is 5 mm. The CT scans were acquired on a GE 9800 using 3-mm-thick sections. Note that soft-tissue and bone detail on CT must be displayed at two different window settings, whereas on MR only one window setting is required. There is to a large extent complete reversal of the gray scale in comparing MR to CT. On MR the cortical bone surrounding the vertebral body is of low signal intensity. The cancellous bone is of intermediate to high signal intensity depending on the age of the patient and relative ratio of fat to marrow. **A:** In the central portion of the body is the basivertebral plexus. Around the periphery of the body are ovoid structures with signal void representing branches of the anterior external venous plexus (*horizontal arrows*). Note how the epidural fat sharply contrasts the internal vertebral veins (*vertical arrows*) and the ganglia within the foramen. The dural sac is easily identified. The lamina are outlined by the signal void from the cortical bone. **B:** On a section through the inferior endplate of the body of L4, a Schmorl's node (*arrow*), which is sclerotic on the CT scan, appears as an area of signal void on the MR scan. The opposing cortical margins of the facet joints are of low signal intensity. Note the ligamentum flavum on the left. Individual nerve roots within the thecal sac are not identified on this patient due to CSF and/or nerve root motion.

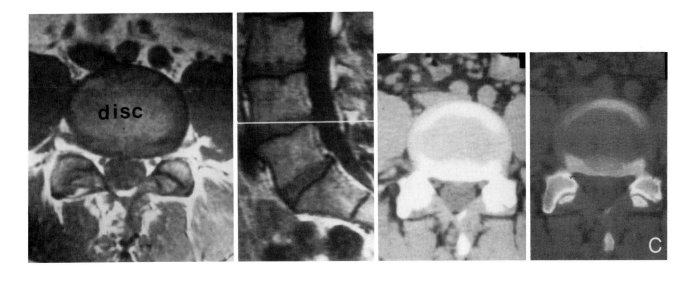

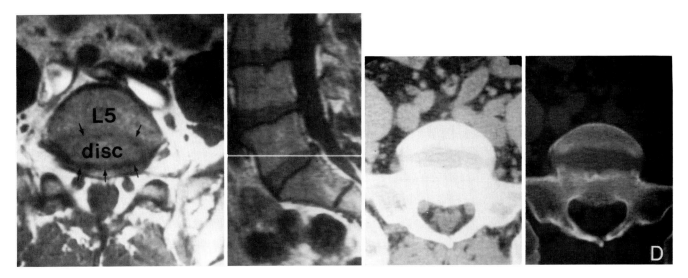

FIG. 1. C: On section through the L4–L5 disc, the L4 nerve roots are identified just medial to the neural foramen. The disc is difficult to characterize on the axial views without the benefit of the sagittal localizer. **D:** A lower section on the same plane is perpendicular to the table top. The scan passes through the body of L5, the inferior cortical end-plate of L5 (*downward-pointing arrows*), the disc, the cephalad end-plate of S1 (*upward-pointing arrows*), and a portion of the cancellous bone of the body of S1. Note the L5 nerve roots medial to the neural foramen. The relationship of the nerve roots to the foramen is more easily identified on MR than on the CT scan.

lowing approach may be used: A relatively T1-weighted sagittal image is first obtained using an asymmetric echo technique (TR = 1,000 msec; TE = 20, 70 msec) (Fig. 2). In this single imaging sequence, the first echo is a T1-weighted image with excellent spatial detail; the second echo has relatively greater T2 weighting, which results in increased CSF signal intensity and permits improved discrimination between subarachnoid space and adjacent ligaments and cortical bone. In most instances, the sagittal sequence is followed by a relatively T1-weighted series of axial images (TR = 1,000 msec; TE = 20 msec). The axial image is obtained with a single echo only. This allows sufficient cephalocaudad coverage, which is usually not possible if two echoes are acquired. It is desirable to use thin sections. With diminished slice thickness there is, however, a decrease in S/N that may result in loss of significant diagnostic information. For this reason, images are currently obtained with

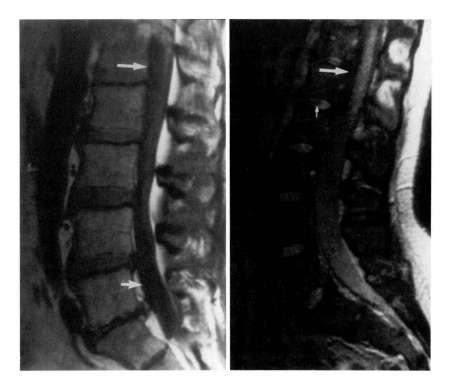

FIG. 2. Sagittal lumbosacral spine examination; asymmetric echo acquisition (TR = 1,000 msec; TE = 20/70 msec). On the first echo (*left*), CSF has a grayish hue. Note that the cortical end-plates are thicker on the cephalad end of the vertebral body in comparison to the caudal end, reflecting chemical shift artifact. On the second echo, CSF has relatively high signal intensity. Note the relative loss of definition between cortical and cancellous bone with fall off of signal from fat and marrow, which occurs with increased TR and TE. On both images, the CSF signal is of greater intensity in the more caudal aspects of the canal (L4, L5, and S1) (*short arrow*) than in the more cephalad portion (*long arrow*). This reflects more rapid flow of CSF in the more cephalad portions of the lumbosacral canal. The *small vertical arrow* on the second echo points to a cleft in the disc, a normal finding, which is more pronounced with increased TR and TE.

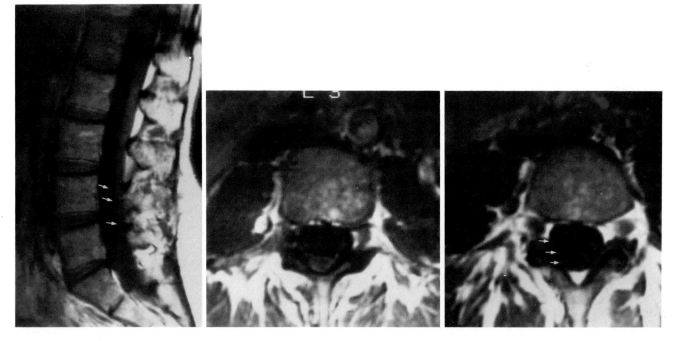

FIG. 3. T1-weighted sagittal image (partial saturation, TR = 600 msec) in a normal patient. The individual roots can be identified on the sagittal view (*arrows*). On the axial view, the nerve roots can be seen to layer posterolaterally at the L3 and L5 levels (*arrows*). Their margins are slightly blurred due to motion.

3-mm-thick sections (six excitations) in the sagittal plane and 5-mm-thick sections (four excitations) in the axial plane. If smaller surface coils are used, a 128 × 256 rather than 256² acquisition matrix can often provide quality diagnostic images with a halving of the acquisition time.

T2-weighted sagittal or axial images are rarely required in evaluation of the lumbar canal and/or discs in patients with degenerative disease. This may not be the case in patients with tumor or infection. In these cases, supplemental T2-weighted images may be useful (*vide infra*).

LUMBAR SPINE AND CANAL: NORMAL ANATOMY

T1-weighted sequences (TR = 600–1,000 msec; TE = 20 msec) provide the best anatomic detail. On midsagittal views, the low-signal cortical bone frames the vertebral body (Fig. 2). The cancellous matrix has a signal intensity that is usually isointense with muscle. The relative signal intensity becomes brighter with increasing age or with spinal radiation (2) due to replacement of marrow by fat. In the posterior midportion of the body, the emissary veins of Batson's plexus may appear as either low or high signal intensity depending on the flow rate and the sequence utilized (Figs. 1 and 2). They have a characteristic morphologic appearance. The intervertebral discs are of slightly less intense signal than cancellous bone and are framed by the cortical end-plates, the cephalad plate appearing thicker than the caudal plate due to chemical shift artifact (Fig. 2). With increasing age and/or degeneration, there is progressive loss in signal intensity due to disc desiccation. The annulus fibrosus is of similar signal intensity to cortical bone and appears as a convex band of signal void contrasted on midline sections, with CSF of intermediate signal intensity, or on parasagittal images, with fat of high signal intensity within the foramina (3). Within the fat-filled foramen, the exiting nerve is seen in the upper third of the foramen. The nerve is midrange in signal intensity. The epidural veins appear as tubular areas of signal void located superior and anterior to the nerve.

It is not possible to distinguish among the posterior cortex, annulus, ligaments, and dura on the sagittal view. They all are of a similar low signal intensity. CSF is also of similar low signal intensity on images acquired with a very short TR (600 msec). On images obtained with longer repetition times (TR = 1,000 msec), CSF acquires a grayish hue.

The signal intensity of the conus is similar to normal discs (Fig. 2). The conus usually terminates at the L1 level. Caudal to the conus, the nerves of the cauda equina appear as a posteriorly situated caudally tapering

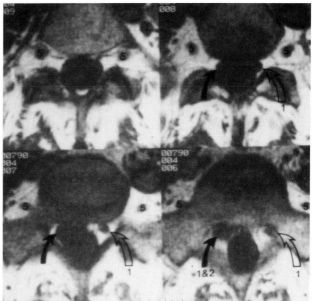
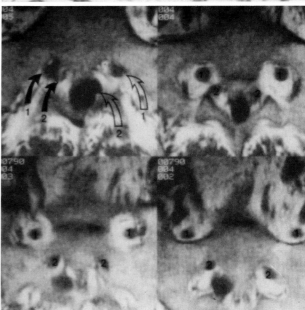

FIG. 4. A series of T1-weighted axial cuts extending from the L5-S1 through the S2 levels. Images should be viewed from left to right and top to bottom. Note normal budding of the left L5, S1, and S2 nerve roots. On the right, a "mass" can be seen (*black arrow*), which, as viewed more caudally, can be appreciated to represent a conjoined nerve root. Note the clarity with which both the S1 and S2 nerve roots can be seen within the sacral foramina. This series of images demonstrates the superiority of MR over CT in defining soft-tissue structures within the foramina.

column with slightly irregular margins (Fig. 3). The dorsal location reflects the fact that the image was obtained with the patient supine.

On T2-weighted images, the vertebral bodies lose sig-

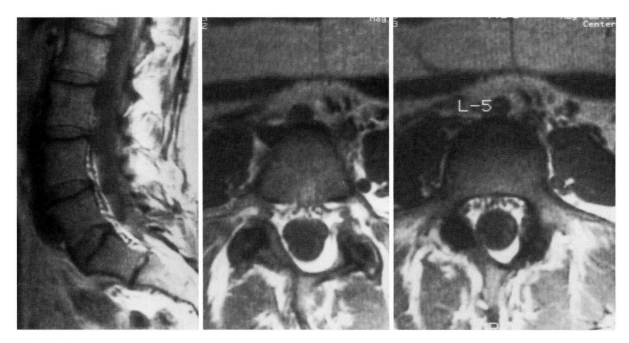

FIG. 5. Prominent epidural veins appear as areas of signal void contrasted with epidural fat on sagittal and axial images (TR = 1,000 msec; TE = 20 msec). These are often more pronounced with disc herniation.

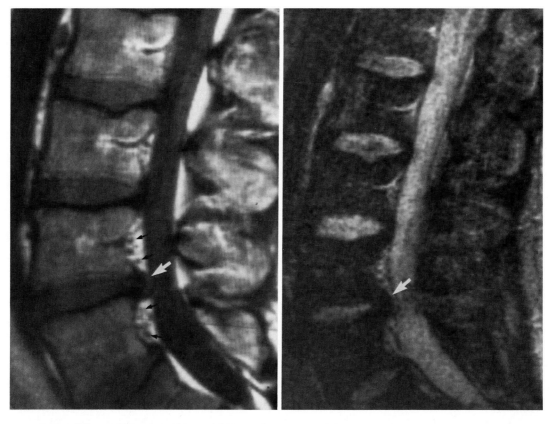

FIG. 6. Herniated disc (TR = 1,000 msec; TE = 20/70 msec) of the L4–L5 level (*white arrow*). There is relative loss of disc signal at both the L4–L5 and L5–S1 levels, indicating desiccation. The epidural veins are engorged above and below the disc (*black arrows*). Compare to the veins at the more cephalad levels.

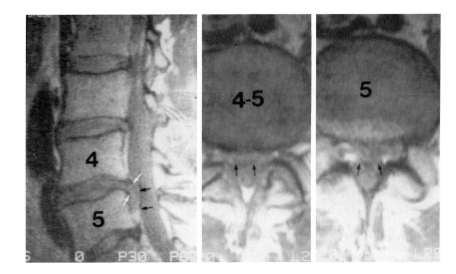

FIG. 7. Herniated disc at the L4–L5 level extending caudally for two-thirds of the height of the body of L5 (*black arrows*) (TR = 1,000 msec; TE = 20 msec). Note disruption of the annulus (*white arrows*). On the axial scans, the central location of the disc herniation is confirmed.

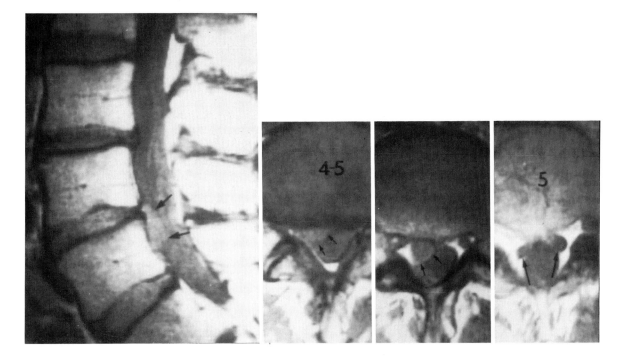

FIG. 8. Sagittal and axial scans demonstrating L4–L5 herniated disc (TR = 600 msec; TE = 20 msec). On the axial exam, the disc is seen to extend to the right-hand side with compression of the thecal sac and displacement of the right L5 nerve root (*arrows*). A large disc extending laterally and caudally is likely to be a free fragment. A free fragment was removed at surgery.

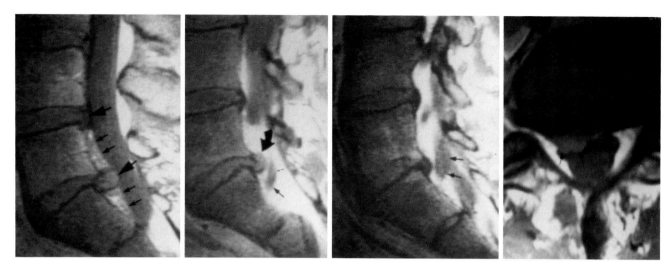

FIG. 9. Herniated disc at the L5–S1 level (TR = 1,000 msec; TE = 20 msec). Note disruption of the annulus on the sagittal image (*lower large arrow*). On the parasagittal images, the relationship of the herniated fragment to the right exiting nerve root can be identified. The axial scan confirms the location of the disc seen on the right parasagittal sections.

nal intensity. The cortex continues to be of lower signal intensity. Emissary veins now appear brightly contrasted as areas of higher signal intensity in the midsagittal sections. The normal hydrated disc is of high signal intensity with a central lower intensity "cleft" on very heavily T2-weighted images in patients over 30 years (Fig. 2). This cleft is thought to represent an invagination of annular lamellae of the annulus into the nucleus (4). Differences in disc hydration are reflected as differences in signal intensity, the desiccated discs being of much lower intensity (Figs. 6 and 11). CSF acquires a very high signal intensity due to its prolonged T2 relaxation times. This high-intensity (white) CSF silhouettes any discs and/or osteophytes that may extend into the canal. Due to flow effects, the signal from the CSF may have an unstructured reticular and/or streak quality that often diminishes the diagnostic utility of the T2-weighted images. Gating during image acquisition can significantly reduce or eliminate these flow artifacts (5).

On T1-weighted axial images, the canal appears as an area of low signal intensity surrounded by bright epidural fat. Nerve roots can frequently be identified within the theca as tubular structures in cross section with signal intensity similar to muscle. Their margins may be indistinct due to motion (Fig. 3). Beyond the dura, exiting nerve roots are clearly identified contrasted by the high signal intensity of epidural fat (Fig. 4). The nerves may be followed laterally as they join to form the ganglion within the foramen. The high contrast between the epidural fat (white) and cortical bone (black) outlines

the foramen. Epidural veins are identified particularly well on axial scans as serpiginous tubular structures of signal void just dorsal to the posterior rim of the cortex of the vertebral body (Fig. 5).

T2-weighted axial lumbar canal images demonstrate increased signal from CSF and with prolonged echoes, diminished signal from epidural fat. Again, CSF motion frequently results in significant degradation of image quality and therefore diagnostic utility.

DEGENERATIVE DISEASE

Intervertebral discs have a variable appearance, depending on their state of hydration and the imaging parameters used. On T1-weighted images, the nucleus is midrange in signal intensity, similar to that of nerve roots. The annulus and adjacent ligaments are of very low signal intensity and cannot be readily distinguished from each other, nor can they be distinguished from adjacent cortical bone. On sagittal images, the cephalad cortical end-plate usually appears much thicker than that of the caudal end-plate. This is the so-called chemical shift artifact that causes the end-plates in the frequency-encoded direction (usually the cephalad end-plate) to appear thicker than the opposite end-plate (Fig. 2). This artifact reflects the differing resonant frequencies of protons in water and fat. It is field-strength related, but in practice no appreciable difference can be detected; for example, between images acquired on

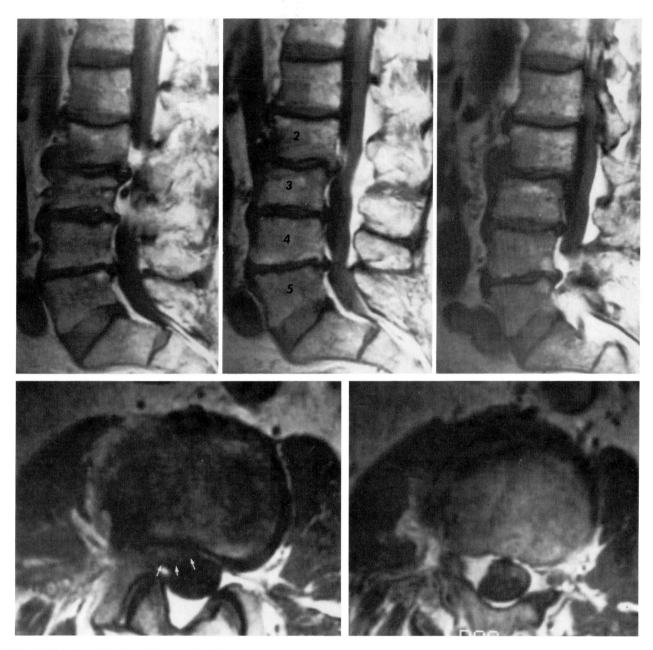

FIG. 10. Herniated lumbar discs at L2–L3, L3–L4, and L4–L5 (TR = 1,000 msec, TE = 20 msec). Herniation is most severe at the L2–L3 level. The disc is seen best in the right paramedian and midline cuts. On the axial cut, the disc fragments are identified in the right gutter (*arrows*). On the more superior axial section, the epidural fat, which has been displaced by the disc, compresses the thecal sac.

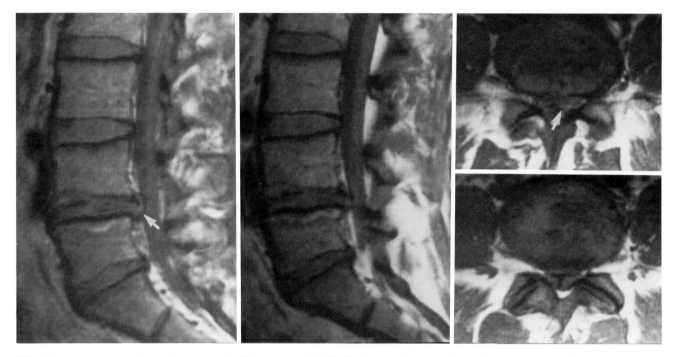

FIG. 11. Severe congenital spinal stenosis. There is an L4–L5 disc herniation, which on the axial cut can be seen to extend primarily to the left (*arrow*). On the axial scans, crowding of the nerve roots can be seen (*lower right*). On the sagittal study (TR = 1,000 msec; TE = 20 msec), there is disruption of the superior portion of the annulus at the L4–L5 level.

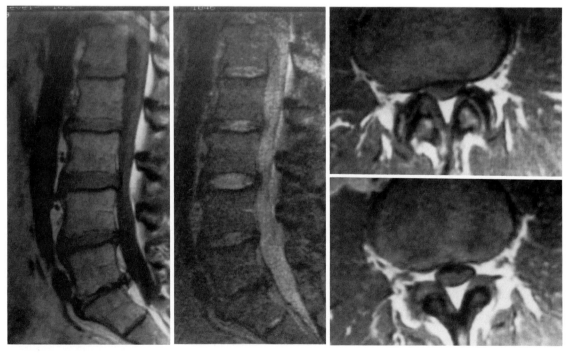

FIG. 12. Small disc herniation at the L5–S1 level and mild bulges at the L3–L4 and L4–L5 levels. The marked narrowing of the anterior-posterior dimensions of the canal are much better appreciated on the more T2-weighted image (TR = 1,000 msec; TE = 70 msec). On the axial scans, the nerve roots appear to fill almost the entire thecal sac.

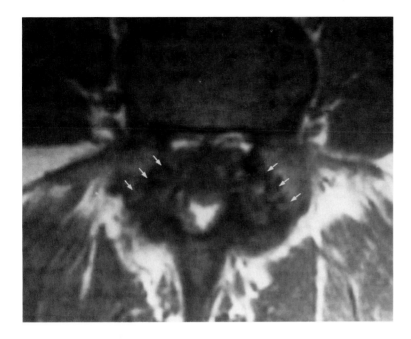

FIG. 13. Grade I spondylolisthesis at the L5–S1 level. Note pars defect on the axial scans (*small arrows*).

FIG. 14. Patient 2 years after lumbar laminectomy and discectomy. Sagittal scans (TR = 1,000 msec; TE = 20/70 msec) show recurrent disc herniation with caudal extension of disc material. More T2-weighted image demonstrates disc desiccation. The axial scan shows absence of the lamina on the left and morphologic appearance of a disc herniation extending to the left. At surgery, a recurrent free fragment was removed.

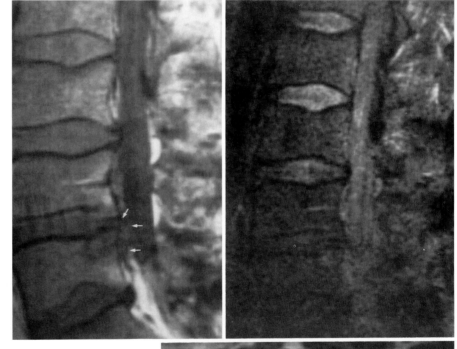

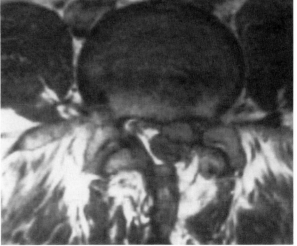

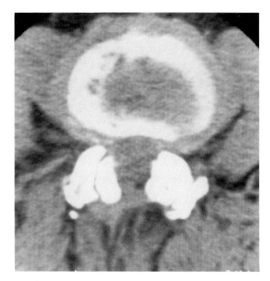

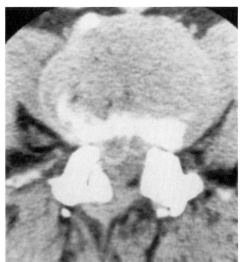

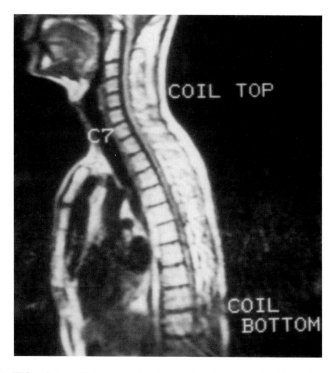

FIG. 16. Localizing scan for thoracic spine examination (TR = 600 msec; one excitation). The cephalocaudad location of the coil can be readily identified. This is a particularly useful technique in imaging the thoracic spine with surface coils because it permits accurate identification of all the vertebral bodies.

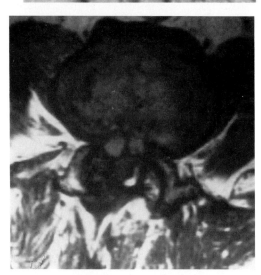

FIG. 15. Pre- and postcontrast CT scan in patient with symptoms of recurrent disc following lumbar laminectomy. On the postcontrast study, a bilobed recurrent disc is outlined by the contrast material. This bilobed disc extrusion is more readily identified on axial MR scan without the aid of any contrast agents (*bottom*).

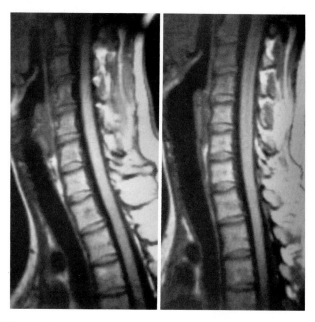

FIG. 17. Normal sagittal cervical spine image (TR = 600 msec; TE = 20 msec) in a 26-year-old woman.

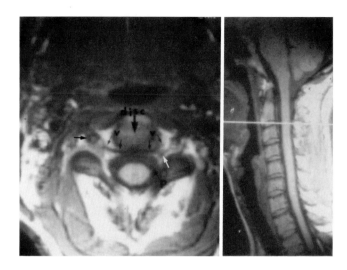

FIG. 18. Axial images (TR = 600 msec; TE = 20 msec) at the C2–C3 interspace demonstrate the epidural veins (v), the dorsal nerve root (p), the ganglia (*diagonal white arrow*), and the vertebral artery (*horizontal black arrow*). The patency of the neural foramina is easily identified due to epidural fat in the normal foramen.

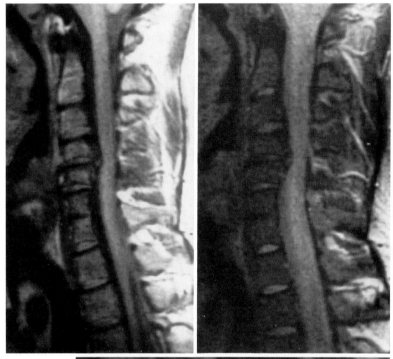

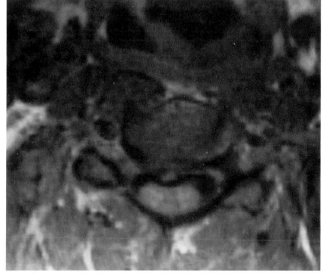

FIG. 19. C4–C5 central disc clearly identified on both T1- (TR = 1,000 msec; TE = 20 msec) and T2- (TR = 1,000 msec; TE = 70 msec) weighted images. The axial section confirms central cord compression.

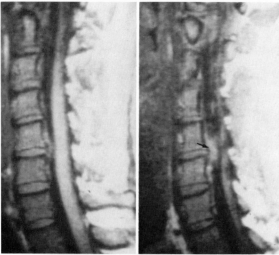

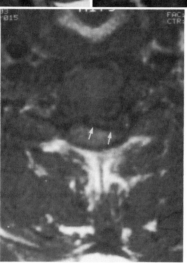

FIG. 20. Midsagittal T1-weighted image (TR = 600 msec; TE = 20 msec) demonstrates disc protrusion at the C5–C6 level, which is much more pronounced on the left parasagittal section. Lateralization of the disc is confirmed by an axial image that demonstrates disc material compressing the cord and extending through the left foramen (*arrows*).

0.5-T and 1.5-T units. It is one of those artifacts that one quickly learns to "see through."

On T2-weighted images, differences in disc hydration become apparent. The normal disc is composed of a central semifluid nucleus pulposus and a peripheral annulus fibrosus. The normal nucleus pulposus in young people is 85% to 90% water. With degeneration or aging or both, fluid content diminishes to 70%. Water content of the fibrous lamellae of the annulus fibrosus is 78% and diminishes to 70% with aging and degeneration. In the aged or desiccated disc, nucleus pulposus and an-

nulus fibrosus can no longer be distinguished (Fig. 6) (6). As T2-weighting increases, CSF signal becomes brighter, whereas signal from cancellous bone diminishes.

On T1-weighted sagittal images, discs and/or osteophytes extending into the epidural space can be readily identified as areas of diminished signal intensity. If the disc is completely desiccated, it is not usually possible to distinguish between disc and osteophyte. Osteophytes may be identified by the presence of fat of high signal intensity that is deposited in the adjacent cancellous bone. It may also be difficult to distinguish between disc herniation and disc bulge. Both, of course, can cause symptoms. Differences in morphology tend to be the most useful signs. Herniation is definitely present when disruption of the annulus with focal disc extrusion can be identified (Fig. 7). A concentric extension of disc material with an intact, but often thin, annulus is regarded as a bulge. Free fragments are portions of disc material that have herniated through the posterior longitudinal ligament (Fig. 8). They are almost always lateral in location because the ligament is so thick in the midline. Often, parasagittal images will demonstrate compression of the exiting nerve root by a lateralized disc (Fig. 9). Axial images are usually more useful in lateralizing a herniated disc. Herniated discs may displace epidural fat. The fat may then compress the thecal sac or adjacent nerve roots (Fig. 10).

Disc pathology can be readily detected on T1-weighted images. T2 weighting provides a myelographic effect and demonstrates desiccation. Signal is degraded by CSF motion. T2-weighted images are most useful for assessing the size of the CSF space. The low-intensity ligaments and cortical bone are silhouetted by the white CSF. In cases of spinal stenosis with or without disc herniation, the intense CSF signal may be especially helpful (Figs. 11 and 12).

It would appear that MR is equivalent to and, in some cases, superior to CT in the detection and localization of disc disease (6–9). The relative sensitivity of CT versus MR in detection and characterization of spondylosis has not been well evaluated. Although MR will often detect the pars defect and slippage, CT appears to be more sensitive in detecting the osseous abnormalities (Fig. 13).

FACET DISEASE

Experience with facet disease is limited. Correlation with clinical symptoms is limited, even with CT. Advanced degenerative changes are readily identified on MR. Cortical bone disruption and/or distortion of facet articular surfaces are usually well delineated both in sagittal and axial planes. CT is certainly superior in providing definition of the facets.

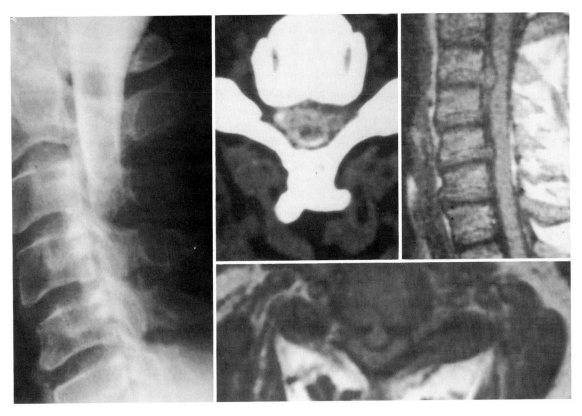

FIG. 21. Water-soluble contrast myelogram. Contrast was introduced at the C1–C2 level. There is partial obstruction to caudal flow at the C3–C4 level compatible with disc disease. Supplemental axial CT shows displacement of contrast in the ventral aspect of the subarachnoid space compatible with herniated disc. A sagittal MR examination (TR = 600 msec; TE = 20 msec) on the same patient demonstrates a large herniated disc at the C3–C4 level extending cephalad and an additional herniated disc at the C5–C6 level. Axial image at the C3–C4 level demonstrates that the disc protrusion is central with secondary deformity of the cord.

POSTOPERATIVE SPINE

The postoperative spine is a difficult diagnostic challenge. Distinction between recurrent disc or scar is elusive by most techniques. Operative confirmation is not always forthcoming. The contrast and spatial detail intrinsic to MR suggest that it will be more specific than CT (Figs. 14 and 15).

CERVICAL AND THORACIC SPINE

The approach to imaging the cervical and thoracic spine is a bit more complicated because patients may present with either myelopathy or radiculopathy.

Imaging Technique

All images are obtained by using surface-receiving coils. When imaging the thoracic spine, a large field of

view sagittal image using the body coil for both transmission and receiving is first obtained with the surface coil in place to localize the coil in the cephalocaudad direction (Fig. 16). T1-weighted sagittal images are then acquired using 3-mm-thick sections (Fig. 17). Axial images are usually acquired, using 5-mm-thick sections (Fig. 18). Thinner sections would be more desirable to obtain improved spatial detail, but reduction in S/N significantly compromises the diagnostic quality of the images.

Radiculopathy

Most disc disease can be identified in the sagittal plane. The sagittal images are usually supplemented with a T1-weighted axial scan (Fig. 19). The axial images assist in lateralization of the offending disc and more reliably identify lesions in the lateral recesses and foramina (Fig. 20). The axial images are more sensitive in

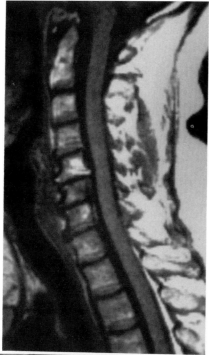

ence of spondylosis may be heralded by the often associated replacement of marrow by fat at the site of the degenerative disease (Fig. 22). Image quality in the thoracic area is somewhat degraded by superimposed artifact from cardiac and respiratory motion as well as flow through the great vessels (Fig. 23). The implementation of both respiratory compensation and cardiac gating may significantly improve the quality of these images. In postoperative spine examinations, an area of signal void may be identified at the operative site. This is usually a paramagnetic artifact associated with metallic fragments that are generated by contact between the drill and the metallic sucker (Fig. 24).

In those patients with radiculopathy in whom both the sagittal and axial scans are interpreted as normal, an intrathecal contrast (ITC) CT may be warranted. The ITC CT is the more sensitive and is possibly more specific. It is usually not performed as the first study of choice because it is (a) invasive, (b) involves exposure to ionizing radiation, and (c) is usually more costly.

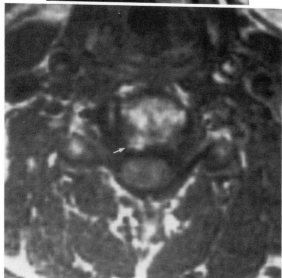

FIG. 22. A 62-year-old man with right-sided radiculopathy. Sagittal image (TR = 600 msec; TE = 25 msec) demonstrates cervical spondylosis at the C5–C6 level. Note bright signal in the osteophyte secondary to replacement of marrow by fat. The osteophyte impresses the ventral aspect of the cord. Axial image localizes the spondolytic process to the right side (*arrow*).

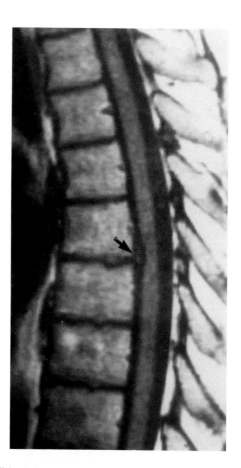

FIG. 23. A 32-year-old man with thoracic radicular pain. Sagittal MR (TR = 1,000 msec; TE = 20 msec) demonstrates thoracic disc compressing the ventral aspect of the cord at the T8–T9 level.

the detection of spondylotic lesions compromise of the neural foramen and ligamentous hypertrophy and/or calcification with secondary cord compression. Rotation, displacement, and compression of the cord are better appreciated in the axial plane (Fig. 21). The pres-

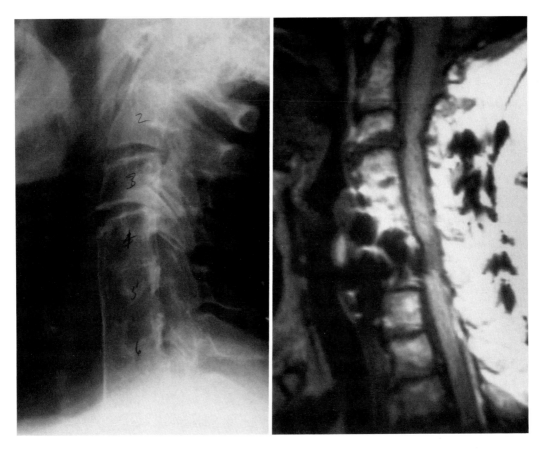

FIG. 24. A 54-year-old man following anterior cervical discectomy and fusion of the C4–C6 levels for cervical myelopathy. Sagittal MR exam (TR = 1,000 msec; TE = 20 msec) shows multiple areas of low signal that appear as artifacts that are usually attributed to metal; yet, there is no evidence of metallic bodies on the plain film. These artifacts are believed to represent metallic fragments left behind during surgical extirpation of the disc and placement of the bone graft. Fragments are probably secondary to the drill coming into contact with the tip of the metallic sucker, with resultant deposition of metallic fragments.

CERVICAL AND THORACIC MYELOPATHY

MR is superior to any other imaging modality in the evaluation of patients with myelopathy (10). The initial acquisition should be a relatively T1-weighted sagittal image (TR = 600–1,000 msec). The sagittal image will almost always demonstrate cord compression, widening, and/or cavitation. This imaging technique is relatively insensitive to lesions that manifest themselves primarily as regions of demyelination. If demyelination is suspect and/or if the T1-weighted image is normal, then a T2-weighted sagittal image is appropriate. An asymmetric echo technique, as described with lumbar disc disease, may serve to provide adequate T1- and T2-weighted images. If cord widening is present, and/or if tumor is suspect and the T1-weighted sagittal MR is negative, then a T2-weighted sagittal image may provide additional information. If cord cavitation is detected, the most caudal aspects of the cavity should be identified, and if an associated tumor is suspect, then T2-weighted imaging techniques may be required to detect alterations in signal intensity that may serve to distin-

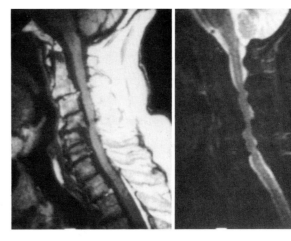

FIG. 25. A 70-year-old woman with cervical myelopathy. Sagittal image (TR = 600 msec; TE = 25 msec) demonstrates advanced degenerative changes in the cervical vertebra with spondylosis most pronounced at the C2–C3, C3–C4, and C5–C6 levels. There is significant cord compression at the C2–C3 and C4–C5 levels. T2-weighted image (TR = 2,000 msec; TE = 25 msec) shows loss of all CSF signal from C2 through C6.

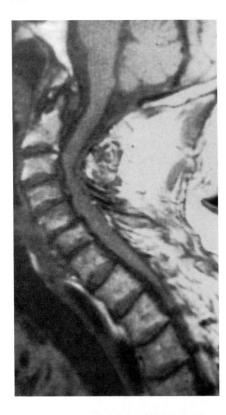

FIG. 26. A 58-year-old man after cervical laminectomy for myelopathy secondary to spinal stenosis. Note continued ventral impression on the cord by herniated disc material and spondylosis at the C3–C4, C4–C5, and C6–C7 levels. MR in the future may serve to focus on the relative benefits of posterior versus anterior approaches for cervical disc disease and/or spondylosis.

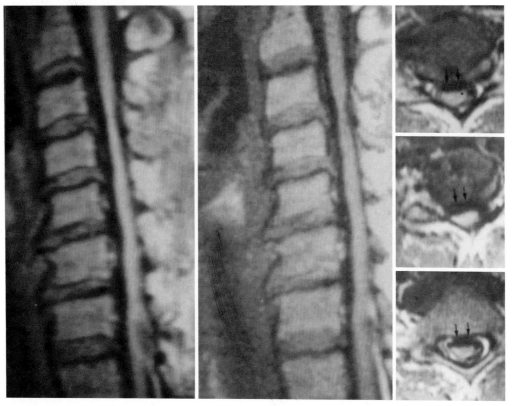

FIG. 27. A 44-year-old man with cervical myelopathy. Sagittal image (TR = 600 msec; TE = 25 msec) shows irregular narrowing of the cord. Careful inspection indicates that there is a longitudinal area of very low signal intensity associated with disc herniations parasagittally. The findings are confirmed on the axial scan in which an ovoid-shaped lesion of very low signal intensity is compressing the cervical cord. If the signal intensity is reversed, the diagnosis of ossification of the posterior longitudinal ligament (OPLL) would have been more readily appreciated. The MR examination is in fact superior to any other imaging study in detecting the abnormality and characterizing its impact on the cervical cord.

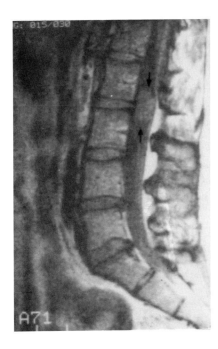

FIG. 28. Sagittal image (TR = 1,000 msec; TE = 20 msec) demonstrating a conus mass (*arrows*) at the L2–L3 level. A tumor at this site is most likely a conus ependymoma. Lesion was proven at surgery.

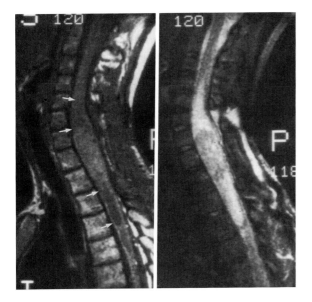

FIG. 29. Cervicothoracic sagittal image (*left*) (TR = 1,000 msec; TE = 20 msec) demonstrates widening of the cervicothoracic cord. The widest portion of the cord is at the C7–T2 levels and is of higher signal intensity on the T1-weighted image than the adjacent cord. Above and below this surgically proven astrocytoma are well-marginated areas of homogeneous low signal intensity representing cysts capping both the cephalad and caudal portions of the tumor (*arrows*), a finding not uncommon in astrocystomas. On the T2-weighted image (*right*) (TR = 2,000 msec; TE = 20 msec), the tumor cysts are now of higher signal intensity than the adjacent solid portion of the lesion. This has occurred because we are beyond the crossover point on the T2 decay curve.

guish the tumor from the associated cyst. In practice, this is rarely necessary.

In those patients in whom the lesion is extramedullary and either intra- or extradural, the T1-weighted sagittal images should be supplemented with a T1-weighted axial scan for improved localization. It is rare that a supplemental T2-weighted image is either required or useful.

SPINAL STENOSIS

Cervical spinal stenosis is usually degenerative in nature, not infrequently with a superimposed congenitally small cervical spinal canal. Canal compression may also be ligamentous. Sagittal MR exams are uniquely sensitive in detection and characterization (Figs. 25–27).

INTRINSIC CORD TUMORS

Ninety percent of intrinsic cord tumors are either ependymomas (60%) or astrocytomas (30%). Ependymomas usually occur in the region of the conus (Fig. 28). A significant number also occur, however, in the cervical region. They are more common in adults. Astrocytomas are more common in the cervicothoracic region and are more frequently seen in children. It is not uncommon for cysts to cap both the cephalad and caudal portions of intrinsic cord tumors. They are noncommunicating and often have an elevated protein content.

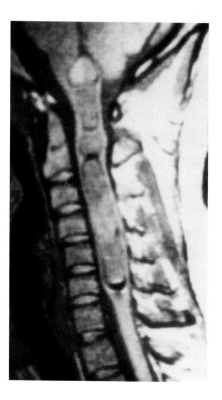

FIG. 30. Cystic intrinsic cervical tumor with contents of mixed signal intensity. The cystic quality is based primarily on smooth margins and fluid-fluid layers. At surgery, biopsy revealed an astrocytoma. The cyst contents were hemorrhagic.

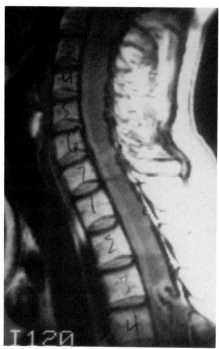
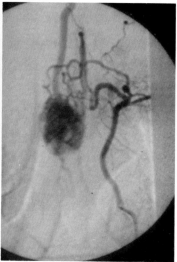

FIG. 31. Cervicothoracic sagittal image (TR = 1,000 msec; TE = 70 msec). The entire cord is wide. A large dorsal draining vein is depicted as a serpiginous structure of very low signal intensity (signal void). At the T3–T4 level, a solid vascular nidus is seen as an area of higher signal intensity interspersed with serpiginous areas of signal void. The widened portion of the cord cephalad to the nidus is cystic based on homogeneity of signal and smooth contours. Spinal angiogram demonstrates a highly vascular tumor supplied by the radicular branch of the left T3 intercostal artery. The dorsal draining vein is midline. Angiographic appearance is specific for hemangioblastoma; so is the MR image.

FIG. 32. A 24-year-old woman with progressive paraparesis and sensory deficit of the lower extremities. A water-soluble myelogram with contrast introduced from above and below indicates an intramedullary lesion approximately one vertebral body in length. Sagittal MR (TR = 1,000 msec; TE = 20 msec) demonstrates partially cystic intramedullary lesion with a focal area of high signal intensity (*arrow*). T2-weighted image (TR = 2,000 msec; TE = 20 msec) demonstrates an area of increased signal intensity surrounding the tumor but loss of the focal area of high signal seen on the T1-weighted image. This sequence of changes in the latter area is most compatible with fat, suggesting either a teratoma or hamartoma. At surgery, histologic specimen con-

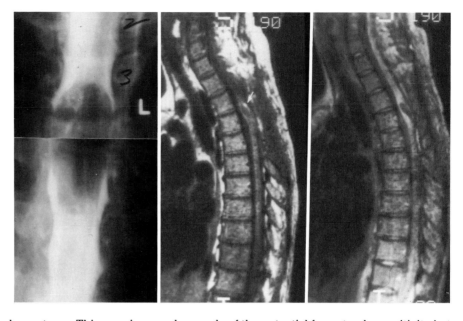

firmed the diagnosis of intramedullary hamartoma. This case is a good example of the potential for not only sensitivity but specificity with MR.

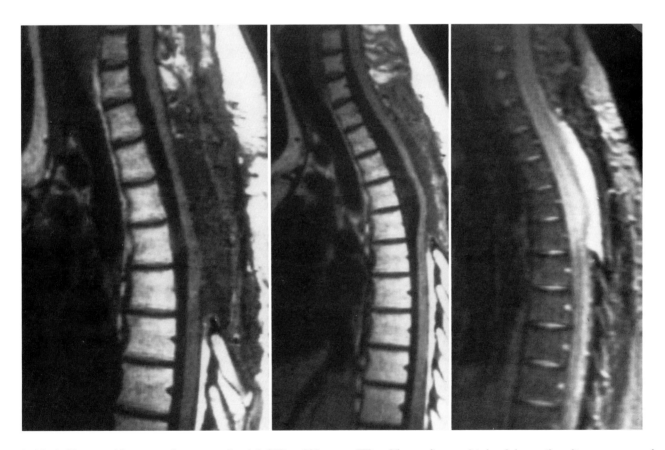

FIG. 33. A 35-year-old woman. Image on the *left* (TR = 600 msec; TE = 25 msec) was obtained 4 months after surgery and radiation therapy for a cervicothoracic ependymoma. Repeat examination (*center*) 1 year later (TR = 600 msec; TE = 25 msec) demonstrates progressive decrease in the cord diameter and tethering of the cord to the posterior aspect of the canal and an outpouching that is a pseudomeningocele. On a T2-weighted image (TR = 2,000 msec; TE = 70 msec), the pseudomeningocele has a higher signal intensity than the adjacent CSF space. This reflects relatively less CSF motion rather than elevated CSF protein content.

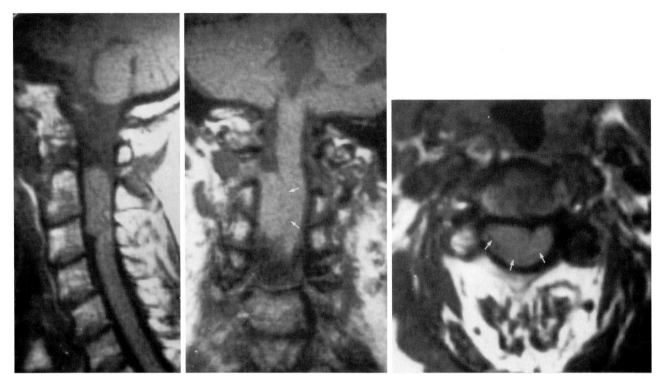

FIG. 34. A 67-year-old woman with upper- and lower-extremity weakness. Sagittal, coronal, and axial MR images (TR = 600 msec; TE = 20 msec) show an isointense mass compressing the lateral aspect of the cord and displacing it to the left. Although there is no difference in signal intensity between the tumor and the cord, high spatial detail provides discrimination between the two (*arrows*). At surgery, a meningioma was removed.

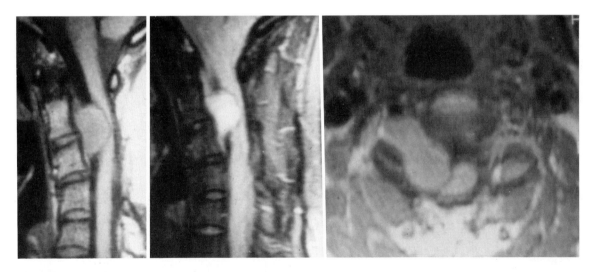

FIG. 35. Patient with known neurofibromatosis presenting with spasticity. Sagittal image (**left**) (TR = 1,000 msec; TE = 20 msec) demonstrates large, well-circumscribed lesion at the C1–C2 level compressing the ventral aspect of the cord. The T2-weighted image (**center**) (TR = 2,000 msec; TE = 20 msec) demonstrates increased signal intensity but provides no additional information. The axial image (**right**) is of more value in that it indicates the dumbbell-shaped nature of the lesion, which extends out through the neural foramen laterally and medially compresses the dural sac and displaces the cord to the left. No additional studies were required prior to surgery.

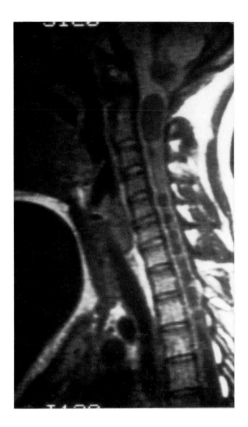

FIG. 36. Hydromyelia associated with Chiari malformation. Note irregular cystic dilatation of the cord extending to the posterior aspect of the fourth ventricle. Synechiae segmenting the hydromyelic cavity are not an uncommon finding.

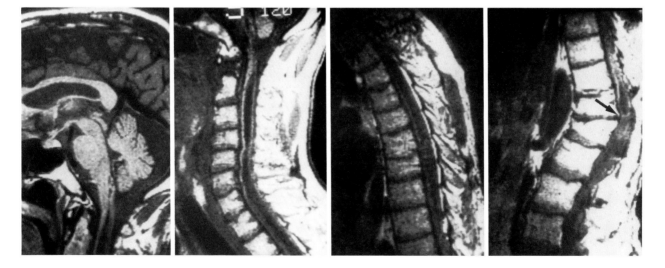

FIG. 37. Post-traumatic syrinx extending from the posterior aspect of the fourth ventricle caudally to the T11–T12 level (*arrow*) at the site of a traumatic compression fracture, which compresses the cord and compromises the subarachnoid space.

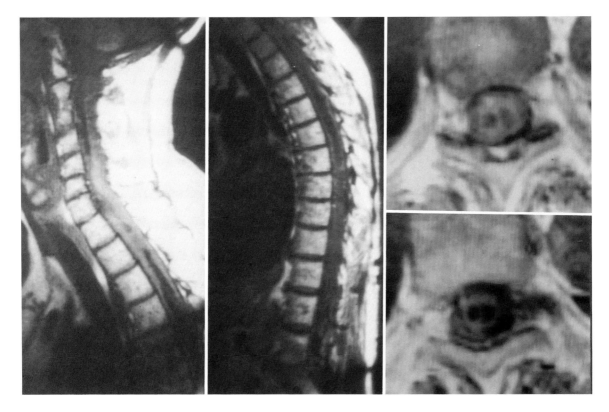

FIG. 38. A 37-year-old patient with long-tract signs 2 years after listeria meningitis. There is obliteration of the normal subarachnoid space and secondary cavitation of the cord identified both on sagittal (TR = 600 msec; TE = 25 msec) and axial (TR = 1,000 msec; TE = 25 msec) sections.

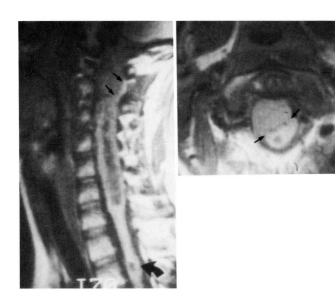

FIG. 39. T1-weighted sagittal image in a patient with spasticity demonstrates a mass ventral to the cord of the C1–C2 level (*arrows*). The cord is draped over the dorsal aspect of the mass. Of interest is a cavity below the level of the mass. The relationships between the extra-axial mass and the cord cavitation are better appreciated on the axial image. At surgery, an extra-axial meningioma was removed. Cord cavitation resulted from interruption of normal CSF pathways.

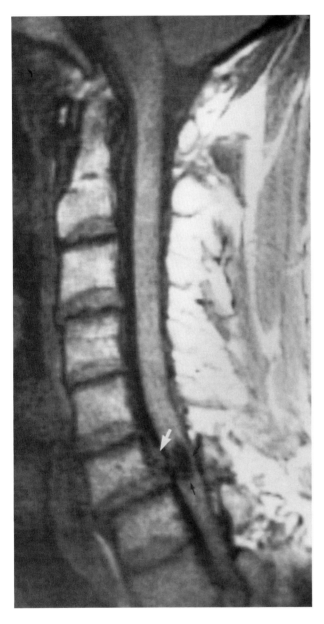

FIG. 40. A 27-year-old patient examined 4 months after traumatic disc herniation (*white arrows*) and development of secondary focal myelomalacia (*black arrows*).

These cysts are more commonly seen in astrocytomas (Figs. 29 and 30). MR readily distinguishes between solid and cystic portions of tumors, in contrast to myelography and/or CT, which rarely accomplish this degree of characterization. On T1-weighted images, the cord will appear as an area of increased diameter. The cyst(s) above and/or below appear as areas that are smooth in contour. Cyst contents usually have a T1 relaxation time equal to or shorter than CSF. The T1

shortening may reflect increased protein content and/or absence or relative paucity of fluid motion.

Other far less common intrinsic cord tumors to be considered within the spinal axis include hemangioblastoma (2.5%) (Fig. 31), metastatic tumor, melanoma, hamartoma (Fig. 32), gliosarcoma, etc. The presence of a small solid lesion with an associated large vessel and a large cyst should strongly favor a diagnosis of hemangioblastoma. The use of paramagnetic contrast agents has proven useful in improving sensitivity in detecting both intrinsic and extrinsic cord tumors (11), especially in lower resolution equipment.

In patients who have been operated on for intrinsic cord tumors and/or who have received radiotherapy, a diminution in cord diameter may ensue. Frequently, the cord becomes tethered to the dorsal aspect of the canal (Fig. 33). There are no known clinical symptoms associated with this tethering. Another finding in the postoperative spine in patients who have had a laminectomy is the development of a pseudomeningocele (Fig. 33). Anatomically, there is an outpouching of the dura and/or subarachnoid space. The signal intensity on T2-weighted images is greater than that of CSF in the remainder of the canal. This increased signal intensity reflects diminished and/or absent flow and does not reflect increased protein. This region of increased signal intensity should not be mistaken for a loculated space.

Extramedullary intradural lesions account for more than 55% of spinal neoplasms. The most common encountered are meningiomas (Fig. 34) and neurinomas (Fig. 35). They are both of similar intensity to the cord on T1-weighted images and may or may not exhibit increased signal intensity on T2-weighted images. Approximately 80% of meningiomas are located in the thoracic region and are in women.

CORD CAVITATION

There are multiple causes of cavitary disease in the cord (12). One of the more common is hydromyelia, which is a dilatation of the central canal lined by ependyma indigenous to the central canal. These hydromyelic cavities are most commonly seen in the Chiari I malformation. The cavity is contiguous with the posterior aspect of the fourth ventricle and often extends through the entire length of the cord. There are often "haustra" and/or synechiae at multiple intervals along the length of the cavity (Fig. 36). There appears to be substantial flow within the hydromyelic cavity (5,13). Protein content is normal, so that the fluid has T1 and T2 relaxation times similar to that of CSF.

Another type of cord cavitation is syringomyelia, which by strict definition develops eccentric to the cen-

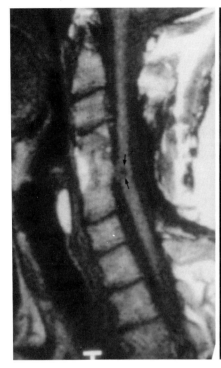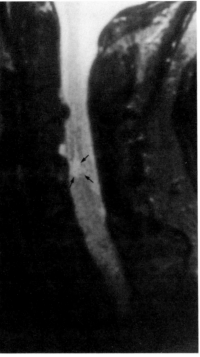

FIG. 41. A 52-year-old man 4 months after anterior discectomy and fusion at the C4–C5 level. Motor symptoms following surgery can be explained by the focal area of myelomalacia (*arrow*) (TR = 600 msec; TE = 25 msec; TR = 2,000 msec; TE = 25 msec).

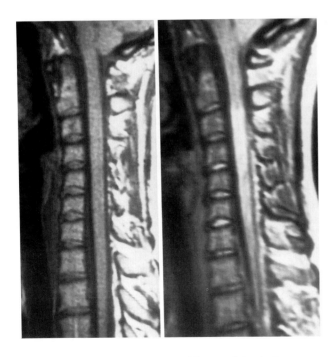

FIG. 42. A 34-year-old woman with spasticity in lower extremities. T1-weighted sagittal MR examination on the *left* (TR = 1,000 msec; TE = 20 msec) shows very subtle increase in cord diameter at the C3–C4 level. More T2-weighted sequence (*right*) (TR = 1,000 msec; TE = 70 msec) shows a definite area of increased signal intensity covering several segments. Patient has clinically definite multiple sclerosis.

tral canal but often communicates with it. The cavity is usually not lined by ependymal cells. Syringomyelia may develop following a vascular, traumatic, or hemorrhagic insult to the cord. Distinction between hydromyelia and syringomyelia may not always be clear or possible, and the terms may be interchanged by many authors. Post-traumatic syringomyelia, for example, is in fact a dilatation of the central canal. It manifests itself as a dilatation of the cord above an obstruction and/or compression of the cord and subarachnoid space secondary to trauma (Fig. 37). Dilatation of the central canal may also be seen following obliteration of the subarachnoid spaces by infection (Fig. 38). Both post-traumatic and postinfectious syringomyelia usually develop 2 to 3 or more years after the initial insult. Widespread availability of improved imaging techniques have made us aware that these lesions are more common than heretofore thought (14). MRI has proven to be invaluable in assessing patients following surgical procedures for correction of cavitary disease (15). Extramedullary intradural masses can also on occasion cause cord cavitation secondary to obstruction of normal CSF pathways (Fig. 39) (16). Trauma to the cord without compromise of the CSF pathways may cause myelomalacia, which may, but rarely, evolve into a syrinx. These post-traumatic cysts and/or cord softening are generically classified clinically as post-traumatic progressive myelopathy (3). These lesions rarely result in cord dilata-

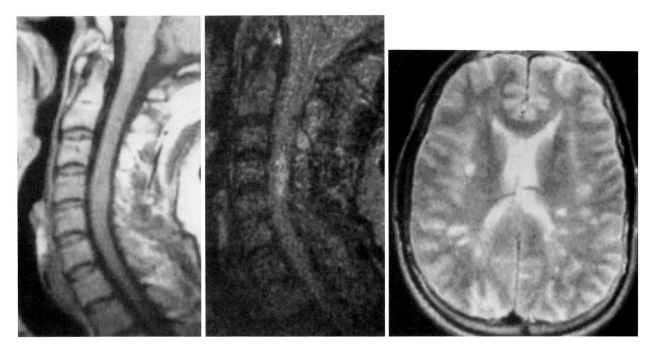

FIG. 43. A 54-year-old man presenting with progressive weakness and decreased sensation of the lower extremities. Sagittal cervical spine examination (TR = 500 msec; TE = 30 msec) demonstrates focal widening of the cord at the C4–C5 level, which increases in relative signal on T2-weighted images (TR = 1,500 msec; TE = 90 msec). The lesion could easily be mistaken for an intramedullary tumor. A T2-weighted brain examination (TR = 2,000 msec; TE = 90 msec) was requested because the cord widening was so focal, an unusual finding for an intrinsic tumor. The brain scan demonstrated multiple areas of increased signal intensity in the white matter, compatible with multiple sclerosis. The patient improved without therapy.

tion. They are not felt by most to improve following shunting procedures (Figs. 40 and 41). Shunting is therefore not appropriate.

Imaging of cord cavitary disease can usually be more than adequately accomplished with T1-weighted sagittal images (5,17). Areas of myelomalacia and/or demyelination are better detected with intermediate weighting (TR 1,500) (14). Placement of the surface coil at multiple levels may be required in order to delineate the full extent of large cavitary lesions.

DEMYELINATING DISEASE

The most common demyelinating process involving the cord is multiple sclerosis. These lesions often cover several segments and have poorly defined margins (Fig. 42). They are well demonstrated on T2-weighted sagittal images (18). There is usually no cord widening. If widening does occur, a mistaken diagnosis of tumor may ensue. If there are any doubts, a T2-weighted head exam should be performed (Fig. 43). The concordance of cord and brain lesions is not known at this time. We have seen a small number of cases in which patients with clinically definite multiple sclerosis have had cord lesions on MR and normal MR exams of the brain.

INFLAMMATORY DISEASE

MR is most effective in delineating subdural or epidural fluid collections. Subdural or epidural inflammatory collections should exhibit T1 relaxation times that are slightly shorter than that of CSF and T2 relaxation times that are prolonged but shorter than T2 relaxation of CSF. In vertebral osteomyelitis, there is displacement of the normal intermediate to bright signal of cancellous bone by inflammatory tissue of low signal intensity on T1-weighted images and on T2-weighted images, a higher signal intensity than normal in the bone marrow. As is characteristic of spine infections, the adjacent endplates and disc are involved. The disc therefore is also of high signal intensity on T2-weighted images (19). There may be involvement of adjacent soft tissues as well (Figs. 44 and 45). Following discectomy or chymopapain injection, the alterations in signal intensity of the vertebral bodies are identical, but the signal emanating from the discs remains low both on T1- and T2-weighted images.

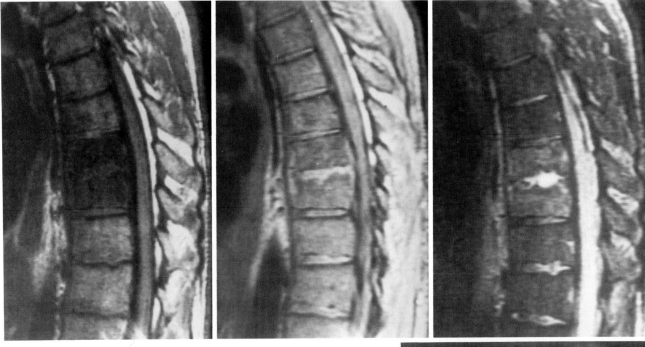

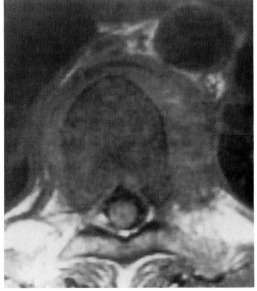

FIG. 44. Bacterial epidural abscess and osteomyelitis in a 27-year-old heroin addict with fever and back pain. Thoracic sagittal image (*left*) (TR = 1,000 msec; TE = 20 msec) demonstrates loss of signal in the T8 and T9 vertebral bodies and loss of definition of adjacent vertebral end-plates. Second echo (*center*) (TR = 1,000 msec; TE = 70 msec) demonstrates marked increase in signal intensity in the intervertebral disc space. Loss of the cortical margins of the vertebral end-plates is more readily appreciated. On the T2-weighted sagittal image (*right*) (TR = 2,000 msec; TE = 20 msec), the involved vertebral bodies and disc spaces exhibit a signal intensity much more intense than the adjacent normal vertebral bodies. This presumably reflects increased water content associated with an inflammatory process. On the axial image, soft-tissue involvement in the form of a "peel" surrounding the vertebral body is easily appreciated. (Courtesy Betsy A. Holland, M.D., Marin General Hospital.)

The vertebral end-plates may be normal or appear slightly irregular. Pathologic correlation is not available. This latter group of findings may represent ischemia of adjacent cancellous bone and/or a sterile inflammatory process (Fig. 46). Another inflammatory disease involving the spinal axis is rheumatoid arthritis (Fig. 47). MR demonstrates the pannus formation of the C1–C2 articulation and may show altered signal in involved vertebral bodies.

Arachnoiditis is not reliably identified on MR. Intrathecal contrast CT examinations are currently more sensitive and are recommended. Pantopaque, which may accompany arachnoiditis, has a characteristic MR appearance (20) (Fig. 48). Experience with imaging of arachnoid adhesions or arachnoiditis is limited.

METASTATIC DISEASE

Metastatic disease is usually blood borne and most commonly involves vertebral bodies and, secondarily, the adjacent canal. Rarely, blood-borne lesions may go

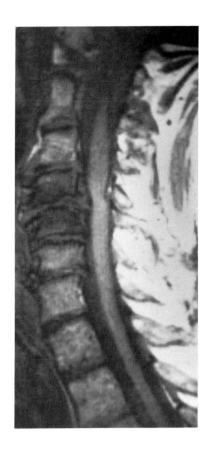

FIG. 45. A 36-year-old woman with neck pain. Sagittal image (TR = 600 msec; TE = 20 msec) demonstrates loss of normal vertebral body signal intensity at the C4 and C5 levels. Adjacent end-plates are eroded. There is a soft-tissue mass ventral to the cord. Involvement of two adjacent vertebral bodies and associated soft-tissue mass is fairly typical of infection. Culture of material removed at surgery revealed coccidioidomycosis.

FIG. 46. A 22-year-old man following L4–L5 discectomy with persistent focal low-back pain. Recurrent disc herniation is present. Note low signal intensity in the cancellous portion of the L4 and the L5 vertebral bodies (*arrows*) adjacent to the interspace (TR = 1,000 msec; TE = 20 msec) and the increased signal intensity in the more T2-weighted image (TR = 1,000 msec; TE = 70 msec). There is no increase in signal intensity in the disc, and the end-plates appear to be within normal limits. Pathologic correlation is not available. Signal changes may represent either focal ischemia and/or a sterile inflammatory process in which the disc is spared.

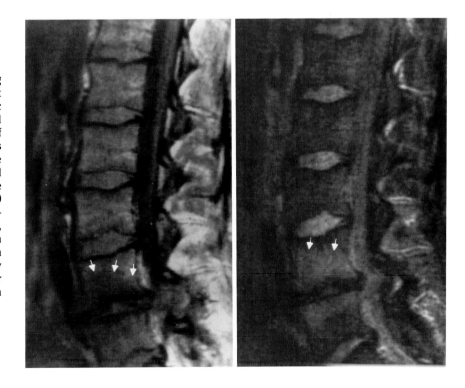

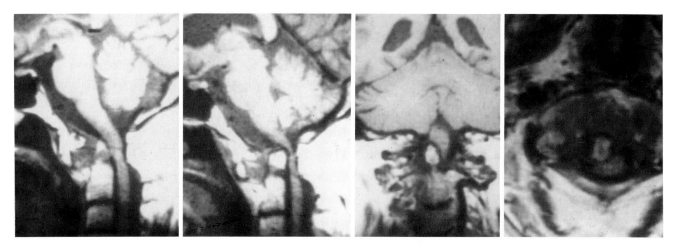

FIG. 47. An elderly female with rheumatoid arthritis and spastic quadriparesis, suggesting a foramen magnum lesion. Sagittal MR (TR = 600 msec; TE = 25 msec) shows marked increase in the distance between the anterior arch of C1 to the dens due to pannus formation. The ventral portion of the cord is compressed by the dens and displaced to the left.

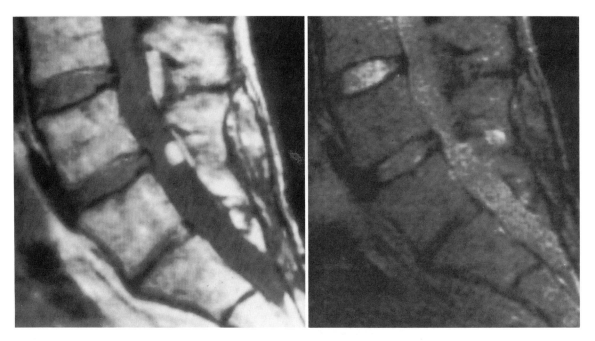

FIG. 48. Focal area of high signal intensity on a T1-weighted sagittal examination (*left*) (TR = 1,000 msec; TE = 20 msec) represents Pantopaque. With increased T2-weighting (TR = 1,000 msec; TE = 70 msec), there was a rapid loss of signal intensity in the same region. Signal from Pantopaque behaves in the same fashion as fat.

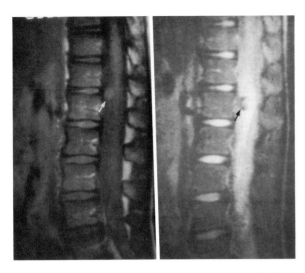

FIG. 49. A 17-year-old man with pinealoma. *Arrow* indicates drop metastasis at the T12–L1 level. The lesion is easily identified on the T1-weighted sagittal image (TR = 1,000 msec; TE = 20 msec). The T2-weighted image (TR = 2,000 msec; TE = 20 msec) provides a myelographic effect but no additional diagnostic information.

directly to the cord. More frequently, lesions that are metastatic to the cord or subarachnoid space are drop metastasis (Figs. 49 and 50). MR is uniquely sensitive to the detection of metastatic lesions. On T1-weighted images, metastases usually appear as areas of decreased signal intensity, displacing the normal high signal in marrow. Disc spaces are typically spared (Fig. 51). Impingement on the subarachnoid space and/or compres-

sion of the cord is readily identified in sagittal images (Fig. 52). On T2-weighted images, there is usually a reversal of signal intensities in which the metastatic lesion appears bright in contrast to the bone marrow, which loses much of its signal intensity in later echoes (Fig. 53). Infiltrative lesions such as neuroblastoma can also be readily detected as altered marrow signal intensity (21). MR should be the first study of choice in dealing with a patient with known or suspected metastatic disease with onset of neurologic symptoms or severe bone pain or both. Myelography should rarely be necessary or indicated. Pathologic fracture can usually be distinguished from osteoporotic compression fracture. In the latter, the normal signal intensity of the vertebral body is maintained (bright on T1 weighting), although vertebral body height is reduced (Fig. 54).

HEMORRHAGE

Although there is limited experience with detection of hemorrhagic lesions in the cord, subacute collections of blood both within the cord substance and/or the subdural or epidural spaces appear as areas of increased signal intensity on both T1- and T2-weighted images (Fig. 55). We have had no experience to date with acute hemorrhage into the cord. There is no reason to suspect that the appearance should be any different from that described within the brain substance. The long-term sequelae of hemorrhage into the cord is identical to that seen with intracranial hemorrhage—a hemosiderin-laden cicatrix (Fig. 56). Vascular malformations appear as serpiginous areas of signal void. On MR, as in angiography, the veins are larger and more distinctive than the

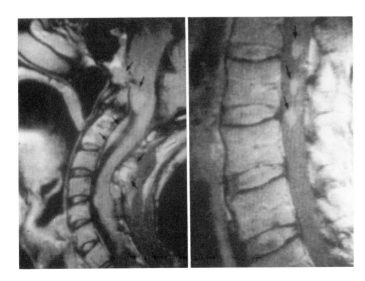

FIG. 50. An unusual case of a 27-year-old woman with a clivus chordoma, the caudal portion of which is compressing the brainstem. Both findings are indicated by the *arrows* in the upper portion of the image on the left. This patient has dural metastasis at the C1–C2 level (*arrows*) and at the C3–C4 level posteriorly (*arrows*). The thoracolumbar image (*right*) demonstrates three additional drop lesions (*arrows*).

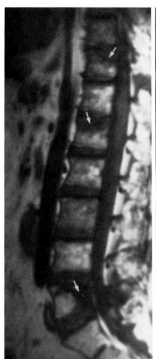
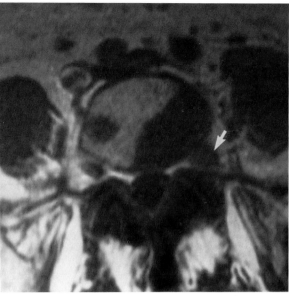

FIG. 51. Patient with known metastatic prostate carcinoma. Sagittal image (TR = 1,000 msec; TE = 20 msec) shows replacement of the normal high signal intensity of cancellous bone by low-signal-intensity metastatic tumor (*arrows*). Axial scan at the L5 level demonstrates involvement of the posterior elements as well as the vertebral body. Note narrowing of the foramen on the left and enlargement of the nerve root (*arrows*) on the left secondary to compression.

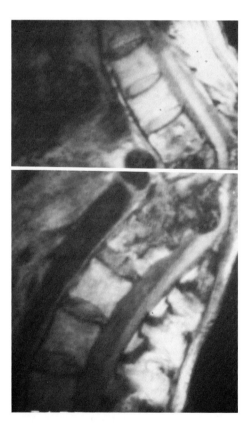

FIG. 52. Patient with known renal cell carcinoma, with metastasis to the thoracolumbar spine. In a single sagittal weighted image (TR = 600 msec; TE = 20 msec), relationships of the tumor to the cord are readily identified. No additional imaging studies were required for either surgery or radiotherapy.

arteries (Fig. 57). MR should prove to be a most sensitive technique for detecting both intramedullary and dural vascular malformations (22). Its sensitivity in comparison to myelography is not established. If high-quality imaging is available, our experience suggests that myelography will be supplanted. Cryptic cord malformations have not heretofore been described, probably due to lack of an adequately sensitive or specific diagnostic modality. Figure 58 illustrates a cryptic malformation of the cervical cord identified on MR. The appearance of a high-intensity methemoglobin-containing central portion and a low-intensity hemosiderin-laden capsule is identical to that described in cryptic malformations in the brain (see Chapter 13).

TRAUMA

Experience with MR in trauma is limited. Once the practical issues of patient handling are addressed, MRI should have a multitude of applications. Deranged relationships of vertebral bodies and/or discs are readily detected. Most important, the relationship of these structures to the adjacent cord and/or nerve roots is elegantly demonstrated by MR (Figs. 59 and 60). The cord integrity, both as the result of acute (Fig. 61) or old (Fig. 62) trauma, can be readily established. Prior to the availability of MRI, early assessment of cord edema, hemorrhage, compression, or cord section was not possi-

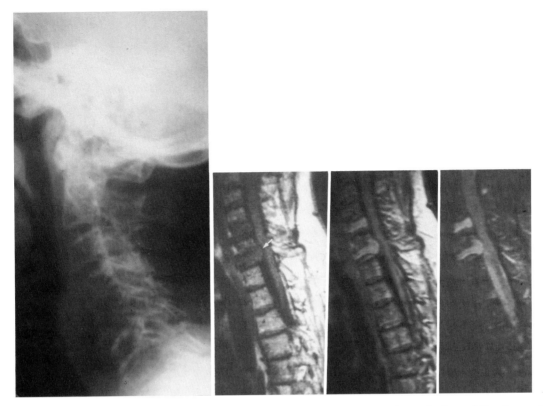

FIG. 53. A 68-year-old patient with known myeloma presents with progressive quadriparesis. Lateral C-spine series demonstrates multiple lytic lesions in the cervical spine that simply confirm the known diagnosis of myeloma. Sagittal T1-weighted (*left*) image shows replacement of the vertebral body at the C5 and C7 levels, with cord compression at the C7 level (*arrow*). The T2-weighted images (*center* and *right*) demonstrate signal reversal but provide little additional information. This case illustrates the lack of utility of plain radiographs in a patient with symptomatic metastatic disease. MR examination should be the first study of choice. It is usually the only examination required.

ble. Issues of spine stability and facet integrity continue to be better addressed with plain films and/or CT.

CONGENITAL SPINE LESIONS

There are a multiplicity of congenital spine lesions. In most clinically significant lesions, the clinician and the radiologist are primarily interested in deranged neural tissue anatomy. Since MRI is the most sensitive technique available for imaging neural elements, it should be the first imaging examination performed. Plain films should be considered supplementary to demonstrate, for example, accompanying vertebral abnormalities.

The most commonly encountered anomaly is the Chiari I malformation in which there is a downward herniation of the tonsils with no displacement of the fourth ventricle or any other posterior fossa structures. On MR, the tonsil is pointed and extends below the foramen magnum (Fig. 63). This should be contrasted with the normal rounded tonsil, which may be seen ex-

tending just below the outer table of the foramen magnum (Fig. 64). Hydromyelia accompanies the Chiari I malformation in as high as 50% of cases. Attention should always be paid to the cervical cord to determine if a cord cavity is present. In patients with gait abnormalities who are examined to screen for multiple sclerosis, a sagittal image should always be obtained to rule out a Chiari I malformation. During a 1-year period, we identified three patients who were being screened for multiple sclerosis and instead were demonstrated to harbor a Chiari I malformation.

Tethering of the cord is another relatively common congenital anomaly. In neonates and children, it is frequently associated with a meningomyelocele. It is usually discovered early in life because of associated overlying cutaneous abnormalities. A T1-weighted sagittal examination is the most useful screening technique. The tethered cord is usually ventral to the overlying lipoma. Accompanying laminar dysraphism can be identified on the axial sections. Tethering of the cord in children may occasionally be associated with more se-

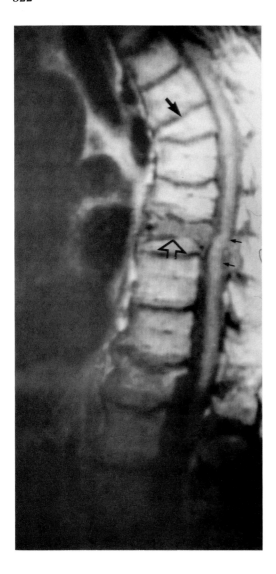

FIG. 54. A 72-year-old woman with known metastatic melanoma who developed symptoms of cord compression. Sagittal MR image (TR = 1,000 msec; TE = 25 msec) demonstrates metastatic tumor replacing most of the body of T9 (*open arrow*). There is cord compression ventrally and dorsally (*small arrows*). *Oblique arrow* points to a compression fracture of the body of T6 due to osteoporosis and not due to tumor. Note that the cancellous bone maintains its normal high signal intensity in contrast to replacement by metastatic tumor, which results in a lower signal intensity.

FIG. 55. A 10-year-old patient with known leukemia and low platelet count presenting with symptoms of spinal subarachnoid hemorrhage. T1-weighted image (TR = 1,000 msec; TE = 20 msec) demonstrates a normal cord anteriorly and a large area of high signal intensity posteriorly. On a more T2-weighted sagittal image (*right*) (TR = 1,000 msec; TE = 70 msec), the posterior aspect of the high-signal-intensity region loses signal, whereas the intensity of the anterior portion remains unchanged. The more posterior low-intensity tissue represents fat. The more anterior area of very high signal intensity represents methemoglobin. (Courtesy of Bent Kjos, Magnetic Imaging Associates, Alta Bates Hospital.)

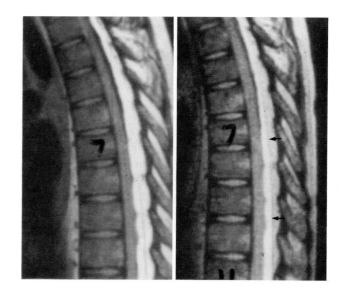

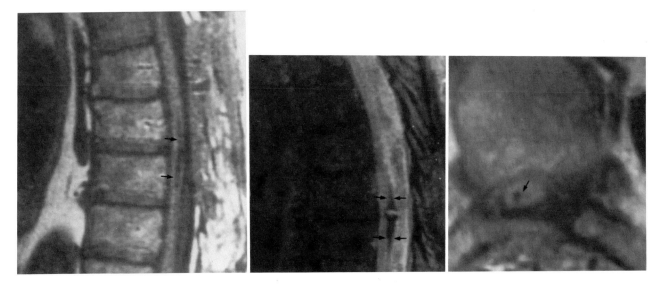

FIG. 56. A 60-year-old man with previously treated vascular malformation of the cord. T1-weighted sagittal image (*left*) (TR = 1,000 msec; TE = 20 msec) demonstrates a slit-like cavity within a partially atrophic cord. This is confirmed on an axial image (*far right*). T2-weighted sagittal image (TR = 2,000 msec; TE = 35 msec) (*center*) shows persistence of low signal intensity within the cord. If this were an area of myelomalacia and/or cyst, high rather than low signal intensity would be expected. Persistence of low signal intensity indicates a preferential T2 shortening. At surgery, a hemosiderin-laden cicatrix was identified. No residual malformation was present.

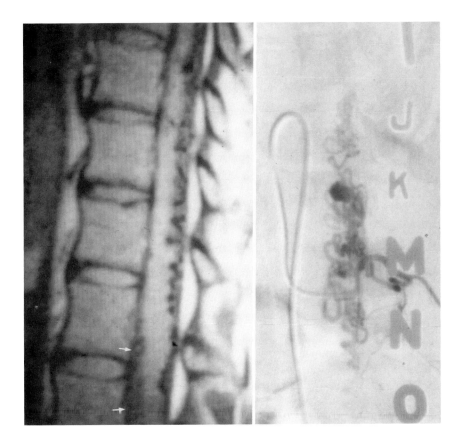

FIG. 57. Cord AVM. Intermediate-weighted sagittal image demonstrates dorsally located serpiginous areas of signal void representing a single, large, draining vein from an intramedullary malformation. In the lower portion of the image, the ventrally located malformation can be identified (*arrows*). The lesion was confirmed angiographically (*right*).

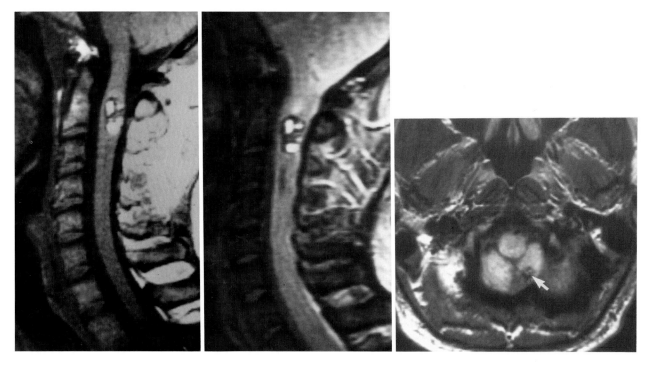

FIG. 58. Cryptic malformation of the cervical cord. High-intensity methemaglobin center and low-intensity hemosiderin capsule are identified on both the T1-weighted image (TR = 600 msec; TE = 25 msec) and the T2-weighted image (TR = 1,500 msec; TE = 35 msec). Axial scan demonstrates a second cryptic malformation in the left tonsil (*arrow*).

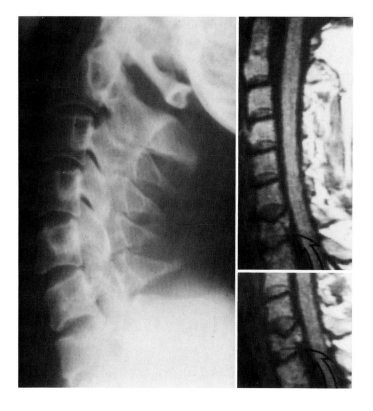

FIG. 59. Lateral cervical spine film following motor vehicle accident is underexposed at the C7 level but is suspicious for an abnormality at that level. Sagittal image (TR = 600 msec; TE = 25 msec) shows fracture of the body of C7 (*arrow*) without cord compression. MR is especially useful in those patients in whom C7 cannot be visualized either due to broad shoulders or inability of the patient to cooperate or both. Issues such as stability are better evaluated with plain films or CT.

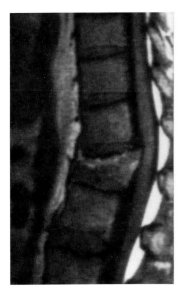

FIG. 60. Seatbelt-compression fracture following a motor vehicle accident. Sagittal image (TR = 1,000 msec; TE = 25 msec) demonstrates compressed vertebral body, expanded intervertebral discs, and compression of the ventral aspect of the cord. Stability of posterior elements is not adequately assessed.

vere anomalies, such as diastematomyelia and scoliosis (Fig. 65). In scoliotic spines, the coronal imaging plane is invaluable (Fig. 65) because it is usually the only plane in which a substantial portion of the spine can be imaged in a single section.

Tethering of the cord may present late in adult life (Fig. 66). These patients usually present with either difficulties with urination or with abnormal gait. In male patients, the initial clinical impression may be that of prostatic hypertrophy. Patients usually do not have overlying cutaneous abnormalities. Myelomeningoceles are uncommon. On T1-weighted sagittal MR images, tethering of the cord is clearly seen. There may or may not be an associated lipoma.

ROLE OF MR IN IMAGING OF THE CORD AND CANAL

One of the most difficult issues in imaging the cord and canal is determining the indications for the imaging examination so that utilization is appropriate. In patients with radiculopathy, plain films, myelograms, and/or CT scans are most valuable in the search for a lesion that is amenable to surgical correction in a patient in whom surgery is a serious consideration. In many instances, imaging examinations are obtained simply to identify the presence of a lesion either to reassure the patient or occasionally for compensation purposes. When it is determined that an imaging study is appro-

FIG. 61. One-month-old infant with flaccid lower extremities following breech forceps delivery. Sagittal (TR = 1,000 msec; TE = 20/70 msec) image shows complete cord transection. Information of this sort is not available with any other imaging technique.

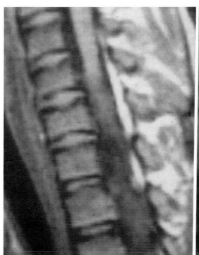
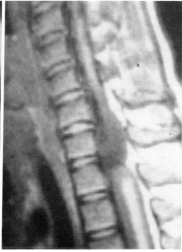

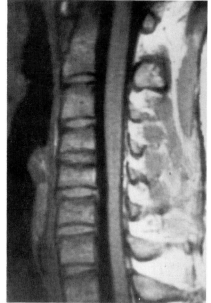

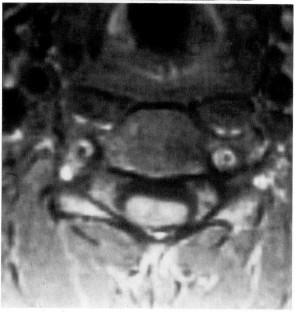

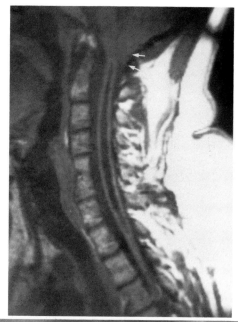

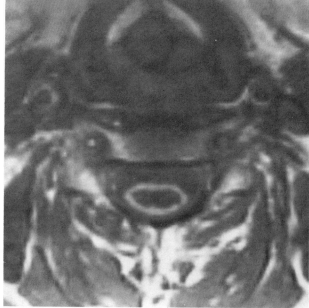

FIG. 62. A 28-year-old man 3 years after motor vehicle accident with residual lower extremity motor weakness. Sagittal image demonstrates a narrowing of the cord at the C5–C6 level with a minimal disc protrusion. Axial image shows loss of cord diameter, more pronounced on the left than the right. This image permits for the first time *in vivo* assessment of focal cord atrophy.

FIG. 63. Young woman with ataxia. Sagittal image (TR = 1,000 msec; TE = 20 msec) demonstrates tonsillar herniation (*arrows*) and hydromyelic cavity extending from the foramen magnum to the T1 level. The axial scan (TR = 1,000 msec; TE = 20 msec) is most useful for confirming the size of the cavity and estimating remaining cord tissue.

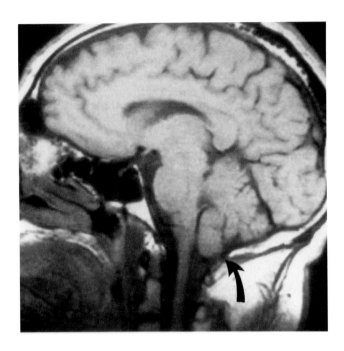

FIG. 64. Normal parasagittal scan (TR = 600 msec; TE = 20 msec). A smoothly rounded tonsil extends slightly below the outer table of the foramen magnum (*arrow*).

priate, MR should, in most patients, be the imaging study of choice, supplanting CT, myelography, or plain films. In contrast to MR, plain films contain little information. Plain films may be better utilized as supplemental examinations in the same fashion that skull films for the past decade have served best as a supplemental examination to head CT studies. CT scans and/or CT supplemented by intrathecal contrast may also in some cases provide important supplemental information. In patients with radiculopathy in whom the MR examination is negative, an intrathecal contrast CT is a most useful examination. In those patients in whom spondylosis is pronounced, CT may again be useful as either a primary or supplementary examination, since high-quality bone detail is often required. There are few indications for myelograms in communities in which high-quality MR is available. Perhaps the strongest indication for myelography at present is in the patient who is suspect for drop metastasis. In this situation, the relative sensitivity of MR has not been established. Myelography continues to be useful in patients with acute or subacute cord compression who are unable to cooperate for an MR examination. In the evaluation of spine stability and/or mobility, MR currently has little if any value.

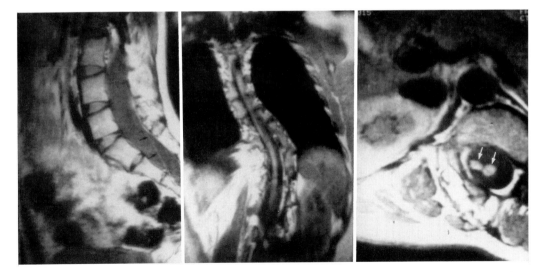

FIG. 65. An 18-month-old child with scoliosis, cord tethering (*arrows*), and splitting of the cord (*white arrow*) associated with diastematomyelia. The fibrous and/or bony septum was not identified on MR but was seen on CT scan.

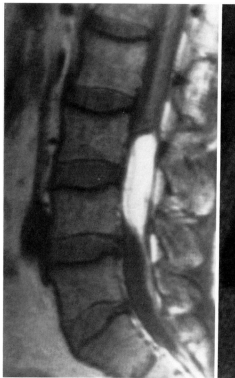 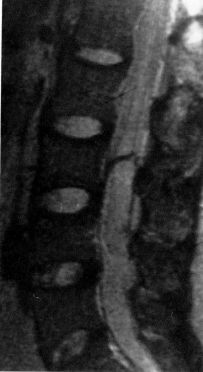

FIG. 66. A 37-year-old woman with a history of several years of urinary retention. Sagittal MR (TR = 1,000 msec; TE = 20/70 msec) demonstrates tethering of the cord with associated sacral lipoma. No vertebral or cutaneous abnormalities are present.

REFERENCES

1. Dooms GC, Fisher MR, Hricak H, Richardson M, Crooks LE, Genant HK. Bone marrow imaging: magnetic resonance studies related to age and sex. *Radiology* 1985;155:429–32.
2. Ramsey RG, Zacharias CE. MR imaging of the spine after radiation therapy: easily recognizable effects. *AJNR* 1985;6:247–51.
3. Pech P, Haughton VM. Lumbar intervertebral disk: correlative MR and anatomic study. *Radiology* 1985;156:699–701.
4. Aguila LA, Piraino DW, Modic MT, Dudley AW, Duchesneau PM, Weinstein MA. The intranuclear cleft of the intervertebral disk: magnetic resonance imaging. *Radiology* 1985;155:155–8.
5. Rubin J, Enzmann D, Silverberg G, Sheuen L. Fluid dynamics within syringomyelic cavities. XIII Symposium Neuroradiologicum, Stockholm, June 23–28, 1986.
6. Modic MT, Pavlicek W, Weinstein MA, Boumphrey F, Ngo F, Hardy R, Duchesneau PM. Magnetic resonance imaging of intervertebral disk disease. Clinical and pulse sequence considerations. *Radiology* 1984;152:103–11.
7. Edelman RR, Shoukimas GM, Stark DD, Davis KR, New PFJ, Saini S, Rosenthal DI, Wismer GL, Brady TJ. High-resolution surface-coil imaging of lumbar disk disease. *AJR* 1985;144:1123–9.
8. Maravilla KR, Lesh P, Weinreb JC, Selby DK, Mooney V. Magnetic resonance imaging of the lumbar spine with CT correlation. *AJNR* 1985;6:237–45.
9. Modic MT, Masaryk T, Boumphrey F, Goormastic M, Bell G. Lumbar herniated disc disease and canal stenosis. *Am J Neuroradiol* 1986;7:709–17.
10. Masaryk TJ, Modic MT, Geisinger MA, Standefer J, Hardy RW, Boumphrey F, Duchesneau PM. Cervical myelopathy: a comparison of magnetic resonance and myelography. *J Comput Assist Tomogr* 1986;10:184–94.
11. Bydder GM, Brown J, Niendorf HP, Young IR. Enhancement of cervical intraspinal tumors in MR imaging with intravenous gadolinium-DTPA. *J Comput Assist Tomogr* 1985;9:847–51.
12. Lee BCP, Zimmerman RD, Manning JJ, Deck MDF. MR imaging of syringomyelia and hydromyelia. *AJNR* 1985;6:221–8.
13. Sherman JL, Barkovich AJ, Citrin CM. The magnetic resonance appearance of syringomyelia: new observations. *AJNR* (*In Press.*)
14. Gebarski SS, Maynard FW, Gabrielsen TO, Knake JE, Latack JT, Hoff JT. Posttraumatic progressive myelopathy. Clinical and radiologic correlation employing MR imaging, delayed CT metrizamide myelography, and intraoperative sonography. *Radiology* 1985;157:379–85.
15. Barkovich AJ, Sherman JL, Citrin CM, Wippold FJ. MRI of post-operative syringomyelia. *AJNR* (*In Press.*)
16. Quencer RM, El Gammal T, Cohen G. Syringomyelia associated with intradural extramedullary masses of the spinal canal. *AJNR* 1986;7:143–8.
17. Pojunas K, Williams AL, Daniels DL, Haughton VM. Syringomyelia and hydromyelia: magnetic resonance evaluation. *Radiology* 1984;153:679–83.
18. Maravilla KR, Weinreb JC, Suss R, Nunnally RL. Magnetic resonance demonstration of multiple sclerosis plaques in the cervical cord. *AJNR* 1984;5:685–9.
19. Modic MT, Feiglin DH, Piraino DW, Boumphrey F, Weinstein MA, Duchesneau PM, Rehm S. Vertebral osteomyelitis: assessment using MR. *Radiology* 1985;157:157–66.
20. Mamourian AC, Briggs RW. Appearance of pantopaque on MR images. *Radiology* 1986;158:457–60.
21. Cohen MD, Klatte EC, Baehner R, Smith JA, Martin-Simmerman P, Carr BE, Provisor AJ, Weetman RM, Coates T, Siddiqui A, Weisman SJ, Berkow R, McKenna S, McGuire WA. Magnetic resonance imaging of bone marrow disease in children. *Radiology* 1984;151:715–8.
22. Di Chiro G, Doppman JL, Dwyer AJ, Patronas NJ, Knop RH, Bairamian D, Vermess M, Oldfield EH. Tumors and arteriovenous malformations of the spinal cord: assessment using MR. *Radiology* 1985;156:689–97.
23. Han JS, Benson JE, Kaufman B, Rekate HL, Alfidi RJ, Bohlman HH, Kaufman B. Demonstration of diastematomyelia and associated abnormalities with MR imaging. *AJNR* 1985;6:215–9.

CHAPTER 19

The Nasopharynx

William P. Dillon

Magnetic resonance (MR) imaging has evolved into the imaging modality of choice for the evaluation of the soft tissue structures of the head and neck (1–5). The chief advantages of MR include the capability of MR for high spatial and soft tissue contrast resolution, multiplanar imaging, the dependence of tissue intensity on several operator-dependent imaging parameters, and an ability to image vessels without the use of intravenous contrast agents.

In this chapter we shall consider the various compartments of the nasopharynx, detailing the normal and pathologic anatomy within each compartment as visualized by MR sequences emphasizing both T1 and T2 relaxation differences.

NORMAL ANATOMY

The nasopharynx occupies the most superior extent of the aerodigestive tract, participating in both nasal respiration and deglutition. Although anatomically a small part of the extracranial head and neck soft tissues, its close proximity to the critical neurovascular anatomy of the skull base gives the nasopharynx special neuroradiologic importance. The jugular fossa (cranial nerves IX–XII), foramen ovale (cranial nerve V₃), carotid canal, sella turcica, cavernous sinus (cranial nerves III–VI), and the clivus all are within close proximity to the nasopharyngeal mucosa. It is thus not surprising that invasive nasopharyngeal pathology frequently results in neurologic symptoms, such as diplopia, trigeminal pain or anesthesia, and jugular fossa syndrome.

The nasopharynx is an open airway lined by squamous epithelial mucosa. The airway is held patent by a firm fascial layer, the pharyngobasilar fascia, which surrounds the mucosa, the superior constrictor muscle, and the levator palatini muscle (Fig. 1). The pharyngobasilar fascia attaches to the clivus just in front of the prevertebral muscles and extends laterally to the carotid canal region, where it turns medially and anterior to insert on the medial pterygoid plates (Fig. 1). This fascial plane is

occasionally detected on MR as a thin band of low signal intensity. It effectively divides the nasopharynx into a superficial "mucosal" compartment and a larger deep compartment containing the muscles of mastication, the carotid sheath vessels and lymphatics, and the intervening fat of the deep fascial planes (Figs. 1 and 2). The deep compartment, also known as the infratemporal fossa, actually consists of several spaces enclosed by portions of the deep cervical fascia (Fig. 2). Through an understanding of the fascial spaces and their contents, pathology may be localized more effectively and a differential diagnosis tailored according to the space in which it originates (Table 1) (6–10).

Superficial (Mucosal) Compartment

The superficial or mucosal compartment of the nasopharynx contains the squamous mucosa, adenoidal (lymphoid) tissue, the superior constrictor muscle, the torus tubarius, and the levator palatini muscle (Figs. 1 and 3–5). These structures lie on the airway side of the pharyngobasilar fascia, which provides an initial barrier to the spread of mucosal disease into the deeper compartments (4).

The mucosa and adenoidal tissue of the nasopharynx have a relatively prolonged T1 and T2 relaxation time, resulting in a low signal intensity on T1-weighted images (Fig. 3C) and a high signal intensity on T2-weighted images (Figs. 4E and F). Adenoidal tissue occupies the superior recesses of the nasopharynx (Fig. 3C). Its presence is largely age dependent. Children and young adults may have prominent adenoidal tissue that fills the superior recesses of the nasopharynx (Figs. 4E and F and 6 and 7). Degenerative or cystic changes can often be identified within the adenoidal tissue on T2-weighted images (Fig. 6B). Gradual involution of the adenoidal tissue begins at puberty, and although large amounts of lymphoid tissue may be seen into the sixth or seventh decade, most adults have lost this tissue by age 30 (Fig 3B). Benign adenoidal tissue is enclosed by the pharyn-

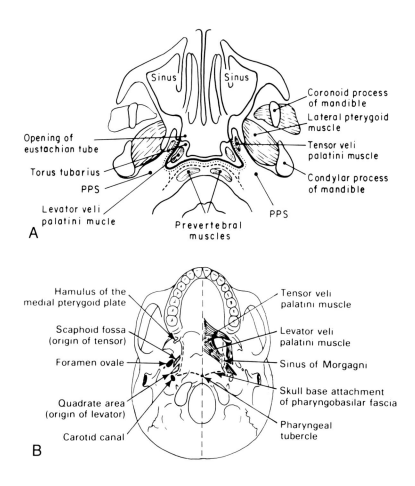

A

B

FIG. 1. A: Axial schematic through the upper nasopharynx. The pharyngobasilar fascia (*dark solid line*) attaches to the medial pterygoid plate and skull base enclosing the nasopharyngeal airway, the torus tubarius, the superior constrictor muscle, and the levator veli palatini muscle. It is occasionally seen on MR scans as a solid band of low intensity. The buccopharyngeal fascia (*dotted line*) is located lateral to the pharyngobasilar fascia. The tensor veli palatini muscle lies outside these fascial layers until the lower aspect of the nasopharynx, where it pierces the pharyngobasilar fascia wrapping around the medial pterygoid plate to insert on the soft palate musculature (see **B**). The prevertebral fascia (*dashed line*) covers the prevertebral muscles. The space between the prevertebral and buccopharyngeal fascia is the retropharyngeal space. **B:** Attachment of the tensor and levator veli palatini muscles to the skull base. The tensor veli palatini muscle originates in the scaphoid fossa medial to the foramen ovale. It courses laterally to the pharyngobasilar fascia and hooks around the medial pterygoid plate to insert on the soft palate musculature. Contraction of this muscle tenses the palate in a lateral direction. The levator veli palatini muscle attaches to the skull base in the quadrate area adjacent to the carotid canal. It courses through the sinus of Morgagni, an opening within the pharyngobasilar fascia, and attaches to the posterior soft palate musculature. Contraction of this muscle elevates the palate and opens the torus tubarius. (From ref. 10.)

gobasilar fascia and lateral recesses of the nasopharynx. It never infiltrates structures deep to the pharyngobasilar fascia (Figs. 1–7). Obliteration of fascial planes deep to the pharyngobasilar fascia indicates invasive pathology.

Other prominent superficial landmarks in the naso-

pharynx include the torus tubarius, the levator palatini muscles, and the lateral pharyngeal recess of Rosenmuller (Figs. 1 and 2). The torus tubarius, the cartilaginous covering for the eustachian tube orifices, protrudes into the upper nasopharyngeal airway and has a high

FIG. 2. Spaces of the nasopharynx. Axial schematic through the lower (*left side*) and upper (*right side*) nasopharynx. The medial (mucosal) compartment of the nasopharynx is enclosed by the pharyngobasilar fascia (*dark solid line*). The soft tissues deep to the pharyngobasilar fascia are compartmentalized by fascial layers. These include the masticator space enclosed by the superficial layer of the deep cervical fascia, the parapharyngeal space (PPS) enclosed by the buccopharyngeal fascia (*dotted line*), and the carotid sheath enclosed by all three layers of the deep cervical fascia (*thin solid line*). The retropharyngeal space is bordered by the buccopharyngeal fascia (*dotted line*) and the prevertebral fascia (*dashed line*). The prevertebral space is enclosed by the prevertebral fascia and contains the longus colli and capitis muscles.

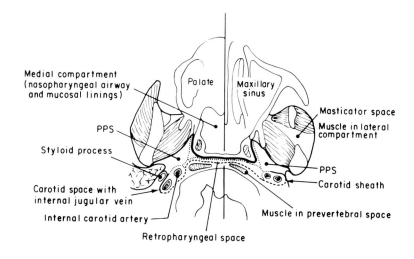

TABLE 1. *Deep compartments of the nasopharynx*

Compartment	Contents	Pathology
Mucosal space	Adenoids Mucosa	Carcinoma, lymphoma Plasmacytoma, melanoma Pediatric rhabdomyosarcoma Juvenile angiofibroma Non-Hodgkin's lymphoma
Parapharyngeal space	Fat Ascending pharyngeal artery Third division of trigeminal nerve V_3 Internal maxillary artery	Minor salivary gland tumors Lipoma Second branchial cleft cyst Schwannoma Cellulitis Abscess (tonsillar)
Carotid space	Carotid artery Jugular vein Cranial nerves IX–XII Sympathetic chain Retropharyngeal nodes	Paragangliomas Schwannomas Extracranial meningiomas Adenopathy Lymphoma Cellulitis Abscess

Masticator space	Mandible
	Medial pterygoid muscle
	Lateral pterygoid muscle
	Temporalis muscle
	Masseter muscle
	Inferior alveolar nerve
		Abscess and cellulitis: odontogenic
		Benign masseteric hypertrophy
		Tumor
		  Benign
		    Lipoma
		    Hemangioma
		    Neurogenic tumors
		  Malignant
		    Minor salivary gland
		    Metastatic to mandible
		    Sarcoma of muscle or mandible
		    Direct spread of squamous Ca
		    Lymphoma

Retropharyngeal space	Fat Nodes	Lymphoma Metastatic adenopathy Lipomas Abscesses or cellulitis
Prevertebral space	Notochord elements Prevertebral muscles	Chordomas Metastatic disease to the spine Osteomyelitis with abscess, cellulitis

intensity signal on T2-weighted images of the nasopharynx (Figs. 4A and 6B). The actual eustachian tube orifices may be identified as smaller recesses just anterior and inferior to each tori (Figs. 4A and 5C). In some children, adenoidal tissue may fill the eustachian tube orifice, resulting in serous or purulent otitis media (Fig. 4E). The lateral pharyngeal recess of Rosenmuller is identified just posterior to the protruding torus tubarius (Figs. 1, 4B, 4F, 5C, and 6B). The fossae of Rosenmuller are the most common site of squamous carcinomas of the nasopharynx.

The posterior aspect of the nasopharyngeal airway rests on the prevertebral muscles, the longus colli, and capitis muscles (Figs. 1–4). The prevertebral muscles are anterior to the upper cervical vertebral bodies and the lower clivus (Fig. 3). Fat within the bone marrow of these osseous structures has a characteristic high signal intensity on T1-weighted images. A thin rim of low-density cortical bone surrounds the medullary cavity of bone (Figs. 3 and 7A).

The levator palatini muscle is identified on axial MR scans as a muscular band located just lateral to the torus tubarius (Figs. 1 and 4A). The levator palatini muscle pierces the upper pharyngobasilar fascia and courses from the skull base to the soft palate. It functions to elevate the soft palate during swallowing (Figs. 1 and 2B). A slip of this muscle also inserts onto the torus tubarius, controlling its opening and closing during

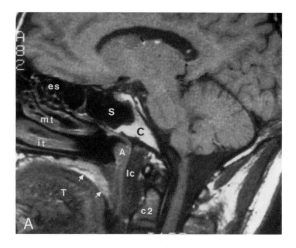

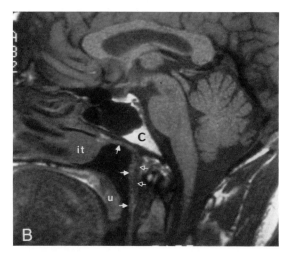

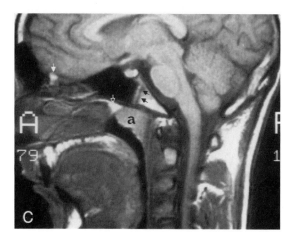

FIG. 3. Normal nasopharynx (sagittal). **A:** Sagittal T1-weighted image 5 mm off midline. This section, lateral to midline, demonstrates the posterior lateral pharyngeal wall structures that represent mucosa and adenoidal tissue (A) resting upon the longus capitis muscle (lc). Increased intensity is seen within the clivus (C) and the marrow-filled hard palate and fat of the soft palate (*white arrows*). Also of note is the aerated sphenoid sinus (S) and ethmoid sinuses (es). The inferior turbinate (it) and middle turbinate (mt) are located lateral to midline within the nasal vault. The intrinsic tongue muscle (t) is interspersed with foci of high signal intensity representing fat separating the muscle bundles. **B:** Midline sagittal T1-weighted image through a normal adult nasopharynx. The midline section demonstrates the normal thickness of the posterior pharyngeal wall. Note that the mucosa (*closed arrows*) is separated from the clivus by only 2–3 mm, whereas the posterior nasopharyngeal wall is 3–4 mm in thickness due to the mucosa and the superior constrictor muscle (*open arrows*). Also noted is the fat within the clivus (c), the posterior aspect of the inferior turbinate (it), and the uvula (u). **C:** Midline sagittal T1-weighted image through the nasopharynx of a young child. Prominent adenoidal tissue is present in the superior recess of the nasopharynx (a). The anterior surface of the adenoidal tissue is irregular and does not extend below the midlevel of the C2 vertebral body or into the clivus or surrounding soft tissues. The posterior pharyngeal wall is below the C2 vertebral body at the midline. Also noted is the residual spheno-occipital suture remnant within the clivus (*black arrows*). The high-intensity signal of marrow within the vomer bone (*open white arrow*) and the crista galli (*solid white arrow*) is a normal finding.

swallowing. The levator palatini muscle is surrounded by fat that separates it from the longus colli and capitis muscles (Figs. 1–5). Infiltration of this fat plane, which is adjacent to the lateral pharyngeal recess, is the first sign of nasopharyngeal carcinoma (4). A second palatal

muscle, the tensor palatini muscle, parallels the course of the levator palatini muscle; however, it lies outside the pharyngobasilar fascia and lateral to the levator (Figs. 1 and 2B). It courses from the skull base inferiorly and is tethered around the medial pterygoid plate, inserting on the lateral aspect of the soft palate (Fig. 2B). Contraction of this muscle places lateral tension on the soft palate, elevating it to appose the pharyngeal musculature during swallowing (Fig. 2B). The tensor palatini muscle can usually be identified on axial and coronal images, embedded within fat lateral to the nasopharyngeal airway and medial to the parapharyngeal space (Figs. 1, 4A and B and 5C).

DEEP TISSUE SPACES

The tissues of the nasopharynx deep to the pharyngobasilar fascia are best divided into spaces compartmentalized by the deep cervical fascia. With an understanding of the anatomic contents of these spaces and the pathologic processes that may occur within them, a differential diagnosis is facilitated for mass lesions occurring in these regions (10).

Parapharyngeal Space

The parapharyngeal space is a triangular fat-filled space lying deep to the pharyngobasilar fascia (Figs. 1, 2, and 4D). It spans the entire head and neck region from the skull base to the submandibular space at the floor of the mouth (Figs. 1–4 and 5B). It contains primarily fat as well as the ascending pharyngeal and internal maxillary arteries and branches of the third division of the fifth cranial nerve (Figs. 4C and 5F). On magnetic resonance imaging, the parapharyngeal space has a high intensity on T1-weighted images and an intermediate to low intensity on heavily T2-weighted images (Figs. 3–5). This is due to the short-T1 and intermediate-T2 relaxation values of fat. Foci of low and high signal intensities represent branches of the ascending pharyngeal artery and slow-flowing pharyngeal veins, respectively (Figs. 4B and D).

Deviation of the parapharyngeal space is always abnormal and often helps to localize the compartment from which mass lesions arise (4,11,12). For instance, lateral deviation of the parapharyngeal space occurs with mucosal lesions, such as carcinomas, whereas medial displacement of the parapharyngeal space is characteristic of lateral compartment masses, such as parotid tumors or masticator space masses. Likewise, jugular fossa lesions or carotid space masses displace the parapharyngeal space anteriorly (see section on pathology of the nasopharynx, *this chapter*).

Carotid Space

The carotid space is enclosed by the carotid sheath, which receives contributions from all three layers of the deep cervical fascia (Fig. 2). The fascia is not visualized by MR; however, signal void due to rapid blood flow within the carotid sheath vessels serves to locate the carotid sheath structures (Fig. 4C). The carotid space spans the neck from the skull base to the aortic arch. In the nasopharynx the carotid sheath contains the internal carotid artery, the internal jugular vein, cranial nerves IX to XII, and the cervical sympathetic plexus (9). On MR, the cranial nerves, particularly the vagus nerve, are occasionally seen as high-intensity foci adjacent and posterior to the carotid artery (Fig. 4D). Small retropharyngeal nodes are often present medial to the carotid artery (Fig. 4F). They are the first-order drainage nodes from the nasopharynx and oropharynx and are commonly enlarged in patients with nasopharyngeal carcinoma or prominent adenoidal tissue (4). Their signal intensity increases on T2-weighted scans, but unfortunately, there is no significant signal difference between metastatic and reactive adenopathy (1,2).

On axial MR scans, the internal carotid artery normally has an absent signal due to the time-of-flight effect of high-velocity blood flow. In most instances, the internal jugular vein also has a low intensity (Fig. 4C). Slow blood flow with a small internal jugular vein will sometimes have a bright signal that undergoes even-echo rephasing (1). The carotid sheath may be difficult to distinguish from the aerated cortical bone of the petrous apex in the upper nasopharynx. It can usually be identified by its position posterior and lateral to the parapharyngeal space (Fig. 4D).

Masticator Space

The masticator space is enveloped by the superficial layer of the deep cervical fascia, which splits at the angle of the mandible to enclose the muscles of mastication, the ramus and posterior body of the mandible, and the pterygoid venous plexus (Fig. 2; Table 1). The muscles of mastication include the lateral and medial pterygoid, the temporalis, and the masseter muscle (Fig. 5). The masticator space provides a route of spread to the skull base for tumors and infections (Fig. 5C) (6). On MR, the contents of the masticator space are rather characteristic. The muscles of mastication have a low signal intensity on both T1 and T2 images due to a relatively prolonged T1 and shortened T2 relaxation value (Fig. 5C). These surround the low signal of the cortical portion of the mandible. The mandible itself may have high signal foci of fat in the medullary cavity. Replacement of the fatty medullary cavity may be seen by tumor or infection involving the mandible (see Fig. 24). Masticator space masses usually are odontogenic in origin, most commonly from dental infections, mandibular osteo-

FIG. 4. Normal axial MR scans through the nasopharynx of an adult and a child. **A–D:** Adult. TR = 2,000 msec; TE = 40 msec (*left*) and 80 msec (*right*). **A:** Axial MR scans through the upper nasopharynx demonstrate the normal symmetric contours of the nasopharyngeal wall. The most prominent features of the nasopharyngeal airway are the bilateral torus tubari, the cartilaginous ends of the eustachian tubes, which are relatively high-intensity structures covered by low-intensity mucosa (*white arrow*). The actual eustachian tube recess is anterior to the tori (*single open arrow*). Lateral and posterior to the torus tubarius is the levator palatine muscle (*double open arrow*). The tensor palatini muscle is identified lateral and slightly anterior to the torus tubari (*open black arrows*). Also noted is the lateral pterygoid muscle (LP), the temporalis muscle (T), the masseter (M), and the clivus (C). Note that fat surrounding the muscles in the subcutaneous region and in the retroantral region decreases in intensity on the 80-msec echo. Likewise, fat surrounding the levator and tensor palatini muscle and within the medullary cavity of the clivus decreases in intensity between the 40-msec and 80-msec

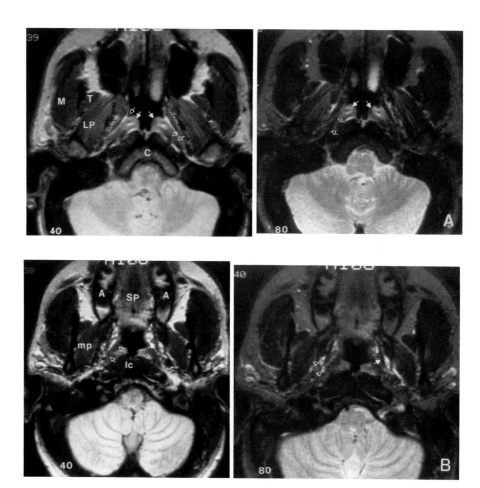

echo. **B:** Axial-5 mm scan through the midnasopharynx inferior to **A.** The levator palatini muscle (*open white arrows*) is identified lateral to the torus tubarius. The parapharyngeal space located just lateral to the tensor veli palatini muscle (*white arrows*) has a high-intensity signal due to fat. The soft palate (sp) is surrounded by the maxillary alveolar ridge (a). Also identified on this section is the longus capitis muscle (lc) and the medial pterygoid muscle (mp). Slowly flowing pharyngeal veins increase in intensity between the first and second (80 msec) echo within the parapharyngeal space (*arrowheads*). **C:** Axial MR scan through the lower nasopharynx. On this section, 5 mm inferior to **B,** the soft palate musculature and the levator and tensor palatini muscles coalesce to form a single muscular band called Passavant's ridge (*open arrows*). Just anterior to Passavant's ridge is the high-intensity signal of lymphatics within the soft palate (sp) and the upper aspect of the tongue (T). Lateral to Passavant's ridge is a high-intensity region that represents pharyngeal vessels and fat within the parapharyngeal space. On the 80-msec echo, the fat within the parapharyngeal space decreases in signal intensity, whereas the slowly flowing blood within the pharyngeal vessels increases its signal intensity due to even-echo rephasing phenomena of slowly flowing blood (*white arrows*). Also identified on this section is the intermediate signal of the parotid gland (P), which swings around the posterior aspect of the mandible. Note that the parotid gland decreases in intensity, similar to fat, on the 80-msec echo. The accessory lobe of the parotid gland (ap) is noted on the right side in its characteristic position lateral to the masseter muscle. The internal carotid artery (*solid black arrow*) and the internal jugular vein (*open black arrow*) are also identified. The buccinator muscle is identified just lateral to the alveolar ridge (b). The parotid gland duct courses around the anterior tip of the masseter muscle and pierces the buccinator muscle to empty into the oral cavity near the upper third molar. **D:** Axial scans through the junction of the nasopharynx and oropharynx. The high-intensity fat-filled parapharyngeal spaces (*black arrows*) are noted just lateral to the musculature surrounding the oronasopharyngeal airway. Note that the parapharyngeal fat decreases in signal intensity on the 80-msec echo. The palatoglossus muscles, which form the anterior tonsillar pillars, course from the tonsillar bed to the lateral aspect of the tongue (*open single white arrows*). The palatine tonsils are atrophic and lie lateral to the oropharyngeal airway (*closed white arrows*). Lying between the tongue (T) and the airway is a high-intensity U-shaped region representing fat within the soft palate. Lateral to the parapharyngeal space is the medial pterygoid muscle, which inserts at the angle of the mandible. Lateral to the mandible (m) is the masseter muscle (M). Posterior to the masseter muscle is the parotid gland (P). At this level, the facial arteries (*open black arrows*) are located within the fatty buccinator space, just lateral to the buccinator muscle (b). Punctate foci of high signal intensity posterior to the internal carotid artery represent the cranial nerves XI–XII (*double open white arrows*). **E,F:** Contiguous axial 5-mm MR scans through the upper and midnasopharynx of a child (TR = 2,000 msec; TE = 40 msec). Adenoidal tissue (a) fills the upper aspect of the nasopharynx and the lateral recesses of Rosenmuller (*black arrows*). The levator palatini muscle (*open black arrow*) is located just lateral to the adenoidal tissue, whereas the tensor palatini muscle (*white arrow*) is located just lateral to the levator. Reactive retropharyngeal nodes (*open white arrow*) are located just medial to the internal carotid artery. These nodes commonly accompany adenoidal tissue. The longus colli and capitis muscles (lc) separate the adenoidal tissue from the anterior arch of the Cl vertebral body.

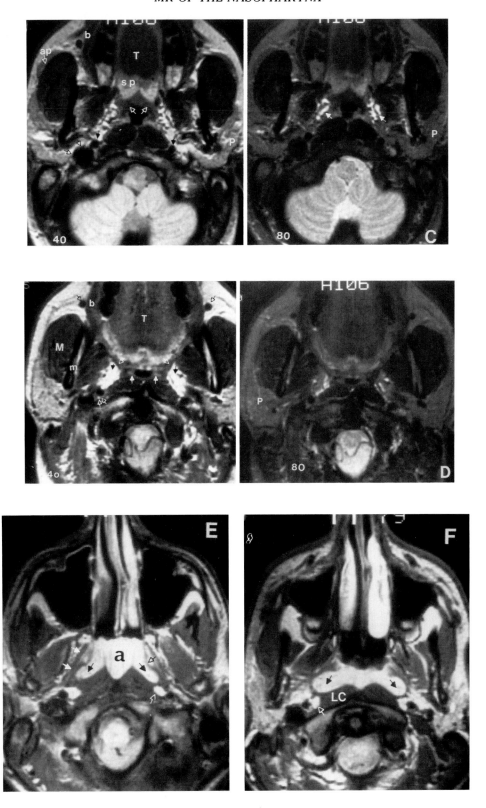

FIG. 4. *(Continued)*

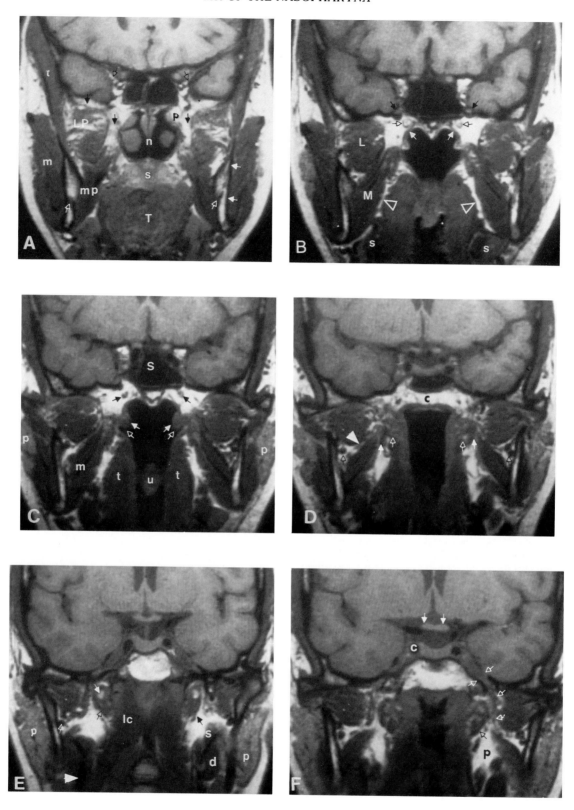

myelitis, and mandibular neoplasms (Table 1). Masses within the masticator space will deviate the parapharyngeal space medially (6).

Retropharyngeal Space

The retropharyngeal space is a potential space that separates the prevertebral muscles and the pharyngeal constrictor muscles. It is bounded anteriorly by the alar fascia (the anterior portion of the deep layer of the cervical fascia) and laterally and posteriorly by the posterior portion of the deep layer of the deep cervical fascia (prevertebral fascia) (Figs. 1 and 2). It extends from the skull base to the level of the third thoracic vertebral body. It contains primarily fat and lymph nodes of the medial retropharyngeal chain (Table 1). Normally, the retropharyngeal space is not a discrete entity on MR or computed tomography (CT) scans; however, inflammatory or postsurgical edema within the retropharyngeal space may enlarge the posterior retropharyngeal space and dissect along its course into the posterior mediastinum (13).

FIG. 5. Normal 5-mm coronal T1-weighted scans through the nasopharynx (TR = 600 msec; TE = 25 msec). **A:** 5-mm coronal section through the anterior nasopharynx and posterior nares (n), soft palate (s), and posterior tongue (T). The masticator space musculature, the temporalis muscle (t), the masseter (m), the lateral pterygoid (lp), and the medial pterygoid (mp) are all identified inserting onto the cortex of the mandible. The masticator muscles are surrounded by the superficial layer of the deep cervical fascia, which encloses the masticator space surrounding the posterior aspect of the mandible and these muscles. The mandible itself is comprised of a low-signal cortical bone surrounding a high-signal marrow cavity (*white arrows*). The inferior alveolar canal carrying the alveolar nerve and vessels is identified as a low-signal intensity focus within the medullary cavity (*open white arrows*). Also identified on this section is fat within the marrow cavity of the skull base and pterygoid plates (*black arrows*), and the superior orbital fissure (*open black arrows*) and the pterygopalatine fossa (p). **B:** 5-mm coronal scan posterior to **A.** The superior constrictor muscle and mucosa surround the nasopharyngeal airway (*closed white arrow*). Lateral to the airway is the high-intensity signal from marrow within the pterygoid plates. Attaching to the pterygoid plates are the lateral pterygoid muscle (l) and medial pterygoid muscle (m). The pterygoid canal (*open black arrows*) courses through the upper medial aspect of the pterygoid plates. This canal carries the pterygoid nerve and vidian artery. The pterygoid nerve carries parasympathetic fibers to the paranasal sinuses and nasopharynx, whereas the vidian artery is a potential communication between the internal maxillary artery and the internal carotid artery. Just superior and lateral to the pterygoid canal is the foramen rotundum containing the second division of the trigeminal nerve (*solid black arrow*). Medial to the medial pterygoid muscle is the fat-filled parapharyngeal space (*open white arrowheads*). The parapharyngeal space separates the medial pterygoid muscle from the tonsillar tissue and constrictor muscles surrounding the airway in the oropharynx. The parapharyngeal space extends from the region of the skull base inferiorly to the submandibular glands (s). **C:** 5 mm scan posterior to **B.** The prominent torus tubarius protrudes into the nasopharyngeal airway (*white arrows*), just superior to the eustachian tube orifice (*open white arrow*). High signal intensity within the marrow of the pterygoid plate and clivus separates the upper aspect of the nasopharynx from the sphenoid sinus (s). Identified within the pterygoid plate is the pterygoid canal (*black arrow*). The soft tissue density lining the airway represents the combined densities of the middle constrictor muscle and the tonsillar tissue (t) surrounding the oropharyngeal airway. The soft tissue density centered within the airway is the uvula. Separating the tonsillar tissue from the medial pterygoid muscle (m) is the parapharyngeal space containing high-intensity fat. Deeply invasive tonsillar carcinoma will initially deviate and then infiltrate the parapharyngeal space lateral to the tonsillar capsule. Deeper invasion infiltrates the medial pterygoid muscle, resulting in the clinical symptom of trismus. Also identified on this section is the intermediate intensity of the parotid gland (p), which rests on the masseter muscle. **D:** 5-mm section posterior to **C.** The section is through the upper nasopharynx and clivus (c). Surrounding the airway is the mixed density of adenoidal tissue and the superior constrictor muscle. Just deep to the constrictor muscle are the muscular elements of the levator (*open arrows*) and tensor (*closed white arrows*) palatini muscles. These two muscles elevate and tense the soft palate during swallowing. They are important landmarks in the assessment of early invasion of nasopharyngeal carcinoma deep to the pharyngobasilar fascia. Early invasion of carcinoma will infiltrate the fat planes surrounding these muscles. Also shown on this section is the internal maxillary artery (*open black arrows*), which is located in the fat-filled space between the mandible and the pterygoid musculature, referred to as the pterygomandibular space. The inferior alveolar and lingual branches of the third division of the trigeminal nerve also course within the pterygomandibular space between the lateral pterygoid muscle and the medial pterygoid muscle (*large white arrowhead*). **E:** 5 mm coronal T1-weighted MR scan posterior to **D.** This section courses through the posterior musculature of the nasopharynx and includes the longus captitis muscle (lc), the tensor veli palatini muscle (*black arrow*), and the levator veli palatini muscle (*open black arrow*). Also noted on this section is the inferior alveolar artery (*open white arrow*), the auditory tube (*closed white arrow*), the internal carotid artery (*large white arrowhead*), the styloglossus muscle (s), and the posterior belly of the digastric muscle (d). **F:** Normal 5-mm MR scan of the nasopharynx and skull base posterior to (**E**). The coronal MR scan is through the level of the foramen ovale. The third division of the trigeminal nerve courses through the foramen ovale and has a characteristic course medial to the lateral pterygoid muscle within the upper parapharyngeal space (*open white arrows*). The trigeminal nerve can be identified on most 5-mm coronal MR sections. Also noted is the optic chiasm (*solid white arrows*), the cavernous carotid artery (c), the tensor palatini muscles (*open black arrows*), and the parapharyngeal space (p).

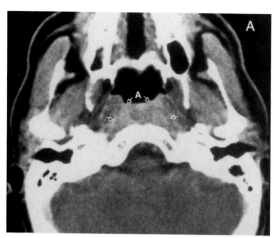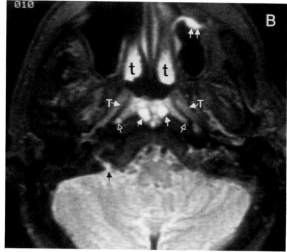

FIG. 6. Adenoidal tissue. **A:** Axial CT scan through the midnasopharynx. Adenoidal tissue fills the superior recess of the nasopharynx (A, *arrows*). Its CT density is similar to muscle, making it difficult to differentiate it from surrounding superficial nasopharyngeal musculature. **B:** Axial T2-weighted MR scan through the midnasopharynx (TR = 2,000 msec; TE = 80 msec). The adenoidal tissue has high signal intensity on this T2-weighted image. Foci of high signal represent cystic degeneration within the adenoidal tissue (*closed white arrow*). These cysts are a normal degenerative occurrence, probably the result of old inflammatory disease. Better identified on the MR scan is the fossa of Rosenmuller (*open white arrows*). The torus tubarii, the cartilaginous portion of the eustachian tube, are identified as bilaterally symmetric protuberances on either side of the nasopharyngeal airway (T). They have high signal intensity due to their cartilaginous component and are often surrounded by low signal intensity muscles. Also noted on this image are the inferior turbinates (t), left maxillary mucosal thickening (*double arrows*), and the normal right hypoglossal nerve (*closed black arrow*).

Prevertebral Space

The prevertebral space contains the vertebral column and prevertebral muscles, the longus colli, and longus capititis (Figs. 1 and 2). It extends from the skull base to the coccyx. This space lies between the deep layer of the cervical fascia and the vertebral bodies, directly posterior to the retropharyngeal space (Figs. 1 and 2). Laterally, the prevertebral space is limited by attachment of the fascia to the transverse process of the vertebral body. Prevertebral space lesions include infections or tumors of the cervical spine. In addition, extension to the prevertebral space may occur from retropharyngeal space tumors or infections (Table 1) (13).

Parotid Space

The parotid gland is routinely imaged on MR scans of the nasopharynx (Figs. 4 and 5). It contains a superficial portion, lateral to the mandible and masseter muscle, and a deep portion that wraps around the posterior aspect of the mandibular ramus (Figs. 3 and 4 and 5B and C). The deep portion abuts the parapharyngeal space in the nasopharynx (Fig. 4D). On MR, the parotid gland normally has a signal intensity slightly lower than fat on T1-weighted images and approaching fat on T2-weighted images (Fig. 4B and C). Differentiation from the parapharyngeal fat is best obtained on spin-density images with a repetition time (TR) in the range of 1 sec and an echo delay time (TE) of 20 to 30 msec. Pathology arising within the deep portion of the parotid gland may deviate the parapharyngeal space medially and present clinically as a primary nasopharyngeal mass (see section on pathology of the nasopharynx, *this chapter*).

NEURAL ANATOMY OF THE NASOPHARYNX

The nerves supplying the motor input to the muscles of the nasopharynx include V_3, IX, and X. These nerves can be routinely imaged on thin-section T1-weighted MR scans (14). On T1-weighted images they appear as intermediate-intensity structures surrounded by fat (Figs. 4D and 5F). Most of the muscular elements of the nasopharyngeal soft tissues are innervated by the third division of cranial nerve V (V_3). The third division of the trigeminal nerve, which exits the foramen ovale, divides into several motor branches within the upper parapharyngeal space (Fig. 5F). The masticator nerve innervates the medial and lateral pterygoid muscles, the temporalis muscle, and the masseter muscle. A separate branch, the mylohyoid nerve, innervates the mylohyoid muscle and anterior belly of the digastric muscle within the floor of

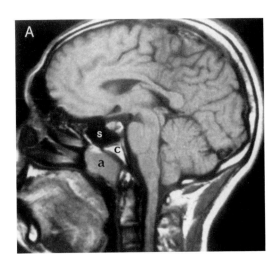

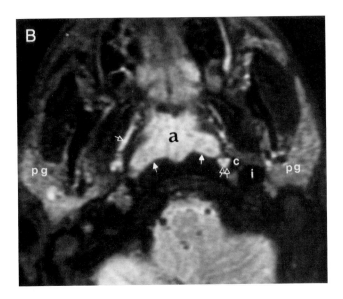

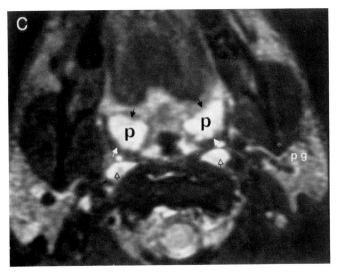

FIG. 7. A 30-year-old man with ARC. **A:** Sagittal T1-weighted image through the nasopharynx demonstrates prominent adenoidal tissue (A), which has muscular intensity. Note that the nasopharyngeal airway is almost completely obscured by this mass of adenoids; however, no deep invasion of the skull base, clivus (c), or sphenoid sinus (s) is present. **B:** Axial T2-weighted MR scan through the midnasopharynx (TR = 2,000 msec; TE = 80 msec). The adenoidal tissue (a) has increased intensity on the T2-weighted examination. Note its interface with the prevertebral muscles (*solid arrows*). In this instance, fat within the parapharyngeal space can still be identified (*single open arrow*). Note also the left retropharyngeal node (*double open arrow*), which is commonly associated with prominent adenoidal masses in ARC: (c) internal carotid artery; (i) internal jugular vein. **C:** Axial T2-weighted image through the oropharynx and tonsils. The palatine tonsils have high signal intensity (p). They are enclosed by the palatoglossus muscle (*black arrows*) and the posterior palatopharyngeus muscle (*white arrows*). Retropharyngeal lymph nodes are noted adjacent to the carotid artery (*open black arrows*). The T2-weighted image demonstrates the parotid gland (pg), which has slightly higher intensity compared to muscle. T1-weighted images demonstrate the parotid gland to be slightly lower in intensity than fat.

the mouth. The third division of the trigeminal nerve also provides motor innervation to the levator palati muscle and sensory branches to the anterior two-thirds of the tongue via the lingual nerve, and the lower face and the lower teeth via the inferior alveolar nerve (15).

The first and second divisions of the trigeminal nerve also have a characteristic course. The first division (V_1) exits the cavernous sinus and enters the superior orbital fissure. It becomes the superior orbital nerve, a sensory branch supplying the upper forehead and lower scalp. The second division passes through the foramen rotundum to enter the pterygopalatine fossa (Fig. 5B and C). The pterygopalatine fossa, between the posterior wall of the maxillary sinus and the pterygoid plate, contains the terminal branches of the internal maxillary artery, the second division of the trigeminal nerve, the sphenopalatine ganglion, and the infraorbital nerve. These structures are embedded within high-intensity fat. Infiltration of the fat within the pterygopalatine fossa is always abnormal and may be seen with tumor, infection, pseudotumor of the orbit, and trauma (see section on pterygopalatine fossa, *this chapter*) (see Fig. 14).

The vagus nerve (X) supplies the motor fibers of the superior and middle pharyngeal constrictor muscles and the soft palate, including the tensor palatini muscle. The glossopharyngeal nerve (IX) supplies motor input to the stylopharyngeus muscle, which is not routinely imaged on MR scans. The spinal accessory nerve (XI) innervates the trapezius and sternocleidomastoid muscles. It exits the jugular foramen with the ninth and tenth cranial nerves, then travels within the posterior cervical triangle accompanied by spinal accessory lymph nodes.

PATHOLOGY OF THE NASOPHARYNX

Displacement or infiltration of the deep musculofascial fat planes localize nasopharyngeal masses to the various spaces described above. Once a mass is localized to a particular space, the differential diagnosis is facilitated by knowledge of the pathologic entities developing in that space. As a general rule, T1-weighted MR images (TR ≤ 600 msec; TE = 25 msec) best outline musculofascial anatomy (Figs. 3–5), whereas heavily T2-weighted images (TR ≥ 2,000 msec; TE ≥ 70 msec) best identify signal intensity differences between normal and pathologic anatomy. T2-weighted imaging sequences highlight areas of increased water content present in most head and neck tumors, edematous fluid, cystic and necrotic tissue, reactive and metastatic adenopathy, and submucosal or intramuscular pathology (1).

Usually, a sagittal T1-weighted "localizing" sequence is obtained to reference subsequent coronal and axial scans (Fig. 3). Subsequently, an axial spin-echo T2-weighted sequence is then obtained through the naso-pharynx to highlight intensity differences as described above. Coronal 5-mm T1-weighted images are then obtained through the area of pathology. Coronal views of the skull base are mandatory in every patient with suspected nasopharyngeal pathology in order to detect early bone and intracranial invasion.

MUCOSAL SPACE LESIONS

Mucosal space lesions arise on the airway side of the pharyngobasilar fascia. Although most are malignant, it is important to identify those benign lesions that can be left untouched by the surgeon's hand.

BENIGN LESIONS

Benign primary mucosal masses of the nasopharynx are rarely symptomatic. They include variations of adenoidal tissue and the congenital Thornwald's cyst. Other benign lesions from tissues surrounding the nasopharynx, such as frontoethmoidal encephaloceles, invasive pituitary neoplasms, nasal polyps, and malignant otitis externa, may encroach on the mucosal space. Their site of origin is usually clear from their vector of growth. Adenoidal tissue is prominent in children and young adults, appearing as a homogeneous superficial mass of soft tissue occupying the superior and lateral recesses of the nasopharynx (Figs. 3C and 4E and F). Adenoidal lymphatic tissue regresses with age; however, small superficial tags of adenoidal tissue may be present at any age. Residual adenoidal tissue may be impossible to differentiate from superficial noninvasive carcinomas of the nasopharynx.

Adenoidal tissue has a high spin density and relatively long T1 and T2 relaxation times (1). These factors result in a signal intensity quite similar to muscle on T1-weighted images (Fig. 7A) but a high signal intensity on T2-weighted images (Figs. 6B and 7B). Occasionally, small foci of higher signal intensity may be detected within the adenoidal bed on T2-weighted images (Fig. 6B). These represent degenerative cysts probably due to prior infections. Adenoidal tissue never infiltrates the soft tissue planes deep to the mucosa or the pharyngobasilar fascia (4); however, its signal characteristics are quite similar to most nasopharyngeal malignancies, making the exclusion of superficial, noninvasive nasopharyngeal carcinoma quite difficult in patients with residual nasopharyngeal adenoidal tissue. Reactive cervical adenopathy often accompanies prominent adenoidal tissue in children; in adults with the acquired immunodeficiency syndrome (AIDS)-related complex (ARC) syndrome (Fig. 7B).

Thornwald's cyst is present in 4% of normal autopsy specimens and develops from an ectopic portion of no-

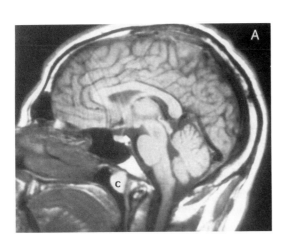
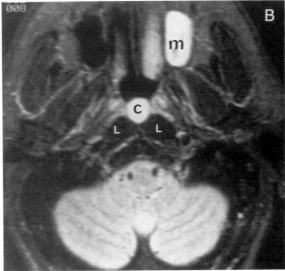

FIG. 8: Thornwald's cyst. **A:** Sagittal T1-weighted MR sequence (TR = 600 msec; TE = 20 msec). A high-intensity mass within the midline of the upper nasopharynx represents a Thornwald cyst. It has a characteristic position beneath the clivus and posterior to the vertical plane of the pituitary infundibulum. The cyst (c) has a high intensity on T1-weighted images as a result of proteinaceous or hemorrhagic debris. **B:** T2-weighted axial image through the upper nasopharynx (TR = 2,000 msec; TE = 80 msec). The Thornwald cyst (c) increases in intensity similar to CSF and the fluid within the left maxillary sinus (m). Note its characteristic position in the midline between the longus capitis muscles (L). Extension off the midline has only been seen in one of our cases due to a Thornwald's abscess.

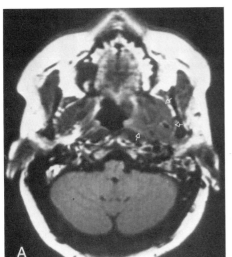
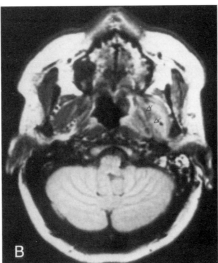
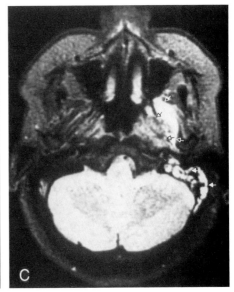

FIG. 9. Nasopharyngeal squamous cell carcinoma. **A–C:** Axial sections through the midnasopharynx. **A:** T1-weighted image (TR = 600 msec; TE = 25 msec). Infiltration of the left parapharyngeal space and medial peterygoid muscle has occurred from a deeply invasive nasopharyngeal carcinoma (*arrows*). On T1-weighted sequences such as this, tumor infiltration of fat planes is quite evident; however, intensity differences between tumor and surrounding muscle is poor. **B,C:** 40-msec echo (**B**) and 80-msec echo (**C**) from a TR = 2,000-msec spin-echo series. The left nasopharyngeal carcinoma increases in intensity with progressive T2-weighting. Edema of the left medial pterygoid muscle is best evident on the 80-msec echo (*open white arrows*). The carcinoma infiltrates the muscle but has slightly lower intensity than the edematous muscle (*open black arrows*). Note also the increased signal from the left mastoid air cells, filled with fluid secondary to eustachian tube dysfunction or obstruction (*solid white arrows*).

tochordal remnants in the nasopharynx. The notochordal remnants occasionally give rise to an epithelial tract that empties into the midline of the nasopharynx. This tract may close over and result in a midline cyst, which on occasion may become infected. The cyst is located in the midline of the nasopharynx nestled in the pharyngeal bursa between the longus capitis muscles (Fig. 8). The cyst varies from 1 mm to 5 mm in diameter and has a high signal intensity on T1- and T2-weighted images, probably due to either proteinaceous or hemorrhagic contents (Fig. 8). Occasionally, Thornwald's cyst may become infected, leading to a syndrome consisting of prevertebral muscular spasm with head motion, postnasal discharge, and foul breath. Thornwald's abscess must be surgically drained to prevent retropharyngeal abscess.

Malignant Mucosal Tumors

More than 98% of malignancies in the nasopharynx are carcinomas. Eighty percent are squamous cell carcinomas, whereas 18% are adenocarcinomas or minor salivary gland carcinomas, such as adenoid cystic carcinoma and mucoepidermoid carcinoma (16). Non-Hodgkin's lymphoma and sarcomas represent a small minority of malignancies in the adult; however, they are the most common histologies in children (5,16).

The clinical symptomatology and MR signal characteristics of most carcinomas are indistinguishable from each other. Most patients present to their physician with one or more of the following complaints:

1. an asymptomatic neck mass representing a metastatic cervical node, usually within the posterior triangle;
2. serous otitis media produced by obstruction or dysfunction of the eustachian tube;
3. symptoms related to cavernous sinus invasion or other cranial neuropathies;
4. trismus due to pterygoid muscle involvement; and
5. nasal obstruction or epistaxis.

Since nasopharyngeal carcinoma represents most nasopharyngeal lesions, it is considered in detail.

Squamous cell carcinoma of the nasopharynx is rare in most countries of the world, with an incidence in the Caucasian population of less than 1 per 100,000 people per year (16). This tumor is more prevalent in Asian countries, particularly in the southern provinces of China, where an incidence as high as 18 to 20 cases per 100,000 people per year have been reported. Squamous cell carcinoma can develop in any age group; however, it favors the middle-aged and older patients. Tobacco and alcohol abuse are associated with the development of nasopharyngeal carcinoma; however, both environmental and genetic factors appear to play a role in Chinese

patients. IGA antibodies to the Epstein-Barr virus have been associated with undifferentiated carcinoma of the nasopharynx and can be used as a marker for tumor in patients with this specific histology (16).

Squamous carcinoma of the nasopharynx most often develops in the lateral pharyngeal recess of Rosenmuller (Figs. 9 and 10). Invasion of the deep musculofascial planes around the levator and tensor palatini muscles is the most frequent appearance on MR (Figs. 9 and 13), although exophytic or superficial spreading mucosal carcinomas occasionally occur (Fig. 10). Invasion of the levator palati muscle results in eustachian tube dysfunction and rapid serous otitis media (Fig. 9C). Ipsilateral mastoid opacification and serous otitis media are a very common finding with nasopharyngeal carcinoma (Fig. 9). As the tumor invades laterally, it may initially displace and then invade the parapharyngeal fat plane (Fig. 11). At this point, the tumor may grow in a caudal or cranial direction along the muscular planes deep to the nasopharyngeal mucosa (Fig. 11). Tumor may extend to the soft palate inferiorly (Fig. 11C) or through the skull base foramina superiorly, eventually involving the cavernous sinus. Anterior extension to the nares may result in nasal congestion and epistaxis.

Direct coronal MR images will demonstrate skull base erosion by replacement of the normal cortical and marrow bone by signal similar to tumor. These changes may be more subtle on MR than CT; however, if one pays particular attention to the normal appearance of the skull base, early skull base erosion may also be detected by MR imaging. In rare cases, sclerotic foci adjacent to a nasopharyngeal carcinoma have been detected in the skull base. These probably represent reactive bone changes and not tumor invasion, although both may coexist in the same patient.

Carcinoma may also spread along nerves, vessels, or within lymphatics (15,16). The nasopharynx has a rich cross-network of lymphatics first draining to retropharyngeal nodal chains that lie just medial to the carotid artery (Figs. 4E and 12). This so-called lateral retropharyngeal group, or node of Rouviere, is the sentinel node of nasopharyngeal carcinoma (Fig. 12A and B). Drainage from this group occurs inferiorly along the retropharyngeal chain, then laterally to the posterior triangle nodes deep to the sternocleidomastoid muscle, and finally, anteriorly along the internal jugular vein (Fig. 12). In general, adenopathy has a homogeneous low signal intensity on T1-weighted images and a high signal intensity on T2-weighted images (Figs. 4E and 12). Node necrosis can best be identified on heavily T2-weighted images as foci of very bright signal intensity (Fig. 12E–G).

Perineural tumor growth may occur from any head and neck malignancy, especially adenoid cystic carci-

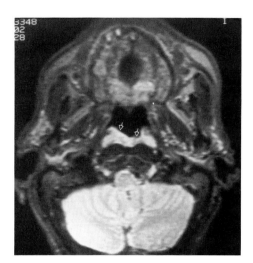

FIG. 10. Superficial squamous cell carcinoma of the naso-pharynx. Axial image through the nasopharynx (TR = 2,000 msec; TE = 80 msec). This patient had palpable cervical adenopathy (not shown). MR scan was undertaken to eval-uate for an unknown primary site. Increase in signal within the nasopharyngeal airway is demonstrated (*open white arrows*); however, this signal appears similar to adenoidal tissue. Biopsy of this region revealed squamous cell carci-noma that had not infiltrated deep into the pharyngobasi-lar fascia. This cannot be differentiated from residual adenoidal tissue.

nomas, squamous cell carcinomas, and lymphomas (16). Perineural spread of tumor may be detected on MR in either a direct or indirect manner. Direct findings of perineural spread include enlargement of a cranial nerve or neural foramina near the skull base with occa-sional extension into the cavernous sinus. Indirect evi-dence of perineural tumor or neural compromise is indicated by muscular denervation atrophy (15). Intra-vascular spread of tumor is most unusual, occurring through invasion of the internal jugular vein. This may lead to thrombosis of the vessel.

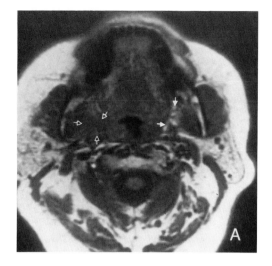

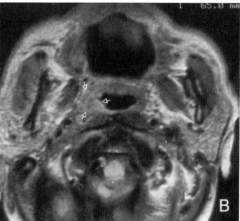

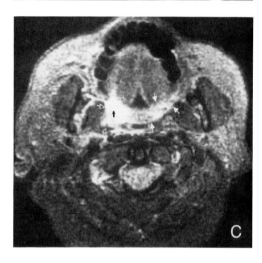

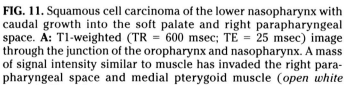

FIG. 11. Squamous cell carcinoma of the lower nasopharynx with caudal growth into the soft palate and right parapharyngeal space. **A:** T1-weighted (TR = 600 msec; TE = 25 msec) image through the junction of the oropharynx and nasopharynx. A mass of signal intensity similar to muscle has invaded the right para-pharyngeal space and medial pterygoid muscle (*open white arrows*). Note the normal parapharyngeal fat separating the tonsillar bed from the medial pterygoid on the left (*white arrows*). **B:** Spin-density image (TR = 2,000 msec; TE = 40 msec) at the junction of the nasopharynx and oropharynx. Thickening of the right pharyngeal wall and effacement of the right parapharyngeal space is evident (*open white arrows*). Signal intensity differences between the tumor and surrounding musculature are minimal. The tumor from the nasopharynx has grown inferiorly along the superior and middle constrictor muscles to involve the tonsillar region. **C:** T2-weighted image (TR = 2,000 msec; TE = 80 msec) through the soft palate and tonsillar region. The carcinoma has increased in signal intensity (*open white arrows*). The high-intensity signal of the normal soft palate glandular tissue (*solid white arrows*) makes the medial aspect of the nasopharyngeal tumor (t) difficult to assess.

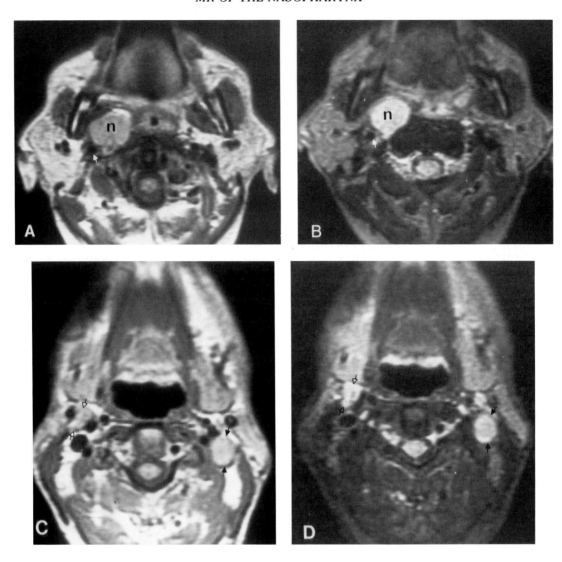

In most instances of perineural tumor, a primary tumor grows around a distal branch of one of the cranial nerves in a retrograde direction toward the skull base. Neurologic symptoms may thus relate to either skull base erosion, cavernous sinus invasion, or isolated cranial neuropathy. The most common nerves involved by upper aerodigestive tract tumors are the second and third division of the trigeminal nerve, the facial nerve and the hypoglossal nerve; however, every combination of every cranial nerve can be involved by perineural tumor growth. Involvement of the trigeminal nerve results in sensory changes along the face or inner aspect of the mouth. If the third division of the trigeminal nerve is involved, the motor supply to the masticator muscles

may be compromised (Fig. 13). In this instance, MR may show fatty replacement and atrophy of those muscles (Fig. 13B).

Pterygopalatine Fossa

The pterygopalatine fossa (PPF) is a particularly important region to assess when looking for perineural tumor, especially in those patients with symptoms related to the second division of the trigeminal nerve. This space is located between the pterygoid plates and the posterior maxillary sinus wall (Fig. 14). It normally contains fat and the terminal branches of the internal maxillary artery. The sphenopalatine ganglion is also located

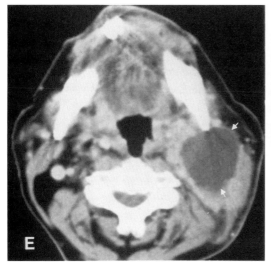

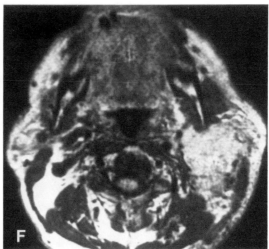

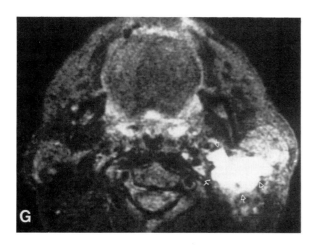

FIG. 12. Adenopathy from nasopharyngeal carcinoma. **A,B:** TR = 2,000 msec; TE = 40 msec (**A**) and 80 msec (**B**) through the lower nasopharynx. Adenopathy from a squamous cell carcinoma of the nasopharynx has involved the medial retropharyngeal node of Rouviere (n). Just as with normal lymphatics and reactive nodes, metastatic adenopathy increases in signal intensity on the heavily T2-weighted image. Subtle foci of inhomogeneity probably relate to areas of normal node interspersed with tumor. Necrosis has not occurred in this example. Note that MR provides good contrast between the patent internal carotid artery (*arrow*) and the node. In this example the node is separated from the lumen of the carotid artery by surrounding musculature. **C,D:** TR = 2,000 msec; TE = 40 msec (**C**) and 80 msec (**D**). Axial MR images through the upper neck reveal bilateral cervical adenopathy from the patient's nasopharyngeal carcinoma. The right anterior internal jugular node (*open black arrow*) is present between the internal carotid artery and the external carotid artery. The left posterior triangle (spinal accessory) node lies deep to the sternocleidomastoid muscle within the fat-filled posterior triangle space (*closed black arrow*). Neither node is greater than 1.5 cm in diameter, and their signal intensities are similar to those of reactive nodes (see Fig. 7B). Fine-needle aspiration biopsy would be necessary to confirm metastatic disease; however, in light of the very large retropharyngeal node in **A**, these nodes are presumed metastatic. **E:** CT scan through the midoropharynx in a patient (different patient from **A–D**) with a left neck mass and nasopharyngeal carcinoma. CT scan demonstrates an area of low signal density posterior to the left mandible consistent with a necrotic lymph node. **F,G:** Axial MR scans through the same region as **E**. TR = 2,000 msec; TE = 40 msec (**F**) and 80 msec (**G**). The necrotic center is best identified as a very bright signal intensity on the heavily T2-weighted image (*open white arrows*).

within the PPF, receiving the V$_2$ nerve from the foramen rotundum, the pterygoid nerve (parasympathetic supply to the paranasal sinus) via the pterygoid canal (Fig. 14A), and giving off the infraorbital nerve (V$_2$), which supplies sensation to the midface. Retrograde perineural spread of tumor along branches of the V$_2$ nerve may result in infiltration of the PPF and cavernous sinus invasion (Fig. 14). The PPF may also be involved by intracranial or cavernous sinus tumors, which grow antegrade along the second division of the trigeminal nerve (Fig. 15), or by juvenile angiofibromas.

Deep Compartment Masses

Deep compartment masses can usually be localized by their characteristic displacement of the fat-filled parapharyngeal space. The mass may reside within the carotid space, the retropharyngeal space, the parotid space, the masticator space, or within the parapharyngeal space itself. Retropharyngeal masses are detected by their characteristic displacement of the mucosa anteriorly and the prevertebral muscles posteriorly.

It is important to remember that MR may not differ-

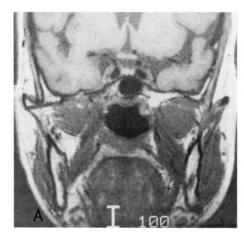
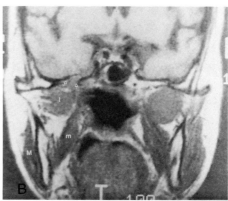

FIG. 13. Perineural spread of nasopharyngeal carcinoma along the right third division of the trigeminal nerve. This patient had been treated for nasopharyngeal carcinoma 4 years prior to this study and presents with new symptoms of right lower facial pain and numbness. **A:** Coronal T1-weighted image through the nasopharynx (TR = 600 msec; TE = 25 msec). Fat planes around the right upper skull base and nasopharynx have been obliterated by the infiltrating carcinoma (*open white arrows*). **B:** Coronal T1-weighted section 5 mm posterior to **A.** The infiltration has occurred along the proximal branch of the third division of the trigeminal nerve widening the foramen ovale (*open white arrows*). Also note atrophy of the lateral pterygoid (l), medial pterygoid (m), and masseter muscle (M), which are innervated by the motor division of the third division of the trigeminal nerve.

entiate between infiltrative inflammatory lesions and tumor. For instance, mucormycosis of the paranasal sinuses or malignant otitis external may extend into the nasopharynx and appear similar in MR and CT appearance to primary nasopharyngeal carcinoma (Fig. 16). In these instances, involvement of the sinuses and/or the external ear canal may lead one to the appropriate diagnosis.

Carotid Space Masses

The carotid space is created by fascial contributions from all layers of the deep cervical fascia (9). In the nasopharynx it includes the internal carotid artery and internal jugular vein, the cranial nerves IX to XII, the cervical sympathetic plexus, and the retropharyngeal nodes, which surround the carotid sheath and can be

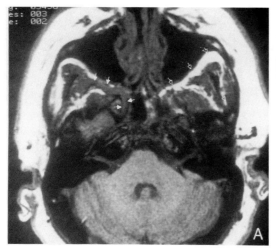
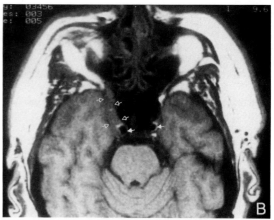

FIG. 14. Infiltration of the pterygopalatine fossa (PPF) by adenocarcinoma. **A:** 5-mm T1-weighted (TR = 600 msec; TE = 25 msec) scan through the pterygopalatine fossa. The normal left fat-filled PPF is located posterior to the aerated maxillary sinus and anterior to the musculature of the infratemporal fossa (*open white arrows*). The right PPF has been infiltrated by a tumor growing in a retrograde fashion along the infraorbital nerve. The tumor can be seen growing within the PPF and in a retrograde fashion through the pterygoid canal (*white arrows*) (see text). **B:** 5-mm T1-weighted MR scan superior to **A** (TR = 600 msec; TE = 25 msec). The right cavernous sinus has been infiltrated by tumor growing retrograde along the second division of the trigeminal nerve in **A** (*open white arrows*). Note the normal cavernous carotid artery (*solid white arrows*) located just lateral to the aerated sphenoid sinus.

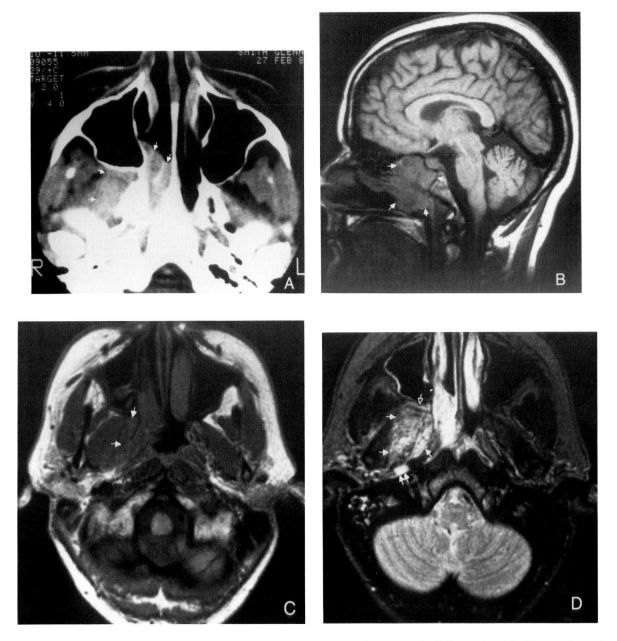

FIG. 15. Cavernous sinus meningioma growing into the PPF and posterior nares. **A:** Enhanced axial CT scan through the pterygopalatine fossa reveals an enhancing mass infiltrating the right pterygoid palatine fossa and growing into the posterior nares and the medial infratemporal fossa (*white arrows*). **B:** Sagittal T1-weighted image through the midline (TR = 600 msec; TE = 25 msec). The homogeneous mass of low signal intensity has replaced the sphenoid sinus and infiltrated the upper nasopharynx (*arrows*). **C:** Axial T1-weighted image through the pterygopalatine fossa and midnasopharynx (TR = 600 msec; TE = 25 msec). The mass has a similar intensity to muscle and is only recognized by its infiltration of fat planes around the medial pterygoid and pterygopalatine fossa (*arrows*). **D:** T2-weighted image at the same plane as **C** (TR = 2,000 msec; TE = 80 msec). The meningioma has increased in signal intensity (*arrows*) and can be recognized infiltrating the pterygopalatine fossa (*open white arrow*). Note also a probably reactive lateral retropharyngeal lymph node (*double white arrows*).

considered within the carotid space. These tissues may give rise to a variety of lesions including vascular masses, such as paragangliomas, neurogenic tumors, and lymph node pathology. Jugular foramen masses, such as jugulotympanic paragangliomas, extracranial meningiomas, skull base metastatic disease, and chor-

doma, may grow inferiorly into the upper nasopharynx and also present as carotid space masses.

Paragangliomas are benign vascular lesions arising from paraganglion cells along the carotid artery or jugular vein (16). The most common sites of origin include the carotid bifurcation, the internal jugular bulb, the

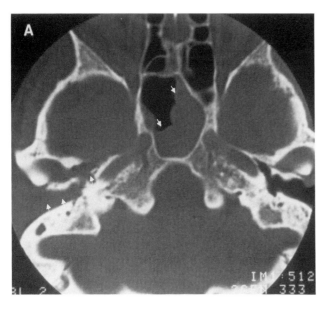

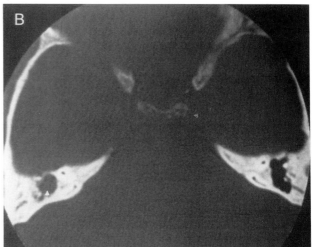

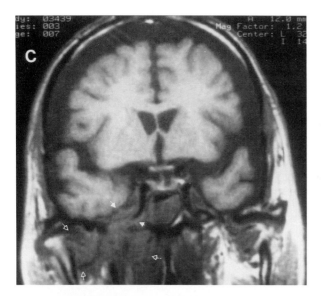

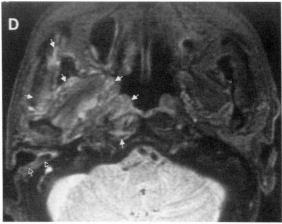

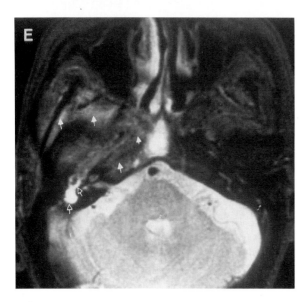

FIG. 16. Malignant otitis externa infiltrating the nasopharynx. This elderly diabetic man presented with several months of external ear canal drainage, headache, and jugular foramen cranial nerve palsies. **A:** Axial CT scan through the skull base and external canal. Soft tissue density infiltrates the right external canal and middle ear. Soft tissue is present within the sphenoid sinus (*white arrows*). **B:** Axial CT scan through the petrous apex and middle ear reveals opacification and expansion of the epitympanic recess of the right middle ear (*arrow*). This has the appearance of a cholesteatoma, which was present at surgery. **C:** Coronal T1-weighted image through the nasopharynx and skull base (TR = 600 msec; TE = 25 msec). Infiltration of the fat planes surrounding the skull base and right temporomandibular joint has occurred secondary to a soft tissue mass (*open white arrows*). There has also been erosion and enlargement of the foramen ovale and invasion of the inferior right cavernous sinus (*white arrows*). **D:** T2-weighted axial MR scan through the midnasopharynx (TR = 2,000 msec; TE = 80 msec). Subtle increase in signal intensity is present within the right mucosa of the nasopharynx, right prevertebral muscle, and right infratemporal fossa (*arrows*). In addition, increased signal intensity lines the external canal and middle ear (*open arrows*). This proved to be an extensive inflammatory mass from the patient's otitis externa. The

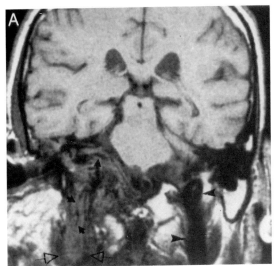

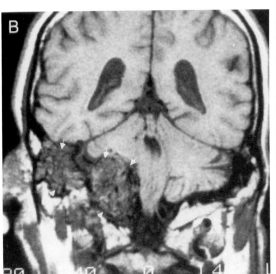

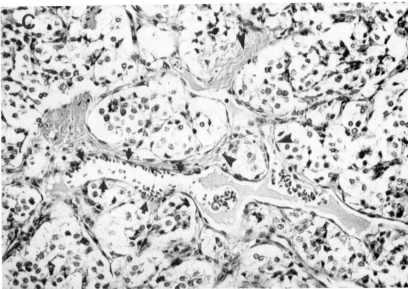

FIG. 17. A: Jugulotympanic paraganglioma. Coronal T1-weighted MR scan (TR = 600 msec; TE = 25 msec). A heterogeneous mass is present in the right posterior nasopharynx, infiltrating the right skull base and jugular foramen region. Serpiginous areas of high-velocity signal loss representing arterial feeding vessels are indicated (*small black arrows*). Invasion down the right jugular vein (*open black arrows*) has occurred and in common with jugulotympanic paragangliomas. The normal left internal jugular vein is indicated (*solid arrowheads*). **B:** Coronal T1-weighted MR scan posterior to **A**. The paraganglioma has infiltrated the left cerebellopontine angle, displacing the right cerebellar hemisphere and pons superiorly and medially. The tumor has invaded the right temporal bone and mastoid air cells (*arrows*). Again identified are foci of high-velocity signal loss amid a heterogeneous tumor matrix, probably secondary to fibrous stroma (see **C**). **C:** Histologic appearance of paraganglioma. Photomicrograph of the paraganglioma demonstrates cellular nests separated by fibrous stroma (*arrowheads*) and vascular lumina (*arrows*), contributing to the heterogeneous quality on MR.

middle ear, and along the nodosa ganglion of the vagus nerve. In the nasopharynx, paragangliomas usually have a jugular fossa component that produces pulsatile tinnitus, but occasionally, a patient may present with a neck mass with bruits, cranial neuropathy, or jugular fossa syndrome. On MR, paragangliomas 2 cm or greater in size have a specific heterogeneous appearance consisting of foci of high and low intensity on T2-weighted sequences. The low signal probably reflects the dense fibrous matrix separating higher signal intensity of cellular nests (Figs. 17 and 18). T1-weighted sequences may demonstrate foci of high-velocity signal loss within vessels supplying the tumor (Fig. 17). Extension through the jugular foramen into the temporal bone and middle

signal intensity simulates that of nasopharyngeal carcinoma; however, a diffuse infiltration of musculature within the retropharyngeal and infratemporal fossa regions would be distinctly unusual for nasopharyngeal carcinoma. Nasopharyngeal carcinoma generally grows in a mass-like fashion from the mucosa laterally into the infratemporal fossa, displacing structures rather than infiltrating in a diffuse fashion. **E:** Axial T2-weighted image through the posterior fossa and right middle ear (TR = 2,000 msec; TE = 80 msec). Increase in signal intensity is seen in the upper nasopharynx and infiltrating the base of skull (*white arrows*). This represents subperiosteal abscess and inflammatory disease from the otitis externa. Very bright signal intensity within the middle ear is detected, consistent with the patient's diagnosis of associated cholesteatoma (*open white arrows*).

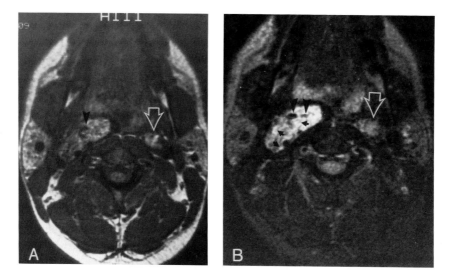

FIG. 18. Bilateral carotid space paragangliomas. **A,B:** Axial T2-weighted scans [TR = 2,000 msec; TE = 40 msec (**A**) and 80 msec (**B**)]. The 40-msec echo demonstrates bilateral masses of heterogeneous signal intensity. The right mass deviates the internal carotid and jugular vein posteriorly and contains foci of high-velocity signal loss within vessels supplying the tumor (*black arrowhead*). Foci of even-echo rephasing, indicating slow blood flow within the tumor, is indicated on the 80-msec echo (*small black arrows*). The smaller left carotid space paraganglioma has a more homogeneous intensity on the T2-weighted image (*open white arrow*), although several foci of low signal in supplying vessels can be identified. These signal features are distinctly different from other carotid space masses.

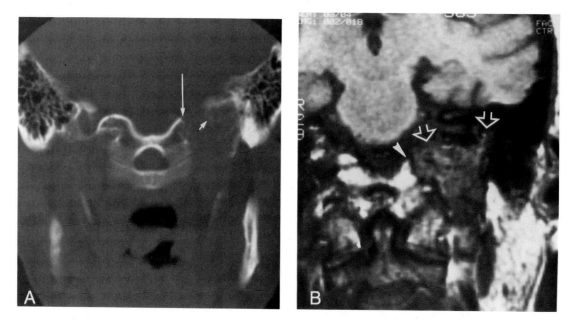

FIG. 19. Jugulotympanic paraganglioma. **A:** Coronal CT scan with bone review demonstrates erosion of the left jugular foramen (*small arrow*) and truncation of the left jugular tubercle (*long arrow*). **B:** Coronal T1-weighted MR scan through the posterior nasopharynx and jugular foramen (TR = 600 msec; TE = 25 msec). The left jugulotympanic paraganglioma of mixed signal intensity invades the inferior aspect of the left temporal bone (*open white arrow*) and truncates the medial left jugular tubercle (*arrowhead*) (compare with **A**).

ear may be seen with larger lesions (Fig. 17). The heterogeneous appearance differentiates these lesions from other metastatic and neurogenic lesions of the carotid space. Extension within the internal jugular vein may be detected in some patients (Figs. 17 and 19).

Our approach to paragangliomas includes an initial diagnostic MR study. The patient may be referred to angiography if surgical therapy or embolotherapy is planned. Alternatively, we feel confident about the MR

diagnosis such that radiation therapy may be given on the basis of the MR findings alone.

Schwannomas are benign tumors that arise from the Schwann cell encircling the axon of a peripheral nerve. Schwannomas are more common in the third to sixth decade. Male and female incidence is equal. They have a predilection for developing in the head and neck region, particularly from the spinal cord rootlets, the vagus nerve, or from the cervical sympathetics. The tumor

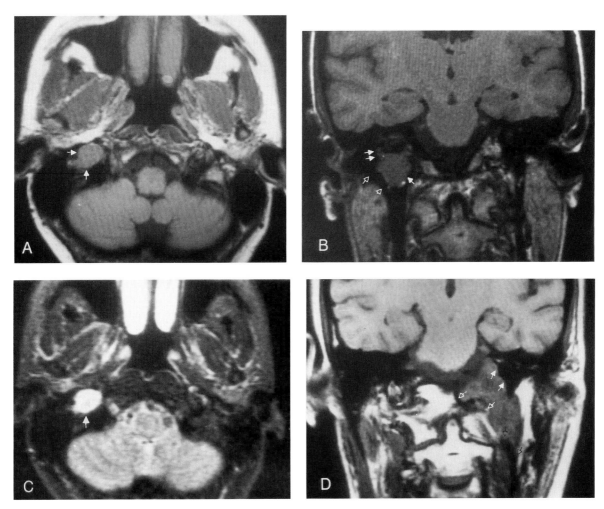

FIG. 20. Schwannomas of the jugular foramen. **A:** Tenth nerve schwannoma. T1-weighted axial image (TR = 600 msec; TE = 25 msec) through the region of the jugular foramen demonstrates a homogeneous mass equal in intensity to cerebellar gray matter (*white arrows*). Note that the internal signal is homogeneous and does not contain vascular channels like paragangliomas (Fig. 18). **B:** Coronal T1-weighted image through the jugular foramen (TR = 600 msec; TE = 25 msec). The right jugular foramen schwannoma (*white arrows*) is positioned medial to the patent jugular vein (*open arrows*). Note the tongues of soft tissue extending into the jugular foramen and into the middle ear (*double white arrows*). **C:** T2-weighted axial image through jugular foramen (TR = 2,000 msec; TE = 80 msec). The right jugular foramen schwannoma has homogeneous increase in signal intensity similar to CSF. Signal intensity increases greater than most meningiomas and is more homogeneous than the paragangliomas previously illustrated (Figs. 18 and 19). **D:** Jugular foramen schwannoma (different patient from A–C). T1-weighted coronal image through the left jugular foramen (TR = 600 msec; TE = 25 msec). The schwannoma has a low signal intensity, is homogeneous, and expands the left jugular foramen (*white arrows*). The mass has smoothly eroded the cortex of the skull base and C1 vertebral body (*open white arrows*) and grows inferiorly along the carotid sheath, obliterating the jugular vein. The jugular vein reconstitutes at the inferior margin of the tumor (*open black arrows*).

may be silent for many months or years until local symptoms of pain or cranial neuropathy present. The schwannoma or neurilemmoma is encapsulated and may consist of two distinct histologic components: a cellular component (Antoni A area) and a loose or myxoid component (Antoni B area). This histologic feature differentiates schwannomas from the very heterogeneous neurofibroma.

On MR, schwannomas usually have a homogeneous signal intensity that increases with progressive T2 weighting (Fig. 20). Internal necrosis or cystic degeneration is a feature of larger lesions and is best assessed on T1-weighted images. Smooth bony expansion and erosion may be detected. The lesion is suggested in cases of soft tissue homogeneous neoplasms in and about the jugular foramen. It may be difficult to differentiate a small schwannoma from a carotid space retropharyngeal node.

Retropharyngeal adenopathy may present as a carotid space mass, although anatomically these nodes are located just outside the carotid fascia. Retropharyngeal adenopathy may occur from metastatic disease (Fig. 12A and B) or lymphoproliferative disorders, such as non-Hodgkin's lymphoma and benign conditions [such as ARC (Fig. 7)], or in young children with recurrent adenoidal infections (Fig. 4E). Lymph nodes have a prolonged T1 and T2 relaxation time, resulting in a muscular density on T1-weighted images and a hyperintense signal on T2-weighted images (Fig. 12). Carotid space nodes are homogeneous unless necrotic. Necrosis is recognized by a foci of hyperintense signal on T2-weighted images (Fig. 12G).

Unusual jugular foramen lesions include chordoma and extracranial meningioma (17). Extracranial meningioma may descend from the jugular fossa to involve the carotid space (Fig. 15). Meningioma has a signal charac-

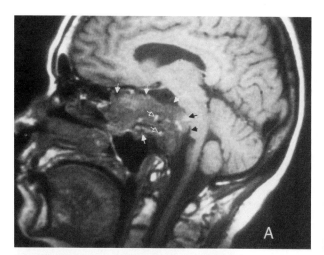

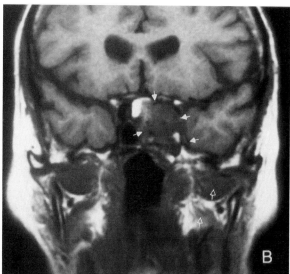

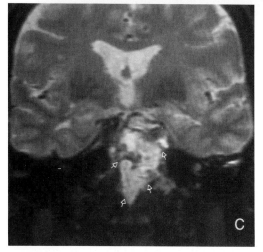

FIG. 21. Skull base chordoma. Young female patient complaining of pain and anesthesia over the lower aspect of her face. Long-tract signs with weakness of both lower extremities were present for several months. A: Sagittal T1-weighted (TR = 600 msec; TE = 25 msec) image through the skull base. A soft tissue mass of heterogeneous intensity (*white arrows*) has destroyed the normal features of the clivus and sella. The mass extends posteriorly into the prepontine cistern, displacing the pons posteriorly (*arrows*). Chordoma often extends anteriorly into the upper nasopharynx where it may at first push mucosa anteriorly and inferiorly. Residual islands of bone can be seen within the tumor as foci of high-signal-intensity fatty marrow (*open arrows*). B: Coronal T1-weighted image through the nasopharynx and sphenoid sinus (TR = 600 msec; TE = 25 msec). The chordoma has filled the sphenoid sinus and invaded the left cavernous sinus (*arrows*). Involvement of the third division of the trigeminal nerve has resulted in atrophy of the left masticator muscles (*open arrows*). The left lateral pterygoid and medial pterygoid muscles are diminished in size compared to the right (*open arrows*). C: Coronal T2-weighted image through the posterior nasopharynx and skull base (TR = 2,000 msec; TE = 80 msec). The chordoma has increased in signal intensity (*open arrows*) relative to surrounding bone and muscle.

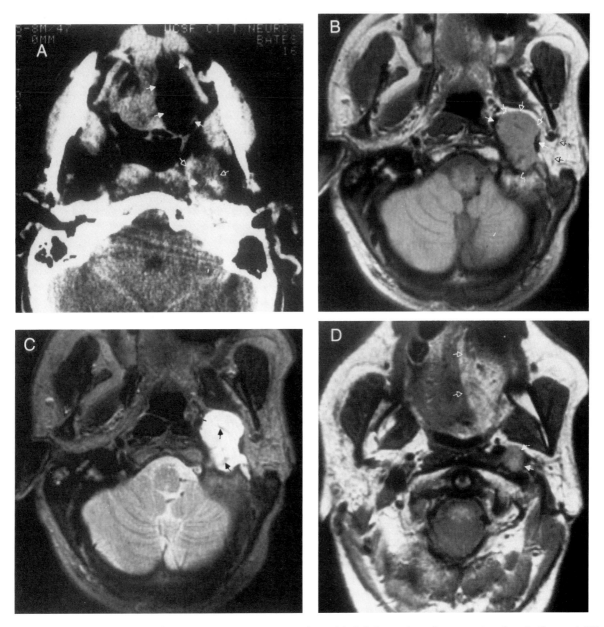

FIG. 22. Jugular fossa chordoma; 30-year-old woman presenting with left hypoglossal nerve atrophy. **A:** Coronal CT scan demonstrates a mass in the region of the left jugular fossa (*open arrows*). Hemiatrophy of the left side of the tongue is evident by fatty replacement of the left intrinsic tongue muscle, genioglossus, and geniohyoid muscles (*closed arrows*). **B:** Axial T1-weighted image through the lower nasopharynx (TR = 2,000 msec; TE = 40 msec). The chordoma is present in the left carotid space, deviating the parapharyngeal space anteriorly (*open white arrows*). The mass separates the internal carotid from the internal jugular vein (*solid arrows*) and deviates both vessels anteriorly, indicating its carotid space location. Also note the plane of the facial nerve within the left parotid gland (*open black arrows*). The facial nerve courses from the region of the stylomastoid foramen medial to the mastoid tip, just lateral to the retromandibular vein within the parotid gland. **C:** T2-weighted image at the same level as **B** (TR = 2,000 msec; TE = 80 msec). The mass has increased in signal intensity on the heavily T2-weighted image. Foci of lower signal within the mass represent calcifications (*arrows*). The signal intensity and position are similar for jugular foramen schwannomas. In this case, the initial diagnosis was schwannoma until biopsy revealed chordoma. **D:** Axial T1-weighted image through the oropharynx. The inferior aspect of the left jugular foramen chordoma is present (*arrows*). Hypoglossal nerve palsy is indicated by fatty replacement of the left half of the tongue (*open arrows*).

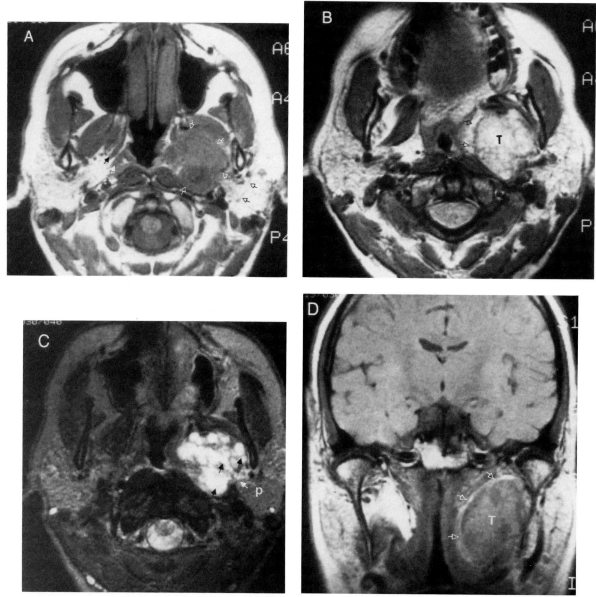

FIG. 23. Benign mixed-cell tumor of the deep lobe of the parotid gland **A:** T1-weighted axial MR scan through the midnaso-pharynx (TR = 600 msec; TE = 25 msec). A homogeneous low-intensity mass arises from either the deep lobe of the parotid or the left parapharyngeal space (*open arrows*). The medial pterygoid muscle is deviated anteriorly, the carotid vessels are deviated posteriorly and laterally, and the nasopharyngeal mucosa is deviated medially. Note the normal appearance of the levator palatini muscle (*closed white arrow*) and the tensor palatini muscle (*black arrows*). Also of note is the plane of the left facial nerve within the parotid gland coursing just lateral to the retromandibular vein (*open black arrows*). **B,C:** Axial T2-weighted images through the midnasopharynx [TR = 2,000 msec; TE = 40 msec (**B**) and 80 msec (**C**)]. The left parapha-ryngeal space tumor has increased in signal intensity, with foci of high signal intensity separated by areas of lower signal intensity fibrous tissue. The foci of high signal intensity correlate with islands of myxoid matrix, which separate areas of fibrotic and cellular tissue in benign mixed-cell tumors. This same "bubbly" appearance may be seen with malignant mixed-cell tumors but appears fairly specific for the mixed-cell tumor histology. The actual site of origin of this tumor is difficult to assess and could either be a primary parapharyngeal space mass or a deep lobe of the parotid mass; however, deviation of the carotid vessels posteriorly definitely separates this lesion from the carotid space masses (see Fig. 22). Note the islands of high signal intensity (*black arrows*) abutting the deep lobe of the parotid gland (p) (*white arrow*). Note also the deviation of the parapharyngeal space (*open black arrows*) by the tumor (t). **D:** Coronal T1-weighted image through the nasopharynx (TR = 600 msec; TE = 25 msec). The mass (t) involves the left lateral aspect of the nasopharyngeal compart-ment, deviating the parapharyngeal space medially (*open white arrows*). This identifies the mass as extrinsic to the para-pharyngeal space rather than within the parapharyngeal space. If the parapharyngeal fat encircles the tumor, then it can be considered a primary parapharyngeal space mass. The mass is well circumscribed, which is in keeping with a benign histology.

teristic similar to gray matter on T1-weighted images (Fig. 15C). Progressive T2 weighting may demonstrate either isointense or slight hyperintensity of the tumor, compared to gray matter (Fig. 15D). Meningiomas can usually be differentiated from schwannomas on the basis of the latter's prolonged T2 relaxation time.

Chordoma is a benign, relentless tumor of the notochordal remnant and usually involves the midline of the clivus, resulting in skull base erosion and a nasopharyngeal mass (Fig. 21). Rarely, the chordoma may extend through the jugular foramen, just as the extracranial meningioma, and produce a carotid space mass (Fig. 22). Cranial neuropathy is a common feature and may occasionally be manifested as denervation atrophy and fatty replacement of a muscle (Figs. 21B and 22D). Foci of low signal intensity may be seen in up to 50% of these patients who have calcification within the chordoma. On T2-weighted images, chordoma may either be homogeneous in signal intensity or have foci of myxoid elements with higher signal intensity similar to benign mixed-cell tumors (*vide infra*).

Parotid Space Masses

Tumors of the deep portion of the parotid gland produce an infratemporal fossa or nasopharyngeal submucosal mass (Fig. 23). MR is useful in localizing the mass to the parotid gland. Larger masses characteristically displace the parapharyngeal space medially (Fig. 23A). Benign lesions are usually well circumscribed (Fig. 23), whereas malignant masses tend to infiltrate the gland and extend outside its capsule into surrounding fat. There is, however, some overlap in the appearance of benign and malignant parotid tumors (18). Low-grade malignancy of the parotid gland may sometimes appear well circumscribed, whereas benign tumors and inflammatory processes may occasionally appear well defined. Thus, it is imperative that parotid masses be biopsied prior to exploration, since malignant lesions necessitate more radical resections. In the hands of expert cytologists, fine-needle aspiration biopsy techniques are reliable in defining the histologic component of parotid lesions. For nonpalpable masses, a biopsy is best performed with CT guidance.

MR is useful in the localization of a mass within the parotid, assessing the histology (*vide supra*), and determining the relationship of the facial nerve to the mass prior to biopsy. The relationship of a parotid mass to the facial nerve is imperative in the preoperative planning. MR can localize the position of a tumor in relationship to the main trunk of the facial nerve in most instances (14). The main trunk of the facial nerve exits the stylo-

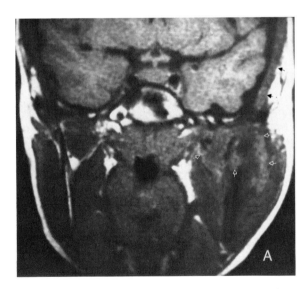
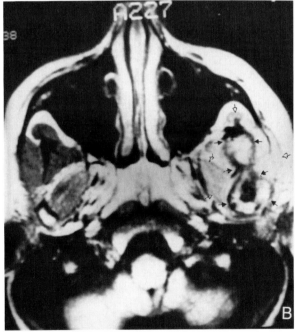

FIG. 24. Actinomycosis of the masticator space. **A:** Coronal T1-weighted MR scan through the nasopharynx and mandible (TR = 600 msec; TE = 25 msec). An inhomogeneous mass (*white arrows*) has infiltrated the left mandibular marrow cavity and extended lateral and medial to the mandible to involve the masseter and lateral pterygoid muscles within the masticator space. Thickening and slight increase in intensity of the left temporalis muscle are also consistent with the masticator space infection (*black arrows*). **B:** Axial T2-weighted MR scan through the nasopharynx (TR = 2,000 msec; TE = 40 msec). Expansion of the mandibular cortex (*black arrows*) and enlargement of the medullary cavity by an inflammatory component are indicative of either tumor or osteomyelitis. There has been infiltration of the surrounding muscles of the masticator space (*open black arrows*). This appearance is most consistent with mandibular osteomyelitis; however, mandibular metastasis with extramandibular spread of tumor can appear very similar.

mastoid foramen near the mastoid tip and courses in a 45° oblique plane within the parotid gland, just lateral to the retromandibular vein and external carotid artery (Figs. 22B and 23A). Benign tumors that are superficial to the facial nerve may usually be resected through a superficial parotidectomy, whereas tumors deep to the facial nerve usually require a total parotidectomy.

The normal parotid gland has a signal intensity that closely parallels that of subcutaneous fat (Fig. 23A and C); however, parotid gland tumors have a signal intensity much lower than fat and are best visualized (Fig. 4D) on intermediate-weighted images (TR = ~2,000 msec; TE = 40 msec). Masses of the parotid gland generally have long T1 and T2 relaxation times. This accounts for their high contrast with normal parotid tissue on T1- (Fig. 23A) and T2-weighted images (Fig. 23C). Thus, although parotid tissue is not optimally differentiated from subcutaneous fat on T1-weighted images, the tumors are best differentiated from normal parotid tissue on this short-TR sequence. Likewise, heavily T2-weighted images do not optimally differentiate the parotid tissue from subcutaneous fat (Fig. 23C); however, tumors have a high degree of contrast with surrounding parotid gland on this sequence. Therefore, we recommend a heavily T1- and T2-weighted image sequence for delineation of parotid lesions from surrounding normal parotid glands.

It is well to remember that calcifications, which are often present in inflammatory and calculous disease of the parotid, will not be as sensitively imaged with MR as with CT. Thus, in a patient with acute swelling of the parotid gland or suspected calculous disease, CT is still recommended as the imaging modality of choice.

Masticator Space

The masticator space is enveloped by the superficial layer of the deep cervical fascia and contains anatomy on both sides of the mandibular ramus (Fig. 2). It includes the lateral and medial pterygoid muscles, the masseter muscle, the temporalis muscle, the inferior alveolar branch of the third division of the fifth cranial nerve, the ramus and body of the mandible, and the pterygoid venous plexus (6,7). Masses involving the masticator space are usually inflammatory processes or neoplasms. Most masticator space infections result from osteomyelitis of the mandible due to uncontrolled dental infection (Fig. 24). Other causes also include hematogenous osteomyelitis of the mandible and, rarely, fungal infections of the mandible, such as actinomycosis (Fig. 24). Masticator space infections may be differentiated from tumors by the surrounding soft tissue inflammatory cellulitis and the clinical history.

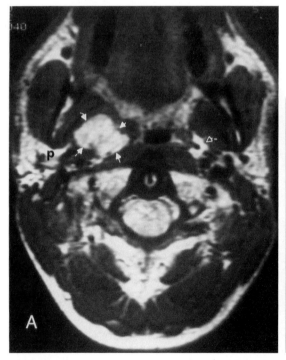
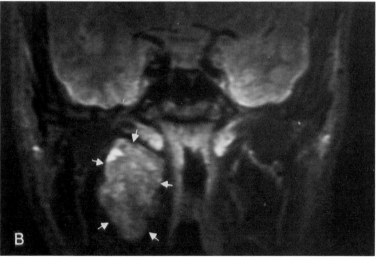

FIG. 25. Primary hemangiopericytoma of the parapharyngeal space. **A:** Axial T2-weighted image through the oropharynx (TR = 2,000 msec; TE = 40 msec). A high-intensity mass is present in the right parapharyngeal space (*white arrows*). Note the normal parapharyngeal space (*open white arrow*). The mass is homogeneous; however, foci of high-velocity vessels surround the mass, indicating its vascular supply. Note that the mass deviates the medial pterygoid muscle anteriorly, the prevertebral muscle posteriorly, and is separate from the parotid gland (p). **B:** Coronal T2-weighted image through the nasopharynx (TR = 2,000 msec; TE = 80 msec). The hemangiopericytoma has slight inhomogeneity on the T2-weighted image but does not have the heterogeneous signal typical of paraganglioma (Figs. 19 and 20) (*white arrows*).

Tumors of the masticator space include benign and malignant lesions (Table 1). Benign lesions of the masticator space include hemangiomas of the masseter muscle, benign osseous lesions of the mandible, lipoma, and benign neural tumors related to the distal branches of the fifth cranial nerve. Malignant lesions of the masticator space include minor salivary gland tumors, malignant neurogenic lesions, lymphoma of the mandible, metastatic or sarcomatous lesions of the mandible or surrounding soft tissues, and, occasionally, spread of squamous carcinomas from the oral cavity to the masticator space. Neuroblastoma metastatic to the mandible may also lead to masticator space masses in children. Tumors generally have an asymptomatic course until destruction of the mandible leads to pain or neurologic (V_3) compromise; however, they may be difficult to differentiate from indolent infections of the mandible (Fig. 24).

PARAPHARYNGEAL SPACE MASSES

Masses of the parapharyngeal space are present clinically with inward bulging of the intact nasopharyngeal mucosa. In this situation, the parapharyngeal space mass must be differentiated from a mass of the deep lobe of the parotid gland. The surgical approach to these two tumors is quite different: A parapharyngeal space mass is approached intraorally, whereas the deep lobe of the parotid mass is often approached through a parotidectomy (11,12).

Primary lesions of the parapharyngeal space may be benign or malignant. Benign lesions are uncommon but include benign mixed tumors of the minor salivary glands, lipomas, an occasional atypical branchial cleft cyst, schwannomas from the third division of the trigeminal nerve, and extension of a tonsillar abscess (7,10). Hemangiopericytoma is a rare vascular parapharyngeal mass lesion that arises from vascular elements supplied by the ascending pharyngeal artery (Fig. 25).

Malignant lesions of the parapharyngeal space are also uncommon. These include malignant classes of minor salivary gland tumors, such as adenoid cystic carcinoma and mucoepidermoid carcinoma, liposarcoma, metastatic disease to nodes contained near the parapharyngeal space, and malignant degeneration of neurogenic neoplasms. MR may be quite useful in localizing masses to the parapharyngeal space. A primary parapharyngeal space mass deviates the medial pterygoid muscle anteriorly, the nasopharyngeal constrictor muscles medially, the prevertebral muscles posteriorly, and

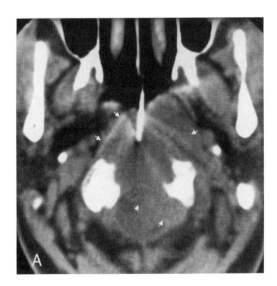
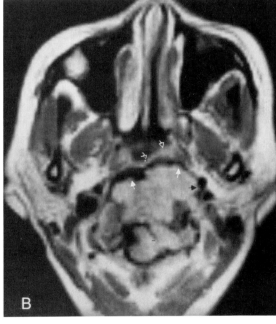

FIG. 26. Retropharyngeal breast metastasis; 40-year-old Black woman with known breast carcinoma 4 years prior to the development of a retropharyngeal mass. **A:** Axial CT scan through the upper nasopharynx during transnasal biopsy. A large retropharyngeal mass lesion has eroded the C2 vertebral body and extended into the upper cervical epidural space (*white arrows*). This CT scan was obtained during transnasal biopsy of the soft tissue mass, revealing breast carcinoma. **B:** Axial T2-weighted MR scan (TR = 2.0 sec; TE = 56 msec) through the upper nasopharynx. The metastasis has a homogeneous high signal intensity. Its retropharyngeal position is indicated by displacement of the prevertebral musculature anteriorly (*solid white arrows*), the internal carotid artery laterally (*black arrow*), and extension into the epidural space. Note the normal mucosal signal anterior to the prevertebral muscles (*open white arrows*). This scan helped tailor the biopsy (see **A**) because it permitted better soft tissue detail and localization of the abnormal mass. In addition, the MR confidentally identified the position of the carotid vessels in relationship to the mass, permitting a safe biopsy transnasally.

is separate from the deep lobe of the parotid gland (Fig. 25). In addition, parapharyngeal space fat may surround the entire lesion, documenting its origin within this space.

RETROPARAPHARYNGEAL SPACE MASSES

The retropharyngeal space is a potential space delineated by the buccopharyngeal fascia and the prevertebral fascia (Fig. 2). Normally, it is not visualized as a discrete space on MR or CT. It contains fat, lymph nodes, and lymphatics; however, it is only imaged as a discrete space in pathologic conditions. Retropharyngeal nodes drain the nasopharynx, the oropharynx, and the paranasal sinuses. Inflammatory or neoplastic involvement of these sites may result in retropharyngeal adenopathy. The retropharyngeal nodes usually involve the lateral retropharyngeal chain just medial to the internal carotid artery (Fig. 12). Occasionally, lymphoproliferative disorders, such as ARC or lymphoma, may involve the medial retropharyngeal chain directly posterior to the pharyngeal wall. Metastasis from malignancies of the upper aerodigestive tract may also course to the retropharyngeal nodes (Fig. 12A and B). Metastasis to the spine and skull base may result in retropharyngeal masses (Fig. 26). Inflammatory lesions may involve the retropharyngeal space, either from iatrogenic or traumatic perforation of the posterior pharyngeal wall or from osteomyelitis extending anteriorly from the spine. In the latter instance, a fluid collection will then be present posterior to the superior constrictor muscle and anterior to the prevertebral muscles. We have seen such examples in patients with coccidioidomycosis, tuberculosis, and suppurative infections of the spine, as well as extension from tonsillar infection and retropharyngitis. Extension of inflammatory lesions to the retropharyngeal space is particularly ominous because this space communicates with the posterior mediastinum to the level of the third thoracic vertebral body (13).

CONCLUSION

The enhanced soft tissue contrast provided by high-resolution MR scanning permits more optimal localization and tissue characterization of nasopharyngeal masses than presently available by CT scanning. Other advantages of MR include better delineation of vascular structures and the vascular matrix of tumors, such as paraganglioma and hemangiopericytoma, without the additional need for intravenously administered contrast agents. In addition, the fibrous component of tumor, such as fibrosarcoma, or treated neoplasms, such as nasopharyngeal carcinoma, may also be more precisely assessed by MR scans (see Chapter 19). Precise compartmental localization assists in the approach to differential diagnosis of nasopharyangeal masses. Once a mass is localized, its signal characteristics may permit a precise diagnosis and in many instances obviate the need for further invasive procedures.

REFERENCES

1. Dillon WP, Mills CM, Kjos B, et al. Magnetic resonance image of the nasopharynx. *Radiology* 1984;152:731–5.
2. Dooms GC, Hricak H, Moseley ME, et al. Characterization of lymphadenopathy by magnetic resonance relaxation times: preliminary results. *Radiology* 1985;155:691–7.
3. Lufkin R, Hanafee W, Worthan D, Hoover L. MRI of the tongue and oropharynx using surface coils. *Radiology* (in press).
4. Mancuso AA, Hanafee WN. *Computed tomography and magnetic resonance imaging of the head and neck.* Baltimore: Williams and Wilkins, 1985.
5. Scotti G, Harwood-Nash DC. Computed tomography of rhabdomyosarcomas of the skull base in children. *J Comput Assist Tomogr* 1982;6:33–9.
6. Hardin CW, Harnsberger HR, Osborn AG. Infection and tumor of the masticator space: CT evaluation. *Radiology* 1985;157:413–7.
7. Hardin CW, Harnsberger R, Osborn AG, Smoker W. CT in the evaluation of normal and diseased oral cavity and oropharynx. *Semin Ultrasound, CT, MR* 1986;7:133–53.
8. Silver AJ, Mawad M, Hilal S, et al. Computed tomography of the nasopharynx and related spaces. *Radiology* 1983;147:725–31.
9. Silver AJ, Mawad M, Hilal S, et al. Computed tomography of the carotid space and related cervical spaces. Pt I: Anatomy. *Radiology* 1984;150:723–8.
10. Smoker WRK, Gentry LR. Computed tomography of the nasopharynx and related spaces. *Semin Ultrasound, CT, MR* 1986;7:107–30.
11. Som PM. The parapharyngeal space. In: Bergeron RT, Osborn AG, Som PM, eds. *Head and neck imaging excluding the brain.* St. Louis: Mosby, 1984;235–50.
12. Som PM, Miller HF, Lawson W, et al. Parapharyngeal space masses: an updated protocol based on 104 cases. *Radiology* 1984;153:149–56.
13. Everts EC, and Ecatvarria J. Diseases of the pharynx and deep neck infections. In: Paparella M, Shumrick D, eds. *Otolaryngology.* Philadelphia: WB Saunders Company, 1980.
14. Teresi L, Lufkin R, Hanafee W, et al. MR of the normal infratemporal facial nerve. *AJNR* (in press).
15. Harnsberger HR, Dillon WP. Major motor atrophic patterns in the face and neck: CT evaluation. *Radiology* 1985;155:665–70.
16. Batsakis JG. *Tumors of the head and neck: clinical and pathologic considerations.* 2nd ed. Baltimore: Williams and Wilkins, 1979.
17. Geoffray A, Lee YY, Ging BS, Wallace S. Extracranial meningiomas of the head and neck. *AJNR* 1984;5:599–604.
18. Bryan RN, Miller RH, Ferreyo RI, et al. Computed tomography of the major salivary glands. *AJR* 1982;139:547–54.

CHAPTER 20

The Neck

David D. Stark, Robert B. Lufkin, and William N. Hanafee

Cross-sectional imaging has become indispensable in the evaluation of diseases of the tongue base, oropharynx, hypopharynx, larynx, thyroid and parathyroid glands, and thoracic inlet. The majority of imaging studies are performed for the detection or evaluation of masses. Evaluation of the airway following trauma or infection is a less common indication. Imaging studies rarely allow a specific tissue diagnosis but are essential in detecting pathologic masses, narrowing the diagnostic differential, and guiding biopsies or excisional surgery. The selection of sonography, X-ray computed tomography (CT), or magnetic resonance (MR) imaging depends upon the anatomic region of interest, the nature of the suspected pathology, and the availability of relevant technology.

MR is a promising technique for imaging the neck because of its freedom from artifacts, multiplanar capabilities, and excellent soft tissue contrast. This chapter will review the recent development of the applications of MR to neck imaging, including normal anatomy of the neck as visualized by various MR techniques, and illustrate application of MR to diverse pathologic processes.

MR TECHNIQUES

Magnet Design

Images of the neck have been obtained in MR imaging systems operating at field strengths from 0.15 to 1.5 tesla (T). Low field systems appear to suffer from reduced signal-to-noise levels, particularly when conventional, circumferential "body" radio-frequency (RF) coils are used. Most of the images in this chapter have been performed using systems operating at 0.3 T (Fonar) and 0.35 T (Diasonics). The Fonar system contains a permanent magnet with a vertical main (B_0) magnetic field. The Diasonics system utilizes a conventional (Oxford) superconducting magnet with a solenoidal configuration.

High field systems (1.5 T) offer improved signal-to-noise ratios under some conditions but have been susceptible to motion-induced "ghost" artifacts. It is obvious that expected refinements in both instrumentation and software will greatly improve image quality in the near future by comparison with that given by all current-day MR imagers.

Radio-frequency Coils

For MR applications in the torso, body coils allow the large field of view appropriate for the anatomic region. Although images of reasonable quality can be produced using the conventional "saddle" configuration body coils, these coils (also known as antennas or probes) are often inefficient because of poor coupling between the coils and the small size of the region of interest. Surface coils have been shown to bridge the gap between RF coils of large diameter and small anatomic sites (Fig. 1), and have been used to good advantage for a variety of anatomic applications, e.g., to the lumbar spine, extremities, and some abdominal viscera. The neck is ideally suited to the use of surface coils because of its small size and the suprficial location of the organs of interest. Dramatic improvements in image quality have been shown in all imaging systems when surface coils are used.

Surface coils are generally used selectively as receivers while the larger circumferential "body" coil remains in place as an RF transmitter. The surface coils are made of a conductive material, usually copper, and configured in a loop. As the axis of a coil must be perpendicular to the main (B_0) magnetic field, the orientation of the surface coil is determined by magnet design. For example, conventional superconducting magnets have B_0 parallel to the patient's spine and therefore the surface coil loop must be applied like a pancake to the front, rear, or side of the neck. Obviously, this will create some problems because of the shoulders or curvature of the neck. The use of flexible materials and partial or half "saddle" configurations have allowed better conformity with the

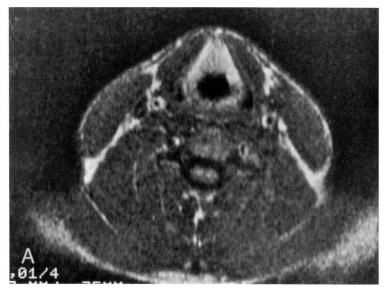

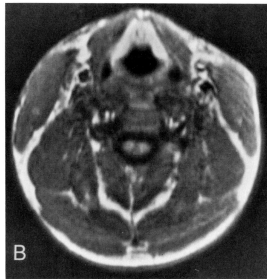

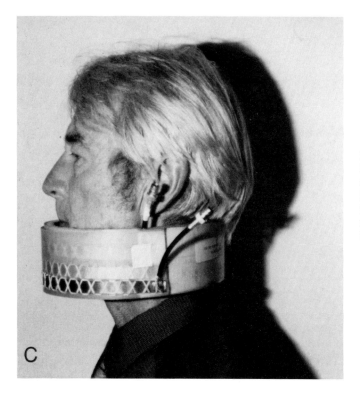

FIG. 1. Normal neck, transverse plane of section at the level of the piriform sinuses. **A:** 0.3 T, SE 1,000/28, body coil. **B:** 0.3 T, SE 1,000/28, surface coil. Note improved resolution of the normal neck in transverse section provided by the surface coil. As this solenoidal coil encircles the neck, no signal intensity "fall-off" is seen (cf. Figs. 10B and 11B). **C:** Solenoidal surface coil in place.

tubular shape of the neck. Vertical magnetic field orientations of some imagers (e.g. the Fonar permanent magnet system) allow utilization of solenoidal surface coils which may consist of multiple windings of copper applied circumferentially around the neck (Fig. 1C). This configuration offers improved RF homogeneity and maximizes signal-to-noise ratios for deeper structures (1). Solenoidal coil configurations may also be inherently more sensitive than single loop configurations.

Image Geometry

As with CT, each MR image offers a full cross-sectional field of view and a series (stack) of images provides a permanent record of the entire examination. Both CT and MR have this distinct advantage over real-time sonography, which has a limited field of view and rarely allows achievement of a complete anatomic examination. Therefore, sonography has the disadvantage of being "operator dependent" and requires recognition of pathology at the time of the examination. On the other hand, MR resembles sonography by allowing imaging in multiple planes of section, but is inferior in that the plane of section must be selected in advance and

that only a limited number of planes can be imaged within a reasonable amount of time (Figs. 2–4). This multiplanar capability is a significant advantage of both MR and sonography over CT, which is effectively limited to the transverse plane of section.

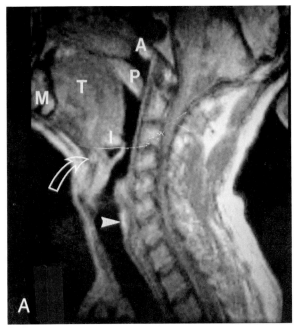

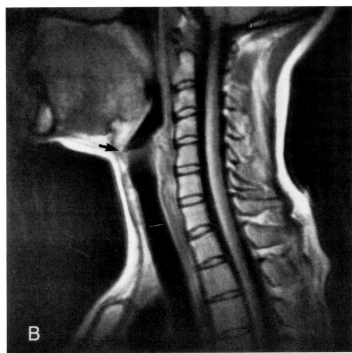

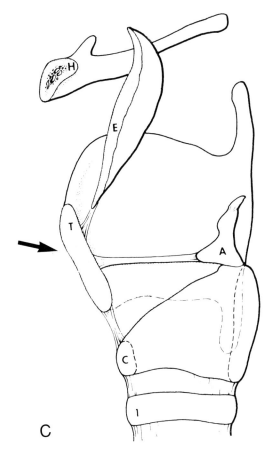

FIG. 2. Normal midline sagittal plane of section. **A:** 0.35 T body coil image, SE 1,500/28. The marrow within the hyoid bone has a high intensity (*open arrow*). Fatty preepiglottic and paralaryngeal tissues are seen caudal to the hyoid bone. The cervical esophagus is seen below the level of the posterior cricoid lamina (*arrowhead*). Mandible (M), tongue (T), soft palate (P), adenoids (A), lingual tonsil (l). **B:** Surface coil image, SE 500/28. The anterior part of the true vocal cord and laryngeal ventricle (*arrow*) is in this plane of section. **C:** Anatomic drawing showing the laryngeal skeleton, lateral view, midline sagittal plane of section. Hyoid bone (H) and epiglottis (E), thyroid (T), arytenoid (A), cricoid (anterior lamina C), and first tracheal ring (1) cartilages are shown. The vocal ligament is seen extending from the thyroid cartilage to the arytenoid cartilage at the level of the arrow.

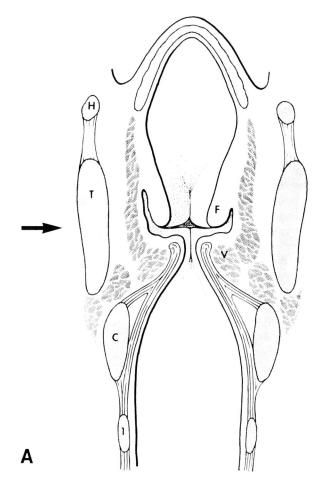

A

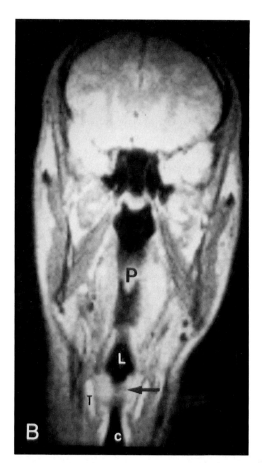

B

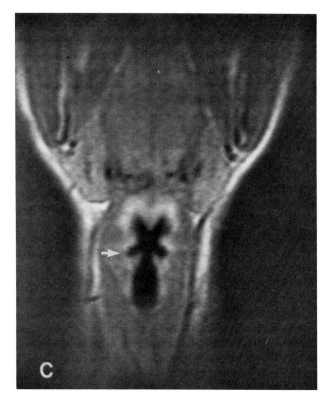

C

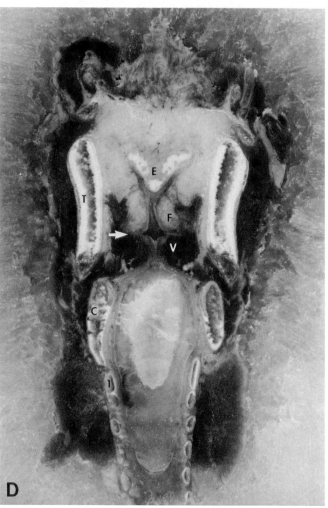

D

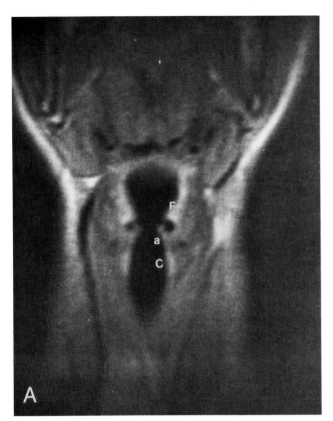

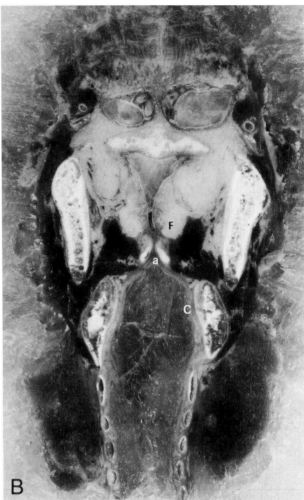

FIG. 4. **A:** Coronal image 7 mm dorsal to Fig. 3C at the level of the arytenoid cartilages (a). **B:** Corresponding cadaver section. False vocal cord (F) and cricoid cartilage (C) also shown.

Artifacts introduced by metal and dental amalgam, surgical clips, or other hardware severely limit CT. Furthermore, beam hardening and "overshoot" reconstruction artifacts which are caused by air–tissue interfaces severely limit CT in the region of the mandible and oropharynx.

MR images are not degraded by dental amalgam or by the dense bone of the mandible. And not all metals cause artifacts on MR images, in contrast to the case with CT. Only the subset of metals which are ferromagnetic cause artifacts on MR. Although dental amalgam produces no artifact, root canal prostheses or metal bridge work may occasionally do so. However, most alloys are nonferromagnetic; even stainless steel usually contains sufficient nickel to minimize ferromagnetism (2). Ferromagnetic materials result in image distortion that is usually limited to the immediate area of the offending material without producing the streak artifacts and global image disruption that occur with CT.

Sonography is limited to structures away from bone and air by the necessity of acoustic transmission. Although sonography is excellent for the thyroid and

FIG. 3. **A:** Normal coronal section through the larynx (labels correspond to those in Fig. 2C). Fatty paralaryngeal tissues within the false vocal cords (F) are separated by the air-filled laryngeal ventricle from the true vocal cords and vocalis muscle (V). **B:** Coronal body coil image with a 7 mm slice thickness shows the vocal cords (*arrow*) but fails to delineate the laryngeal ventricle. The uvula of the soft palate (P), medullary cavity of the thyroid cartilage (T), and laryngeal vestibule (L) are also shown. **C:** Coronal surface coil image using a 4 mm slice thickness. The laryngeal ventricle (*arrow*) is now easily identified. The sharp free margin of the muscular true vocal cord is well defined. **D:** Corresponding cadaver section. The epiglottis (E) is angled much further posteriorly than would occur in a living patient. Intrinsic muscle bundles are thicker in general because of their relaxed state.

parathyroid glands, it is useless for the oropharynx, larynx, airway, and unoperated spine.

Image Plane Selection

The transverse plane of section is well suited to delineate the entire anatomy of the neck. The coronal plane of section is particularly useful in delineating the relationship of the true cords, ventricles, and false cords (Figs. 3 and 4). Either the coronal or the sagittal plane is complementary to the transverse images for delineating the craniocaudal extent of lesions. Because of gaps between slices, transverse images alone may be inadequate.

The sagittal plane of section is best for evaluating the anterior and posterior walls of the airway, the tongue base, the epiglottis and preepiglottic space, and the anterior commissure of the vocal cords (Fig. 2). Demonstration of mucosal abnormalities is good but does not approach that of the clinician's endoscopic examination. Therefore, even with the introduction of surface coil MR techniques, cross-sectional imaging will remain a complementary procedure in staging aerodigestive tract neoplasms. For example, identification of tumor spread across the anterior commissure and definition of cephalocaudal margins are extremely important for precise planning of voice conservation surgery or radiation therapy portals. For this reason, transverse and either sagittal or coronal images are recommended for all patients with cancer of the neck.

Pulse Sequences

The greatest advantage of MR is its flexibility in manipulating soft tissue contrast over a wide range. Utilization of "T1-weighted" or "T2-weighted" pulse sequences allows distinction of pathology from fatty tissue planes or skeletal muscle, respectively. Pulse sequence selection also has impact on image signal-to-noise ratios and thereby influences the operator's choice of image matrix, section thickness, and/or imaging time. Although short TR spin echo images are useful in eliminating motion artifacts, they may also limit the number of images (sections) that can be simultaneously acquired, requiring additional trade-offs between anatomic coverage, slice thickness, and/or imaging time. Indeed, as with all clinical applications of MR, time is the currency that must be exchanged for image contrast, signal-to-noise ratios, spatial resolution, and anatomic coverage. CT and ultrasound are much simpler examinations to plan, as additional views can be obtained without a substantial time penalty.

MR Scanning Technique

Most neck examinations are now conducted using surface coils applied to the region of interest. Specialized coils are becoming available for the tongue, larynx, and thoracic inlet. Initial localization is confirmed by obtaining preliminary images in 1 to 4 min with a short TR/short TE spin echo (SE) technique, relatively thick slices, and low in-plane spatial resolution. Once the coil is centered over the region of suspected pathology, slice thickness is decreased to the desired minimum, and in-plane spatial resolution (pixel size) can be reduced to 0.8 × 0.8 mm or less. Patients are instructed to breathe normally and refrain from moving their tongues or swallowing. High resolution transverse images are obtained using the short TR/short TE spin echo technique. Depending on the geometry of the lesion, either sagittal or coronal images are next obtained. For example, coronal images are particularly useful in demonstrating lateral pharyngeal wall masses, whereas sagittal images are better for posterior pharyngeal wall pathology. For thyroid and parathyroid examinations the transverse plane of section is used exclusively.

The T1-weighted short TR/short TE spin echo images offer the best anatomic resolution because they have the greatest signal-to-noise ratios per unit time and because of their relative freedom from motion artifacts. When pathology is adjacent to strap muscles or involves the tongue muscles, T2-weighted images offer improved tissue contrast and may allow improved visualization of the tumor. Selection of pulse sequences for apropriate tissue contrast is relatively straightforward: all tumors have long T1 and T2 relaxation times, whereas fatty tissue planes have short T1 and intermediate T2 relaxation times and therefore show the greatest image signal intensity difference (contrast) relative to tumor when a "T1-weighted" technique is used. Similarly, muscle has long T1 and short T2 relaxation times and therefore shows the greatest contrast relative to tumor when "T2-weighted" images are used. Tumor will be dark on T1-weighted images and bright on T2-weighted images. In the MR examination of the neck, pulse sequences are selected solely to optimize delineation of pathology. No tissue specificity has been reported in the neck using currently available MR imaging techniques.

As a general rule, the fast "T1-weighted" spin echo techniques are used to localize the abnormality and select the optimal plane of section. This plane of section is then used to obtain a single "T2-weighted" sequence (SE 2,000/30–120) in order to obtain complementary tissue contrast information. As the T2-weighted sequences are inherently slower and have lower signal-to-noise levels per unit time, slice thickness and/or in-plane spatial resolution is often sacrificed to improve image quality and save time. Despite these trade-offs, it is

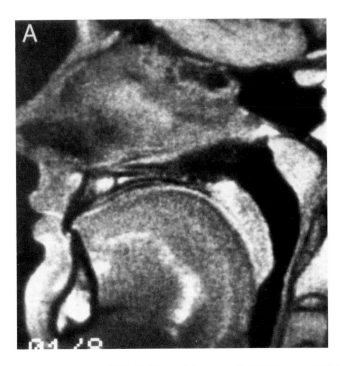
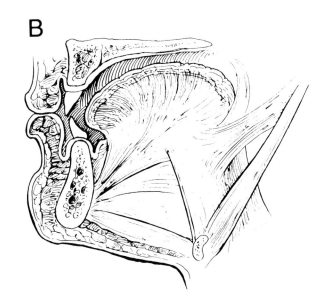

FIG. 5. Normal tongue. **A:** Midline sagittal image. **B:** Corresponding anatomical diagram.

common to spend 9 or 18 min acquiring only two or four T2-weighted data sets, respectively. Inversion recovery sequences have not enjoyed routine use in MR imaging of the neck because they share the inefficient use of time inherent to all long TR techniques and offer no advantage in tissue contrast over the faster short TR/short TE spin echo techniques.

NORMAL ANATOMY

Oropharynx

Both the branchial arches and the occipital and upper cervical myotomes contribute to the diverse embryological origins of the muscle groups that form the pharyngeal constrictor muscles, tongue, and floor of the mouth. These structures appear on both T1- and T2-weighted MR images as intermediate intensity tissue outlined by the high signal intensity of adjacent fat (3).

Three pharyngeal constrictors form the oropharynx and make up its posterolateral margins. The palatoglossus and palatopharyngeus muscles entend inferiorly from the soft palate to form the tonsillar pillars which border the palatine tonsils. Tonsillar tissue is of intermediate signal intensity on T1-weighted images and relatively high intensity on T2-weighted images (Fig. 2).

The tongue is made of paired sets of intrinsic and extrinsic muscles on either side of a fibrous lingual sep-

tum (4). The septum or midline raphe has a high signal on MR images, presumably because of its high fat content. The intrinsic muscles consist of four interdigitating bundles of muscle fibers with characteristic orientations that appear on MR images as low signal intensity striations in various orientations with interspersed high signal of fat (Fig. 5). The superior and inferior longitudinal fibers run from the tongue tip to the base. The vertical fibers extend from the mucosa downward. The transverse fibers attach to the fiber septa and extend laterally; on transverse views these may be mistaken for a mass in the posterior tongue. Because of improved soft tissue contrast and the ability to perform direct sagittal plane images, intrinsic musculature is better seen by MR than by CT or other techniques (5–7).

The extrinsic tongue muscles consist of three groups. They are the genioglossus, hyoglossus, and styloglossus muscles, which are attached to the genial tubercle of the mandible, the hyoid bone, and styloid process, respectively. The genioglossus muscles are paramedian and make up the bulk of the tongue. The two other groups interdigitate to form the major portion of the lateral border of the tongue and are well seen as low signal intensity structures on T2-weighted MR images.

The main supporting structure of the floor of the mouth is the mylohyoid muscle, which originates along the mylohyoid line of the mandible and joins its partner in a midline raphe with posterior attachment to the hyoid bone. Deep to the mylohyoid muscle is the geniohyoid muscle, extending from the mandible to the hyoid bone. Superficial to the mylohyoid muscle is the anterior belly of the digastric muscle, extending from the midline mandible to the hyoid bone. Innervation to the tongue is provided by the hypoglossal (motor) and lingual (sensory) nerves which pass along the oral surface of the mylohyoid muscle to penetrate the tongue base. Blood supply to the tongue is via the lingual artery and veins which course between the interdigitation of the hyoglossus, styloglossus, and genioglossus muscles. Because of flow void effects, the vascular structures often appear as regions of low signal intensity on MR images.

Neck

The neck is defined as the anatomic region of the body lying below the plane demarcated by the lower margin of the mandible and the superior nuchal line of the occipital bone. The lower margin of the neck is the plane demarcated by the suprasternal notch and the top of the first thoracic vertebral body. Fascial planes divide the neck into several compartments. For the interpretation of transverse images it is useful to define three anatomic compartments: visceral, posterior, and lateral.

The visceral compartment of the neck is the most anterior and contains structures of the aerodigestive tract, including the larynx, trachea, and esophagus. The thyroid and parathyroid glands also lie within the visceral compartment. Sternocleidomastoid and pharyngeal constrictor muscles form the lateral and posterior

boundaries, respectively, of the visceral compartment (Fig. 6) (31,40).

LARYNX

The main function of the larynx is to act as a sphincter rather than as an organ for producing sound. Keeping this function in mind simplifies an understanding of the anatomical physiology of the larynx. In addition to its role as a sphincter, the larynx is involved in respiration, deglutition, and phonation. Several cartilages (cricoid, thyroid, epiglottic, arytenoid, corniculate, cuneiform) and a single bone (hyoid) form the foundation of the larynx. Numerous ligaments and folds attach to this skeleton (Figs. 6–12).

Cricoid cartilage

The signet ring-shaped cricoid cartilage lies at the base of the larynx above the first tracheal ring (Fig. 11). It is the only complete cartilage encircling the airway. It has a narrow anterior arch and a wider, higher posterior lamina. At the junction of the arch and lamina, the cricoid cartilage articulates with the inferior cornu of the thyroid cartilage, forming synovial cricothyroid joints bilaterally. A scan at this level corresponds to the infraglottic or subglottic region. In older patients the cricoid, arytenoid, and thyroid cartilages have peripheral calcification which appears as a zone of high density on CT and low signal intensity on MR images. The central zone is a medullary cavity that contains a fatty marrow

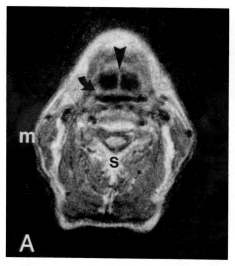
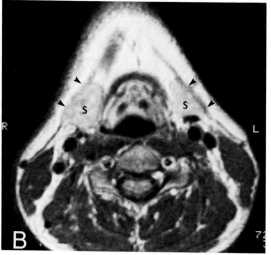

FIG. 6. Transverse image near the level of the hyoid bone, 0.35 T. **A:** The median glossoepiglottic fold (*arrowhead*) and lateral glossopharyngeal folds (*curved arrow*) border the air-filled paired valleculae and the hypopharynx which lies posterior to the epiglottis. The sternocleidomastoid muscles (m) have an intermediate signal intensity and are seen immediately caudal to their insertion into the mastoid process of the temporal bone. Extensor muscles are seen posterior to the cervical spine (S), separated by high intensity adipose tissue. TR 2.0; TE 28. **B:** 1 cm further caudal, at the inferior tip of the valleculae. Note the submandibular salivary glands (S) bilaterally within the anterior neck bounded laterally by the platysma muscle (*arrowheads*). TR 1.0; TE 40.

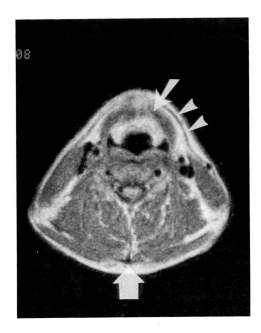

FIG. 7. At the base of the epiglottis and aryepiglottic folds and preepiglottic soft tissues have a slightly lower intensity than subcutaneous fat. The constrictor muscles of the hypopharynx are immediately anterior to the cervical spine and have an intermediate intensity, similar to the sternocleidomastoid muscles. The lateral entrances to the piriform sinuses are also seen at this level. The platysma (*white arrowheads*) and infrahyoid strap muscles (*small white arrow*) are seen within the subcutaneous fat. The nuchal ligament (*large white arrow*) also has a low intensity. TR 2.0; TE 28.

and appears as a zone of low density on CT and high signal intensity on MR images (10–12). In younger patients these cartilages are usually isointense with surrounding fatty tissue planes. The mucosa of the subglottic larynx is imperceptibly thin in normal patients; imaging of this region is important to detect pathologic thickening by subglottic extension of laryngeal cancer. The two vocal cords lie at the level of the glottis, at the highest portion of the cricoid lamina (Fig. 10).

Thyroid cartilage

The shield-shaped thyroid cartilage is superior to the cricoid cartilage and is attached anteriorly by the cricothyroid membrane (Figs. 9 and 10). The midline fusion of two laminae gives the thyroid cartilage its characteristic appearance. It is the largest laryngeal cartilage and provides anterior shelter for the vocal cords which attach to it at the anterior commissure. One centimeter above the anterior commissure is the thyroid notch, which appears as a narrow space between the laminae. In addition to the inferior cornu, each thyroid lamina has a superior cornu which often extends to the greater horns of the hyoid bone.

Hyoid bone

The tripartite hyoid bone (a central body with two wings) suspends the thyroid cartilage via the thyrohyoid membrane and is in turn suspended from the mandible and styloid process via the suprahyoid muscles. The cortical bone of the hyoid is low signal surrounding a higher signal narrow space on MR images of patients of all ages.

Epiglottis

The leaf-shaped epiglottis consists of a perforated elastic cartilage which rarely calcifies and maintains an appearance of intermediate signal intensity on MR images of patients of all ages (Figs. 2 and 6). The epiglottis lies in the coronal plane and is posterior to the thyroid cartilage and hyoid bone. It is connected to the thyroid cartilage at its inferior tip (petiole) by the thyroepiglottic ligament. Superiorly, the hyoepiglottic ligament links the body of the epiglottis to the hyoid bone.

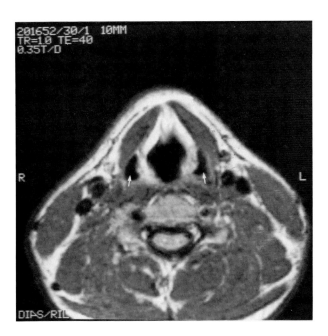

FIG. 8. Caudal to Fig. 7, the piriform sinus apices (*arrows*) are surrounded by fatty paralaryngeal tissues. TR 1.0; TE 40.

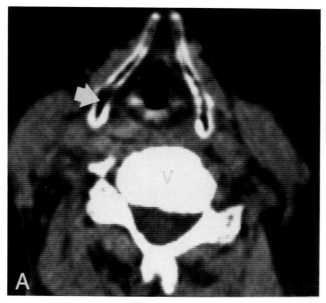
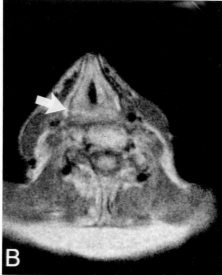

FIG. 9. **A:** CT scan at the level of the false vocal cords. The calcified thyroid cartilage (arrow) is seen as a peripherally calcified structure with a fatty medullary cavity. The thyroid cartilage forms the lateral borders of the fatty paralaryngeal tissues. **B:** MR shows the medullary cavity of the thyroid cartilage (*arrow*) as a high signal intensity, presumably due to its fat content. The calcified portions of the thyroid cartilage have a low signal intensity. The false vocal cords are contiguous with the fatty connective tissue of the aryepiglottic folds (Figs. 7 and 8) and paralaryngeal tissues. TR 2.0; TE 28.

The high signal intensity fatty tissues of the preepiglottic space are divided in the midline by the low intensity hyoepiglottic ligament. The free margin of the epiglottis lies above the hyoid and posterior to the vallecula. Here it is attached to the lateral hypopharynx and the tongue base by the pharyngoepiglottic and median glossoepiglottic folds, respectively (Fig. 6).

Arytenoid, corniculate, and cuneiform cartilages

The paired, pyramidal arytenoids rest on the posterior cricoid lamina (Figs. 4 and 10). Each arytenoid has a lateral muscular process and an interior vocal process. During respiration the arytenoids are laterally located; the muscular processes closely approximate the thyroid laminae. During phonation the arytenoids glide supramedially and rotate to adduct the vocal cords. An MR scan at the glottic level will visualize the vocal processes of the arytenoids, the posterior lamina of the cricoid, and of course, the vocal cords. On the other hand, a scan through the superior processes of the arytenoids is at the level of the false vocal cords. At the apex of the arytenoids are the nodular, paired, corniculate cartilages. These paired cuneiform cartilages lie in the aryepiglottic folds slightly superior and interior to the corniculate cartilages.

Laryngeal soft tissues

CT and MR excel in delineation of the deep soft tissues of the larynx because of the interspersion of fatty

tissue planes in the muscles in the preepiglottic, paralaryngeal, and deep infraglottic spaces. The paired aryepiglottic folds extend from the corniculate and arytenoid cartilages to the lateral margins of the epiglottis in a superior and anterolateral fashion. The aryepiglottic folds separate the laryngeal vestibule (endolarynx) from the piriform sinuses (hypopharynx) (Figs. 7 and 8).

Piriform sinuses

The piriform sinuses are intimately related to the larynx, although they are actually part of the digestive tract. They serve as conduits for food from the oropharynx to the cervical esophagus. Superiorly, the piriform sinuses are posterior to the vallecula, separated from them by the pharyngoepiglottic folds. Slightly inferiorly, the aryepiglottic folds separate the piriform sinuses and the laryngeal vestibule. The piriform sinuses lie just beneath the ala of the thyroid cartilage. The fatty areolar tissues of the paralaryngeal spaces provide room for the piriform sinuses to expand when swallowing a bolus of food. Posterior to the cricoid cartilage the piriform sinuses unite to become the cervical esophagus.

True and false vocal cords

The true vocal cord level can be identified by the vocal processes of the arytenoid, which corresponds to the superior margin of the cricoid lamina and somewhat triangular airway (Fig. 10). On MR images, the true

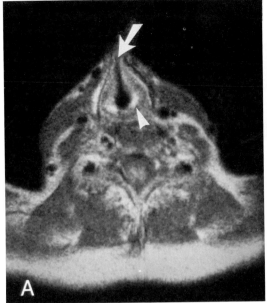

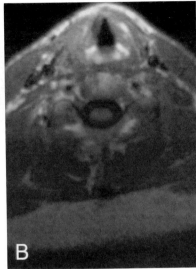

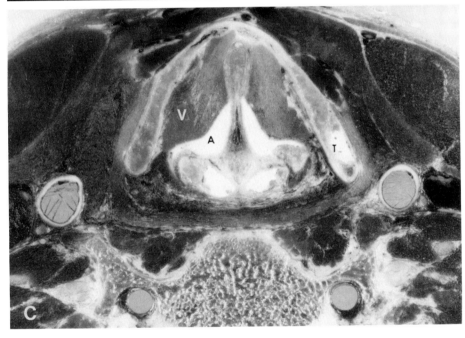

FIG. 10. A: True vocal cords. The true vocal cords are separated by the anterior commissure (*arrow*). The true vocal cords are lower in signal intensity than the false vocal cords because of the vocalis muscle. The arytenoid cartilages (*arrowhead*) have a fatty marrow cavity similar to the thyroid cartilage (Fig. 9) and cricoid cartilage. **B:** Surface coil image, using a single loop antenna applied to the anterior neck. Note fall-off in signal intensity away from the coil (cf. Fig. 1B). **C:** Corresponding cadaver section. Vocalis muscle (V), vocal process of the arytenoid cartilage (A), and thyroid cartilage (T) are indicated.

cords are intermediate in intensity because of the vocalis muscle, as compared to the high signal intensity of the fatty false vocal cords (Fig. 9). The airway between the true vocal cords is named the rima glottis. The true vocal cords have smooth medial margins. At the anterior commissure, no significant soft density is normally present between the airway and the inner surface of the thyroid cartilage. (The maximum soft-tissue thickness here is less than 1 mm).

The true and false vocal cords are separated bilaterally by the laryngeal ventricles. These small, lateral, air-filled outpouchings may be best seen on coronal scans. On sagittal scans, the appendix, a small structure originating from the anterior laryngeal ventricle, is visualized in the anterior false vocal cord. The false vocal cords are just superior to the laryngeal ventricles. This level can be recognized by identifying the superior processes of the arytenoids and the high signal fatty areolar tissue that is characteristic of false cords.

Preepiglottic, paralaryngeal, and infraglottic spaces

The preepiglottic and paralaryngeal spaces are composed predominantly of fat and therefore are of low density on CT and high signal intensity on MR images. The midline preepiglottic space extends downward from the hyoid bone to the anterior commissure, it can be traced as a continuum with the lateral paralaryngeal

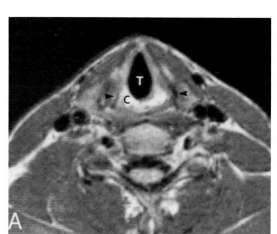

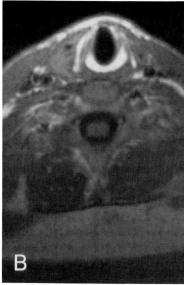

FIG. 11. Posterior cricoid lamina. **A:** Body coil image shows high intensity marrow of the posterior cricoid lamina (C) and inferior cornua of the thyroid cartilage (*arrowheads*). Note the very thin mucosal tissue separating cricoid cartilage from the trachea (T). **B:** Surface coil image.

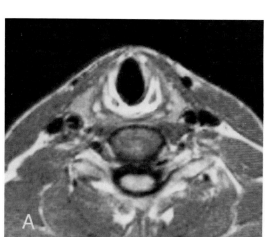

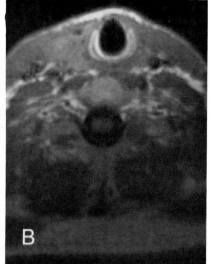

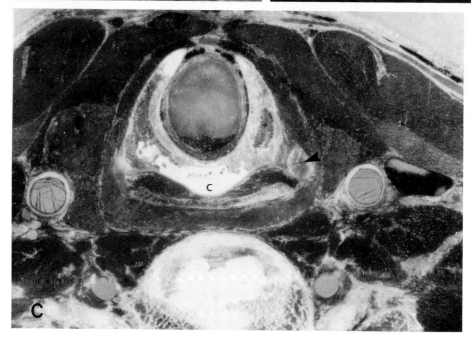

FIG. 12. A: 7 mm caudal to Fig. 11, through the body of the cricoid cartilage. TR = 1.0; TE = 40. **B:** Surface coil image. **C:** Corresponding cadaver section.

spaces, which are immediately medial to the thyroid cartilage, and contain the intrinsic muscles of the larynx (see below). In the normal infraglottic region no significant soft tissue is present between the airway and the cricoid cartilage. The conus elasticus originates from the cricoid cartilage and spreads upward to the free margin of the true vocal cords, thereby forming the vocal ligaments. As will be described later, the conus elasticus affects infraglottic tumor spread.

Intrinsic laryngeal musculature

Unlike CT, MR routinely visualizes the intrinsic musculature of the larynx. This can be attributed to increased tissue contrast and the ability to obtain direct coronal images. The muscles appear as vertical bands of moderate signal intensity surrounded by fatty tissue planes of high signal intensity (Fig. 3A). The paired intrinsic muscles act as a sphincter during swallowing. A superior group consisting of the aryepiglottic and thyroepiglottic muscles forms a protective cap over the aperture of the laryngeal airway by acting to invert the epiglottis during swallowing. The muscles of the vocal folds complete the sphincter inferiorly, and can be subdivided into those muscles that open or close and others that lengthen or shorten the sphincter. The posterior cricoarytenoid muscles act to open the vocal cords and are in fact the only dilator muscles of this group. Their action is opposed by the lateral cricoarytenoid and interarytenoid muscles which tend to close the vocal folds. The vocal folds are lengthened by the action of the cricothyroid muscles and shortened by the thyroarytenoid and vocalis muscles.

Lymphatic drainage

The lymphatic drainage of the larynx determines the spread of mucosal carcinoma. Embryologically, the larynx can be divided superiorly and inferiorly at the level of the laryngeal ventricles. Lymphatic drainage follows these embryologic origins. Above the ventricles, lymphatics drain over the top of the thyroid cartilages because the supraglottic larynx is embryologically related to the oral cavity. Inferiorly, the lymphatics of the true vocal cords and subglottis drain inferiorly, posteriorly, and occasionally anteriorly through the cricothyroid membrane because this portion of the larynx is derived from tracheobronchial anlage.

Thyroid

The normal thyroid gland is readily distinguished from the sternothyroid and sternocleidomastoid muscles because of its greater signal intensity on T2-weighted images (Figs. 13 and 14). The thyroid gland is located inferior to the thyroid cartilage and extends over a 3 to 5 cm craniocaudal distance as a symmetric, homogeneous, wedge-shaped structure on either side of the trachea. The thyroid isthmus crosses anterior to the trachea and bridges the inferior portion of the right and left thyroid lobes. Transverse images alone are sufficient to examine the thyroid gland. When craniocaudal relationships must be delineated, the coronal plane-of-section is favored because of the symmetry of the thyroid gland in this plane.

Parathyroid Glands

Four glands as upper and lower bilateral pairs normally exist posterior to the thyroid lobes in the tracheoesophageal groove. However, normal parathyroid glands are smaller than 5 mm in their largest (craniocaudal) dimension and are not routinely imaged by sonography, CT, or MR.

Thymus Gland

The normal thymus is located in the mediastinum but is embryologically derived from neck structures and frequently has a "tongue" of remnant tissue extending to the inferior thyroid margin. Although the thymus is a prominent structure in children, in adults both the thymus and its superior tongue are atrophic and difficult to visualize by MR. T1-weighted techniques are best suited to separate normal thymic tissue from surrounding mediastinal fat (Figs. 15 and 16). The thymus is of interest primarily when imaging the necks of patients with hyperparathyroidism as ectopic parathyroid glands are commonly located in the thymus, occasionally as low as the level of the tracheal carina.

Lateral Compartments

The lateral compartments of the neck contain the carotid sheaths. The cervical carotid arteries and jugular veins are easily distinguished from adjacent fat, muscle, and lymph nodes because of the low signal intensity of flowing blood, which is black on the MR image gray scale (Figs. 13A and 15). Because of the inherently superior contrast of blood vessels and the absence of streak artifacts, MR is superior to CT for delineation of vessels at the thoracic inlet. Small branches of major cervical vessels can easily be traced from section to section on transverse images. Images obtained in the coronal or oblique-coronal planes-of-section are particularly suitable for delineation of cervical vascular anatomy. Lymph nodes are best seen with MR when T1 imaging techniques are selected. Lymph nodes are similar to thyroid and thymic tissue in having relatively long T1 and T2 times, allowing discrimination from fatty tissues

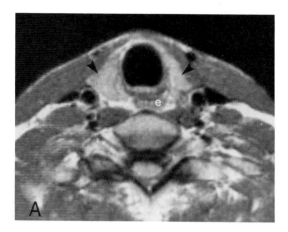

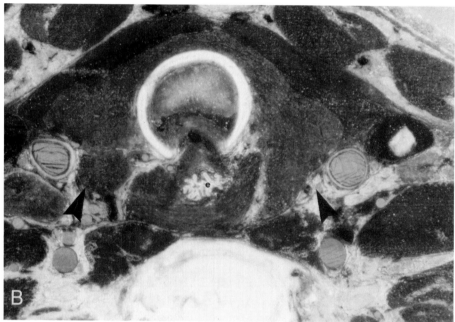

FIG. 13. A: Body coil high resolution image, pixel size 0.8 × 0.8 mm (cf. Fig. 14). The thyroid gland (*arrowheads*) is seen immediately posterior to the sternothyroid muscle. Thyroid tissue has greater intensity than muscle on this SE image, TR = 2 sec, TE = 28 msec, because of its longer T2. The spinal cord is seen surrounded by cerebrospinal fluid that has a low intensity because of an extremely long T1. The carotid arteries and jugular veins, lateral to the thyroid gland, have low intensity because of blood flow. The esophagus (e) is also shown. **B:** Corresponding cadaver section.

on T1-weighted images and from muscle on T2-weighted images.

POSTERIOR COMPARTMENT

The posterior compartment of the neck includes the cervical vertebrae, posterior extensor muscles, and anterior flexor muscles, including the scalenes, longus capitus, and longus colli muscles. These muscle groups have the same intermediate signal intensity as that of muscle in the tongue and paralaryngeal structures because they have similar MR tissue characteristics (long T1, short T2 relaxation times). The fibrous tissue of the nuchal ligament has a low intensity similar to that of dense cortical bone in the vertebral bodies, posterior elements, and ribs. Hematopoietic and fatty marrow within cancellous bone has a high signal intensity on both T1- and T2-weighted pulse sequences, approaching the intensity of subcutaneous fat.

PATHOLOGY

Cancer of the Tongue and Oropharynx

T2-weighted MR images optimize contrast between muscle and carcinoma, and are more useful than T1-weighted images for delineating the extent of tumor (Figs. 17 and 18). MR can delineate the relationship of tumors to the midline of the tongue and mandible, identifying margins for surgical resection. Identification of the lingual artery and hypoglossal nerve is also important as at least one artery and nerve must be preserved in order to permit a partial glossectomy. Many surgeons feel that a total glossectomy is incompatible with a satisfactory quality of life. T1-weighted images are useful for detecting nodal disease which affects staging of the tumor, overall prognosis, and whether a nodal dissection is performed with the primary surgical resection. High in the neck and deep to the sternocleidomas-

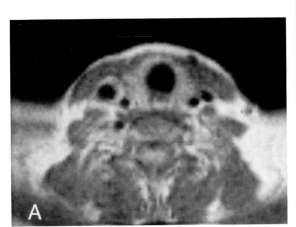
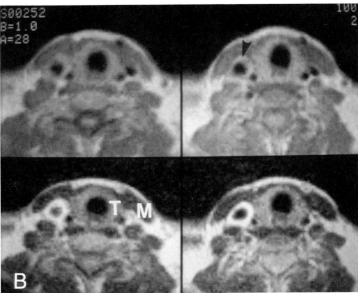

FIG. 14. A: Standard resolution image, pixel size 1.7 × 1.7 mm (cf. Fig. 13). TR 2.0; TE 28. **B:** Normal thyroid tissue (T) increases in intensity (**bottom right**) at longer TR and TE relative to the sternocleidomastoid muscle (M) because of the longer T1 and T2 values of thyroid tissue. Signal from the periphery of the right jugular vein (*arrowhead*) is related to laminar blood flow and increases markedly on the second echo images. **Top left,** TR = 1.0 sec, TE = 28 msec; **top right,** TR = 2.0 sec, TE = 28 msec; **bottom left,** TR = 1.0 sec, TE = 56 msec; **bottom right,** TR = 2.0 sec, TE = 56 msec.

toid muscle, adenopathy can be inaccessible to palpation and is best evaluated with cross-sectional imaging. A major advantage of MR imaging over CT is in distinguishing adenopathy from blood vessels without bolus injection of contrast material. Unfortunately, the interpretation of adenopathy on MR images still relies on the size and morphologic criteria used with CT. MR tissue characteristics (T1 and T2) derived by comparing different pulse sequence techniques cannot differentiate enlarged malignant nodes from enlarged reactive nodes. In patients who have had previous surgery or radiation therapy, both MR and CT are nonspecific in distinguishing scar tissue and inflammatory changes from recurrent tumor.

OROPHARYNX

Extension of mucosal tumors into the preepiglottic space, valleculae, or tonsilar bed can be readily detected by either CT or T1-weighted MR imaging techniques. Deep extension of tumor requires laryngectomy and/or partial pharyngectomy for a curative resection. Involvement of the carotid artery is a relative contraindication to surgery and can be excluded when the normal fatty tissue plane of high signal intensity is shown to surround the vessel.

Involvement of the mandible can be detected equally well by MR and CT. Loss of the normal low signal intensity of mandibular cortical bone adjacent to a tumor mass indicates invasion.

Normal lymphoid tissue shows increased signal intensity, similar to tumor, relative to muscle on T2-weighted images. T1 and T2 values for malignant tumors overlie the relaxation times of normal lymphoid tissue, benign tumors, and inflammatory lesions of the tongue, so that absolute T1 and T2 values are of no clinical value (Fig. 19).

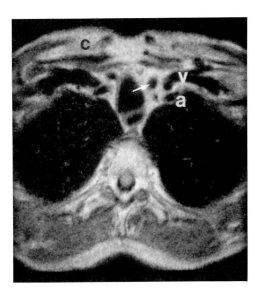

FIG. 15. MR at the level of the clavicular heads; a high signal intensity as seen from fat in the medullary cavity (c) surrounded by a low intensity rim of cortical bone. Subclavian vein (v) and artery (a); carotid artery (*arrow*). The thoracic spinal cord is seen ventral to low intensity CSF.

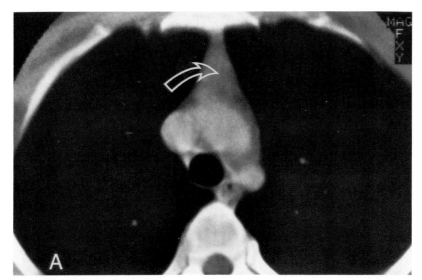
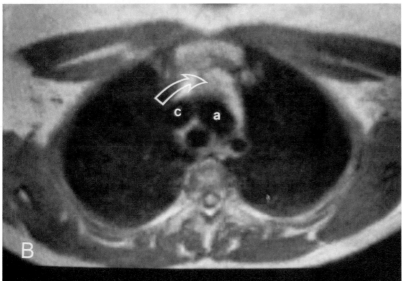

FIG. 16. Thymus gland. **A:** CT scan shows soft tissue density (*arrow*) within the mediastinal fat anterior to the aortic arch. **B:** MR imaging shows the thymus gland as a low signal intensity tissue (*arrow*) relative to surrounding mediastinal fat. The aortic arch (a) and superior vena cava (c) have very low signal intensities because of flow. The mediastinum is stretched in the CT scan as a result of breath holding and is relatively rounded on the MR exam which was obtained during quiet breathing.

Laryngeal Carcinoma

As in other areas of the head and neck, the primary role of CT or MR in imaging the larynx and hypopharynx is to define the extent of disease (Figs. 20–22) (13–16). Although laryngoscopy can show mucosal surfaces and masses involving the lumen, deep extensions are difficult to detect and have profound implications in the management of disease. Planning for conservation laryngeal surgery depends on accurate knowledge of the extent of disease within the larynx. Specifically, all techniques require an intact cricoid cartilage on which to construct a functional voice box. A total laryngectomy results in a devastating loss of natural voice function. The accurate delineation of tumor extension in two planes of section by MR may allow more precise planning of conservation surgery.

CT and MR may detect the deep extent of tumors that have normal overlying mucosa and are not detectable on endoscopy. Sometimes large, bulky, proximal lesions obscure the view of endoscopists, who may also have difficulty in viewing the infraglottic region and the apices (inferior tips) of the piriform sinuses. Occult tumor involvement of lymph nodes may be detected by imaging techniques. The head and neck surgeon and radiation oncologist become better able to decide the appropriate surgery and/or radiation therapy by using CT and/or MR for staging (17). In some cases, partial laryngectomy with preservation of glottic function may be possible instead of total laryngectomy. In others, tumor invasion of the laryngeal cartilages, preepiglottic space, or infraglottic region may exclude radiation therapy as the sole treatment. Later, posttreatment scans may detect recurrent disease, especially in nonpalpable lymph nodes.

CT and MR can provide vital information about a laryngeal tumor in several areas (18–20):

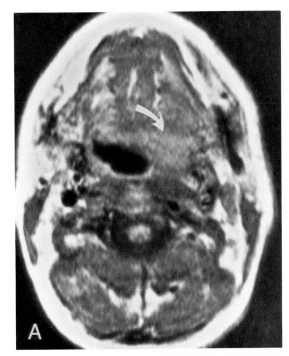

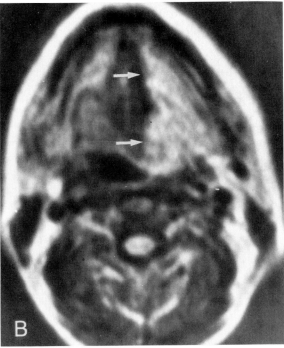

FIG. 17. Squamous carcinoma of the tongue base. **A:** Transverse T1-weighted images show the mass (*arrow*) extending posterior to the lateral pharyngeal wall. **B:** T2-weighted image shows more extensive involvement of the tongue. Reduced anatomic resolution is the result of the lower signal-to-noise ratios achieved with longer echo delays.

1. Anterior and posterior commissure
2. Supraglottic extension (preepiglottic space, paralaryngeal spaces, piriform sinuses, vallecula)
3. Infraglottic extension
4. Vocal cord fixation
5. Extralaryngeal spread (soft tissues of the neck, tongue base, postcricoid region)
6. Cervical adenopathy
7. Cartilage invasion
8. Carotid artery involvement.

Laryngeal cancers are classified into four groups based on origin: supraglottic, glottic, infraglottic or subglottic, and transglottic. Each tumor type has a characteristic pattern and rapidity of spread. For instance, metastatic disease to the lymph nodes is more common in supraglottic and infraglottic tumors than in glottic lesions. Tumors of the piriform sinus will be included in the discussion because of their close relation to the supraglottic lesions. A brief mention of transglottic tumors will also be included.

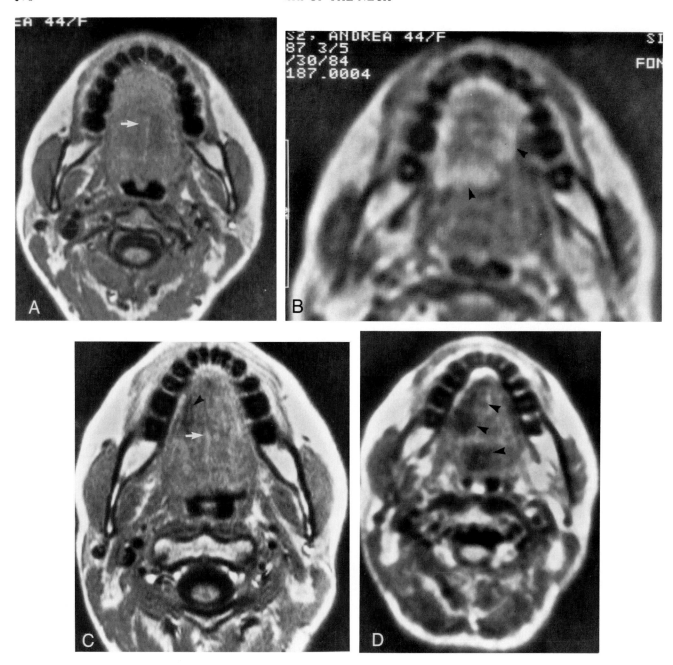

FIG. 18. Floor of mouth carcinoma. **A:** T1-weighted scan shows only a slight mass effect deviating the midline septum (*arrow*). **B:** T2-weighted sequence shows extensive infiltration of the tongue by tumor crossing the midline (*arrowheads*). **C:** Following radiation therapy, the T1-weighted image shows reduction of mass effect and restoration of the tongue septum to the midline (*arrow*). A small region of low signal intensity is seen in the irradiated region (*arrowhead*). **D:** Posttreatment T2-weighted image shows larger areas of low signal intensity, indicating a dramatic reduction in the T2 relaxation time of tissues in the region of the tumor.

Histologically, more than 90% of laryngopharyngeal cancers are of squamous cell origin. Other types of malignancies found in the larynx and hypopharynx include pseudosarcoma, adenocarcinoma, "spindle cell" carcinoma, oat cell carcinoma, and basal cell carcinoma. Laryngeal cancers of connective tissue and hematopoietic elements have also been documented; examples include chrondrosarcoma, fibrosarcoma, reticulosarcoma, and lymphosarcoma.

SUPRAGLOTTIC CANCERS

Supraglottic tumors, arising anywhere from the false vocal cords to the epiglottis, comprise 20 to 35% of laryngeal cancers (Fig. 21). Supraglottic tumors tend to spread to lymph nodes high in the neck, involving the internal jugular chain and often the jugulo-digastric node because of the abundant lymphatics. Consequently, supraglottic cancers often present as more ad-

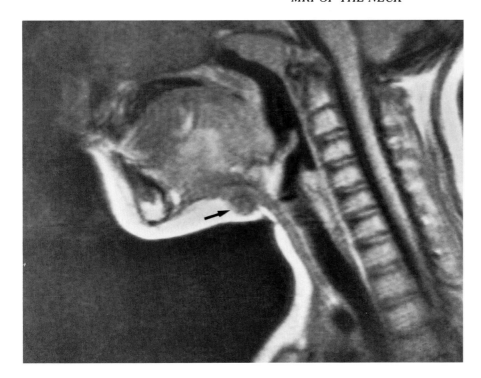

FIG. 19. Thyroglossal duct cyst. A cystic dilatation may occur anywhere along the course of the midline thyroglossal duct which extends from the foramen cecum to the thyroid gland. This 6-year-old female shows a small mass with a low signal intensity (*arrow*) inferior to the level of the hyoid bone (SE 500/28 image).

vanced tumors than glottic lesions. Thyroid cartilage invasion is not a common finding unless the tumor extends to the anterior commissure. The hyoid bone is usually displaced by tumor, not destroyed.

Carcinomas of the supraglottic region can be subdivided into two groups: *anterior,* i.e., carcinomas arising in the epiglottis or preepiglottic space, and *posterolateral,* i.e., carcinomas found in the aryepiglottic folds and the paralaryngeal spaces (marginal tumors). Anterior supraglottic tumors have a better prognosis than those of the posterolateral supraglottis. Suprahyoid epiglottic cancers can initially present as thickening of the free margin and can be treated by surgery or radiation therapy. More advanced lesions may spread to the pharyngoepiglottic folds, lateral pharyngeal walls, vallecula, or base of the tongue. On the other hand, infrahyoid epiglottic cancers often extend into the preepiglottic space, which then loses its normal fatty appearance.

Abnormality of the preepiglottic space may also result from edema, blood, or inflammation. Advanced infrahyoid epiglottic cancers frequently cross the midline with the paralaryngeal lymphatics and extend into the paramedial portions of the thyroid cartilage, just above the anterior commissure level.

Posterolateral supraglottic tumors appear as thickened aryepiglottic folds and a mass in the paralaryngeal space. Their natural tendency is to grow posteriorly and inferiorly to the arytenoids, rather than anteriorly to the preepiglottic space. Marginal tumors can cross the midline via the preepiglottic space. Advanced piriform sinus carcinomas can often resemble supraglottic marginal lesions.

GLOTTIC CANCERS

Glottic tumors, arising from the true cords, are the most common laryngeal cancers. They comprise 50 to 70% of laryngeal malignancies and are usually well-differentiated, slow-growing lesions. Seventy-five percent of these tumors involve the anterior half of the true vocal cord. Nodal spread is rare in the case of early lesions because there is an absence of lymphatics along the free margin of the vocal cords. However, advanced lesions with a fixed cord have a higher incidence of lymphatic involvement.

Glottic tumors may extend to the anterior commissure. From there they may grow into the infraglottic or supraglottic (preepiglottic space) regions, into the contralateral vocal cord, or into the thyroid cartilage and cricothyroid membrane. Alternatively, tumor may grow posteriorly to the posterior commissure, arytenoids, and cricoarytenoid joints. From the posterior commissure, continued tumor extension may occur into the contralateral cord or into the soft tissues of the neck. The cricothyroid space may become widened.

Early glottic lesions have an excellent prognosis; the 5-year survival approaches 95% with surgery or radiation therapy. CT or MR of these lesions does not usually add additional information to laryngoscopy. A thickened cord may be secondary to tumor or fibrosis, edema, inflammation, and hemorrhage. Anterior commissure involvement necessitates an "extended" hemilaryngectomy. Occasionally, an abundance of soft tissue density at the anterior commissure is the major clue to pathology despite the symmetrical appearance of the

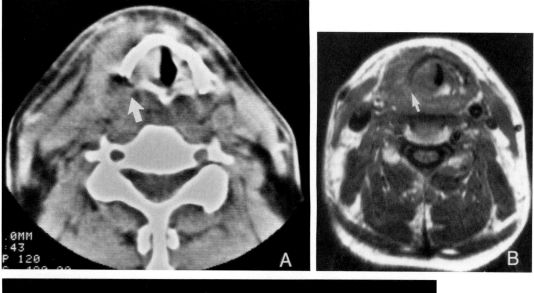

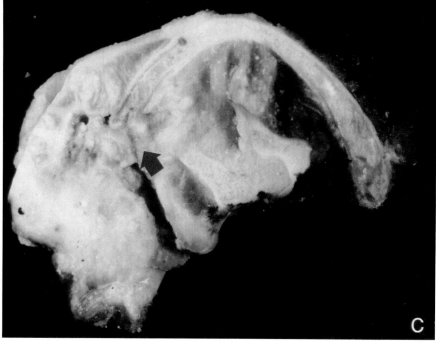

FIG. 20. Piriform sinus carcinoma. This 61-year-old female presented with a sore throat and mild hoarseness which have persisted after 2 months of antibiotic therapy. Endoscopy and biopsy revealed a squamous cell carcinoma of the right piriform sinus. **A:** A preoperative CT scan revealed inferior extension of the tumor with destruction of the thyroid and cricoid cartilages (*arrow*). **B:** Transverse MR scan (SE 500/28, "T1 weighted") shows similar cartilage destruction. **C:** Surgical specimen confirms the imaging findings.

vocal cords. In general, early mucosal disease is best evaluated with endoscopy.

Vocal cord fixation can also be detected by CT or MR. Scans may show an arytenoid cartilage in the median or paramedian position. Cord fixation may be the result of several mechanisms. Tumor may infiltrate the intrinsic laryngeal musculature and fix the cord to the thyroid cartilage; bulky tumor may limit cord mobility by mass effect, or tumor may involve the cricoarytenoid joint.

INFRAGLOTTIC CANCERS

Infraglottic tumors arise between the true vocal cords and the inferior border of the cricoid cartilage and comprise 2 to 6% of laryngeal cancers. True primaries here are rare and spread early to the trachea, thyroid, hypopharynx, and inferior lymph nodes. Infraglottic tumors are more often inferior extensions of glottic (and sometimes supraglottic) cancers.

As mentioned earlier, the conus elasticus separates deep and mucosal tumors since it resists tumor invasion. Tumors infiltrating deep to the conus elasticus (e.g., transglottic) tend to remain on its deep surface (paralaryngeal surface), whereas those beginning on its mucosal side tend to remain mucosal. On scans below the true vocal cords any soft tissue between the cricoid cartilage and the airway is abnormal and may represent subglottic extension.

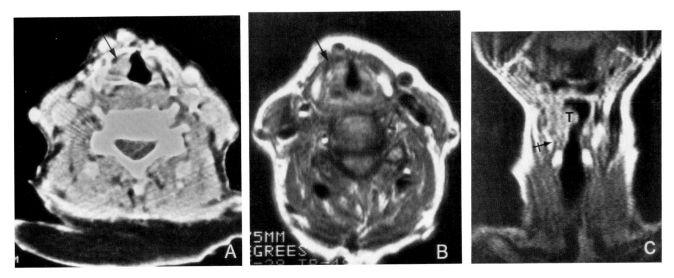

FIG. 21. Squamous cell carcinoma of the larynx. Staging for conservation laryngeal surgery. **A:** CT scan suggests a fullness in the right true vocal cord region (*arrow*). **B:** Transverse SE 500/30 MR image also suggests involvement of the right true vocal cord. **C:** Coronal MR image shows the tumor (T) involving the aryepiglottic folds, above the level of the false vocal cords. The right true vocal cord is separated from the tumor by a fatty tissue plane, indicating that the tumor is entirely supraglottic and that the intrinsic laryngeal musculature can be spared by conservation surgery.

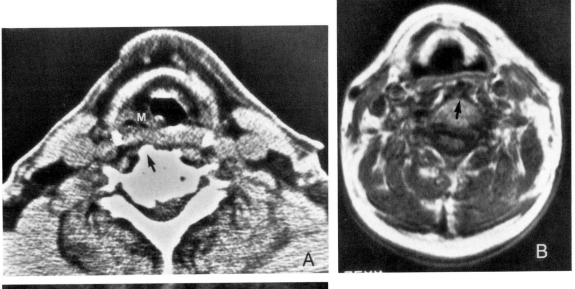

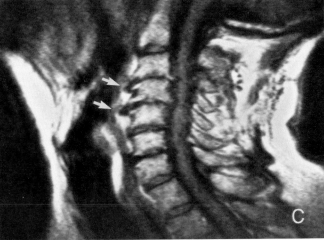

FIG. 22. Severe throat pain with swallowing in a 79-year-old physician. On clinical examination it was difficult to evaluate the left piriform sinus. **A:** CT scan suggests a mass effect in the left piriform sinus (M). Cervical spine osteophytes (*arrow*) are noted. **B:** The MR image shows a normal piriform sinus but a prominent osetophyte of low signal intensity relative to the cancellous bone, which has a higher signal intensity medullary cavity (*arrow*). **C:** Sagittal MR scan shows spondylosis at several levels with dense, low signal intensity osteophytes protruding into the higher signal intensity prevertebral fat (*arrows*). At follow-up examination no tumor was discovered and the patient's dysphagia was attributed to the osteophytes.

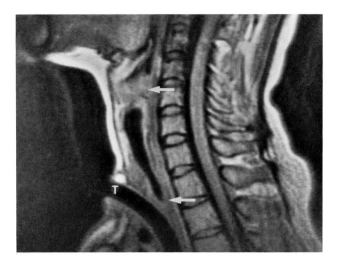

FIG. 23. Tracheal stenosis. The sagittal plane of section is used to evaluate patency of the airway. In this patient with a tracheostomy (T), glottic scarring and adhesions prevented adequate clinical evaluation of her subglottic airway. MR shows obstruction at the level of the tracheostomy (*arrow*) as well as at the glottis (*arrow*).

Generally, if the infraglottic tumor extends more than 1 cm below the true cords, a total laryngectomy is indicated because it is necessary to remove the cricoid cartilage in order to obtain clear margins. With more aggressive voice conservation techniques, parts of the superior rim of the cricoid lamina may be taken while laryngeal function remains intact. In advanced lesions the cricoid cartilage may be eroded and total laryngectomy necessary.

TRANSGLOTTIC CANCERS

Transglottic tumors may be defined as those involving the true cords and subglottic space or those that cross the laryngeal ventricles. Involvement of the true and false vocal cords may cause vocal cord fixation. A few transglottic tumors begin in the laryngeal ventricle; many more originate from the true vocal cord with laryngeal spread. Transglottic tumors have an increased incidence of thyroid cartilage invasion and extension through the cricothyroid membrane. Treatment is usually total laryngectomy with or without radiation therapy.

PIRIFORM SINUS CANCER

Piriform sinus tumors behave more aggressively than endolaryngeal lesions and comprise 10 to 20% of "laryngeal" cancers (25). They are actually cancers of the inferior hypopharynx. Early nodal disease occurs because of the rich lymphatics anterior to the piriform sinuses.

Piriform sinus tumors grow in two major patterns. Those of the lateral wall invade the thyroid cartilage and soft tissues of the neck, forming bulky masses about the piriform sinus. Tumors of the medial wall extend into the paralaryngeal space and vocalis muscle, resembling marginal supraglottic lesions. Less commonly, piriform sinus cancers invade anterior to the preepiglottic space and cross the midline. Tumors of either wall may spread supramedially to the aryepiglottic fold, again simulating marginal supraglottic lesions.

Despite the similarities, piriform sinus tumors have several characteristics that distinguish them from marginal supraglottic lesions. Piriform sinus tumors frequently invade the thyroid cartilage, usually at its posterolateral margins. Also, piriform sinus lesions tend to be unilateral and submucosal. If extensive, these tumors may widen the space between the thyroid and cricoid cartilages. (The tough conus elasticus tends to direct the tumor posterolaterally and inferiorly.)

In the various types of laryngeal cancers, the laryngeal cartilages may be "distorted" by tumor. Distortion can range from mild displacement to frank destruction. When marked, both are easy to recognize on CT or MR (Figs. 21 and 22) (22–23). However, slight asymmetrical deformity and focal infiltrating destruction may be difficult to assess. Normal variations in patterns of cartilage calcification can simulate destruction on MR as well as with CT. Neither CT nor MR can detect microscopic cartilage invasion.

BENIGN LARYNGEAL LESIONS

Most benign lesions have a nonspecific appearance. CT and MR can document their extent very well but cannot always differentiate among neoplastic, inflammatory, traumatic, and degenerative processes.

Laryngocele

A laryngocele is a dilation of the saccule (appendix) of the laryngeal ventricle. Sometimes this appendix extends superiorly in the paralaryngeal space, medial to the thyroid cartilage, where it is known as an internal laryngocele and can present as a submucosal, supraglottic mass. Lateral displacement of the thyroid lamina can occur. If the dilated saccule extends through the thyrohyoid membrane, it is an external laryngocele. The most common type, mixed laryngoceles, combines components of both internal and external laryngoceles.

Laryngoceles are usually unilateral, although they may be bilateral in 25% of cases. Presumably they arise from increased intralaryngeal pressures, as may be caused by glass blowing or playing wind instruments. Laryngoceles present commonly in adulthood; many are asymptomatic.

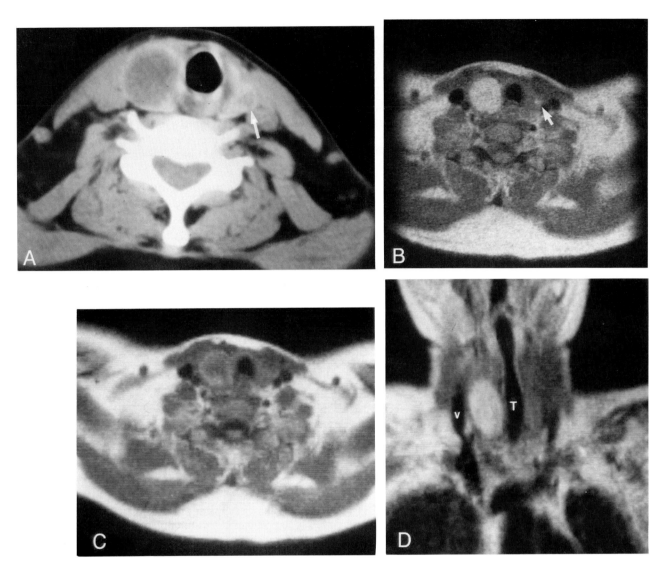

FIG. 24. Palpable thyroid nodule in a woman irradiated 20 years earlier for acne. A single nonfunctioning thyroid nodule was identified by technetium pertechnetate scintigraphy. **A:** CT scan shows a 3 cm mass in the right thyroid lobe and a second unsuspected 8 mm mass in the left thyroid lobe (*arrow*). **B:** SE 2,000/28 MR image, "T2 weighted," shows both thyroid nodules as high signal intensity tissues. At surgery the right lobe nodule was a degenerated thyroid adenoma and the left lobe nodule an 8 mm focus of granulomatous thyroiditis. **C:** SE 500/28 image obtained with lower spatial resolution shows only the right lobe nodule. **D:** Coronal image shows relationships of the right lobe nodule to the trachea (T) and jugular vein (v).

An unobstructed laryngocele is filled with air. With obstruction, fluid accumulates within the dilated appendix. Sometimes a small cancer near the neck of the saccule causes the obstruction and subsequent laryngocele. The lesion is also associated with chronic granulomatous disease, such as tuberculosis. On CT and MR a laryngocele is a well-circumscribed mass extending superiorly from the laryngeal ventricle and false cord into the paralaryngeal space (internal laryngocele) or lateral to the thyrohyoid membrane (external laryngocele) (24–26). In mixed laryngoceles the internal and external features can be identified.

Benign neoplasm

With the exception of papillomas, benign neoplasms of the larynx are rare. Papillomas occur more commonly in children than in adults and are in fact the most common laryngeal tumors in the pediatric age group. Children usually have multiple lesions compared to adults, in whom a single lesion is more common. A characteristic juvenile papilloma originates in the anterior larynx on the true or false vocal cords and extends subglottically. Extension throughout the tracheobronchial tree may follow incomplete removal.

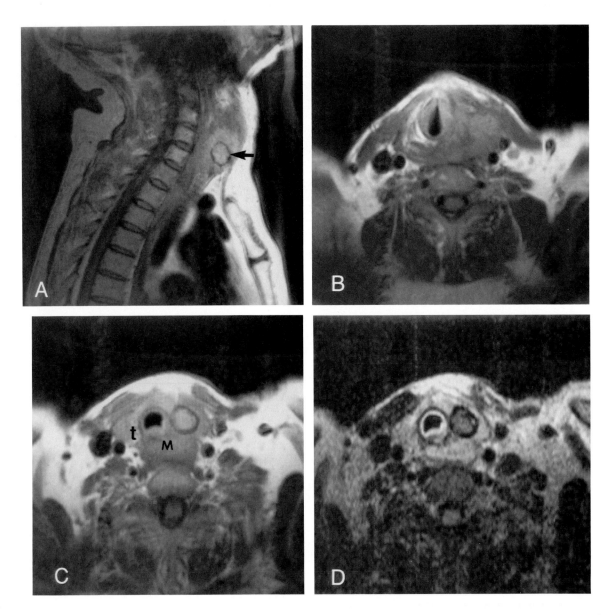

FIG. 25. Calcified thyroid nodule in a patient with multinodular goiter. **A:** Sagittal surface coil image shows a thyroid mass and a low signal intensity ring (*arrow*) corresponding to calcification. **B:** Transverse image (SE 500/30) at the level of the glottis shows a large left thyroid mass. **C:** At the level of the first tracheal ring a normal right thyroid lobe is seen (t). The calcified nodule is seen within a larger left thyroid lobe mass (m) extending behind the trachea. **D:** SE 2,000/60 at the same level shows increased signal intensity of the mass and normal right thyroid lobe relative to subcutaneous fat, indicating that both normal and adenomatous thyroid tissues have long T2 relaxation times. Note the bright tracheal mucosa, indicating an extremely long T2 relaxation time, possibly caused by edema. (From Stark and Bradley (40) with permission.)

Other rare, benign, laryngeal neoplasms include adenomas, chondromas, hemangiomas, neurofibromas, and plasmacytomas. With the exception of chondromas, their CT appearance on scans is not specific. Chondromas arise most frequently from the cricoid cartilage and show matrix calcification. Generally, benign lesions are distinguished from their malignant counterparts by biopsy (Fig. 23). Amyloidosis may also involve the larynx and appear as a mass.

Laryngeal Trauma

Occasionally, posttraumatic changes mimic cancerous masses in the laryngeal cartilages. Most commonly, thyroid cartilage fractures heal in a distorted pattern, causing supraglottic masses. Vocal cord paralysis after trauma may be incorrectly attributed to malignancy.

CT and MR are useful in the study of laryngeal trauma (27). In the acute case, significant injuries should

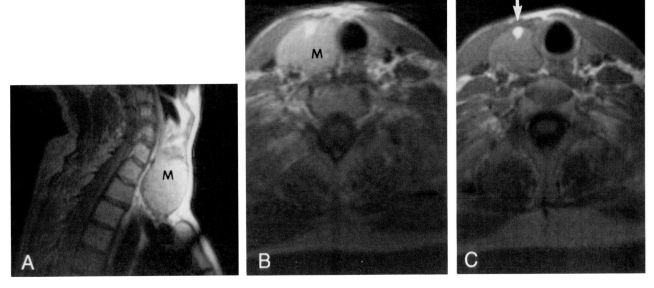

FIG. 26. Hemorrhagic thyroid adenoma. **A:** Sagittal surface coil SE 1,500/30 image shows a prominent thyroid mass (M) near the midline, above the thoracic inlet. **B:** Transverse SE 1,500/30 image shows deviation of the trachea away from the mass. The left thyroid lobe appears normal. **C:** SE 500/20 image shows a region of increased signal intensity (arrow) within the mass. This represents a region of short T1 caused by the paramagnetic effect of old hemorrhage. Nevertheless, a benign diagnosis cannot be established by MR. (From Stark and Bradley (40) with permission.)

be identified and repaired within 7 to 10 days. Delay in the treatment of fractured laryngeal cartilages may lead to posttraumatic laryngeal stenosis. Chronic posttraumatic abnormalities are also easily studied by these techniques. The direct sagittal scanning capability of MR is particularly useful for demonstrating the extent of airway lesions (Fig. 23). This is often the value in planning laryngeal reconstruction. Unsuspected or forgotten old laryngeal trauma presenting as a laryngeal mass may be recognized by the posttraumatic deformity of the cartilages.

Thyroid

Thyroid nodules have prolonged T1 and T2 relaxation times and can be distinguished from normal thyroid tissue by using T2-weighted spin echo images (Figs. 24–29). Unfortunately, functioning and nonfunctioning nodules, cancers, and even cysts have a wide range of relaxation times and these values overlap. No functional MR contrast agent exists for the thyroid gland. By comparison, nuclear medicine scanning studies have the advantage of targeting functioning thyroid nodules with

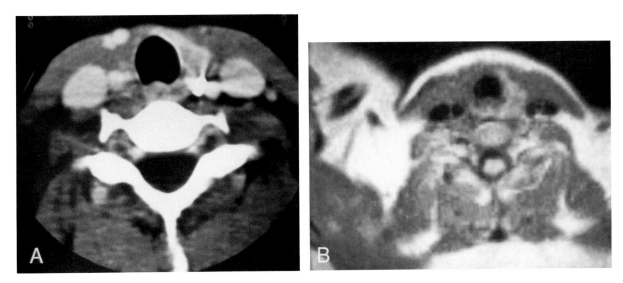

FIG. 27. A: Postoperative changes. CT scan during bolus infusion of contrast material is degraded by streak artifact from surgical clip. Only the left hemithyroid is seen because of a previous right hemithyroidectomy. **B:** MR image is free of artifact. TR = 2.0; TE = 28.

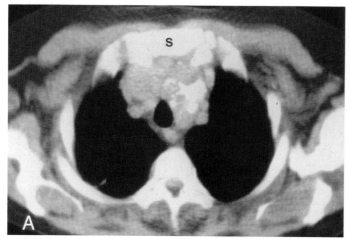

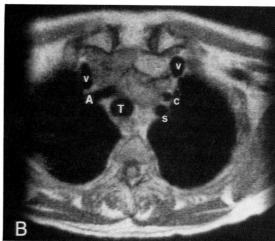

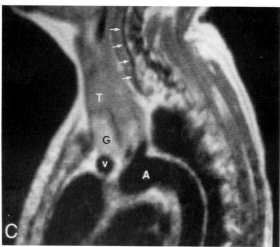

FIG. 28. Intrathoracic extension of multinodular goiter. **A:** CT scan shows retrosternal (s) extension of a calcified mass. Surgical planning for median sternotomy versus a simple "collar" neck incision to excise this goiter depends on its relationship to the great vessels and other mediastinal structures. **B:** MR image shows heterogeneous tissue characteristics of the mass with low intensity septations representing fibrous tissue and calcification. The left subclavian artery (s), carotid artery (c), innominate veins (v), innominate artery (A), and trachea (T) are not encased by the mass, allowing a simple cervical approach. **C:** Sagittal image obtained with a T2-weighted technique (SE 1,500/28) shows the nodular goiter (G) to have a greater signal intensity (longer T2 relaxation time) than the cervical thyroid gland (T). Aortic arch (A), innominate vein (v), and left vertebral artery (arrows) are also shown.

pertechnetate (TcO_4^-). Although permanganate (MnO_4^-) is selectively accumulated by functioning thyroid tissue, manganese in this form is not paramagnetic. Nonspecific extracellular agents such as gadolinium-DTPA are not likely to show tissue-specific differential enhancement. In the absence of a functional contrast agent, MR provides only anatomic information. Although in some cases MR may show more lesions than nuclear medicine techniques, it is unlikely to compete effectively with high resolution ultrasound. In patients with known thyroid carcinoma, MR may substitute for CT in staging cervical lymph nodes or evaluating tumor recurrence. However, sonography will remain the procedure of choice for anatomic imaging of the thyroid gland itself (28).

Parathyroid Glands

Sonography is also an excellent technique for imaging parathyroid adenomas (36,39,42,45). Because of its multiplanar capabilities and excellent spatial resolution,

it is ideally suited to sort out anatomic relationships in the retrothyroidal region. When sonography is obstructed by tracheal air or when intrathoracic extension of parathyroid tumors is suspected, either CT or MR will be useful (Figs. 30 and 31) (33). Although the spatial resolution of body coil MR is slightly inferior to that of high resolution CT, surface coil techniques can be applied to the thoracic inlet and anterior mediastinum, allowing comparable anatomic resolution. The absence of streak artifacts and the ease of identification of blood vessels by MR are significant advantages.

T1-weighted spin echo techniques readily differentiate parathyroid tumors from fat and adjacent vessels. Parathyroid tumors also have a long T2 relaxation time and can be distinguished from muscles on T2-weighted spin echo images. In fact, the T2 relaxation time of parathyroid tumors is longer than the T2 of fat or thyroid gland, allowing parathyroid tumors to stand out with a relatively high signal intensity on heavily T2-weighted images (e.g., SE 2,000/60–120). Parathyroid adenomas appear to have slightly longer relaxation times than hyperplastic glands, but this difference is not

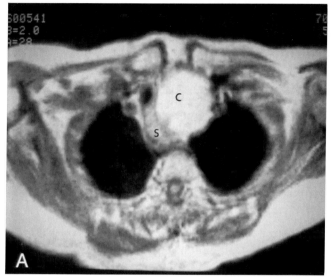

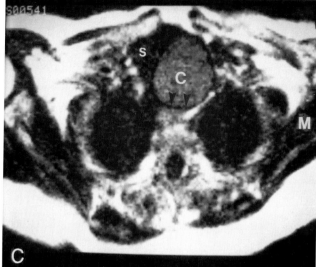

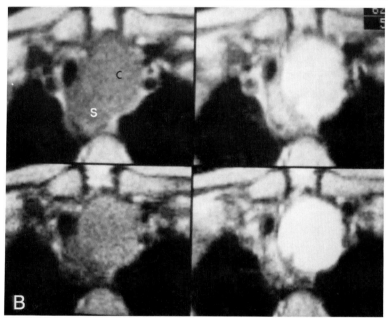

FIG. 29. Intrathoracic goiter with solid and cystic components. **A:** SE 2,000/28 image shows the cystic component (c) to have a high signal intensity because of its long T2 relaxation time. The solid component (s) of the multinodular goiter is lower in signal intensity because of a shorter T2 relaxation time and is heterogeneous because of its nodular, septated components. **B:** MR image obtained using different spin echo techniques. **Top left,** TR = 0.5 sec, TE = 28 msec; **top right,** TR = 2.0 sec, TE = 28 msec; **bottom left,** TR = 0.5 sec, TE = 56 msec; **bottom right,** TR = 2.0 sec, TE = 56 msec. The cyst fluid (c) has the longest T1 and T2 values of all tissues studied and shows the greatest intensity increases with increases in TR and TE. Inhomogeneity of the solid portion of the goiter (s) correlated with histologic findings of intermixed colloid nodules and fibrous bands. **C:** MR inversion recovery image, TR = 1.8 sec and T1 = 278 msec, 1 cm cephalad to **A,B,** shows muscle (M), lung, vessels, trachea, esophagus, goiter, and the fibrous wall of the cyst (*arrowheads*) as structures with similar low intensities. The cyst fluid (c) has a slightly greater intensity than thyroid gland because fluid has exceedingly long T1 and this image is a magnitude reconstruction. Subcutaneous fat has the highest intensity because of its very short T1.

useful in individual cases. As with thyroid adenomas and carcinomas, parathyroid carcinoma shows no significant difference in relaxation times from the much more common adenomas.

Lymph Nodes

Pathologic lymph nodes are detected by MR using morphologic criteria analogous to those used by CT (Figs. 32–34) (34–37). Intensity measurements as well as T1 and T2 relaxation times appear to be similar for normal lymph nodes (less than 1 cm in size) and pathologic lymph nodes (greater than 1.5 cm in size). Lymphadenopathies as a consequence of Hodgkin disease, non-Hodgkin lymphoma, infection, and metastatic cancer all have similar intensities, T1, and T2 values. The T1 and T2 relaxation times of pathologic lymph nodes are only slightly longer than those of thyroid nodules and must be distinguished from thyroid tumors by

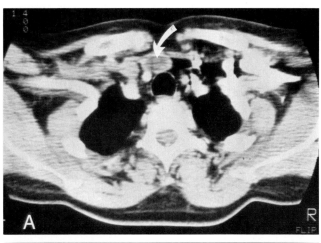

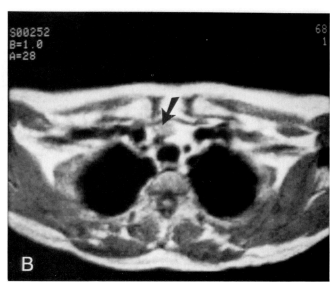

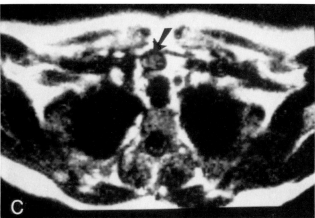

FIG. 30. Parathyroid adenoma. **A:** CT scan following contrast infusion demonstrates an abnormal structure (arrow) at the thoracic inlet. **B:** MR spin echo image (TR = 1.0 sec, TE = 28 msec) identifies this structure as a soft tissue mass (*arrow*) and differentiates adjacent vascular structures. **C:** Inversion recovery image (TR = 1.8 sec, T1 = 278 msec) demonstrates a low intensity rim (arrow) surrounding the central portion of the parathyroid adenoma which has a higher intensity, indicating a difference in T1 between the rim and center of the tumor. Histology showed the rim to be adenomatous parathyroid tissue. The center was an acellular collagenous matrix.

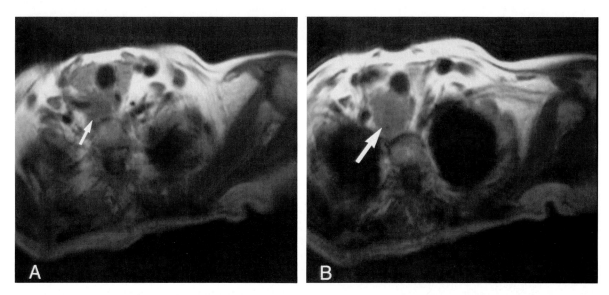

FIG. 31. Parathyroid adenoma in an obtunded, hypercalcemic patient. **A:** Surface coil images degraded by patient motion. A mass is seen in the tracheoesophageal groove at the right lower thyroid pole (arrow). The mass has a lower signal intensity than the thyroid gland on this SE 330/18 image, indicating a longer T1 relaxation time. **B:** Caudally, the mass extends into the mediastinum and enlarges. The degree of hypercalcemia correlates with the size of parathyroid adenomas. In this case the absence of a palpable neck mass led to a delay in diagnosis. (From Stark and Bradley (40), with permission.)

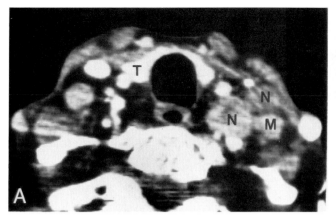
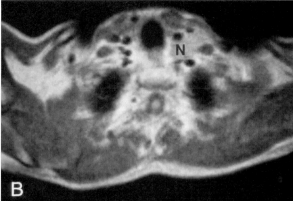

FIG. 32. Non-Hodgkin lymphoma. **A:** CT scan is degraded by streak artifact. The thyroid gland (T) is identified as a high density structure that enhances following bolus administration of intravenous contrast material. Enlarged lymph nodes (N) in a patient with non-Hodgkin lymphoma have an appearance similar to the left anterior scalene muscle (M). **B:** Enlarged lymph nodes (N) are easily differentiated from the anterior scalene muscle. The esophagus is seen indenting the posterior margin of the tracheal air column. TR = 2.0, TE = 28.

delineation of intervening fatty tissue planes. Tissue planes are best demonstrated with short TR/short TE spin echo techniques. T1-weighted images may not allow separation of lymph nodes from muscle as both tissues have relatively long T1 relaxation times. In this instance, complementary T2-weighted images are particularly valuable as muscle will have a low signal intensity relative to lymph nodes.

A major advantage of MR over CT is discrimination of lymph nodes and muscle from tortuous vessels in the

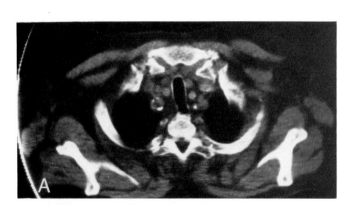
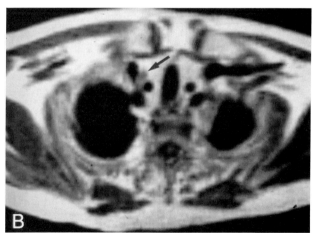
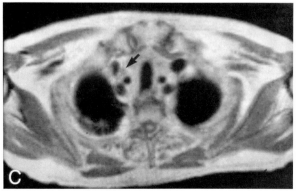

FIG. 33. Malignant adenopathy. **A:** Contrast-enhanced CT scan shows complex vascular anatomy at the thoracic inlet. **B:** SE 500/28 "T1-weighted" MR image clearly distinguishes a 1 cm lymph node (*arrow*) from adjacent vessels. **C:** SE 1,000/28 image suffers from decreased contrast between the lymph node and surrounding mediastinal fat as these tissues have long T2 relaxation times. Furthermore, this image is somewhat degraded by motion-induced blurring. Sequences with long TR have increased sensitivity to motion artifacts.

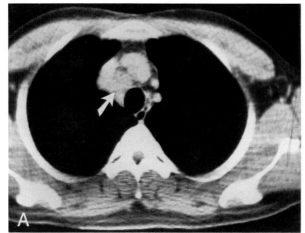

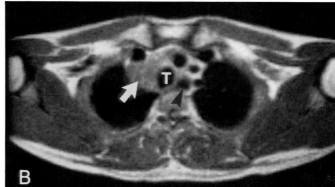

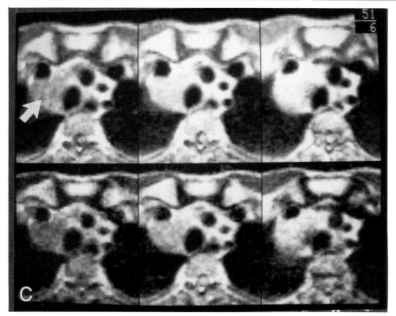

FIG. 34. Inflammatory lymphadenopathy. **A:** CT scan during bolus administration of intravenous contrast material distinguishes lymph nodes (*arrow*) from adjacent vessels. **B:** Standard resolution spin echo image, TR = 0.5 sec, TE = 28 msec, demonstrates the mass as a moderate intensity structure (*arrow*) surrounded by high intensity fat. The trachea (T), esophagus (*arrowhead*), and major vessels are well seen. **C:** The mass has a long T1 compared to fat; therefore, the intensity of the mass increases relative to fat at long TR. **Left** to **right,** TR = 0.5, 1.0, 1.5 sec. The mass has a T2 slightly shorter than fat; therefore, the intensity of the mass decreases slightly relative to fat at long TE. **Top row,** TE = 28 msec; **bottom row,** TE = 56 msec.

neck at the thoracic inlet (38–40). Because of blood flow, vascular structures are usually seen as very low intensity structures. However, when blood flow is abnormally slow or turbulent, particularly in venous structures, increased signal intensity within the vascular lumen may cause some confusion. Blood vessels with regions of increased intraluminal signal intensity can usually be distinguished from other soft tissues by examining adjacent sections to demonstrate continuity with blood vessels or by demonstrating flow effects on even spin echos (second echo rephasing). Magnetic resonance imaging can detect atheromatous plaque or thickening of the vascular wall resulting from inflammatory vascular disease (Fig. 35). Vascular occlusion or thrombosis is seen as regions of high signal intensity without even echo rephasing. However, vascular calcifications are difficult to identify and small calcifications are missed because volume averaging with surrounding tissues of higher signal intensity.

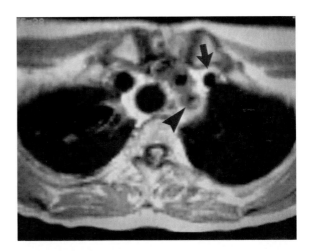

FIG. 35. Takayasu arteritis. MR at the level of the thoracic inlet shows thickening of walls of the major arteries [subclavian artery (*arrowhead*)]. Subclavian veins are not involved (*arrow*).

CONCLUSIONS

Magnetic resonance imaging of the neck combines the advantages of CT and sonography. In evaluation of aerodigestive tract tumors, MR can substitute for CT in evaluating deep extension of mucosal cancers. Tumors of the tongue and supraglottic region are better imaged with surface coil MR techniques than with CT. While CT can better delineate the calcified portions of the laryngeal skeleton, MR imaging provides superior delineation of soft tissue extension of tumors and can better provide information to plan conservation surgery because of its multiplanar imaging capabilities. Where rapid scan times are essential, as in uncooperative patients, CT is superior to MR. A major advantage of MR over CT is the absence of artifacts from the mandible or dental amalgam. Neither CT nor MR are tissue specific and therefore were less effective in the postoperative or postirradiation neck.

Although T2-weighted scans are the most important in evaluating tongue neoplasms, the majority of aerodigestive tract tumors were better staged using T1-weighted techniques because of superior contrast between tumor and fatty tissue planes. Neither MR nor CT is competitive with laryngoscopy for determination of mucosal extension of disease. However, neither technique had any useful degree of tissue specificity. Benign pathologic conditions such as laryngoceles, thyroglossal duct cysts, or laryngeal trauma can also be evaluated by MR.

In evaluating tumors of the thyroid and parathyroid glands, neither MR nor CT can match the low cost, availability, ease of use, and overall effectiveness of sonography. When nodal metastases are suspected, the full cross-sectional field of view of MR has advantages similar to those established for CT. Intrathoracic extension of thyroid goiters or ectopic parathyroid glands can be evaluated to advantage by MR because of the improved delineation of blood vessels and excellent tumor–fat contrast. Suspected adenopathy or vascular pathology in the thoracic inlet is also well delineated by MR.

With further improvements in surface coil technology, improved spatial resolution, faster scan times, and reduction in motion artifacts, MRI will continue to replace CT as the technique of choice for evaluating head and neck cancers. Until a functional contrast agent is developed, scintigraphy will remain the technique of choice for evaluating thyroid nodules.

REFERENCES

1. Lufkin RB, Votruba J, Reicher M, et al. Solenoid surface coils in magnetic resonance imaging. *AJR,* 1986;146:409–12.
2. New PFJ, Rosen BR, Brady TJ, et al. Potential hazards and artifacts of ferromagnetic and nonferromagnetic surgical and dental materials and devices in nuclear magnetic resonance imaging. *Radiology* 1983;147:139–48.
3. Unger JM. The oral cavity and tongue: magnetic resonance imaging. *Radiology* 1985;155:151–3.
4. Rauschning W, Bergstrom K, Pech P. Correlative craniospinal anatomy studies by computed tomography and cryomicrotomy. *J Comput Assist Tomogr* 1983;7:9–13.
5. Larsson S, Mancuso AA, Hanafee W. Computed tomography of the tongue and floor of mouth. *Radiology* 1982;143:493–500.
6. Lufkin RB, Larsson SG, Hanafee WN. NMR anatomy of the larynx and tongue base. *Radiology* 1983;148:173–5.
7. Muraki AS, Mancuso AA, Harnsberger HR, et al. CT of the oropharynx, tongue base, and floor of mouth. *Radiology* 1983;148:725–31.
8. Reede DL, Whelan MA, Bergeron RT. Computed tomography of the infrahyoid neck. Part I. Normal anatomy. *Radiology* 1982;145:389–95. Part II. Pathology. *Radiology* 1982;145:397–402.
9. Stark DD, Moss AA, Gamsu G, et al. Magnetic resonance imaging of the neck. Part I. Normal anatomy. *Radiology* 1983;150:447–54.
10. Lufkin R, Hanafee W. Application of surface coils to MRI anatomy of the larynx. *AJNR* 1985;491–497.
11. Mancuso AA, Calcattera TC, Hanafee WN. Computed tomography of the larynx. *Radiol Clin North Am* 1978;16:195–208.
12. Silverman PM, Korobkin M. High-resolution computed tomography of the normal larynx. *AJR* 1983;140:875–9.
13. Lufkin RB, Hanafee W. *MRI of the head and neck.* New York: M. Decker, 1986: in preparation.
14. Mancuso AA, Hanafee WN, Julliard GF, et al. The role of computed tomography in the management of cancer of the larynx. *Radiology* 1977;124:243–4.
15. Sagel SS, Auf der Heide JF, Aronberg DJ, et al. High resolution computed tomography in the staging of carcinoma of the larynx. *Laryngoscope* 1981;91:292–300.
16. Scott M, Forsted DH, Rominger CJ, et al. Computed tomographic evaluation of laryngeal neoplasms. *Radiology* 1981;140:141–4.
17. Mancuso AA, Hanafee W. A comparative evaluation of computed tomography and laryngography. *Radiology* 1979;133:131–8.
18. Mafee MF, Schild JA, Valvassori GE, et al. Computed tomography of the larynx: correlation with anatomic and pathologic studies in cases of laryngeal carcinomas. *Radiology* 1983;147:122–8.
19. Mancuso AA, Tamakawa Y, Hanafee W. CT of the fixed vocal cord. *AJR* 1980;135:529–34.
20. Mancuso AA, Hanafee WN. *Computed tomography of the head and neck.* Baltimore, Md: Williams & Wilkins, 1982.
21. Mancuso AA, Hanafee W. Elusive head and neck carcinomas beneath intact mucosa. *Laryngoscope* 1983;93:133–9.
22. Gamsu G, Webb WR, Shallit JB, et al. Computed tomography in carcinoma of the larynx and piriform sinus—the value of phonation CT. *AJR* 1981;136:577–84.
23. Gamsu G. Computed tomography of the larynx and piriform sinuses. In: Moss AA, Gamsu G, Genant H, eds. *Computed tomography of the body.* Philadelphia: WB Saunders, 1983:65–143.
24. Glazer HS, Mauro MA, Aronberg DJ, et al. Computed tomography of laryngoceles. *AJR* 1983;140:549–52.
25. Lufkin R, Hanafee W, Wortham D, et al. MRI of the larynx and hypopharynx using surface coils. *Radiology* 1986; in press.
26. Silverman PM, Korobkin M. Computed tomographic evaluation of laryngoceles. *Radiology* 1982;145:104.
27. Mancuso A, Hanafee W. Computed tomography of the injured larynx. *Radiology* 1979;133:139–44.
28. Stark DD, Clark OH, Gooding GAW, et al. Localization of thyroid lesions by high resolution ultrasound and high resolution CT in patients with hyperparathyroidism. *Surgery,* 1983;94:863–8.
29. Simeone JF, Mueller RP, Ferrucci JT Jr, et al. High resolution real-time sonography of the parathyroid. *Radiology* 1981;141:745–51.
30. Stark DD, Gooding GAW, Moss AA, et al. Parathyroid imaging: comparison of high resolution CT and high resolution ultrasound. *AJR* 1983;141:633–8.
31. Stark DD, Gooding GAW, Clark OH. Noninvasive parathyroid imaging. *Semin Ultrasound Comput Tomogr Magn Reson* 1985;6:310–20.
32. Wang C. Parathyroid re-exploration: a clinical and pathological study of 112 cases. *Ann Surg* 1977;186:140–5.

33. Stark DD, Moss AA, Gooding GAW, et al. Parathyroid scanning by computed tomograpy. *Radiology* 1983;148:297–9.

34. Dooms GC, Hricak H, Crooks LE, et al. Magnetic resonance imaging of the lymph nodes: comparison with CT. *Radiology* 1984;153:719–28.

35. Dooms GC, Hricak H, Moseley ME, et al. Characterization of lymphadenopathy by magnetic resonance relaxation times: preliminary results. *Radiology* 1985;155:691–7.

36. Mancuso AA, Maceri D, Rice D, et al. CT of cervical lymph node cancer. *AJR* 1981;136:381–5.

37. Mancuso AA, Harnsberger HR, Muraki AS, et al. Computed tomography of cervical and retropharyngeal lymph nodes: normal anatomy, variants of normal, and applications in staging head and neck cancer. Part I. Normal anatomy. *Radiology* 1983;148:709–14. Part II. Pathology. *Radiology* 1983;148:715–23.

38. Miller EM, Norman D. The role of computed tomography in the evaluation of neck masses. *Radiology* 1979;133:145–9.

39. Stark DD, Moss AA, Gamsu G, et al. Magnetic resonance imaging of the neck. Part II. Pathologic findings. *Radiology* 1983;150:455–61.

40. Stark DD, Bradley WG. *Magnetic resonance imaging.* St Louis: CV Mosby, 1988: in preparation.

Subject Index